Lee McGregor's
Synopsis of

SURGICAL ANATOMY

Lee McGregor's
Synopsis of
SURGICAL ANATOMY

Edited by

G. A. G. Decker
MB, ChB, FRCS

Principal Surgeon and Senior Lecturer,
J. G. Strijdom Hospital and
University of the Witwatersrand, Johannesburg

Assisted by

D. J. du Plessis
ChM, FRCS, FACS (Hon), FCS(SA) (Hon),
LLD (Hon)

formerly Head of the Department of Surgery
(1958–77) and Vice-Chancellor (1978–83) of the
University of the Witwatersrand,
Johannesburg

With a Foreword by

J. A. Myburgh
ChM, FRCS (Eng), FACS (Hon), FRCS (Hon)

Twelfth edition

WRIGHT
BRISTOL
1986

Published by
John Wright & Sons Ltd,
Techno House, Redcliffe Way, Bristol BS1 6NX

First Edition 1932
Second Edition 1934
Third Edition 1936
Reprinted 1937
Fourth Edition 1939
Reprinted 1940, 1942
Fifth Edition 1943
Reprinted 1943, 1944, 1945
Sixth Edition 1946
Reprinted 1947, 1948
Seventh Edition 1950
Reprinted 1952
Eighth Edition 1957
Reprinted 1959, 1961
Ninth Edition 1963
Reprinted 1966
Tenth Edition 1969
Eleventh Edition 1975
Twelfth Edition 1986

British Library Cataloguing in Publication Data
McGregor, Lee
    Lee McGregor's synopsis of surgical anatomy.— 12th ed.
    1. Anatomy, Surgical and topographical
    I. Title   II. Decker, G. A. G.   III. Du Plessis, D. J.
    IV. Du Plessis, D. J. Synopsis of surgical anatomy
    611′.00246171   QM531

    ISBN 0 7236 0801 6

Typeset by Activity Ltd, Salisbury, Wilts
Printed in Great Britain by The Bath Press, Lower Bristol Road,
Bath BA2 3BL.

PREFACE TO THE TWELFTH EDITION

This edition appears after an unusually long interval, which was necessitated by the need for a formal reappraisal of the purpose of the book and how this objective could be reached.

The main aim remains, as before, to provide a source of information for senior students and practitioners. The book is obviously not a formal treatise on anatomy, but aims to give the anatomical background which would assist the practitioner in the diagnosis and treatment of surgical disorders.

While the actual anatomy has not changed, the advances in surgery have introduced new methods of investigation and treatment and have rendered some of the older ones obsolete. These changes in surgical knowledge have required revision of most sections, with the addition of several new chapters and many new illustrations. Some parts have been reduced in length or totally deleted.

With the extensive specialization which has occurred in surgery it has become impossible for one person to undertake such a major revision in all the facets of surgery, and for that reason a number of colleagues were invited to contribute in areas appropriate to their special interests. The contributors are all members of the Joint Staff of the University of the Witwatersrand, Johannesburg, and the Transvaal Provincial Administration, and we are most grateful to them for their valuable assistance. The contributions were edited to conform with the general format of the book and in some instances this required significant reductions and changes in emphasis.

The previous system of separating the anatomy of the normal from the abnormal has been changed. All aspects of a given region have now been brought together and this should make the book easier to use.

The editors wish to express their special appreciation to Professor J. A. Myburgh, Head of the Department of Surgery of the University of the Witwatersrand, for his encouragement and support; Professor L. J. Levien for his very major contribution at the proof-reading stage; the illustrator, Mr C. Richards BA (FA) of the University of the Witwatersrand, for the many new illustrations; Mrs Y. Cohen and Mrs J. A. Cuthbert for valuable secretarial assistance, and to Messrs John Wright & Sons Ltd for their advice and guidance.

G. A. G. DECKER
D. J. DU PLESSIS
Department of Surgery, University of the
Witwatersrand, Johannesburg, South Africa

PREFACE TO THE FIRST EDITION

The book has been written with the object of presenting anatomical facts of practical value to the senior student and practitioner; no attempt has been made to deal exhaustively with the anatomy of the whole body; the classical textbooks are intended for that purpose. The contents of this book are presented as separate essays, any one of which is complete in itself. It is unnecessary, therefore, to read from the beginning of the book to understand any of the subsequent chapters. In the section on development no dates of the various stages have been mentioned; they are of academic value only, and it is my experience that in the effort to remember dates the student forgets the developmental facts which are of value in practice.

I must express my deep indebtedness to my teachers, the late Dr. Ryland ('Daddie') Whitaker, Dr. E. B. Jamieson, Professor Wm Wright, and many others. I must make especial mention of Sir Harold J. Stiles, who taught me the value of a knowledge of anatomy, and I must thank him for the honour he has done in writing a Foreword for this volume. To Professor Raymond Dart I am grateful for the Introduction, for advice, and for constant encouragement. I have endeavoured throughout to mention the authorities whose work I have made use of, but I should like to express here my appreciation of the fact that it is the work of others which gives this book any value it may have.

The illustrations, which form so essential a feature of the work, have been done for me by one of my students, now Dr. E. A. Thomas. I cannot thank him sufficiently for his care and patience with the drawings.

My sincere thanks are due to the publishers, Messrs. John Wright & Sons Ltd., for the great trouble they have taken in the arrangement of the text, and for the remarkable success they have achieved in the reproduction of the drawings.

A. LEE McGREGOR
62 Muller Street, Yeoville,
Johannesburg, South Africa

CONTRIBUTORS

The editors gratefully acknowledge the assistance given by the following contributors from the University of Witwatersrand:

I. ABRAMOWITZ
MB, BCh, FCS(SA), FRCS(Edin)
Surgeon/Lecturer (Part-time), Johannesburg Hospital
(Veins and great lymph vessels; lymph tissue of the head and neck)

J. C. ALLAN
MB, BCh, MD, FRCS(Edin)
Surgeon/Lecturer (Part-time), Johannesburg Hospital
(The scalp)

B. M. BEREZOWSKY
BDS
Clinical Assistant/Junior Lecturer (Full-time), University of the Witwatersrand Dental Hospital
((The mandible and maxilla)

K. D. BOFFARD
MB, BCh, FRCS(Eng)
Surgeon/Senior Lecturer (Full-time), Johannesburg Hospital
(The hand; the anatomy of abdominal incisions)

J. R. BOTHA
MB, ChB, FCS(SA)
Senior Surgeon/Senior Lecturer (Full-time), Johannesburg Hospital
(The thyroid; thymus and parathyroid; veins and great lymph vessels)

S. BRAUN
MB, BCh, FRCS(Edin)
Plastic Surgeon/Lecturer (Part-time), Johannesburg Hospital
(The hand)

C. G. BREMNER
MB, BCh, ChM (Witwatersrand), FRCS(Eng), FRCS(Edin)
Professor and Chief Surgeon, Coronation Hospital
(The oesophagus)

A. A. CONLAN
MB, BCh, FRCS(Eng)
Senior Thoracic Surgeon/Senior Lecturer, Johannesburg Hospital
(The chest wall, lungs and mediastinum)

S. A. R. COOKE
MB, BS, MS, FRCS(Eng), FRCS(Edin)
Surgeon/Lecturer (Part-time), Johannesburg Hospital
(The large bowel, ischiorectal fossa and anal fistulae)

J. B. CRAIG
MB, BCh, FRCS(Edin), FRCS(Glas), FCS(SA)Orth
Senior Orthopaedic Surgeon/Senior Lecturer, J. G. Strijdom Hospital
(Bones and amputations)

K. DAVIDGE-PITTS
MB, BCh, FRCS(Edin), FCS(SA)
ENT Surgeon/Senior Lecturer, Baragwanath Hospital
(The cranial nerves)

M. R. Q. DAVIES
MB, ChB(Pret), FCS(SA), FRCS(Eng), FRCS(Edin)
Professor and Chief Paediatric Surgeon, Johannesburg Hospital
(The anatomy of the child and the developmental anatomy in the various chapters)

J. W. D. DYMOND
MB, BCh, FRCS(Edin), FCS(SA)Orth
Orthopaedic Surgeon/Lecturer, Hillbrow Hospital
(The hip joint; the elbow joint)

R. A. HINDER
MB, BCh, PhD(Med), FRCS(Eng), FRCS(Edin)
Associate Professor of Surgery/Senior Lecturer, Johannesburg Hospital
(Veins and great lymph vessels)

M. KATZEN
MB, BCh, FRCS(Edin)
Paediatric Surgeon/Lecturer (Part-time), Johannesburg Hospital
(The anatomy of the child and developmental anatomy in the various chapters)

R. H. KINSLEY
MB, BCh, FCS(SA), FACC
Professor and Chief Cardiothoracic Surgeon, Johannesburg Hospital
(The heart and great vessels)

A. B. KOLLER
MB, BCh, DipMidCO&G(SA), MRCOG, FCOG(SA)
Obstetrician and Gynaecologist/Lecturer (Part-time), Johannesburg Hospital
(Prolapse of the uterus, vaginal examination and hysterectomy)

M. LANGE
MB, ChB, FRCS(Edin)
Surgeon/Lecturer (Part-time), Johannesburg Hospital
(The breast)

H. H. LAWSON
MB, BCh, ChM, DSc, FRCS(Eng)
Professor and Chief Surgeon, Baragwanath Hospital
(The stomach)

L. J. LEVIEN
MB, BCh, PhD(Med), FCS(SA)
Professor and Chief Surgeon, Hillbrow Hospital
(The autonomic nervous system; collateral circulation and vascular approach)

R. LIPSCHITZ
MB, BCh, PhD(Med), FRCS(Edin)
Professor and Chief Neurosurgeon,
(The scalp; the anatomy of the normal and enlarged pituitary and the meninges; cerebrospinal fluid and the spinal cord)

T. G. LORENTZ
MB, BCh, ChM, FRCS(Eng), FRCS(Edin)
Surgeon/Lecturer (Part-time), Johannesburg Hospital
(The thyroid, thymus and parathyroid glands)

J. F. LOWNIE
BDS, HDipDent, MDent
Professor and Chief Maxillo-facial and Oral Surgeon, Johannesburg Hospital
(The mandible and maxilla)

L. NAINKIN
MB, ChB, FRCS(Edin)
Orthopaedic Surgeon/Lecturer (Part-time), Johannesburg Hospital
(The spinal column)

G. O. READ
MB, BCh, FRCS(Edin), FRCS(Glas), FCS(SA)Orth
Senior Orthopaedic Surgeon/Senior Lecturer (Full-time) Baragwanath Hospital
(The shoulder joint)

I. M. ROGAN
MB, BCh, FRCS(Eng), FRCS(Edin)
Orthopaedic Surgeon/Lecturer (Part-time), Johannesburg Hospital
(The knee joint)

M. STEWART
MB, BS, LRCP, MS, FRCS(Eng)
Senior Surgeon/Senior Lecturer (Full-time), Baragwanath Hospital
(Peripheral nerves)

P. J. P. van BLERK
BSc, MB, BCh, DipSurg
Professor and Chief Urologist, Johannesburg Hospital

(The kidney, ureter and adrenal; the bladder; prostate and urethra)

G. A. VERSFELD
MB, ChB, FCS(SA)Orth
Senior Orthopaedic Surgeon/Senior Lecturer (Full-time), Baragwanath Hospital
(The foot and ankle)

D. H. WALKER
MB, BCh, DipSurg, FRCS(Edin), FRCS(Glas)
Plastic Surgeon/Lecturer (Part-time), Johannesburg Hospital
(The face and branchial arches)

CONTENTS

	Foreword to the twelfth edition	xv
1.	The oesophagus	1
2.	The stomach	10
3.	The rotation of the gut	22
4.	The duodenum, jejunum and ileum	30
5.	The large bowel, and canal and ischiorectal fossa	41
6.	The liver and biliary system	78
7.	The pancreas	102
8.	The spleen	106
9.	The anatomy of abdominal incisions	113
10.	The groin and scrotum	118
11.	The chest wall, lungs and mediastinum	137
12.	The diaphragm	152
13.	The breast	161
14.	Development anomalies of the face and branchial arches	171
15.	The mandible and maxilla	181
16.	Lymph tissue of the head and neck	189
17.	The thyroid, thymus and the parathyroid gland	198
18.	The autonomic nervous system	207
19.	Collateral circulation	224
20.	Vascular approach	239
21.	The veins and great lymph ducts	248
22.	The heart and great vessels	273
23.	The kidneys, ureters and adrenals	289
24.	The bladder, prostate and urethra	314
25.	The scalp	328
26.	The anatomy of the normal and the enlarged pituitary body	333
27.	The meninges, cerebrospinal fluid and spinal cord	340
28.	The cranial nerves	352
29.	Peripheral nerves	375
30.	Prolapse of the uterus, vaginal examination and hysterectomy	395
31.	The anatomy of the child	401
32.	Bones and amputations	407
33.	Shoulder joint	433
34.	The elbow	454
35.	The wrist complex	460
36.	The hand	466
37.	The hip	498
38.	The knee joint	513
39.	The ankle–foot complex	530
40.	The spinal column	547
	Selected further reading	567
	Index	569

FOREWORD TO TWELFTH EDITION

It is a pleasure for me to have the opportunity to welcome this new edition of a book which has made such a remarkable contribution to surgical education for over half of a century.

This edition heralds a new phase in the history of this book because, since the retirement of the previous editor, Professor D. J. du Plessis, the editorial responsibility has been vested in the Department of Surgery of the University of the Witwatersrand, Johannesburg. Mr G. A. G. Decker, Principal Surgeon and Senior Lecturer in the Department, has accepted this responsibility and the new edition is a great tribute to his ability and tenacity. Professor D. J. du Plessis very generously agreed to assist Mr Decker. This not only ensured the necessary continuity between the old and new editors, but was a source of stimulation, guidance and encouragement of inestimable value. The Department of Surgery of the University of the Witwatersrand is proud to be associated with this publication and I am most grateful to the many members of staff who have contributed. We look forward to the further success of this outstanding book.

J. A. Myburgh ChM, FRCS(Eng), FACS (Hon), FRCS (Hon)
Head of the Department of Surgery,
University of the Witwatersrand, Johannesburg

Chapter 1

THE OESOPHAGUS

DEVELOPMENT OF THE OESOPHAGUS

Initially the oesophagus is very short but it elongates rapidly with the growth of the fetus. The epithelium of the oesophagus proliferates and almost obliterates the lumen but recanalization occurs at a later stage.

The respiratory system arises as the laryngotracheal diverticulum from the primitive pharynx. It grows ventrocaudally and becomes separated from the oesophagus by longitudinal ridges (tracheo-oesophageal folds) which fuse to form a partition to divide the laryngotracheal tube ventrally from the oesophagus dorsally.

CONGENITAL ABNORMALITIES

Congenital abnormalities may arise if there is interference with the normal development of the trachea and oesophagus.

Oesophageal atresia and tracheo-oesophageal fistula

This may take the form of an atresia of the oesophagus with or without an accompanying fistulous communication to the trachea. Many variations on this theme are described. Those most commonly encountered are illustrated in *Fig.* 1. An isolated atresia of the oesophagus is found in about 10 per cent of instances—note the large gap between the two oesophageal segments (*Fig.* 1A). An oesophageal atresia with a distal tracheo-oesophageal fistula is shown in *Fig.* 1B. This anatomical arrangement occurs in over 80 per cent of cases. A tracheo-oesophageal fistula may develop without an oesophageal atresia (*Fig.* 1C). The N-shaped fistula usually lies at the level of the thoracic inlet.

Tracheo-oesophageal fistula is one of the commoner neonatal emergencies with a frequency of one per 3000 births. It may be associated with cardiac lesions, duodenal stenosis and imperforate anus.

Tracheo-oesophageal fistula results from incomplete division of the foregut into respiratory and digestive portions. Incomplete fusion of the tracheo-oesophageal folds results in a defective septum leaving a communication between the trachea and the oesophagus.

Stenosis and atresia probably result from unequal partitioning of the foregut into the oesophagus and the trachea, but could also result from the failure of oesophageal recanalization.

Congenital diverticula and enterogenous cysts of the oesophagus

Cysts whose walls reproduce the structure of the oesophagus may be found:

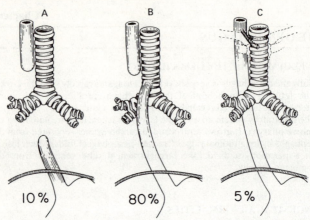

Fig. 1. Expected incidence of **A** an isolated oesophageal atresia; **B** an oesophageal atresia with distal tracheo-oesophageal fistula; **C** a tracheo-oesophageal fistula.

(*a*) in the wall of the oesophagus; (*b*) attached to the oesophagus; (*c*) more or less remote from the oesophagus. They are enterogenous and originated as diverticula. In the developing oesophagus there are normally many bud-like projections from the mucous membrane which contain a cavity communicating with the lumen. If they fail to disappear they may persist as either congenital diverticula or congenital enterogenous cysts.

CONGENITAL DIVERTICULA: They may occur in any part of the gut from the oesophagus to the colon but they are rare.

CONGENITAL ENTEROGENOUS CYSTS: They arise as diverticula of the lumen which later get cut off from the lumen of the oesophagus thus forming a separate cavity. Such a cyst may be, in relation to the oesophageal wall, a submucous, intermuscular or subserous (extramuscular) cyst which may lose its attachment to the oesophagus and be found in a para-oesophageal position, presenting on radiography as a mediastinal tumour. Computerized axial tomography of the mediastinum has proved of great value in differentiating fluid-filled mediastinal tumours from solid tumours.

THE ANATOMY OF THE OESOPHAGUS

The oesophagus commences at the lower edge of the cricoid cartilage (C6 vertebra) and ends at the oesophagogastric junction (T11 vertebra), which is situated posterior to the 7th left costal cartilage about 2·5 cm from the midline. It is closed at the upper end by the cricopharyngeus muscle, the lower edge of which is 18 cm from the incisor teeth, and at the lower end by the lower oesophageal sphincter (LOS). The distance of the LOS from the incisor teeth depends on the height of the patient. In an average-sized person (145 cm height), it lies approximately 40 cm from the incisor teeth (for 132 and 165 cm height—37 and 43 cm from incisors). It has a cervical, thoracic and abdominal course.

Cervical oesophagus

The relationships of the cervical oesophagus are shown in *Fig.* 2. From the surgical point of view it is important to note that the recurrent laryngeal nerves ascend on each side in the groove between the trachea and the oesophagus. The left border of the oesophagus extends beyond the trachea so that the oesophagus is more easily exposed via a left-sided cervical incision.

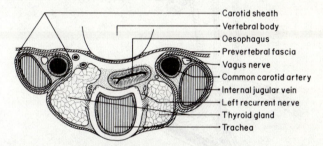

Fig. 2. The cervical oesophagus on cross-section.

Thoracic oesophagus

In the chest, the oesophagus runs through the superior and posterior mediastinum. Below the tracheal bifurcation the oesophagus curves to the right (*Fig.* 3). The descending aorta continues straight down on the left of the vertebral column, so that the oesophagus at first lies more to the right than anterior to the aorta. The right-hand wall of the oesophagus is immediately adjacent to the parietal pleura of the right pleural cavity just behind the hilum of the lung. Perforation of the oesophagus at this point may produce a right-sided pleural effusion. The thoracic duct crosses behind the oesophagus from the 7th to the 5th thoracic vertebrae and then continues up along its left border. Should it be torn during dissection of the oesophagus, as indicated by an escape of milky fluid, its ends should be tied. The lymph finds alternative routes to the venous system and the accident is usually not attended with any dire consequence if it be recognized and dealt with as outlined. Lower down

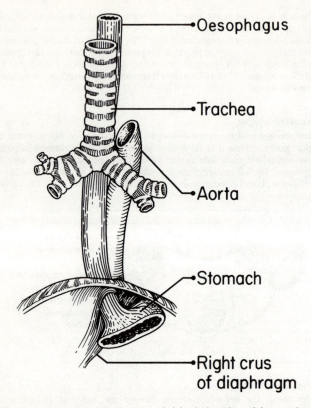

Fig. 3. Anterior view of the thoracic and abdominal portions of the oesophagus.

the oesophagus takes a curve to the left behind the pericardial sac, and passes completely to the left of the midline toward the oesophageal hiatus, crossing anterior to the aorta. Perforations of the lower third of the oesophagus are therefore more likely to result in left-sided pleural effusions.

Abdominal oesophagus

The abdominal part of the oesophagus is about 2·5 cm long and grooves the posterior surface of the left lobe of the liver. It is covered with peritoneum on its front and left side only.

Oesophageal sphincters

There is an anatomical sphincter at the upper end of the oesophagus and a physiological sphincter at the lower end of the oesophagus.

CRICOPHARYNGEUS OR INFERIOR CONSTRICTOR OF THE PHARYNX: This muscle consists of two parts, a lower transverse part (cricopharyngeus) and an upper oblique portion (thyropharyngeus). The lower transverse fibres arise from the cricoid cartilage and pass horizontally backward round the pharynx to be inserted into a median raphe at the back of this tube. Its function is to prevent regurgitation of the oesophageal contents into the pharynx. The upper oblique fibres arise from the cricoid and thyroid cartilages, and encircle the hypopharynx, ending in the median raphe. In the act of swallowing, the upper (oblique) part of this muscle propels the contents downwards and the lower (transverse) part relaxes to allow the contents to pass into the oesophagus. Incoordination of this action, with failure of the cricopharyngeus to relax, will result in increased pressure in the pharynx and production of a pharyngeal diverticulum (*Fig.* 4).

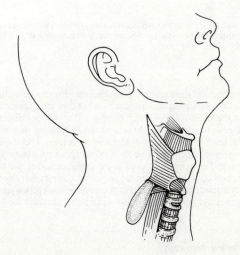

Fig. 4. Anatomic relationship of a pharyngo-oesophageal pouch.

A cricopharyngeal myotomy is performed in conditions associated with incoordination of muscle relaxation (such as in pharyngeal diverticulum). Intraluminal pressure recording demonstrates a high pressure zone of 2–4 cm.

THE OESOPHAGOGASTRIC JUNCTION: Normally gastric contents cannot regurgitate into the oesophagus because of the mechanism at the cardia preventing this (*see* Chapter 12).

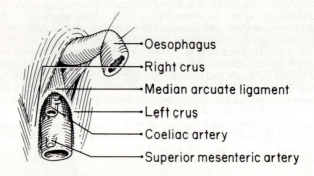

Fig. 5. The oesophageal hiatus and median arcuate ligament. The left and right limb of the right crus encircle the oesophagus. The median arcuate ligament joins the left crus and the left limb of the right crus.

The median arcuate ligament (*Fig.* 5) does not directly contribute to the competence of the oesophagogastric junction but is of importance in surgical procedures in the region. It is a tough fibrous 1–3 mm wide condensation of the medial fibrous borders of the 2 crura of the diaphragm. It is usually at a level just proximal to the origin of the coeliac artery. The coeliac artery origin, however, may be at or above the median arcuate ligament in up to 33 per cent of cases. The ligament is used as the main anchoring site for the Hill antireflux operation. It is important for surgeons to remember that it may be absent or very attenuated. The origin of the phrenic vessels lies just proximal to the coeliac vessels and should be carefully avoided when the ligament is dissected.

Landmarks during endoscopy
In passing a gastroscope one can identify the cricopharyngeal sphincter which

opens and closes intermittently. Left atrial distension may compress the oesophagus and displace it posteriorly. A tumour involving the left main bronchus may also cause narrowing of the oesophagus.

The nerve supply of the oesophagus

The vagi are the motor nerves to the oesophagus. In the body of the oesophagus there are only cholinergic receptors and vagal stimulation results in contraction. In the inferior oesophageal sphincter there are both cholinergic and adrenergic receptors, but innervation is largely adrenergic and vagal stimulation results in relaxation of the sphincter.

Afferent visceral pain impulses pass along the sympathetic nerves which are closely related to the somatic sensory fibres of the phrenic and intercostal nerves in the posterior horn of the spinal cord. Afferent impulses from the oesophagus may thus 'overflow' into adjacent somatic neurones in the posterior horn to give pain referred to the neck, arm, chest, or back. Some pain fibres must be carried in the vagus nerves because occasionally oesophageal pain is referred to the ear, presumably via the auricular branch of the vagus.

ACHALASIA: In this condition there is failure of the inferior oesophageal sphincter to relax during deglutition and an absence of coordinated peristalsis in the body of the oesophagus, resulting in an obstruction at the cardia. By means of electron microscopy, Wallerian degeneration is seen in the vagus nerve, and the oesophageal smooth muscle shows changes of denervation. There is a reduction in the number of cells in the dorsal motor nucleus of the vagus nerve and, in most cases (especially those of long standing), there is degeneration or even absence of myenteric ganglion cells. These findings support the theory that this disease primarily affects the extrinsic neural structures (either the dorsal motor nucleus or the vagus nerve) and that the oesophageal changes are secondary.

DIFFUSE SPASM OF THE OESOPHAGUS: There is a neuromuscular incoordination of the lower two-thirds of the oesophagus in response to deglutition, resulting in simultaneous diffuse contraction of the oesophagus from the aortic arch downwards. This causes intermittent dysphagia and retrosternal pain. The sites of contraction are constant and this later results in hypertrophy of the circular muscle and pulsion diverticula between the areas of hypertrophy.

ACQUIRED DIVERTICULA OF THE THORACIC OESOPHAGUS:
  Pulsion Diverticulum: A pulsion diverticulum is usually situated above the diaphragm (supradiaphragmatic or epiphrenic). It is due to increased pressure in the oesophageal lumen which results in herniation of the

mucosal and submucosal layers through the muscular wall. This diverticulum is due to disease in the oesophagus distal to the diverticulum, such as diffuse spasm, or achalasia. It may produce retrosternal pain and difficulty with swallowing.

Traction Diverticulum: This is caused by the breaking down of diseased lymph nodes lying near the oesophagus. Fibrosis occurs and the consequent retraction of the resulting scar tissue pulls on the oesophagus, forming a pouch. It is a true diverticulum in the sense that its walls are composed of all the coats of the oesophagus.

Leugart's Pouch: There is a fibrous band known as Leugart's ledge passing from the left bronchus to the side of an adjacent vertebra. The oesophagus crosses this ledge. The wall of the oesophagus may prolapse over the ledge and give rise to a small diverticulum. It is a curiosity that may be seen during an X-ray contrast study of the oesophagus and its benign implications should be remembered.

Muscles of the oesophagus

The oesophagus has an inner circular and outer longitudinal layer. The mucosa is easily stripped away from the muscle layer. This feature is evident when the paediatric surgeon performs circumferential myotomies to lengthen a shortened oesophagus after tracheo-oesophageal fistula repair, and by the surgeon who performs a modified Heller's cardiomyotomy for achalasia or diffuse spasm of the oesophagus.

The upper third of the muscle layers consists of striated muscle and the lower two-thirds consist of smooth muscle. There is a short transition zone of both striated and smooth muscle between these segments.

Arteries supplying the oesophagus

The oesophagus is supplied with blood in its upper part by the inferior thyroid artery, by oesophageal branches of the aorta in its main extent, and by branches of the gastric and inferior phrenic arteries in its lower part. It is to be remembered, therefore, that rough handling or wide mobilization of the oesophagus may imperil its blood supply, especially over its main extent where the aortic branches are distributed in a segmental manner (*Fig.* 6). They are slender, tenuous vessels and this makes it possible to mobilize the intrathoracic oesophagus by blind digital dissection from the suprasternal notch above and from the oesophageal hiatus below during certain cases of oesophagectomy.

Venous drainage of the oesophagus

The veins of the cervical oesophagus drain into the inferior thyroid veins and

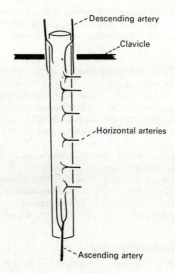

Fig. 6. Schematic presentation of the blood supply of the oesophagus.

then the brachiocephalic veins. The veins on the left side of the thoracic oesophagus drain into the brachiocephalic vein via the left hemiazygos system; on the right side drainage is through the azygos system into the superior vena cava. At the cardio-oesophageal junction venous drainage of the oesophagus may be into the coronary, splenic, retroperitoneal and inferior phrenic veins which connect with the portal and caval systems. In portal hypertension (*see* Chapter 6) the cardio-oesophageal junction is the site of oesophageal varices.

Lymphatic drainage
The lymphatic drainage of the oesophagus is longitudinal rather than segmental.

LYMPHATIC VESSELS: The lymphatic vessels in the submucosa may run for considerable distances up and down the oesophagus before penetrating the muscle layers to join the lymphatics in the adventitia. Although the adventitial lymphatics usually drain into adjacent lymph nodes, these lymphatics also have a longitudinal arrangement. The implication of this is that the first lymph node to be involved in cancer may be distant from the primary tumour, but this does not necessarily mean that the primary lesion is unresectable.

THE LYMPH NODES: The lymph nodes of the oesophagus consist of three parallel and interconnected chains (*Fig.* 7).

> *The Para-oesophageal Nodes:* These are situated on the wall of the oesophagus and include the cervical, upper, middle and lower thoracic para-oesophageal nodes and the paracardial nodes.
>
> *The Peri-oesophageal Nodes:* These are located on structures immediately adjacent to the oesophagus; they include the deep cervical, scalene, paratracheal, subcarinal, posterior mediastinal, diaphragmatic, left gastric, lesser curvature and coeliac nodes.
>
> *The Lateral Oesophageal Nodes:* These are found lateral to the oesophagus and receive lymph from the para- and peri-oesophageal nodes. They include posterior triangle (or lateral cervical), hilar, suprapyloric, common hepatic and greater curvature lymph nodes.

SURGERY OF THE OESOPHAGUS

In patients in whom a diagnosis of carcinoma of the oesophagus has been made, computerized tomography (CT) is an excellent non-invasive method of detecting extra-oesophageal spread of malignancy. Mediastinal infiltration obliterates the peri-oesophageal fat planes in relation to the tumour and loss of these fat planes, which separate the involved oesophagus from the tracheobronchial tree, the pericardium, aorta and azygos veins, can be clearly seen on CT scan.

Anastomosis of the oesophagus to another portion of the gastrointestinal tract, such as stomach, small bowel or colon, is prone to leakage from the suture line. This is because of its poor blood supply, the absence of a serosal covering and the friability of the muscular layers. It is particularly important to include the mucosal layer in suturing the oesophagus. Most surgeons use an 'all coats' interrupted suture when anastomosing the oesophagus.

Chapter 2

THE STOMACH

Due to its reservoir function the stomach has a variable shape depending on the volume of fluid or food it contains. The position of the stomach varies, depending upon whether the patient is in the erect or supine position.

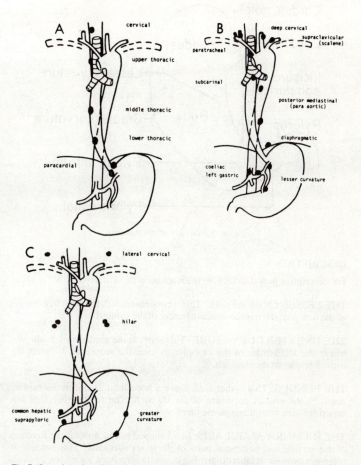

Fig. 7. Lymph nodes of the oesophagus. A, Para-oesophageal; B, peri-oesophageal; C, lateral oesophageal. (Reproduced with permission from A. Mannell 'Carcinoma of the esophagus', in M. M. Ravitch et al. (eds): *Current Problems in Surgery*. Copyright 1982 by Year Book Medical Publishers, Inc., Chicago.)

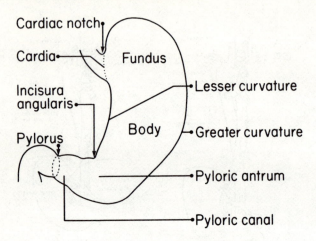

Fig. 8. Subdivision of the stomach.

DESCRIPTION

For descriptive purposes (*Fig.* 8) the stomach is divided into:

THE LESSER CURVATURE: This is continuous with the right free border of the oesophagus; it is the concave border of the stomach.

THE GREATER CURVATURE: This starts at the cardiac notch (the site where the left border of the oesophagus joins the stomach). It forms the convex border of the stomach.

THE FUNDUS: This is that area above a horizontal line from the cardiac notch to the greater curvature of the stomach. The fundus therefore lies superior to the oesophagogastric junction.

THE INCISURA ANGULARIS: In a J-shaped stomach this is the junction of the vertical and horizontal parts of the lesser curvature. This junction is often not obvious at laparotomy, but is clearly seen from within the stomach at the time of gastroscopy.

THE BODY: This is that portion of stomach lying between the fundus and the pyloric portion of the stomach.

THE PYLORIC PORTION: Approximately the distal one-fifth of the stomach consists of the pyloric antrum, canal and sphincter. The pyloro-duodenal junction is identified by the vein of Mayo.

HISTOLOGY

Histologically three types of gastric mucosa can be recognized:

THE CARDIA: A small area of stomach around the oesophagogastric junction. It contains mucus-secreting glands only.

FUNDIC GLAND AREA: This lies between the pyloric gland area and the cardia. The gastric crypts are shallow and the mucosa contains parietal (acid-secreting) and chief (pepsin-secreting) cells. It is badly named because it includes the mucosa of both the fundus and body of the stomach.

PYLORIC GLAND AREA: This forms the mucosa of the pylorus. This area has deep gastric pits and contains mucus-secreting cells. Gastrin-secreting cells can be detected only on immunofluorescence. The pyloric gland area extends higher on the lesser curve than on the greater curve.

PYLORIC SPHINCTER

The circular muscle of the pyloric canal is a triangular-shaped muscle in the position of an inverted V with the apex at the pyloric end of the lesser curvature and the two limbs spreading out towards the greater curvature. This specialized circular muscle extends along the greater curvature for about 5 cm, but is bunched up on the lesser curvature to form a thick mass about 2 cm long (muscle torus). The right edge of this muscle is thickened to form the pylorus.

On the outside of this circular muscle there is the longitudinal muscle which partly extends over the pylorus to be continuous with the longitudinal muscle of the duodenum and is partly inserted into the circular muscle at the pylorus and the submucosa in the area.

These circular and longitudinal muscles form a functional entity, contracting concentrically to form the emptying mechanism of the stomach. The narrow lumen of the distal limb of the circular muscle acts as a filter resulting in regurgitation of solid material back into the stomach, so slowing down gastric emptying. At the end of this concentric contraction the canal is shortened and closed, thus preventing regurgitation of duodenal contents during duodenal contractions.

Abnormalities of the pyloric sphincter

HYPERTROPHIC PYLORIC STENOSIS IN THE INFANT: There is pyloric obstruction from the second week of life. Medical measures may overcome this obstruction but division of the hypertrophied muscle (the Ramstedt operation) may be necessary.

SPASM AND SECONDARY HYPERTROPHY: This often follows other gastrointestinal disorders, e.g. peptic ulcer, hiatus hernia, cholelithiasis and appendicitis.

PRIMARY HYPERTROPHIC PYLORIC STENOSIS: This occurs in the adult due to ineffectual contractions of the circular muscle as a result of a deficiency of the longitudinal muscle.

THE BLOOD VESSELS AND LYMPHATICS OF THE STOMACH

Arteries

There are four main arteries to the stomach (*Fig.* 9).

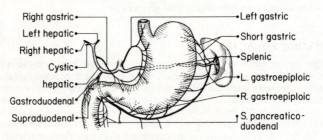

Fig. 9. Blood supply of the stomach.

THE LEFT GASTRIC ARTERY: This arises from the coeliac axis and divides into an ascending (oesophageal) branch and a descending branch.

The descending branch, lying between the layers of the lesser omentum, is closely opposed to the lesser curvature and sends branches to the stomach.

THE RIGHT GASTRIC ARTERY: The right gastric artery, arising from the common hepatic artery, also divides into a number of branches to the stomach (and duodenum) along the lesser curvature and anastomoses with the left gastric.

THE RIGHT GASTRO-EPIPLOIC ARTERY: This arises from the gastroduodenal artery, and anastomoses with the left gastro-epiploic vessel with which it forms an arcade supplying the greater curvature.

The gastroduodenal artery arises from the hepatic artery, and passes down behind the duodenum. It is often this artery that is eroded and is the source of bleeding in duodenal ulceration.

THE LEFT GASTRO-EPIPLOIC ARTERY: This arises from the splenic artery and contributes to the arterial arcade along the greater curvature. Five to seven small branches arise from the splenic artery to supply the fundus (short gastric arteries).

THE BLOOD SUPPLY OF THE GREATER OMENTUM: This comes from the right and left gastro-epiploic arteries which form an arcade along the greater curvature of the stomach. The right epiploic (omental) artery (from the right gastro-epiploic artery) and the left epiploic artery (from the left gastro-epiploic artery) form an anastomotic (epiploic) arcade in the lower part of the omentum which is joined by accessory epiploic arteries (from the two gastro-epiploic arteries), and provide a rich blood supply to the omentum (*Fig.* 10). When mobilizing the greater omentum from the greater curvature of the stomach, it is therefore not necessary to preserve the gastro-epiploic arcade provided the epiploic arcade is preserved.

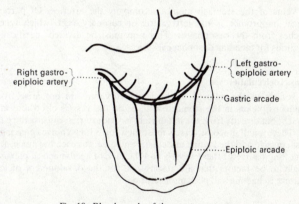

Right gastro-epiploic artery

Left gastro-epiploic artery

Gastric arcade

Epiploic arcade

Fig. 10. Blood supply of the greater omentum.

In 2–9 per cent of people, the anastomosis between the two main epiploic arteries takes place 2–3 cm from the gastro-epiploic arch (*Fig.* 11). In such cases this epiploic arcade may be ligated during mobilization of the omentum and this may result in necrosis of part of the greater omentum if the right or left epiploic artery is also ligated.

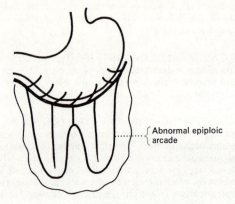

Fig. 11. Abnormal position of the epiploic arcade in the greater omentum.

Veins

The veins of the stomach mainly accompany the arteries. Of particular surgical importance is the left gastric or coronary vein, which receives branches from the oesophagus. This vein must be divided specifically in operations for bleeding oesophageal varices.

The microcirculation

The vessels to the mucosa of the lesser curvature do not arise from a submucous plexus in the stomach wall, as do the vessels elsewhere in the stomach, but directly from the left or right gastric arteries, outside the gastric wall. These small mucosal vessels must then run a long course, piercing the serosa, muscle and the lamina muscularis mucosae, to reach the mucosa.

The long course of these vessels and the lack of a submucosal plexus are thought to be factors that are responsible for the development of lesser curvature ischaemia and perhaps ulceration.

Lymph drainage of the stomach

Each of the three branches of the coeliac axis takes a share in the arterial supply of the stomach which may be divided into three lymphatic areas corresponding fairly closely to the arterial territories. Divide the stomach by a line in its long axis, two-thirds of the stomach being to the right of this line, one-third to the left. Divide that left third into two by a line at the junction of its upper third and lower two-thirds. This marks out the three lymph

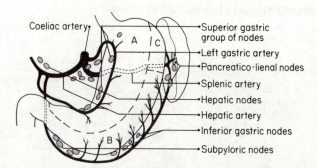

Fig. 12. The lymph territories of the stomach are indicated by the letters A, B and C. A drains to the superior gastric nodes; B drains to the inferior gastric nodes; C drains to pancreaticolienal nodes.

territories of the organ (*Fig.* 12). The efferents from all these nodes go to the lymph nodes around the coeliac axis in front of the aorta, i.e. the coeliac group of pre-aortic nodes.

The lymph nodes concerned in the drainage of the stomach are:

HEPATIC GROUP: These lymph nodes lie in the lesser omentum along the bile ducts and receive lymph from the liver and gallbladder. An outlying member is in relation to the neck of the gallbladder along the cystic artery; this is the cystic node.

THE SUBPYLORIC NODES: These lie in the angle between the first and second parts of the duodenum on the head of the pancreas in relation to the bifurcation of the gastroduodenal artery. They receive the lymph from the right two-thirds of the greater curvature of the stomach which comes through the inferior gastric nodes.

GASTRIC GROUP: These lymph nodes consist of (*a*) superior and (*b*) inferior sets.
  a. Superior Nodes: These lie along the left gastric artery and the paracardial nodes are grouped around the cardia of the stomach.
  b. Inferior Nodes: These lie along the pyloric half of the greater curvature of the stomach between the layers of greater omentum.

PANCREATICOLIENAL GROUP: These lymph nodes lie along the splenic artery in relation to the upper border of the pancreas. Some occur in the gastrosplenic ligament in relation to the short gastric branches.

PERITONEAL REFLECTIONS OF THE STOMACH

The gastrolienal (gastrosplenic) and lienorenal (splenorenal) ligaments are of particular surgical importance with reference to splenectomy (*Fig.* 13).

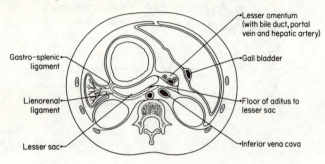

Fig. 13. The peritoneal reflection of the stomach.

The lienorenal ligament consists of two layers (*Fig.* 13) and the splenic artery with its branches runs between the layers. By dividing the lateral or outer layer of the lienorenal ligament, the surgeon exposes the main blood supply to the spleen, and can mobilize the organ sufficiently to make it a midline structure.

The short gastric vessels (vasa brevia) lie in the gastrosplenic ligament. As the name implies, the vessels are short and care must be taken to avoid damaging the wall of the stomach when mobilizing the greater curvature. A number of avascular fibrous bands, in the position of the lowermost vasa brevia, pass directly from the stomach to the spleen and excessive traction on these bands during mobilization of the greater curvature may lead to tearing of the splenic capsule.

The splenic artery lies behind the stomach and lesser sac, and it can therefore be approached by opening into the lesser sac. This is best achieved by approaching the lesser sac from outside the epiploic arch. When the surgeon enters the lesser sac through the gastrocolic ligament, this should be done well to the left of the midline. The gastrocolic ligament here is longer, thinner and avascular. If an attempt is made to enter the lesser sac to the right, the middle colic vessels may be damaged, because in this area embryological fusion has occurred between the gastrocolic ligament and the transverse mesocolon.

THE ABDOMINAL COURSE OF THE VAGUS

The vagi enter the abdomen through the oesophageal hiatus, the left vagus anterior and the right vagus posterior to the oesophagus. The vagi divide into branches at the cardia of the stomach but this division may occur higher, in which case the vagi at the level of the diaphragm will appear as multiple trunks.

The anterior vagus nerve

Soon after entering the abdomen, the anterior vagus (*Fig.* 14) gives off one or more hepatic branches, which run in the lesser omentum to the portal fissure to supply the liver and gallbladder, and ultimately also a branch to the pyloric antrum. The vagus also gives off branches to the fundus and proceeds in the lesser omentum 10–15 mm from the lesser curvature of the stomach as the nerve of Latarjet, giving off branches to the acid- and pepsin-secreting areas of the stomach.

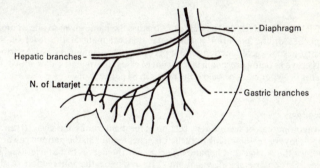

Fig. 14. The anterior vagus.

At a point 5–7 cm proximal to the pylorus which is defined by the presence of the vein of Mayo, the anterior vagus nerve usually divides into branches and the appearance of this division has been described as the 'crow's foot', most of the branches supplying the pyloric antrum.

The posterior vagus nerve

Like the anterior it lies between the leaves of the lesser omentum, and follows much the same course distally in relation to the lesser curvature posterior to the anterior nerve (*Fig.* 15).

Distally, the posterior nerve gives off a coeliac branch to the coeliac ganglion and usually also a branch to supply the antrum, but this is not always the case. Often antral branches of the posterior vagus nerve are less clearly defined than those of the anterior nerve.

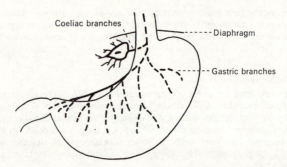

Fig. 15. The posterior vagus.

NERVE OF GRASSI: The nerve of Grassi is the name given to one or more branches of the posterior vagus nerve that originate at the level of the gastro-oesophageal junction, and supply the gastric fundus. Grassi describes this nerve as being present in 90 per cent of cases. It originates at or above the hiatus in 16 per cent, or below the hiatus in 84 per cent of cases.

Vagotomy

A vagotomy can be achieved by section of the main trunks of the vagi (truncal vagotomy) or by sectioning only the branches leading to the parietal cell area and not the coeliac and hepatic branches nor the nerves of Latarjet (highly selective or parietal cell vagotomy). By retaining the innervation of the pyloric antrum in a highly selective vagotomy, there is no functional gastric outlet obstruction. After a truncal vagotomy the entire stomach becomes atonic and, to ensure gastric emptying, it is necessary to do a pyloroplasty (which destroys the pyloric sphincter) or a gastrojejunostomy (as a result of which food can bypass the pyloric sphincter). A highly selective vagotomy is regarded by many as the operation of choice in the surgical treatment of a duodenal ulcer.

At the level of the diaphragmatic hiatus, the anterior vagus nerve lies behind the peritoneum and phreno-oesophageal ligament, and is closely applied to the anterior surface of the oesophagus. It is approached by mobilizing the left lobe of the liver, having divided the left triangular ligament, the peritoneum over the anterior aspect of the oesophagus at the gastro-oesophageal junction, and the underlying connective tissue forming the phreno-oesophageal ligament. The nerve usually consists of a single large trunk, but there may be more than one trunk at the level of the diaphragm in

30 per cent of cases. It is often easier to identify the nerve by palpation, with slight tension on the oesophagus, than it is to see it at this stage. It is attached to the oesophagus by a vascular mesovagus which only becomes apparent as the anterior trunk is mobilized. Often a branch passes to the stomach at a point 5–7 cm above the cardio-oesophageal junction, so that this length of nerve must be mobilized to identify any branch passing to the left.

The posterior vagus nerve is not applied to the oesophagus, but is separated from it by about 10 mm. It is slightly more to the patient's right than the anterior nerve, and is identified by passing the index finger of the right hand behind the oesophagus. It can be felt as a thick cord, usually thicker than the anterior nerve, well posterior to the oesophagus. The posterior vagus nerve at the level of the diaphragm may be present as more than one trunk in 10 per cent of cases. The nerve of Grassi may pass to the stomach at a point 5–6 cm above the cardio-oesophageal junction. For this reason, 5–6 cm of the nerve must be mobilized from the oesophagus and any branch to the left identified.

By keeping to the left side of both main vagal trunks in a highly selective vagotomy, the surgeon will avoid damaging the hepatic branch of the anterior vagus and coeliac branch of the posterior vagus nerve. Both these branches arise from the right side of their respective parent trunks within the lesser omentum. Damage to either branch may be an important factor in the development of postvagotomy diarrhoea.

The parietal area of the stomach is denervated in a highly selective vagotomy by meticulously dividing the small vessels and nerves running from the lesser omentum onto the lesser curvature. The denervation of the lesser curvature is continued down to the 'crow's foot'. Should a branch of the 'crow's foot' supply an area of the stomach situated more than 7 cm proximal to the vein of Mayo, it is divided. The fundic gland mucosa is considered to start at a point 7 cm proximal to the vein of Mayo.

THE STOMACH AS OESOPHAGEAL REPLACEMENT

The stomach has a lesser curve which is short and relatively immobile because of fixation by the left gastric artery and its branches. When this vessel is cut there is considerable mobility of this curvature. If the stomach is now freed from its omental and ligamentous ties and diaphragmatic attachments, and the duodenum is fully mobilized, it can be brought up to the neck. The blood supply is adequately maintained if the two arteries entering from the right are preserved—the large right gastro-epiploic and the small right gastric. It is necessary however to preserve the vascular arcades to ensure a free passage for the collateral circulation (*Fig.* 16).

In carcinoma of the oesophagus, the stomach is used in preference to the small bowel and colon to replace the resected oesophagus.

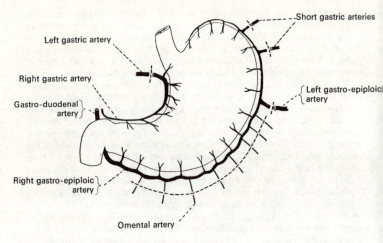

Fig. 16. The sites of division of the blood supply to the stomach when it is used to replace the oesophagus.

Chapter 3

THE ROTATION OF THE GUT

At an early stage of development the alimentary canal is represented by a tube suspended in the midline of the abdominal cavity by a ventral and dorsal mesentery. It consists of three portions, each of which has it own artery, and each of which is destined for a specific function (*see Table* 1).

Table 1

Name	Extent	Artery	Function
Foregut	Stomach and duodenum as far as the entry of the bile duct	Coeliac axis	Digestive
Midgut	From the ampulla of Vater to the junction of the middle with the left third of the transverse colon	Superior mesenteric	Absorptive
Hindgut	The left colon	Inferior mesenteric	Excretory

Departures from the normal situation of the component parts of the foregut and hindgut are exceedingly rare. Errors in the location of the alimentary canal are almost entirely confined to the midgut loop because of the extreme complexity attending its development.

DISPOSITION OF THE GUT BEFORE ROTATION COMMENCES

See Fig. 17.

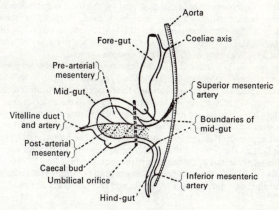

Fig. 17. Alimentary canal before rotation. The midgut loop has herniated into the umbilical cord. The dorsal mesentery, suspending the gut from midline of posterior abdominal wall, is not shown. (After Dott.)

Foregut

The upper part of the alimentary tube soon bulges to form the stomach. The developing pancreas bulges the dorsal mesentery of the duodenum, which thus takes on the normal curvature of its upper part, at the same time becoming fixed in place by the fusion of its mesentery with the peritoneum of the posterior abdominal wall.

Hindgut

The upper end of this part of the tube is fixed to the abdominal wall near the origin of the superior mesenteric artery by a condensed part of the dorsal mesentery. Thus a fixed point is formed where the mid- and hindgut join (the colic angle). It will be noticed that the extremities of the midgut are firmly anchored by the fixed points in the duodenum above and the fixed colic angle below. These two points are quite close together, forming the 'duodenocolic isthmus'.

Midgut

There exists at this time a portion of the coelomic (future peritoneal) cavity in the umbilical cord, known as the 'extra-embryonic coelom'. The midgut forms a loop convex forward. It grows so rapidly that the intra-embryonic coelom is too small to accommodate it, so that part of the loop is extruded into the extra-embryonic coelom in the umbilical cord, forming a temporary physiological hernia. Persistence of this extrusion at birth is called an exomphalos. It is covered from without in by amnion, a thin layer of Wharton's jelly and an inner lining of parietal peritoneum.

At the apex of the extruded gut is the former site of the vitello-intestinal duct (as it is already obliterated). The artery of the midgut loop (superior mesenteric) runs from the aorta through the duodenocolic isthmus to the apex of the extruded gut, sending off branches forwards to the anterior segment of the midgut loop, and backwards to its posterior segment. The midgut loop and its mesentery still lie in the sagittal plane. The part of the gut in front of the artery is the pre-arterial segment, and its mesentery the pre-arterial mesentery. The gut behind the artery is the post-arterial segment, and its mesentery the post-arterial mesentery. During the fifth week the bud for the caecum and appendix appears on the post-arterial segment of the loop. This is the state of affairs at the beginning of the fifth week, and rotation is about to begin.

CHRONOLOGY OF ROTATION OF THE MIDGUT LOOP

Rotation takes place in three stages.

First stage of rotation

This occurs while the loop lies in the umbilical cord, between the fifth and the tenth weeks. It is largely brought about by the development of the liver. The growth of the right lobe of the liver carries this organ downward and to the right, taking the left umbilical vein (future ligamentum teres) with it (*Fig*. 18). This exerts pressure on the base of the pre-arterial segment of the midgut loop so that this segment is pushed down and to the right. As the pre- and post-arterial segments lie side by side within the narrow confines of the umbilical hernia, the movement of the pre-arterial portion down and to the right forces the post-arterial segment upwards and to the left. The first stage of rotation is complete when the midgut loop has rotated through 90 degrees in an anticlockwise direction (*Fig*. 19). (Recent studies suggest that growth in length

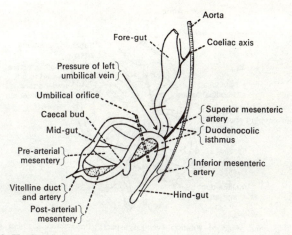

Fig. 18. The first stage of rotation is occurring. Arrow indicates pressure being exerted by left umbilical vein upon the pre-arterial segment of the loop, forcing it down and to the right. (After Dott.)

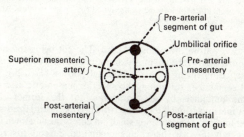

Fig. 19. Diagrammatic representation of first stage rotation, showing rotation of midgut loop through 90° in an anticlockwise direction. Dotted lines show position of gut and its mesentery at completion of first stage of rotation.

of the small bowel causes 180 degrees of anticlockwise rotation before the return of the bowel to the abdomen.)

Second stage of rotation
This occurs at the tenth to eleventh week.

About the beginning of the tenth week the midgut loop returns to the

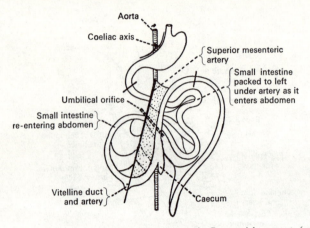

Fig. 20. Second stage of rotation (ventral aspect). Pre-arterial segment (small intestine) of midgut loop has increased in length disproportionately to post-arterial segment. Caecum and ascending colon have become relatively thick. The physiological umbilical hernia is reducing. Small gut is re-entering abdomen on right side of superior mesenteric vessels and passing to the left side of abdomen behind the mesenteric vessels. The vessels are held forward to the umbilicus by the caecum, which still lies outside the umbilicus. (After Dott.)

abdominal cavity from the umbilical cord. The gut being too bulky to be returned *en masse*, it retreats in a definite order. The pre-arterial portion returns first, commencing with its proximal portion (*Fig.* 20). While the pre-arterial segment is returning, the superior mesenteric artery is firmly fixed to the umbilicus by its termination (at the former site of the vitello-intestinal duct), and is therefore stretched like a cord from commencement to termination. The returning small gut enters the abdomen to the right of the artery, but, the space here being too limited, the coils first reduced are pushed to the left behind the taut artery by those following on. By their passage to the left they displace the dorsal mesentery of the hindgut (which occupies the midline) before them, so that the descending colon comes to occupy the left flank and the colic angle is pushed up to form the future splenic flexure. The last coil of the ileum carries the superior mesenteric artery with it as it is reduced.

The caecum still lies in the umbilical cord on a plane anterior to the small intestine and its artery. The caecum and right half of the colon now reduce, passing upward and to the right, the colon crossing the pedicle of the small gut at the point of origin of the superior mesenteric artery from the aorta, and the caecum comes to lie under the liver. The subsequent growth elongation of the

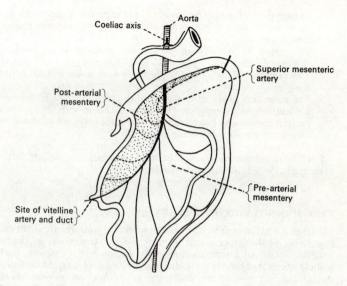

Fig. 21. Completion of second stage of rotation. Caecum is in contact with posterior abdominal wall in right loin. Midgut loop has rotated on axis of superior mesenteric vessels through 270° from its original plane. The essentials of the permanent disposition of the viscera have been attained. (After Dott.)

colon pushes the caecum into the right loin. Now the second stage of rotation is complete (*Fig.* 21).

Note that:

1. The duodenum crosses behind the upper part of the superior mesenteric artery.
2. The transverse colon crosses in front of the same part of this vessel.
3. The descending colon has been pushed into the left flank.
4. The caecum is in the right loin.
5. The coils of small gut range from left upper to right lower segments of the abdomen.

Third stage of rotation

This occurs between the eleventh week and shortly after birth.

During this stage:

1. The caecum descends further, reaching the right iliac fossa.

2. Certain parts of the gut become fixed to the posterior abdominal wall by fusion of their primitive mesenteries with the posterior parietal peritoneum.
3. The mesentery of the small gut becomes adherent to the posterior abdominal wall.
4. The post-arterial mesentery of the transverse colon persists as the transverse mesocolon.
5. The mesentery of the caecum, ascending colon, hepatic flexure, and hindgut becomes completely obliterated by fusion with the posterior parietal peritoneum, excepting in the case of the pelvic colon, where the mesentery persists as the future mesocolon.

It will be noted that the 'function' of the third stage is the efficient fixation of the gut to the posterior abdominal wall.

ERRORS IN ROTATION OF THE GUT

The interest that the rotation of the gut has for the surgeon arises from the fact that errors in this process lead to grave surgical conditions. In clinical practice, rotational errors are commonly encountered in patients with malformations that involve the abdominal wall. Examples are exomphalos, the abdominal musculature deficiency syndromes, and posterolateral diaphragmatic hernia.

The first stage of rotation is never interfered with except in a group of conditions classified under the term 'exomphalos'.

The second stage of rotation consists essentially of the reduction of the physiological hernia in orderly sequence. Abnormalities of the second stage are due to a departure from this sequence. The bulk of the caecum is an important factor in ensuring that it remains outside the abdomen until the remaining gut is reduced.

During the third or fixation stage of rotation, errors may lead to imperfect fixation.

Classification of rotation errors

1. Derangements of the first stage of rotation:
   i. Exomphalos major.
2. Derangements of the second stage of rotation:
   i. Non-rotation of the midgut loop.
   ii. Reversed rotation of the midgut loop.
   iii. Malrotation of the midgut loop.
3. Derangements of the third stage of rotation:
   i. Subphrenic caecum.
   ii. Right lumbar caecum.

iii. Pelvic caecum.
iv. Mobile proximal colon.
v. Volvulus and torsion.

Derangements of second stage of rotation

NON-ROTATION OF THE MIDGUT LOOP: In this condition the umbilical ring is lax. The colon and caecum are the first constituents of the physiological hernia to reduce. The small gut which follows displaces the colon and the superior mesenteric artery to the left.
1. The small gut lies chiefly to the right of the midline.
2. The duodenum descends from its normally fixed upper part down along the right side of the superior mesenteric artery.
3. The terminal ileum may cross the midline to reach a left iliac caecum, entering the caecum from its right instead of from its left or may terminate in the midline in a pelvic caecum.
4. The colon is confined to the left side of the abdomen.
5. Though the gut may become fixed in these abnormal positions, on the other hand no fixative adhesions may occur, so that the whole midgut loop may be suspended in the abdominal cavity by an extremely narrow pedicle (the duodenocolic isthmus).

REVERSED ROTATION OF THE MIDGUT LOOP: In this condition (*Fig*. 22) the caecum and ascending colon reduce first, passing behind the superior mesenteric vessels. The small gut therefore reduces in front of the vessels. As a result:
1. The transverse colon crosses behind the superior mesenteric artery.
2. The duodenum crosses in front of the superior mesenteric artery.

MALROTATION OF THE MIDGUT LOOP: This term is used to imply irregular and mixed defects of rotation.

Derangements of third stage of rotation

CAECUM: Too early fixation causes imperfect descent of the organ, which may be subhepatic or right lumbar.
   Deficient fixation causes the caecum to be pelvic.

PROXIMAL COLON: Deficient fixation of the post-arterial mesentery causes a mobile proximal colon.

Pathological consequences of anomalies of rotation
The following facts are noteworthy:

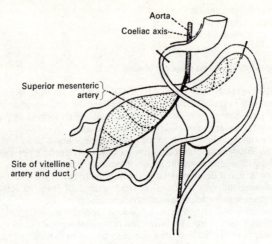

Fig. 22. Reversed rotation of midgut loop. The midgut has rotated in a clockwise direction through 90° from the original sagittal plane. Thus the colon comes to lie behind the mesenteric vessels and the duodenum in front of them. (After Dott.)

1. No functional disturbance may result from abnormal fixation.
2. Excessive fixation may cause interference with mobility, kinks, and compression of the bowel.
3. Deficient fixation may cause ptosis, torsion, volvulus.
4. Abnormal rotation predisposes to volvulus which causes intestinal obstruction. Such obstruction is particularly likely to occur within the first few days of life (volvulus neonatorum). The extent of the twisted gut is from the duodenum above to the transverse colon below.
5. Volvulus of the ileocaecal segment is the typical lesion in later life resulting from imperfect rotation or deficient fixation of the gut.

Chapter 4

THE DUODENUM, JEJUNUM AND ILEUM

DUODENUM

The duodenum is 25 cm long. It makes a C-shaped bend which embraces the head of the pancreas. It consists of three parts.

FIRST PART: Extends up, backwards, and to the right to the level of the upper border of the first lumbar vertebra. It is 5 cm long.

SECOND PART: Extends downwards to the level of the lower border of the 3rd lumbar vertebra. It is 7·5 cm long.

THIRD PART: Extends to the left, then upwards (also called the fourth part) to the level of the left side of the 2nd lumbar vertebra. It is 12·5 cm long.

Relations

FIRST PART:
Anterior: Quadrate lobe of the liver.
Posterior: Portal vein, gastroduodenal artery, and bile duct. The vena cava is behind these.
Superior: Epiploic foramen and hepatic artery (horizontal part).
Inferior: Head of the pancreas.

SECOND PART:
Anterior: Gallbladder, transverse colon, and small gut.
Posterior: Renal vessels, the pelvis of the kidney, and the kidney.
Right: Hepatic flexure of the colon.
Left: Head of the pancreas. It is pierced about the middle by the bile and pancreatic ducts.

THIRD PART:
Anterior: Superior mesenteric vessels, the root of the mesentery, the transverse colon and mesocolon.
Posterior: Inferior vena cava, aorta, spermatic vessels of both sides, the left sympathetic trunk, and the left psoas.
Superior: Head of the pancreas.
Inferior: Small gut.

Peritoneal relations

In general, the C which this part of the gut makes is covered anteriorly and on its convexity by the peritoneum except where the transverse colon crosses the second part and holds the peritoneum away (*Fig.* 23). The posterior surface and concavity of the C are devoid of peritoneum.

The first 2–5 cm of the first part is entirely covered by peritoneum except for a small part above and behind. Duodenal ulcers usually occur in this part of the duodenum. When the ulcer is situated on the posterior wall of the duodenum it causes adhesions between the duodenum and pancreas which may form the base of the ulcer; posterior ulcers penetrate. Massive bleeding

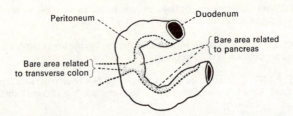

Fig. 23. Peritoneal relations of the duodenum. The stippled area is uncovered by peritoneum and is in relation to the pancreas in the concavity of the gut and in relation to the transverse colon where this crosses the descending portion of duodenum.

may occur if it erodes the gastroduodenal artery. Ulcers situated on the anterior wall may perforate and cause generalized peritonitis.

The ulcer-bearing area of the duodenum is referred to as the duodenal bulb or cap by the radiologists. A barium meal study of this part of the duodenum resembles a cap (*Fig.* 24), probably because there are no folds in this part of the duodenum. As a result of distortion of the duodenal wall by ulceration, pseudodiverticula may occur in this part of the duodenum.

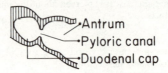

Fig. 24. The duodenal cap.

In the region where the bile duct enters the second part, a congenital diverticulum of the duodenum may occur. It owes its existence to the fact that at a very early developmental stage more than one outgrowth from the gut takes place to form the liver. Usually all except one (the permanent bile duct) disappear. Parts of a second outgrowth may remain, forming a blind protrusion from the bowel. Such a diverticulum is devoid of peritoneal covering. This is of surgical importance, as its removal would be attended by risks of peritonitis since the retroperitoneal tissues have little resistance to infection and the suturing of bowel without a peritoneal coat is less secure.

The cystogastrocolic band is a fold which stretches from the gallbladder across the pylorus to the transverse colon. It may produce symptoms, dating from birth, of partial obstruction to the pyloric outlet from the stomach.

Duodenojejunal flexure

The duodenojejunal flexure is at the left side of the 2nd lumbar vertebra just below the pancreas. It is a fixed part of the gut and easily found. It is supported by a ligament containing unstriped muscle which passes to it from the region of the left crus of the diaphragm and the tissue about the coeliac plexus. This is the suspensory ligament of the duodenum (ligament of Treitz).

Duodenal fossae

PARADUODENAL FOSSA: This fossa (*Fig.* 25) lies to the left of the duodenojejunal flexure and is open to the right and upwards. It occurs in 20 per cent of persons. It never exists together with other types of duodenal fossae.

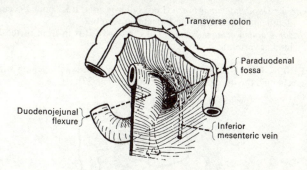

Fig. 25. The paraduodenal fossa.

Boundaries:
   Above: Pancreas and renal vessels.
   Right: Aorta.
   Left: Kidney.
   Anterior: The inferior mesenteric vein runs in the anterior wall of the fossa.
   Should the fossa be the site of strangulated gut, its surgical enlargement can be effected in a downward direction, to avoid injury to the inferior mesenteric vein.

SUPERIOR AND INFERIOR DUODENOJEJUNAL FOSSAE: These often exist (*Fig.* 26). They are formed, when present, by two peritoneal folds running to the left from the region of the termination of the duodenum.

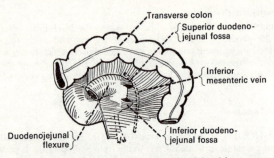

Fig. 26. The superior and inferior duodenojejunal fossae.

Superior Duodenojejunal Fossa: Looks downwards. It is about 2–5 cm in depth and is in front of the 2nd lumbar vertebra.

Inferior Duodenojejunal Fossa: Looks upwards. It is in front of the 3rd lumbar vertebra.

INFERIOR DUODENAL FOSSA: This is an occasional opening which extends behind the third part of the duodenum (*Fig.* 27).

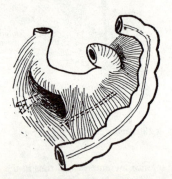

Fig. 27. The inferior duodenal fossa.

MESENTERICOPARIETAL FOSSA OF WALDEYER: The most usual position of this fossa is in the first part of the mesojejunum, immediately behind the superior mesenteric artery, and immediately below the duodenum. The fossa varies considerably in size. The fossa has its orifice looking to the left, its blind extremity to the right and downwards. In front it is bounded by the superior mesenteric artery (or its continuation, the ileocolic artery), and behind by the lumbar vertebrae. The peritoneum of the left leaf of the mesentery lines the fossa; that of the right covers the blind end, and is then continued directly into the posterior parietal peritoneum.

Herniae into this fossa are rare (*Fig.* 28).

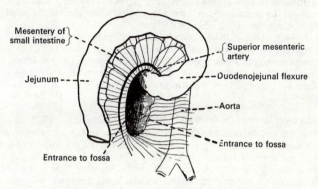

Fig. 28. The mesentericoparietal fossa of Waldeyer.

Mobilization of the duodenum

The first part of the duodenum is mobilized during a subtotal gastrectomy to facilitate closure of the duodenal stump or for anastomosis to the gastric remnant. The bowel has a rich blood supply through small arterial twigs from the right gastric artery which supply the superior border, twigs from the gastroduodenal artery which supply the posterior surface and from the right gastro-epiploic artery to the inferior border of the duodenum.

The second part of the duodenum is mobilized by dividing the peritoneal reflection from the convexity of the C onto the posterior abdominal wall. The loose areolar tissue between the head of the pancreas and aorta is divided. With extensive mobilization of the second part of the duodenum, the pylorus can be made to reach the oesophageal hiatus.

The third (and the fourth) part of the duodenum is mobilized by dividing the peritoneum between the aorta and inferior mesenteric vein. The aorta is exposed by reflecting the duodenum upward and to the right.

SMALL INTESTINE (JEJUNUM AND ILEUM)

The average length of this part of the intestine is 7 m. The upper two-fifths are jejunum, the lower three-fifths are ileum. It is entirely surrounded by peritoneum. It is important to note that the length of the small gut is variable, the extremes being 4 and 9 m.

The small gut is suspended by its mesentery which extends from the left side of the 2nd lumbar vertebra to the right iliac fossa, crossing the third part of the duodenum, aorta, vena cava, and right ureter in its course. It is 1·5 m in length along this line of attachment, but along its free border it is as long as the small gut. Its depth is 15 cm, except in relation to the parts of the small gut which occupy the pelvis, where it is 20 cm.

The parts of the small intestine which lie in the pelvis are the terminal ileum (except the last 5 cm which are fixed in the right iliac fossa), and about 1·5 m of small gut beginning at a point 1·8 m from the duodenojejunal flexure to a point 3·4 m from the flexure. These portions of the small gut are likely to be affected in pelvic peritonitis and irradiation of the pelvis.

Differences between the ileum and jejunum

These are well known. The only distinction of use to the operating surgeon who wants to be sure at a glance whether a part of the gut is upper or lower small gut depends on the blood supply (*Fig*. 29). Jejunum: one or two arterial arcades in the mesentery with parallel vessels 3·7 cm long going to the gut. Ileum: two or three arterial arcades in the mesentery with parallel vessels 1·2 cm long going to the gut.

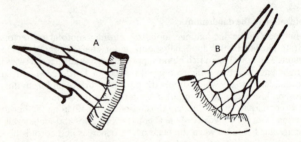

Fig. 29. Arrangement of arteries of small intestine. A, Jejunum; B, ileum.

Blood supply of small bowel

There is no collateral circulation beyond the terminal arcades in the small gut. There is thus no communication between the vasa recta or between the branches they give off to the bowel wall, but there is a rich submucosal anastomosis which ensures an adequate blood supply after small bowel anastomosis, provided that the vasa recta are not damaged too extensively (*Fig*. 30).

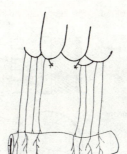

Fig. 30. Small intestine anastomosis. Preparing for the resection.

Congenital abnormalities in the region of the junction of the fore- and midgut

The gut, at a very early stage in its history, is centrally suspended in the abdominal cavity, being attached to the anterior abdominal wall by the ventral mesentery, and to the posterior abdominal wall by the dorsal mesentery.

The liver is formed from a bud which grows out from the gut at the junction of the foregut and the midgut; this bud grows into and distends the ventral mesentery. As the liver increases in size it extends up into the right region of the abdomen and pulls the ventral mesentery over with it, also the duodenum. The falciform ligament is part of this ventral mesentery, so too are the coronary ligament of the liver and the lesser omentum. The rest of the ventral mesentery disappears (*Fig.* 31).

CONGENITAL OBSTRUCTION OF THE DUODENUM: These are classified into two groups—extrinsic and intrinsic forms.

Extrinsic:

1. *Persistence of ventral mesentery:* Embryological remnants, such as the cystogastrocolic fold (*Fig.* 32), are common but are seldom of clinical importance.
2. *Volvulus neonatorum:* Where the duodenum and midgut loops have undergone malrotation with persistence of the duodenocolic isthmus, clockwise rotation around the superior mesenteric vascular pedicle may occur, with occlusion of the distal part of the duodenum by external pressure. In these cases fibrous bands (Ladd's bands) run laterally across the duodenum, attaching the malplaced colon or its mesentery to the ipsilateral kidney. In exceptional circumstances these bands, in the absence of a volvulus, may cause duodenal obstruction and, therefore at operation for volvulus neonatorum,

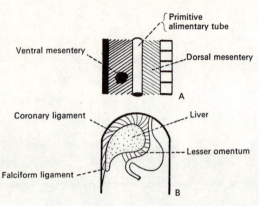

Fig. 31. A, The primitive alimentary canal suspended by ventral and dorsal mesenteries; B, remains of ventral mesentery (mesogastrium).

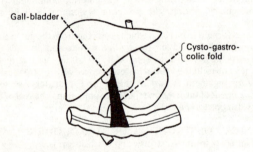

Fig. 32. The cystogastrocolic fold.

these bands have to be looked for and if present they should be divided.

3. *Isolated anomalies of duodenal rotation:* Compression or kinking of the duodenum by bands is rarely encountered in patients with incomplete rotation of the duodenal C loop. The obstruction usually involves the third or fourth part of the duodenum and may be associated with situs inversus abdominalis.

4. *Preduodenal portal vein:* This is usually a chance anatomical finding. When detected in a patient with duodenal obstruction, a second intrinsic anomaly and reason for the obstruction, are usually found.

Intrinsic: At the site where the bile duct grows out to form the liver, atresia or stenosis of the duodenum may occur. Developmental errors tend to occur at the site of an embryological event. In the second month of development, the passage from the stomach to the duodenum is completely blocked by proliferation of the epithelium. Vacuoles appear in this epithelium and then septa stretch across the lumen which ultimately disappear, thus re-establishing the channel. Should development be arrested before vacuolation occurs the intestine remains a solid cord. If development stops before the breaking down is complete, septa occur. Either of these two abnormalities produces obstruction (atresias).

In contradistinction to this type of obstruction, atresias that occur elsewhere in the intestinal tract are due to episodes of intestinal infarction occurring during intra-uterine life.

In cases of duodenal atresia at the level of the ampulla, bile is usually found both proximal and distal to the site of complete obstruction. This infers that an anomaly of the distal common bile duct, i.e. a bifid duct, must be present in these instances.

Remnants of the vitello-intestinal duct

The midgut communicates at an early developmental stage with the yolk sac. This communication is the vitello-intestinal duct also called the omphalo-mesenteric duct. Normally it entirely disappears. Vestiges of it may persist (*Fig.* 33). They are:

1. PATENT VITELLO-INTESTINAL DUCT: The duct entirely fails to close, small intestinal content being discharged at the umbilicus, once the umbilical cord separates.

2. MECKEL'S DIVERTICULUM: The duct closes at its umbilical end but remains open at the intestinal end. This is called a Meckel's diverticulum and occurs in 2 per cent of people. The diverticulum is 5 cm (2 inches) long and is found 60 cm (2 feet) from the ileocaecal valve. In 2 per cent of cases, accessory pancreatic tissue occurs in the vestige. A diverticulum with a broad base may cause intussusception. It is a true diverticulum which is attached to the antimesenteric border of the ileum. It may or may not possess a mesentery which, if present, arises from the mesentery of the small gut. Its apex may be free or attached by a fibrous band to the umbilicus, or to the mesentery, in which case it can cause intestinal obstruction. Bands of other origin, i.e. remnants of the vitelline vessels and not of the duct, occur and attach the mesentery of the ileum at Meckel's point to the inner surface of the umbilicus. Where the diverticulum has a narrow neck, stasis of its contents may precipitate the development of a diverticulitis, causing symptoms indistinguishable from those of appendicitis, but more dangerous because its walls are

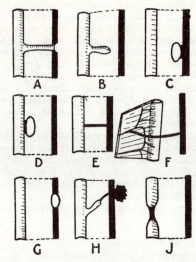

Fig. 33. The vitelline system and its vestiges. A, Patent vitelline duct; B, Meckel's diverticulum; C, enteratoma; D, enterocystocoele; E, fibrous remnant of Meckel's diverticulum; F, remnant of vitelline vessels; G, cysts of umbilicus; H, vitelline sinus; J, obliteration of lumen of the gut at the region of attachment of the vitello-intestinal duct.

thinner and it therefore perforates more easily, and because it is in the middle of the peritoneal cavity where inflammation is more likely to spread.

Gastric-like epithelium with acid-secreting properties is found in a Meckel's diverticulum in 12 per cent of cases and peptic ulceration with its associated dangers of haemorrhage and perforation may occur. Such heterotopic gastric mucosa may occur at the neck of the diverticulum, which can usually be detected by careful palpation. Removal of the diverticulum should therefore include a portion of the adjacent ileum.

A Meckel's diverticulum may enter a hernia sac (Littre's hernia).

3. VITELLINE CYSTS: The duct closes at both ends but remains patent in part. This may cause cysts behind the umbilicus called enterotomata (*Fig*. 33C).

4. VITELLINE SINUS: The duct remains open at its umbilical end and appears as a raspberry red mass at the umbilicus because it becomes turned inside out by intra-abdominal pressure (*Fig*. 33H).

5. THE DUCT: This entirely disappears but a fibrous band remains. This represents the remains of the duct or the vessels of the duct (vitelline) and passes from the umbilicus to the mesentery or to the small gut. Its importance is that it may act as a band under which a loop of gut may be compressed or as a fulcrum around which torsion producing a volvulus occurs, causing obstruction (*Fig.* 33E and F).

Chapter 5

THE LARGE BOWEL, ANAL CANAL AND ISCHIO-RECTAL FOSSA

The large intestine is a muscular tube which extends from the end of the ileum to the anus and is comprised of caecum and appendix, colon, rectum and anal canal. It is approximately 135 cm long. The circular muscle layer is continuous, but the longitudinal muscle is arranged in three bands, the taeniae coli, as far as the rectum where these bands fuse to form a continuous layer. The voluminous large bowel is 'gathered' by the taeniae coli to form the characteristic sacculated appearance.

Those parts with mesenteries (transverse colon, pelvic colon, and appendix) are completely surrounded by peritoneum except for a narrow band between the two layers of the mesenteric attachment. The other parts are devoid of peritoneum posteriorly. The caecum is completely surrounded by peritoneum, except a small part posteriorly and superiorly.

THE APPENDIX

The appendix lies at the commencement of the large gut and has the same basic structure. Its wall contains much lymphoid tissue. The appendix is approximately 9 cm long.

Embryology of the appendix

At an early embryonic stage it has the same calibre as the caecum and is in line with it. It is formed by excessive growth of the right wall of the caecum which pushes the appendix to the inner side (*Fig.* 34).

Congenital absence of the appendix is extremely rare.

Mesentery of the appendix

The appendicular artery reaches the appendix in the edge of this mesentery. If the mesentery is incomplete, the artery lies on the wall of the appendix in its distal part and may become thrombosed in acute appendicitis.

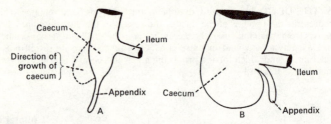

Fig. 34. Development of the appendix. A, Caecum at an early developmental stage showing the future appendix below. The dotted line shows how the appendix is pushed medially by the outgrowth of the right wall of the caecum. B, The adult condition.

Position of the appendix

The location of the base of the appendix is dependent on the position of the caecum. The caecum usually lies in the right iliac fossa, but in incomplete rotation of the bowel it may lie at a higher level beneath the liver in relation to the duodenum and gallbladder. In this position, the symptoms and signs of acute appendicitis may mimic acute cholecystitis. When the caecum is long and mobile the appendix may lie in the pelvis, in which case the tenderness in acute appendicitis is found maximally on pelvic examination. The caecum may even lie in the left iliac fossa and then tenderness to palpation due to appendicitis is similar to that found in acute diverticulitis of the sigmoid colon. The position of the tip of the appendix in relation to the caecum is variable and has been likened to the hands of a clock (*Fig.* 35).

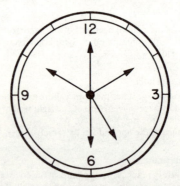

Fig. 35. Positions of the appendix: 12 o'clock—retrocaecal; 2 o'clock—retro-ileal; 5 o'clock—pelvic; 6 o'clock—inguinal position; 10 o'clock—paracolic.

10 AND 12 O'CLOCK POSITIONS: The appendix passes upwards, and may be to the outer side [paracolic (10)] or directly behind the caecum [retrocolic (12)]. The organ may be partly or entirely behind the peritoneum. It is sometimes in front of the kidney.

2 O'CLOCK POSITION: The organ is entirely intraperitoneal and lies behind or in front of the terminal ileum. If inflamed it may affect this part of the ileum and cause incomplete obstruction of the small gut.

5 O'CLOCK OR PELVIC POSITION: The appendix hangs over the pelvic brim into the true pelvis. If inflamed it may cause irritation of the rectum and bladder.

6 O'CLOCK POSITION: Appendix passes down towards the middle of the inguinal ligament.

Appendicectomy

A transverse incision is made over the point of maximal tenderness which is usually at the junction of the outer and middle thirds of a line joining the anterior superior iliac spine with the umbilicus. In advanced pregnancy, the gravid uterus displaces the caecum and appendix so that the site of maximal tenderness is higher.

The aponeurosis of the external oblique is cut in the direction of its fibres. Laterally, the muscle itself may need to be divided. The internal oblique and transversus abdominis muscles are split in the direction of their fibres. The peritoneum is stripped off the back of the transversus muscle before incising it, to facilitate subsequent suture of the peritoneum. The peritoneum is incised at the medial end of the incision, because a laterally placed peritoneal incision may damage the caecum or result in a dissection into the extraperitoneal space.

The caecum should be identified by the faintly bluish colour of its wall and the taeniae coli. If one of these taeniae is followed inferiorly it leads to the base of the appendix. The appendix is mobilized by gently breaking down inflammatory adhesions from the lateral side of the appendix. The appendix is delivered onto the anterior abdominal wall and the meso-appendix is ligated and divided. The base of the appendix is then divided and the appendiceal stump is invaginated with a purse-string suture.

Should the appendix be retrocaecal or adherent to the posterior parietal peritoneum a retrograde procedure can be followed. The caecum is gently delivered into the wound, the base of the appendix is transected, the stump is invaginated and the caecum is returned to the peritoneal cavity. With the caecum within the peritoneal cavity there is now more room available and the vessels in the meso-appendix are carefully divided by working towards the tip of the appendix.

The incision in the abdominal wall can be enlarged medially by dividing the anterior and posterior rectus sheaths and retracting the rectus muscle medially.

An incisional hernia is infrequent after this incision which passes through three layers of muscle with overlapping fibres.

The ilio-inguinal and iliohypogastric nerves, which are both motor and sensory nerves to the inguinal region, run between the internal oblique and transversus muscles from just medial to the anterior superior iliac spine to the inguinal canal. Damage to these nerves may result in paralysis of the conjoint tendon of the inguinal canal (*see* p. 126), with the subsequent formation of an inguinal hernia.

Fossae in relation to the caecum
See Fig. 36.

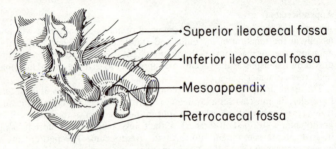

Fig. 36. Fossae associated with the caecum and terminal part of ileum.

ILEOCOLIC OR SUPERIOR ILEOCAECAL FOSSA: This is formed by a fold of peritoneum produced by the anterior caecal artery.
  Boundaries:
    Anterior: The ileocolic fold contains the ileocaecal artery and vein.
    Posterior: Ileum and its mesentery.
    Right: Ascending colon.

The fossa is open to the left.

INFERIOR ILEOCAECAL FOSSA: This is formed by the ileocaecal or bloodless fold of Treves, which extends from the terminal ileum and caecum to the mesentery of the appendix. It should not be confused with the meso-appendix which contains the appendicular artery.

Boundaries:
  Anterior and inferior: Ileocaecal fold.
  Superior: Posterior surface of the ileum and its mesentery.
  Posterior: Mesentery of the appendix.

RETRO- OR SUBCAECAL FOSSA: This is posterior to the caecum.
  Boundaries:
    Anterior: Posterior surface of the caecum.
    Right: Peritoneum of the right colic gutter.
    Left: Mesentery.
    Posterior: The iliac fossa covered by parietal peritoneum.

It often contains the appendix.

THE LARGE BOWEL

Mesenteries of the large gut

TRANSVERSE MESOCOLON: It is a double fold of peritoneum which suspends the transverse colon from the anterior border of the pancreas. The middle colic artery runs in the mesocolon (*Fig.* 37).

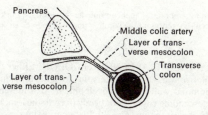

Fig. 37. The attachment of the transverse mesocolon to the anterior border of the pancreas.

Adhesions are frequently present between the superior fold of transverse mesocolon and the posterior wall of the gastric antrum which have to be divided during the course of a subtotal gastrectomy. During this part of the dissection, the middle colic vessels may be damaged. In the operation of radical gastrectomy for cancer, the greater omentum is detached from the transverse colon together with a thin layer of peritoneum representing the fusion of the greater omentum to the transverse mesocolon and its extension over the pancreas.

PELVIC MESOCOLON: It has an inverted V-shaped attachment. The left limb is attached to the brim of the left side of the pelvis. The right limb passes from the apex down to the third piece of sacrum. The apex of the V is situated exactly over the left ureter where it crosses the pelvic brim. This is the surgeon's guide to the left ureter. The mesocolon carries the superior rectal vessels.

JACKSON'S MEMBRANE: This is a fold of peritoneum (*Fig.* 38), thin and diaphanous, which extends from the posterior abdominal wall in the region to the right of the ascending colon, in a direction downwards and inwards, and is attached to the anterior longitudinal band of the ascending colon or caecum. It may even extend from the hepatic flexure to the caecum, or over only part of this segment of the gut. The blood vessels are thin, long and parallel, as shown in *Fig.* 38.

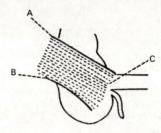

Fig. 38. Jackson's membrane. The membrane lies between the thick lines (A) and (B). The lines between (C), represent the parallel, fine blood vessels so characteristic of this membrane.

MESENTERY TO THE ASCENDING COLON: Either the ascending or descending colon may have a mesentery due to faulty fixation of the gut to the posterior abdominal wall during development. If a mesentery exists, the ascending or descending colon is not firmly fixed to the loin, but is dependent from it by a fold of peritoneum (*Fig.* 39). In the case of the descending colon this is not common and is of little significance. In the case of the ascending colon it is of significance, because when supplied with a mesentery the ascending colon falls away from the loin and drags the caecum and hepatic flexure with it. Though the possession of such a mesentery may never render its owner uncomfortable, it plays an important part in volvulus of the caecum and ileocaecal intussusception.

    Volvulus of the Caecum: The caecum becomes twisted around its own long axis. This cannot occur if the gut is firmly fixed to the abdominal wall.

    Intussusception: The ileum normally projects very slightly into the caecum at the ileocaecal valve. This may, under certain conditions, form the starting point of an invagination of the gut into the caecum. When this

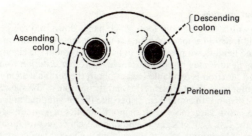

Fig. 39. A diagrammatic transverse section through the abdomen showing the normal relation of the ascending colon and the descending colon to the peritoneum.

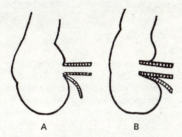

Fig. 40. A, Shows the normal slight invagination of ileum into caecum at the valve. An exaggeration of this is the first stage of intussusception of the ileocaecal variety (B).

occurs the condition is progressive and the invaginated gut travels into the ascending colon, dragging the caecum and appendix with it (*Fig.* 40). This condition is more likely to occur if the caecum is not firmly anchored to the posterior abdominal wall and the existence of a mesentery to the ascending colon and caecum makes it possible for a great degree of invagination of the caecum to occur.

Venous drainage of the colon

The venous drainage corresponds to the arterial supply, with a marginal anastomosis joining the ileocolic, midcolic and left colic veins. However, in 20 per cent of people, there is a defective marginal anastomosis between the major veins of the right and transverse portions of the colon. This is a cause of colonic venous infarction after surgical interruption of one of the main veins.

On the left side, however, there is always an excellent marginal vein and the left colon is recommended for oesophageal replacement in preference to the right to avoid venous infarction of the bowel.

Rectosigmoid junction

In patients with a long sigmoid loop which hangs down into the pelvis, the rectosigmoid junction is marked by a distinct flexure. At operation with the patient in the head-down position or in patients in whom the sigmoid colon is short, this flexure may not be noticeable. No other criterion to mark the rectosigmoid junction is available because both the terminal sigmoid colon and the rectum have short mesenteries and the taeniae of the sigmoid colon blend over a distance of about 8 cm to become the longitudinal muscle of the rectum. To most surgeons, 'rectosigmoid' implies a segment of bowel comprising the last 7 cm of sigmoid and upper 5 cm of rectum rather than a precise point. The promontory of the sacrum is a useful landmark to which tumours of the rectum can be related. If the tumour is situated entirely below the promontory it is said to be a rectal tumour. On sigmoidoscopic examination, the rectosigmoid junction is taken to be a point 15 cm from the anal verge.

Course of the rectum

The rectum proceeds downwards and forwards, closely applied to the concavity of the sacrum and coccyx. It ends 2–3 cm in front and below the tip of the coccyx by turning abruptly downwards and backwards through the levator ani muscle to become the anal canal almost 4 cm from the anal verge.

Peritoneal reflections of the rectum

The upper third of the rectum is covered on its front and sides by peritoneum (*Fig.* 41). The middle third is covered on the front only and the lower third is extraperitoneal. From the middle third of the rectum, the peritoneum is reflected onto the seminal vesicle and bladder in the male and the posterior fornix of the vagina in the female. The peritoneal reflections form the rectovesical pouch in the male and the recto-uterine pouch of Douglas in the female. The point of anterior peritoneal reflection shows considerable variation: in the male it is 8–9 cm from the perineal skin and in the female 5–8 cm. On rectal examination it may be possible to feel a secondary deposit of growth in the rectovesical or recto-uterine pouch.

PELVIC ABSCESSES: Pelvic abscesses form in the rectovesical or recto-uterine pouches because these are the most dependent portions of the peritoneal cavity, into which infected fluid or blood can drain by gravity. It not infrequently happens that a pelvic abscess drains spontaneously into the rectum or vagina.

Usually, pelvic abscesses require to be drained either through an abdominal incision or by opening the abscess through the rectum or posterior vaginal fornix.

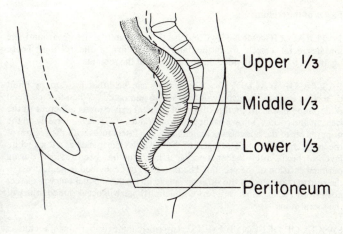

Fig. 41. Peritoneal relations of the rectum.

Abdominal Drainage of a Pelvic Abscess: This route can be used if the abscess is so large that it is also palpable in the lower abdomen. The patient is catheterized to ensure that the bladder is empty and a midline incision is made over the mass. The abscess is entered without contaminating the rest of the peritoneal cavity.

Drainage through the Rectum or Vagina: This is only used if the abscess is palpable through the rectum or posterior vaginal fornix. If there is minimal anal sphincter tone, and a constant discharge of mucus through the anus, the abscess can be drained through the rectum because at this stage there will be no loops of small bowel lying against the rectum. The presence of pus can be confirmed by inserting a needle into the abscess and then a sinus forceps is inserted into the abscess which is allowed to drain.

Venous drainage of the rectum

There is a free anastomosis between the tributaries of the venous system. A submucous plexus of veins drains into a venous plexus around the rectum which also communicates with the venous plexus in the base of the broad ligament in the female and vesical plexus in the male. The rectal plexus drains across the pelvis into the internal iliac veins (systemic circulation) and upwards in the superior rectal vein (portal circulation)

Fascia of the rectum

LATERAL LIGAMENTS: Condensations of areolar tissue around the middle rectal vessels form the lateral ligaments of the rectum. These ligaments have to be divided during excision of the rectum.

FASCIA OF WALDEYER: The rectum can be lifted forward by blunt dissection from the concavity of the sacrum and coccyx. When this has been done, one finds a strong thick layer of parietal pelvic fascia adherent to the sacrum and coccyx, known as the fascia of Waldeyer. Traced inferiorly on the upper layer of the anococcygeal ligament, the fascia fuses with the rectum at the anorectal junction. The fascia of Waldeyer is clearly seen as a thick white layer of fascia after the anococcygeal ligament has been divided during perineal excision of the rectum. The fascia has to be divided to gain access to the retrorectal space. If the surgeon fails to incise this ligament he will dissect posterior to it, in which case serious haemorrhage will occur due to injury of the sacral veins.

FASCIA OF DENONVILLIERS: Anteriorly the extraperitoneal rectum is covered with a closely adherent layer of visceral pelvic fascia which extends from the anterior peritoneal reflection above to the superior layer of the urogenital diaphragm below and laterally becomes continuous with the lateral ligaments of the rectum. This fascia is the fascia of Denonvilliers (*Fig. 251*). During excision of the rectum for cancer, this fascia together with the rectum is separated from the anteriorly placed seminal vesicles in the male and the vagina in the female. At the level of the base of the prostate, the fascia of Denonvilliers is incised transversely to develop a plane of dissection between it and the rectum. The fascia of Denonvilliers remains adherent to the posterior aspect of the prostate gland.

Prolapse of the rectum

This is a circumferential descent of the bowel through the anus. It is important to recognize two degrees of prolapse:
  a. Incomplete or mucosal prolapse where only the mucosa is extruded (more commonly found in the first two years of life and more common in boys).
  b. Complete prolapse (*Fig.* 42) or procidentia where all layers of the bowel are extruded through the anus (more commonly found in elderly females). The rectum may pull the peritoneal sac out of the anus to form a cul-de-sac of peritoneum which may contain coils of small bowel. In this position the small bowel may be damaged during manipulation of the fully prolapsed rectum.

SUPPORTS OF THE RECTUM: The end gut is held in position by:

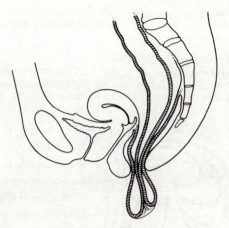

Fig. 42. Rectal prolapse (complete).

1. The attachments of the levatores ani between the internal and external sphincters.
2. The visceral layer of the pelvic fascia.
3. The recto-urethralis muscle which attaches it to the urogenital diaphragm and perineal body.
4. The rectal stalk or lateral ligament. On each side of the back of the rectum, 2–5 cm above the levator, is a dense fibrous cord running from the third piece of the sacrum to the rectal wall. It contains the nervi erigentes (S2, 3) and the middle rectal arteries, and is an important structure in holding up the rectum. The surgeon cannot draw down the rectum in the operation of perineal excision till this 'stalk' is divided.
5. The fatty tissue of the pelvis and ischiorectal fossae.
6. The sacral curve, which is not well marked in the infant and child.

MECHANISM OF PROLAPSE: There is some dispute as to whether complete prolapse is basically a form of sliding hernia (the pouch of Douglas being the hernial sac which presses the anterior wall of the rectum down into the anal canal) or whether it is an intussusception of the rectum. Cineradiographic studies favour the theory of an intussusception when its starting point is about 6–8 cm from the anal verge.

SURGERY OF COMPLETE PROLAPSE: A great many procedures have been described for the correction of prolapse, but probably the most effective is that of posterior rectopexy. After full mobilization, the rectum is fixed in an elevated position to the fascia on the front of the sacrum, either by a simple non-absorbable suture or by a sling of polyvinyl alcohol (Ivalon) sponge.

Arterial blood supply to the large bowel

Arterial blood is supplied by the superior and inferior mesenteric arteries (*Fig.* 43). The internal iliac supplies the important middle and inferior rectal arteries to the anus and rectum. There are numerous important variations.

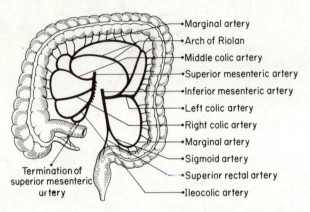

- Marginal artery
- Arch of Riolan
- Middle colic artery
- Superior mesenteric artery
- Inferior mesenteric artery
- Left colic artery
- Right colic artery
- Marginal artery
- Sigmoid artery
- Superior rectal artery
- Ileocolic artery

Termination of superior mesenteric artery

Fig. 43. Blood supply of the colon showing the marginal artery and the arch of Riolan.

THE SUPERIOR MESENTERIC ARTERY: The superior mesenteric artery, which supplies the right and transverse colons, is usually described as giving off three colic arteries: middle, right and ileocolic (23·8 per cent). In about the same percentage of cases the ileocolic artery is constant, but the right colic arises from it (22·7 per cent) or from the middle colic (21·5 per cent).

Less commonly vessels may be duplicated or absent, e.g. the middle colic artery. The right and middle colic arteries may be absent, and the entire colon is supplied by the inferior mesenteric artery which anastomoses via the marginal artery with the ileocolic branch of the superior mesenteric artery.

If, for any reason (arteriosclerosis, vascular anomaly etc.), the collateral circulation to the left colon is deficient, then ligature of the inferior mesenteric artery at its origin may cause ischaemia or gangrene of part of the gut supplied by it.

The artery has to be ligated in some cases of cancer of the colon or aneurysmectomy. The application of a bulldog clamp at the origin of the inferior mesenteric artery at an early stage of an operation will demonstrate the adequacy of the superior mesenteric supply.

THE INFERIOR MESENTERIC ARTERY: The inferior mesenteric artery arises from the aorta 3·8 cm proximal to its bifurcation and supplies the colon from the splenic flexure to the rectum. It is almost never absent but rarely its origin may be higher, behind the duodenum or pancreas. It soon (3·8 cm) gives off the large left colic artery which passes up and to the left at an acute angle (not transversely), being crossed by the inferior mesenteric vein, the left ureter being deep to this transit. The vessel bifurcates near the splenic flexure where one of the branches passes to the right in the transverse mesocolon, to anastomose with a similar branch of the middle colic artery to form the arch of Riolan.

These vessels play an important part in supplementing the marginal artery which is sometimes poor near the flexure. In the 6 per cent of cases in which the left colic artery is absent, the marginal arterial arrangements are good. The inferior mesenteric artery supplies several arteries to the pelvic colon and ends as the superior rectal artery to the rectum.

THE MARGINAL ARTERY: The marginal artery is the paracolic vessel of anastomosis between colic arteries from which arise the terminal arteries to the colon (vasa recta). The vessel extends from the ascending colon to the end of the pelvic colon. It is made up by the succession of terminal arterial arcades formed by the arteries to the colon. It lies 2·5–3·8 cm from the bowel wall.

The anastomosis between middle and left colic arteries is absent in 5 per cent of cases, hence the need to maintain the bifurcation of the left colic artery in resections of the left colon.

It is apparent that the integrity of the marginal artery is vital in cases where the inferior mesenteric artery is ligated at its origin and part of the colon supplied by it is not removed, or when for some reason an arterial trunk must be tied. Even in making a loop colostomy, the colostomy rod must be passed through the mesentery immediately adjacent to the colon so that the marginal artery is not damaged (*Fig.* 44A).

The vasa recta are the terminal arteries to the colon. They arise from the marginal artery and penetrate the bowel wall. The collateral circulation in the bowel wall is not well developed. The long vasa recta encircle the bowel wall and anastomose with each other on the antimesocolic border of the bowel. They send arterial twigs of supply to the antimesocolic taeniae. The short vasa recta supply the mesocolic half of the bowel circumference.

In cases where intestinal anastomosis is intended, and one or both of the bowel ends is dependent for its blood supply on the marginal artery, the mesentery containing the artery should be divided in such a manner as to maintain the integrity of the vasa recta (*Fig.* 44B).

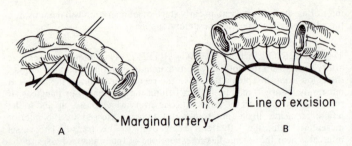

Fig. 44. Protecting the marginal artery. A, The correct situation of a colostomy rod. B, Method of dividing the mesentery of the colon at X. (By courtesy of Morgan and Griffiths.)

There is an abundant and constant anastomosis between the superior and middle rectal arteries. They are branches of the internal iliac, the inferior rectal coming from its internal pudendal branch.

The middle rectal vessels (there may be more than one on each side) are important contributors to the blood supply of the rectum and pelvic colon. They run in the lateral ligaments of the rectum (rectal stalks), which structures should therefore be preserved in high anterior resections of the rectum. These arteries, together with the inferior rectal arteries, are responsible for the blood supply of the terminal colon after ligature of the inferior mesenteric artery at its origin.

Practical Applications:

1. The veins, lymphatic vessels, and lymph nodes draining a part of the large bowel converge on the aortic origin of the vessel supplying that part. The extent of bowel resection in carcinoma is thus determined by the length of bowel supplied by the arterial trunk to the area involved by the disease. The vessel is divided proximally so that the resected bowel and mesentery contain the whole of the related lymphatic apparatus including the proximal lymph node group.

2. In view of the variations in the origin and arrangements of the colic arteries, these vessels should be visualized prior to division of arterial trunks. Transillumination is of great assistance.

3. If an appendix epiploica is sacrificed (which should be avoided if possible), strong traction on an artery forceps in tying it off may draw the loop formed by the long vasa recta into the artery forceps and so damage the blood supply to the cut end of the bowel (*Fig.* 45).

4. If pulsatile flow is observed within a centimetre of the bowel to be anastomosed, the blood supply is almost certainly sufficient.

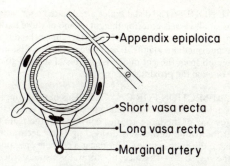

Fig. 45. The vasa recta: traction with an artery forceps may damage these vessels.

Lymph drainage of the large intestine

The nodes are arranged on a plan common to all parts of the large and small intestine. They are very numerous and arranged in three groups: (*a*) proximal; (*b*) intermediate; (*c*) distal (*Fig.* 46).

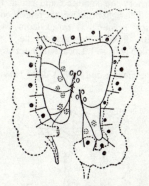

Fig. 46. Arrangement of the lymph glands of the colon. Clear circles: proximal group. Stippled circles: intermediate group. Black circles: distal group.

THE PROXIMAL NODES: The proximal nodes are situated on the main blood vessels to the gut, i.e. superior mesenteric, ileocolic, right colic, left colic, middle colic, inferior mesenteric, superior rectal, sigmoid.

THE INTERMEDIATE NODES: The intermediate nodes are situated along the larger branches of the above-named vessels.

THE DISTAL NODES: The distal nodes are situated near the gut between the numerous small vessels entering the gut. Some of these nodes lie on the gut. The lymph goes for the most part from the gut to the distal nodes and thence to the intermediate glands. It is, however, of the first importance to realize that lymph from the gut may miss the distal set and go direct to the intermediate or even the proximal set.

SURGICAL RESECTION FOR CANCER: This plan of lymph drainage is the same throughout the large and small intestines. The lymphatics from the territory of any one of the large arteries converge on the main trunk of the vessel so that the lymph drainage is divided up fairly accurately into areas corresponding to the main arteries. This fact governs the operative treatment of cancer of the gut, so that if a cancer occurs at, for instance, the caecum, the whole of the gut supplied by the ileocolic and right colic arteries, together with these arteries and their branches and the related peritoneum, is removed to ensure the removal of the whole lymph territory which converges on these vessels. Typical resections are as follows:

  Cancer of Caecum and Ascending Colon:

  Blood vessels to the area for resection: Ileocolic, right colic, and the right branch of the middle colic. The two branches of the superior mesenteric artery are ligatured and cut at their origin from the parent trunk. The right branch of the middle colic is tied at its origin.

  Resection necessary: Terminal 15 cm of ileum, caecum, and ascending colon, hepatic flexure, to include the proximal third of the transverse colon (*Fig.* 47). Local lymph territory into which this gut drains.

  Cancer of the Hepatic Flexure and Right Side of Transverse Colon:

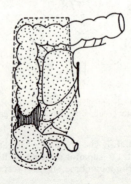

Fig. 47. The stippled area indicates resection necessary in carcinoma of the caecum or ascending colon. (By courtesy of Lawrence Abel.)

Blood vessels to the area for resection: Ileocolic, right colic, and middle colic.

Resection necessary: As for cancer of the ascending colon and caecum together with that part of the transverse colon supplied by the left branch of the middle colic artery (*Fig.* 48).

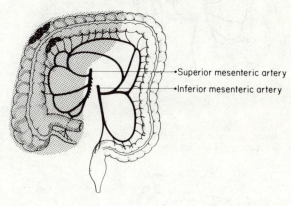

•Superior mesenteric artery
•Inferior mesenteric artery

Fig. 48. Resection for carcinoma of the hepatic flexure and right side of transverse colon.

Cancer of the Transverse Colon and Splenic Flexure:

Blood vessels to the area for resection: The middle colic artery and the left colic branch of the inferior mesenteric.

Resection necessary: The bowel is removed from the middle of the ascending colon to the beginning of the pelvic colon (*Fig.* 49). Lymphatic field draining the area.

Descending and Pelvic Colon:

Blood vessel to the part: Inferior mesenteric artery.

Resection necessary: Descending and pelvic colon with the related lymphatic field. The colon just distal to the splenic flexure is anastomosed to the rectum (*Fig.* 50).

The left colic artery is divided proximal to its bifurcation for carcinoma of the pelvic or rectosigmoid area and the mesentery of the descending colon is divided medial to the marginal artery. This essential vessel may not always be palpable. In such cases the division of the mesentery should be 5 cm from its colonic attachment. The appearance of the bowel is the best guide to its viability. The colon is then divided at the selected point above, and through the upper part of the rectum below, and an end-to-end anastomosis effected (*Fig.*

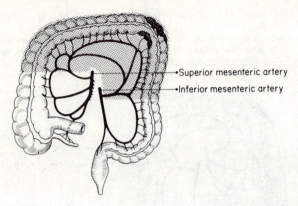

Fig. 49. Resection necessary for carcinoma of distal transverse colon and splenic flexure. (By courtesy of Lawrence Abel.)

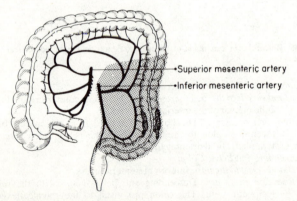

Fig. 50. Resection necessary for carcinoma of the descending and the pelvic colon.

51). This procedure ensures the widest lymphatic ablation that can be surgically obtained.

Cancer of the Rectum: The lymph vessels pass from the rectum:

Downwards to the ischiorectal fossa and to the inguinal nodes (if other lymphatics are blocked); laterally, across the upper surface of the levator ani to the internal iliac nodes; posteriorly to nodes behind the rectum (sacral nodes); upwards along the superior rectal vessels to

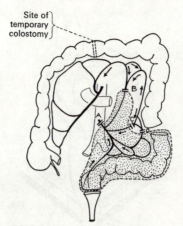

Site of
temporary
colostomy

Fig. 51. High ligation of the inferior mesenteric artery (A), for carcinoma of the sigmoid colon or rectum. B, C, D, Indicate the sites of division of branches of this vessel which protect the marginal anastomosis. The arrow shows the direction of lymph flow (modified). (By courtesy of Morgan and Griffiths.)

the pelvic mesocolon, and so to nodes at the bifurcation of the left common iliac artery, and thence to nodes along the big vessels up to the nodes at the origin of the inferior mesenteric.

Cancer of the rectum may spread in one of three directions depending on the site of the original tumour (*Fig.* 52).

1. *Downward:* Involving perianal skin, ischiorectal fat, and external sphincter ani.

2. *Lateral:* Involving levatores ani muscles, sacral and internal iliac nodes, base of bladder, and seminal vesicles. In women the posterior vaginal wall, cervix, and base of the broad ligament are involved also.

3. *Upward:* Involves the pelvic peritoneum, the whole of the pelvic mesocolon and nodes along the inferior mesenteric artery.

Resection necessary: Tumours of the lower third of the rectum may spread in any of these three directions of lymphatic spread so the resection is extensive. *Fig.* 53 shows the scope of this abdominoperineal resection as advocated by Miles. It will be seen that there are removed: the pelvic colon with its mesocolon, the rectum and anus with the surrounding skin, the fat of the ischiorectal fossa, and the levatores ani with their related fasciae. A permanent colostomy is of course necessary. The total extent of the operation is shown in *Fig.* 54.

Tumours of the upper and middle thirds of the rectum can be treated by anterior (or restorative) resection of the rectum, because it

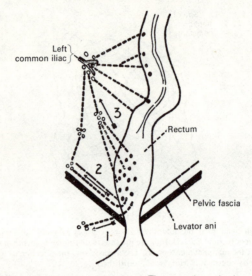

Fig. 52. The lymphatic drainage of the rectum. The arrow shows the three directions in which the efferent lymphatics from the rectum pass: (1) downward flow through ischiorectal fossa; (2) lateral flow between levator ani and pelvic fascia; (3) upward flow in pelvic mesocolon. (After Miles.)

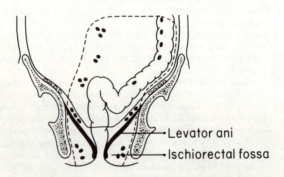

Fig. 53. Carcinoma of the lower rectum. The extent of operative resection as advised by Miles is indicated by the dotted line. The black dots are lymph nodes.

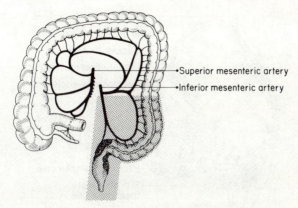

Fig. 54. Resection for carcinoma of the rectum.

has been shown that in such cases downward lymphatic spread does not occur. In this operation the bowel is sectioned well clear of the growth below, but the lower rectum and sphincteric apparatus are not interfered with. The middle and inferior rectal arteries are capable of nourishing the distal rectal stump up to a point 8–10 cm above the peritoneal reflection. Even when the middle rectal artery has been divided, a rectal stump at the level of the peritoneal reflection still has a good blood supply from the inferior rectal artery. If difficulty is experienced in approximating the descending colon to the rectal stump, high ligation of the inferior mesenteric artery where it arises from the aorta will overcome the tethering effect this artery and its left colic branch have on the descending colon.

THE ANAL CANAL

Anatomy

The muscular anal canal forms a sphincter at the distal end of the gastrointestinal tract. The adult canal is about 4 cm long. Posteriorly, the canal is separated from the tip of the coccyx by fibrofatty and muscle tissue known as the anococcygeal ligament. The ischiorectal fossae lie on either side of the anal canal and are continuous with each other via the retrosphincteric space situated between the coccygeal attachments of the external sphincter below and the levator ani above. Anteriorly, the perineal body or central

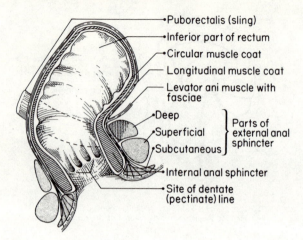

Fig. 55. The lower rectum and anal canal.

tendon of the perineum separates the canal from the lower end of the vagina or from the membranous urethra and bulb.

The dentate (pectinate) line (*Fig.* 55) represents the former site of the embryonic anal membrane.

The lining of the canal above the dentate line is columnar epithelium continuous with that of rectum, and below is skin.

In the upper anal canal, longitudinal folds of columnar epithelium run down to the dentate line level and cover vascular submucosal connective tissue to form 'anal cushions', which, when abnormally enlarged, form haemorrhoids. When the anal canal is opened from its usually closed position using a dilator or retractor, stretching will largely obliterate the anal cushions.

At the dentate line level, transverse folds of mucosa form a ring of anal valves immediately above which are shallow pockets (the anal sinuses or crypts). The anal glands open into the crypts through ducts which have a glandular lining. The anal glands, 5–10 in number, either branch in the submucosal plane or, more frequently, penetrate the internal sphincter to end by branching in the intersphincteric plane between internal and external sphincter muscles. They are of considerable surgical significance in the development of anal abscesses and fistulae.

ANATOMICAL AND SURGICAL IMPORTANCE OF THE DENTATE (PECTINATE) LINE:

1. It forms the embryological watershed between visceral structures above and somatic structures below the line.

2. The mucosa above the line has an autonomic nerve supply and is thus insensitive to cutting and pricking, whereas the skin below is supplied by the inferior rectal branch of the pudendal nerve and is acutely sensitive to these stimuli.
3. The venous drainage of the mucosa is upwards into the inferior mesenteric and portal circulation, whereas that of the skin below is to the systemic venous circulation. This is relevant to the spread of malignant tumours.
4. The lymphatic drainage above the dentate line is upwards and similar to that of the rectum, whereas below lymph drains down and out to the inguinal lymph nodes. The lymphatic spread of malignant tumours and of infections in this area will thus differ.
5. Internal haemorrhoids develop just above this line.
6. The anal glands open into the anal sinuses above the anal valves at this level, and infection in an anal gland may lead to an anal abscess which may extend into the ischiorectal space or the peri-anal space.
7. A crack or fissure in the skin of the anal canal extending from the dentate line to the anal verge, and usually lying in the midline, is associated with local inflammation and spasm of the sphincter, causing severe pain on defaecation in this sensitive area with its rich somatic nerve supply. A fissure-in-ano is sometimes caused by rupture of one of the anal valves.
8. In the finer control of continence, stimulation of nerve endings in the region of the dentate line may initiate reflex or voluntary changes in sphincter tone.

THE ANAL SPHINCTERS: The internal and external sphincters together form the sphincter mechanism of the anal canal. The internal sphincter is a downward extension of the circular layer of the rectal muscle wall and is thus a smooth muscle tube under control of the autonomic system. The external sphincter surrounds the internal and is continuous with the fibres of the levator ani muscle; it forms a skeletal muscle extension of the pelvic floor (*Fig.* 56).

The upper part of the external sphincter, at the level of the anorectal junction, is the puborectalis muscle which forms a sling around the anorectal junction being attached anteriorly to the back of the pubis (*Fig.* 57). In the resting state, the anorectal tube is angled forward at this level, and contraction of the puborectalis sling will increase this angle, an important factor in the continence mechanism (*Fig.* 58). The anorectal ring is palpable on rectal examination.

While the internal sphincter is a well-developed downward extension of the circular muscle layer of the rectum, the longitudinal layer contributes a far less discrete component. Partly muscle and partly fibrous tissue, it runs down to end as fibrous bands passing through the peri-anal fat and lower part of the

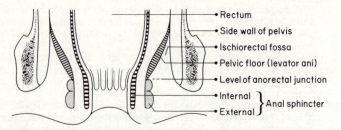

Fig. 56. The anal sphincter in schematic coronal section.

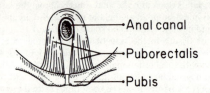

Fig. 57. The plan of the puborectalis muscle sling.

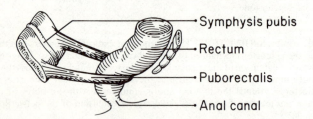

Fig. 58. To show how the anorectal junction is angulated by the sling formed by the puborectalis muscles.

external sphincter, to be attached to the skin. The fat of the peri-anal space is thus broken up into small loculi.

Under anaesthesia or when the anus is stretched, the lower end of the internal sphincter lies lower than the external sphincter. The internal sphincter fibres are light in colour, resembling chicken meat, and this sphincter is the muscle which is divided in a sphincterotomy for anal fissure and is also the muscle exposed during a haemorrhoidectomy.

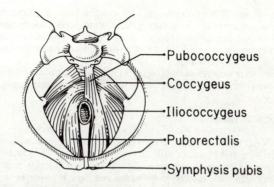

Fig. 59. The floor of the pelvis seen from above to show the levatores ani. (Modified from Milligan and Morgan.)

THE LEVATORES ANI: The levatores ani form the pelvic diaphragm supporting the pelvic viscera (*Fig.* 59). The structures passing through the pelvic diaphragm lie within the sling of the puborectalis. The levatores arise in continuity from the pelvic bone in front and from a thickening of the obturator fascia and the spine of the ischium laterally. They are inserted into the coccyx and anococcygeal ligament posteriorly. The coccygeus muscle forms the posterior part of the pelvic floor, its under surface being continuous with the sacrococcygeal ligament as seen from the perineal aspect. The nerve supply of the levator ani is from the 3rd and 4th sacral segments.

THE INTERSPHINCTERIC SPACE: The interval between the internal and external sphincters is known as the intersphincteric space. The anal intramuscular glands, which open into the anal crypts, pass through this space before penetrating the internal sphincter.

No essential nerves or blood vessels cross the space and a plane of dissection is fairly easily developed between the internal and external sphincters in an intersphincteric excision of the rectum. In this operation, all the anal external sphincters are conserved as well as the puborectalis and levator ani muscle and the somatic and autonomic nerves responsible for erection of the penis and ejaculation.

SURGICAL SIGNIFICANCE OF THE ANAL MUSCULATURE: Continence depends on the integrity of the sphincter mechanism and its nerve supply, and on maintenance of the anorectal angle. Distension of the rectum initiates an anorectal reflex, which results in relaxation of the anal sphincter mechanism and of the puborectalis with straightening out of the anorectal angle and passage of the bolus during defaecation. Reflex contraction of the sphincters and pelvic floor (during coughing) and voluntary contraction prevent incontinence, probably by accessory sphincter tone and partly by increasing the anorectal angle.

Incontinence may result from injury to the pudendal nerve or damage to the sphincter by overzealous stretching, injury or surgical incisions.

Haemorrhoids (piles)

INTERNAL HAEMORRHOIDS: These are associated with dilatation of the superior rectal plexus of veins in the anal columns. The superior rectal veins (portal) communicate with the middle and inferior rectal veins (systemic) (*Fig.* 60); they have no valves and back pressure in the portal venous systems will therefore fill the haemorrhoidal plexus.

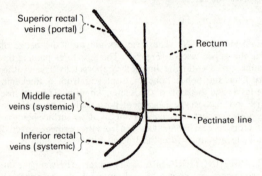

Fig. 60. Showing the portal–systemic anastomosis in the lower rectum.

Internal haemorrhoids are covered by columnar mucosa and lie above the pectinate line. The mucosa over the internal haemorrhoidal plexus is lax and the submucous space is easily distensible by the submucous injection of a sclerosant solution in the treatment of haemorrhoids.

The internal haemorrhoidal plexuses are situated in the left lateral, right anterior and right posterior positions or at 3, 7 and 11 on a clock face with the patient in the lithotomy position.

Rectal bleeding is the main symptom of internal haemorrhoids. The blood is characteristically bright red, like arterial blood. It has been suggested that the internal haemorrhoidal plexus is like a corpus cavernosum with direct arteriovenous communications. The blood acts mainly as a filler without a metabolic role and therefore remains arterial. Prolapse of the haemorrhoidal plexus through the anal orifice occurs with straining. Strangulation (*Fig.* 61) occurs when the haemorrhoids prolapse and the internal sphincter goes into spasm. The strangulated mass of piles consists of an internal and external component divided by a groove due to the binding down of the skin at the dentate line by its attachments to the fibro-elastic extensions of the longitudinal muscle.

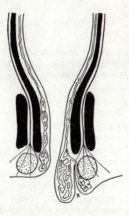

Fig. 61. Diagrammatic representation of a strangulated pile. The X shows the deep fissure between internal and external rectal plexuses produced by the attachment of the fibro-elastic extensions of the longitudinal muscle to the skin. (After Milligan and Morgan.)

EXTERNAL HAEMORRHOIDS: These occur in the lower one-third of the anal canal at the anal orifice itself and form a bluish skin-covered cushion around the anus. The internal and external haemorrhoidal plexuses are connected by small veins crossing beneath the skin. Increased pressure in the internal plexus may therefore be transmitted to the external plexus to produce external (skin-covered) haemorrhoids. They are of little surgical importance.

False External Hamorrhoids: Unlike internal haemorrhoids false external haemorrhoids are usually covered by skin with normal sensation and can be extremely painful.

False external haemorrhoids may be:
    a. One type is properly styled haematoma of the anus (thrombo-tic pile), and is due to straining causing rupture of one of the

small peri-anal veins; it appears clinically as a bluish swelling of variable size at the anal verge.

b. This type is not venous, but merely a tag of skin at the anus. These tags are formed as a result of 'attacks of piles'. Thrombophlebitis of a haemorrhoidal vein causes an area of swelling and oedema of the related segment of the anal skin; subsidence of the oedema leaves a dog-eared tag of skin.

c. A 'sentinel' pile is a tag formed by a ruptured anal valve in some cases of fissure-in-ano.

Anorectal anomalies

EMBRYOLOGY: The rectum is developed from the entodermal cloaca and the anal canal from the ectodermal cloaca. The hindgut is continuous with the entodermal cloaca which is divided into an anterior urogenital and a posterior rectal portion by the downgrowths of the urorectal septum from above and the folds of Rathke from the sides (*Fig.* 62).

ANORECTAL ANOMALIES CAN ARISE AS THE RESULT OF:
1. Overfusion of the labioscrotal folds or the anal tubercles at their posterior ends. This can cause a microscopic anus or membranous occlusion at the normal anal site.
2. Incomplete migration (*Fig.* 63) in which normal division of the cloaca into its urinary and alimentary parts, with subsequent migration of the anus back along the perineum, fails to occur. This results in an anterior perineal ectopic anus in either sex and a vulval or vestibular anus in the female. A more marked failure of division of the cloaca results in rectal agenesis with a recto-urethral or rectovesical fistula in the male. In the female a similar mechanism results in rectovaginal fistula (*Fig.* 64).

In rectal atresia there is a normally formed anal canal with atresia at the lower end of the rectum.

Anatomical assessment:
1. The position of the 'blind end' of the bowel relative to the puborectalis sling. If the 'blind end' is above the puborectalis sling (supralevator), the prognosis for faecal continence after surgery is bad. The reverse is true in the low (translevator) anomalies.
2. The presence or absence of a fistula from the bowel.
3. The course of any fistula and the structure to which it is connected.

Diagnosis:
1. A full clinical examination is made. Covered anus and ectopic anus in the perineum, vulva or vestibule can be diagnosed on inspection. If no visible orifice, is seen, a high anomaly is suspected. In a female, meconium may be seen coming from within the vagina above the hymen. In a male the urine may be meconium stained.

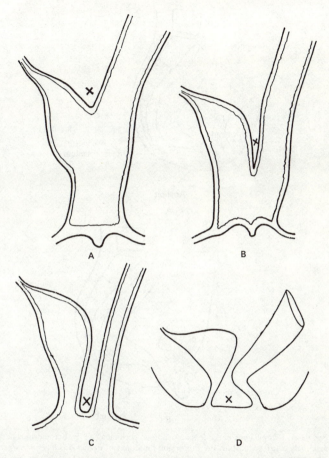

Fig. 62. The figures demonstrate the development of the perineum by the proliferation of mesoderm and the downgrowth of the urorectal septum dividing the entodermal cloaca into the urogenital and rectal cavities. A. The entodermal cloaca. The urorectal septum is indicated by the X. B, The subdivision continues. C, The division is complete. D, The mesodermal proliferation has developed the perineum and pushed the rectum backwards. (After Stephens.)

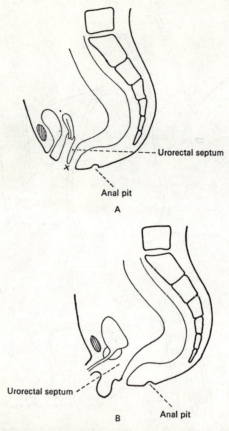

Fig. 63 A, Ectopic anus in the female—shotgun perineum (X). B, Ectopic anus in the male. (By courtesy of Muir, the Editor and Publishers of *Recent Advances in Surgery*, 4th ed.)

2. Inversion X-ray of the infant can be done to determine the relationship of the gas in the rectal pouch to an imaginary line running from the top of the pubis to the sacrococcygeal junction. If the gas bubble is between this line and a radio-opaque marker placed on the skin where the anus should have been, it suggests

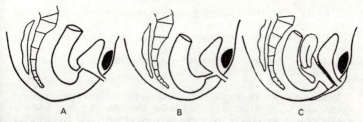

Fig. 64. Abnormal communications between rectum and some other tube. A, Rectovesical fistula; B, recto-urethral fistula; C, rectovaginal fistula.

that the infant has a translevator anomaly. Unfortunately this test may be unreliable because straining by the baby or paralysis of the pelvic floor may also give rise to a low-lying gas shadow. The X-ray may show associated sacral agenesis. If only three or less sacral segments are seen, there is a neurological deficit involving bladder as well as bowel.

3. Excretory urogram. About half the high anomalies and about a quarter of the low anomalies have an associated urological abnormality.

4. Barium study of the distal loop is done after a colostomy for a supralevator anomaly.

CONGENITAL AGANGLIONIC MEGACOLON (HIRSCHSPRUNG'S DISEASE): There is a congenital absence of ganglia of the intramural plexus of the anus and rectum, which reaches proximally for a varying extent. The neural crest cells which give rise to ganglia fail to migrate into the colon. Because of a functional obstruction the normal proximal colon is dilated. The diagnosis is confirmed by doing a rectal biopsy and demonstrating the absence of ganglion cells.

ISCHIORECTAL FOSSA

Anatomy
The ischiorectal fossa is lateral to the anus lying between the skin of the anal region and the levator ani. The two fossae communicate with each other behind the anal canal.

This fossa is pyramidal in shape. It is 5 cm deep, and 2·5 cm wide.
Boundaries:
Lateral: The fascia covering the obturator internus muscle and the ischial tuberosity.

Medial: The fascia covering the levator ani muscle; the external sphincter of the anus.

Posterior: Sacrotuberous ligament, on the posterior surface of which is the gluteus maximus.

Anterior: Urogenital diaphragm (triangular ligament).

Floor: skin.

Under the skin is a large pad of fat filling the fossa. There is here no deep fascia such as exists elsewhere just under the skin. The deep fascia is separated from the skin by the whole thickness of the pad of fat filling the fossa. This fascia is named the 'fascia lunata' (*Fig.* 65).

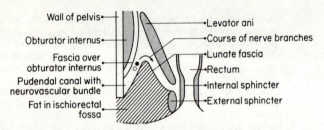

Fig. 65. Coronal section of the ischiorectal fossa. Note the lunate fossa, the pudendal canal, and the course which branches of the pudendal nerve take in relation to the roof of the ischiorectal fossa, *en route* to perineal structures which they supply.

FASCIA LUNATA:
Relations:
Medial: It covers the fascia on the levator (anal fascia) and ends at the lower end of the levator.
Lateral: Covers fascia on obturator internus (obturator fascia) and is attached to ischium. The internal pudendal vessels and nerves are between these two layers which form the pudendal canal.
Anterior: The fascia fuses with the urogenital diaphragm.
Superior: The upper arched portion of the fascia is called the tegmentum. There is a space between this tegmentum and the apex of the fossa, which space is the suprategmental space and contains fat.

THE PUDENDAL CANAL: The pudendal canal (*Fig.* 65) runs forward on the lateral wall of the fossa 3·8 cm above the lower border of the ischial tuberosity, leading from the lesser sciatic foramen posteriorly to the perineal membrane anteriorly. It contains the internal pudendal vessels and puden-

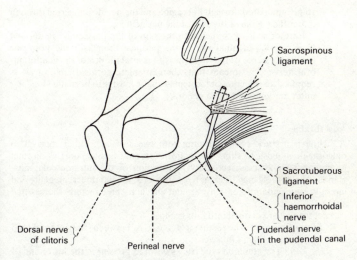

Fig. 66. The anatomy of the pudendal nerve block. The dotted square is the site of injection. (By courtesy of Huntingford and the Editor of the *Journal of Obstetrics and Gynaecology of the British Empire.*)

dal nerve. The artery gives off the inferior rectal branch at the posterior part of the canal and the perineal branch at the anterior end.

THE PUDENDAL NERVE: The pudendal nerve (derived from S2, 3 and 4; *Fig.* 66) leaves the pelvis medial to the sciatic nerve through the greater sciatic foramen. It then crosses the external surface of the ischial spine and re-enters the pelvis through the lesser sciatic notch and passes along the lateral wall of the ischiorectal fossa.

Branches of the pudendal nerve:
  i. The inferior rectal nerve supplies the external sphincter, levator ani and skin of the anal canal and anus. The latter is also supplied by the perineal branch of the 4th sacral nerve, perforating cutaneous branches of the 2nd and 3rd sacral nerves, and gluteal branches of the posterior cutaneous nerve of the thigh.
  ii. Perineal nerve which gives off labial or scrotal branches and continues to supply the muscles of the urogenital diaphragm.
  iii. Dorsal nerve of clitoris or penis which is a sensory nerve.

Pudendal Nerve Block: The pudendal nerve is infiltrated with local anaesthetic where it crosses the ischial spine (*Fig.* 66). The ischial spine is palpated through the vagina and the needle is inserted through either the vagina or the skin of the perineum.

Further sensory branches to the skin of the perineum are derived from the ilio-inguinal nerve, the perineal branch of the posterior cutaneous nerve of the thigh and the genital branch of the genitofemoral nerve. This means that when complete perineal anaesthesia is required an injection of local anaesthetic must also be made along the outer margin of the labia majora.

Anal fistulae

A fistula is a track communicating with two surfaces, either mucosa to mucosa, or mucosa to skin. The majority of anal fistulae start as an anal intersphincteric abscess secondary to infection of the intramuscular anal glands. The abscess may track in five directions: up and down, medially and laterally, and circumferentially around the anus and rectum (horse-shoe abscess).

Anal fistulae are divided into four groups:

1. *Intersphincteric:* The fistula (*Fig.* 67) is between the internal and external sphincter muscles:

    a. The common type tracks down to present at the lower end of the internal sphincter muscle as a perianal abscess.

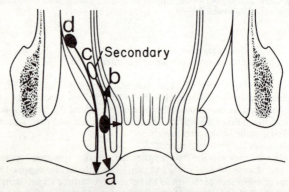

Fig. 67. Extensions of the intersphincteric abscess. (a) Common type of fistula; (b) intersphincteric abscess opening into the rectum; (c) secondary extension into the pelvirectal space; (d) pelvirectal abscess presenting at the anus.

    b. Sometimes it tracks upwards and forms a second opening in the anus or rectum above that of the anal intramuscular glands. The track joining the two openings is not submucous, as was formerly thought, but intersphincteric.

c. The track may extend upwards into the pelvirectal space (space between the pelvic peritoneum and upper surface of levator ani).

d. Infrequently pelvic infection such as a diverticular abscess may extend down the intersphincteric plane and present as a peri-anal abscess.

2. *Trans-sphincteric: See Fig.* 68.

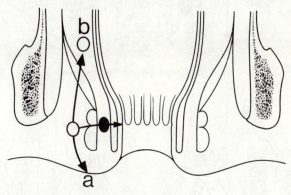

Fig. 68. Trans-sphincteric abscess. (a) Secondary abscess in ischiorectal fossa; (b) extension through the levator ani to form a pelvic abscess.

a. The infection extends from the intersphincteric plane at midanal canal level through the external sphincter into the ischiorectal fossa where it forms an abscess which then ruptures on to the perineal skin.

b. A secondary tract may extend upward through the levator ani and produce a pelvic abscess. On rectal examination, induration is felt at the level of the anorectal ring.

3. *Suprasphincteric:* A pelvic extension of an intersphincteric abscess discharges through levator ani into the ischiorectal fossa (*Fig.* 69). The tract curves above the puborectal sling.

4. *Extrasphincteric:* The track lies outside both the internal and external sphincter muscles (*Fig.* 70):

a. It may be caused by a trans-sphincteric fistula which has entered the rectum at a higher level.

b. It may be a sequel to direct trauma to the perineum.

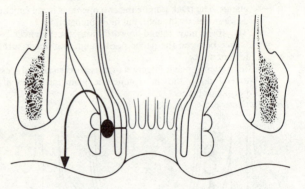

Fig. 69. Extension of suprasphincteric abscess.

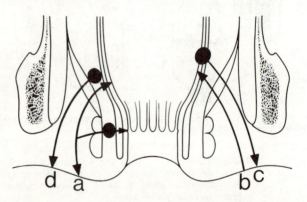

Fig. 70. Extrasphincteric fistula. (a) Extension of trans-sphincteric fistula; (b) trauma to the perineum; (c) disease of the rectum; (d) pelvic abscess.

> c. Specific anorectal disease, such as Crohn's disease, or a carcinoma of the rectum may result in an extrasphincteric fistula.
> d. Secondary to pelvic inflammation which has spread through the levator ani to present in the perineum.

TREATMENT: Certain general principles are applicable to the management of all anal fistulae. Careful examination and gentle probing, with special attention to the relation of the internal opening to the anorectal ring, are essential. The fistulous track must be laid open thereby draining the infected intramuscular gland. Total division of the internal and external sphincters will usually result in incontinence. Curettings from the fistulous track should always be sent for histology to exclude Crohn's disease or carcinoma of the rectum.

Rectal examination

Examination of the abdomen is incomplete unless the peri-anal area has been inspected and a digital examination of the rectum has been performed.

INSPECTION OF THE PERI-ANAL AREA: Look for:
1. Skin tags of external haemorrhoids..
2. Prolapsed internal haemorrhoids.
3. An anal fissure.
4. A fistulous opening.
5. The redness and swelling of an abscess.
6. Excoriation of the peri-anal skin.
7. Loss of anal tone (patulous anus).
8. A pilonidal sinus in the natal cleft.

PALPATION OF THE PERI-ANAL SKIN: Take note of:
1. Tenderness which, together with a swelling, suggests an abscess.
2. Induration around a chronic anal fistula.

PALPATION OF THE ANAL CANAL AND RECTUM: (It should be noted that the anus of the newborn infant admits the little finger.)
  a. In the Lumen and in the Wall:
1. The lower edge of the internal and external sphincter, with the anal intermuscular groove between them, can be felt.
2. The anorectal ring formed by the upper end of the canal sphincters lies about 3 cm from the anal verge. It is felt posteriorly.
3. The tone of the anal sphincter is determined by the patient voluntarily contracting the anal sphincter.
4. A rectal tumour may be felt. More than half the carcinomas of the rectum are palpable on rectal examination.
5. Normal rectal mucosa is smooth: in ulcerative colitis it feels granular.
  b. Extrarectal:
1. In the male the prostate and seminal vesicles are felt anteriorly.
2. Inflamed bulbo-urethral (Cowper's) gland may be felt in the region of the bulbous urethra between the index finger in the rectum and the thumb on the perineum.
3. In the female the cervix and uterus are felt anteriorly.

4. A more proximal tumour in the colon or rectum or faeces may be felt through the rectal wall.
5. A deposit of tumour tissue may be felt in the rectovesical or the recto-uterine pouch.
6. Uterosacral ligaments may be infiltrated with tumour tissue in patients with a carcinoma of the cervix. This type of spread is best assessed on rectal examination.
7. The sacrum and coccyx are felt posteriorly.

Chapter 6

THE LIVER AND BILIARY SYSTEM

THE LIVER

The liver sits astride the portal circulation so that nutrients absorbed from the gastrointestinal tract have to pass through the liver. Long-chain fatty acids are an exception as these are absorbed by lymphatics and travel via the thoracic duct.

Embryology

The liver, gallbladder and bile ducts arise as a ventral bud (hepatic diverticulum) from the most caudal part of the foregut. The hepatic diverticulum extends into the septum transversum and expands the ventral mesentery.

The hepatic diverticulum divides into:
1. A large cranial part which gives rise to interlacing cords of liver cells and the intra-epithelial lining of the intrahepatic portion of the biliary apparatus. The liver cells anastomose around pre-existing endothelium-lined spaces which will become the hepatic sinusoids. The fibrous, haemopoietic and Kupffer cells are derived from the mesenchyme of the septum transversum.
2. A small caudal part which expands to form the gallbladder; its stalk becomes the cystic duct. Initially the extrahepatic biliary apparatus is occluded with endodermal cells, but it is later recanalized. The stalk connecting the hepatic and cystic ducts to the duodenum becomes the common bile duct.

Histology

The liver (*Fig.* 71) is enveloped by a connective tissue capsule which is invaginated at the porta hepatis by the hepatic artery, portal vein and bile

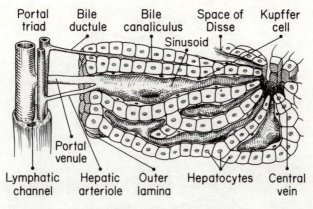

Portal triad   Bile ductule   Bile canaliculus   Space of Disse   Kupffer cell

Sinusoid

Portal venule

Lymphatic channel   Hepatic arteriole   Outer lamina   Hepatocytes   Central vein

Fig. 71. The histology of a liver lobule.

ducts to form sheaths (interlobular septa) around these structures in their intrahepatic course. In the liver, small branches of the portal vein, hepatic artery and bile ducts form the hepatic triad which, together with lymphatics and nerves, lies at the periphery of the lobule in the interlobular septa.

The liver lobule, which is 1–2 mm in diameter, is the basic functional unit of the liver. The liver lobule is constructed around a central (intralobular) vein. Plates (laminae) of hepatic cells or hepatocytes, usually two cells thick, radiate from the central vein to the periphery of the lobule like the spokes of a wheel, but these laminae also branch and anastomose with each other.

The laminae of hepatic cells are separated by vascular spaces called 'sinusoids' which open into the central vein. The sinusoids are lined by endothelial cells and Kupffer cells. The latter form part of the reticulo-endothelial system. The endothelial cells have large pores which allow plasma but no blood cells into the perisinusoidal space of Disse. This is a narrow space between the endothelial cells and the hepatocytes, which connects with lymphatics in the interlobular septa so that an excess of fluid in this space is removed through the lymphatics.

The sinusoids are separated from the hepatic triads by a solid lamina of hepatic cells (the limiting lamina) and distributing venules and arterioles have to penetrate this lamina to gain access to the sinusoids. Blood flows from the periphery of the sinusoid to the central vein because the portal venous pressure is higher than that in the central vein. The hepatocytes at the periphery of a lobule have a better supply of oxygen and nutrients.

Bile formed in liver cells drain, through canaliculi ramifying between the hepatocytes, into interlobular bile ducts in the hepatic triads.

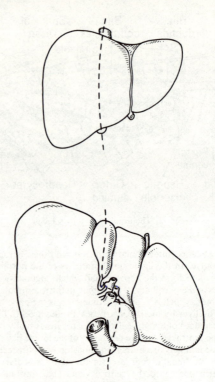

Fig. 72. The principal plane of the liver.

Lobes and segments of the liver

The true division between the right and left lobes of the liver is not at the falciform ligament but at a line (the principal plane) through the bed of the gallbladder projecting posteriorly towards the inferior vena cava (*Fig.* 72). This line divides the liver into two portions of almost equal mass. Note that the caudate lobe is equally shared between the right and left lobes of the liver. Each lobe is divided into two segments (*Fig.* 73); the right lobe into anterior and posterior by an oblique line running anteroposteriorly and the left lobe into medial and lateral segments by the insertion of the ligamentum teres and ligamentum venosum.

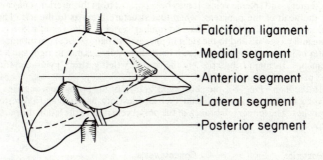

Fig. 73. The segments of the liver.

Blood supply

In man, resting blood flow to the liver is 25 per cent of the cardiac output. Almost two-thirds is provided by portal flow and the remaining third by the hepatic artery.

PORTAL VEIN: The portal system is unique in that it starts and ends in capillaries. The portal vein (*Fig.* 74) is formed in front of the inferior vena cava and behind the neck of the pancreas by the union of the superior

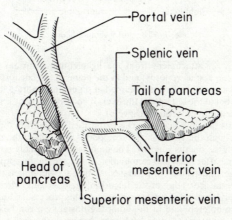

Fig. 74. The portal vein.

mesenteric and splenic veins. It may be separated from the inferior vena cava by the head of the pancreas, when that structure projects to the left. This union occurs at the level of the 2nd lumbar vertebra. The vessel is 5–8 cm long and passes up and to the right in the gastrohepatic (lesser) omentum, to enter the hilum of the liver, where it immediately divides into its right and left branches. Its main tributaries are the coronary (left gastric), pyloric, cystic, and pancreaticoduodenal veins.

In the liver (*Fig*. 75), the short right branch of the portal vein supplies a branch to the caudate lobe and then divides into anterior and posterior branches. The longer left branch of the portal vein runs to the left in the porta hepatis.

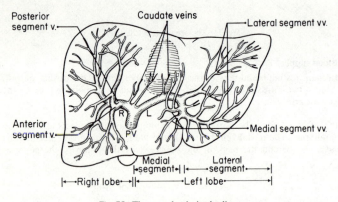

Fig. 75. The portal vein in the liver.

It receives an attachment from the ligamentum venosum (the fibrous remnant of the ductus venosus) and in the plane of the falciform ligament it curves caudally supplying both the medial segment (quadrate lobe) and the lateral segment of the left lobe of the liver. It ends by receiving the attachment of the ligamentum teres (umbilical vein).

In the fetus the umbilical vein carries purified blood from the placenta to the liver through the left branch of the portal vein and to the inferior vena cava through the ductus venosus. The umbilical vein usually remains patent for some time after birth and cannulation of the vein in the cord can be used for exchange transfusions in neonates. Within the abdomen, the umbilical vein runs in the free edge of the falciform ligament and, when it becomes obliterated, it forms the ligamentum teres. In this process the lumen does not disappear completely and in the adult the portal vein can be catheterized through the 'obliterated' umbilical vein. Access to the vein is obtained by probing its obliterated portion (ligamentum teres) through an extraperitoneal upper abdominal incision. This route has been used for portohepatography, and for the infusion of chemotherapeutic agents in the treatment of hepatic tumours.

Preduodenal Portal Vein: In the early embryo the vitelline veins anastomose together across the ventral and dorsal sides of the developing duodenum. The ventral part of this venous plexus usually disappears, the dorsal section forming the portal vein. If the ventral part persists, the portal vein may lie anterior to the pancreas and duodenum (*Fig.* 76).

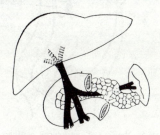

Fig. 76. Preduodenal portal vein.

Portal Hypertension: The portal vein has no valves; the normal pressure in the portal vein is 7–10 cm of saline and, at the junction of the hepatic veins and inferior vena cava, it is zero. Portal hypertension is indicative of an abnormally high pressure within all or part of the portal venous system, either due to increased resistance to flow or uncommonly as the result of increased flow. Anatomically, obstruction to flow can occur at three levels: (*a*) hepatic veins (Budd–Chiari syndrome), (*b*) intrahepatic (cirrhosis, metastatic tumours), and (*c*) portal vein (thrombosis, tumour involvement). Collateral channels enlarge in an attempt to bypass the site of obstruction and carry the portal blood to the systemic circulation. These channels are the anastomoses normally present between the portal and systemic circulations but are inadequate to relieve the back pressure. The sites of portosystemic anastomoses are seen in *Fig.* 77.

1. *At the lower end of the oesophagus:* The veins of the stomach (draining to the portal) communicate with the oesophageal veins (draining to the azygos and vena cava). In portal obstruction these veins often become varicose and burst into the oesophagus, causing vomiting of blood and often fatal haemorrhage.
2. *Around the umbilicus:* Veins pass along the falciform ligament to the

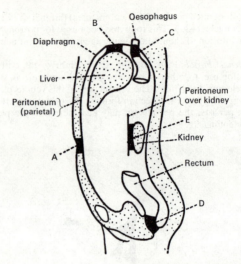

Fig. 77. The black areas are the sites of anastomosis between the portal and systemic circulations. They occur: A, at umbilicus; B, at bare area of liver; C, at lower end of oesophagus; D, at lower end of rectum; E, in the tissue between kidney and peritoneum.

umbilicus, connecting the veins of the liver (portal) with the veins around the umbilicus (epigastric veins which are systemic). Enlargement of these may produce a bunch of veins radiating from the umbilicus, which is called the caput Medusae (*Fig.* 78).

3. *At the lower end of the rectum:* One must distinguish between anorectal varices and haemorrhoids. Haemorrhoids do occur in patients with portal hypertension but are no more common than in the rest of the population. Anorectal varices are the result of portal hypertension. They are dilated submucosal veins formed when the communicating veins that connect the superior rectal with the middle and inferior rectal veins become enlarged in portal hypertension. The collaterals may be seen underlying the mucosa of the rectum and anal canal. They extend upwards well above the level of the haemorrhoids and are easily compressible. Sometimes they extend away from the anus reaching the buttock, perineum and thigh. When these anorectal varices bleed they can be treated by a locking suture extending from the anal margin into the rectum for about 7 cm.

4. *At the back of the colon:* In front of the kidney small vessels unite the

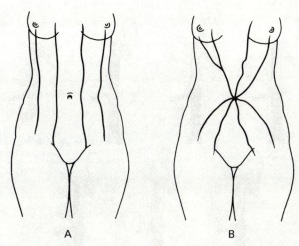

Fig. 78. The subcutaneous collateral circulation in: **A**, inferior vena caval obstruction; **B**, portal obstruction (caput Medusae).

      vessels of the peritoneum and colon (portal) with the vessels of the kidney (systemic).
   5. *Bare area of the liver:* Small vessels unite the diaphragmatic veins (systemic) with the liver veins (portal).
   Surgery for Portal Hypertension: Portal hypertension can be relieved surgically by diverting portal blood into the systemic circulation by anastomosing the portal vein or one of its tributaries to the inferior vena cava or renal vein (*Fig.* 79). The Inokuchi shunt is an anastomosis of the coronary (left gastric) vein to the inferior vena cava which selectively decompresses the veins of the lower end of the oesophagus.

THE HEPATIC ARTERY: It first pursues a horizontal course and then bends sharply at right-angles to run upwards in the lesser omentum to the left of the bile duct and in front of the portal vein. The common hepatic artery gives off the gastroduodenal, right gastric and cystic arteries.

    The frequent variations of the vessel or its branches are in sharp contrast to the stable anatomy of the portal vein. In over 90 per cent of cases, the hepatic artery arises from the coeliac axis. It may come from the superior mesenteric or from the aorta directly..

    The vessel divides near the liver into right and left branches which supply the respective lobes. One or other of these vessels may arise anomalously, e.g. from superior mesenteric, aorta, or left gastric. Such vessels may have

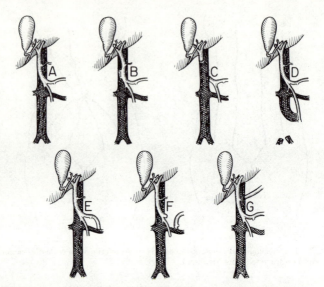

Fig. 79. Types of portasystemic shunts. A, Normal; B, side-to-side portacaval; C, end-to-side portacaval; D, mesocaval; E, central splenorenal; F, distal splenorenal (Warren); G, left gastric to inferior vena cava (Inokuchi).

unusual relationships in the right free border of the lesser omentum and present hazards in cholecystectomy.

Accessory right or left hepatic arteries may occur. In ligature of the left gastric artery in gastrectomy, it is wise to look for a large vessel which this artery sometimes supplies to the liver. This may be an accessory left hepatic artery; alternatively it may be the only artery of supply to the left lobe.

In the surgery of major hepatic injuries, the right or left hepatic arteries can be ligated. The hepatic arteries are not end arteries; four weeks after arterial interruption collateral circulation is visible. There is collateral flow between the lobes when either the right or left hepatic artery has been ligated. Phrenic arteries running through the suspensory ligaments of the liver also contribute to collateral flow; therefore these ligaments should not be divided when hepatic artery interruption is essential.

THE HEPATIC VEINS: The hepatic veins (*Fig.* 80) are formed by the union of the central veins of the lobules. There are three hepatic veins which enter the inferior vena cava just below the diaphragm. These veins lie between the liver lobes and cross the portal triads. There are, therefore, no truly avascular

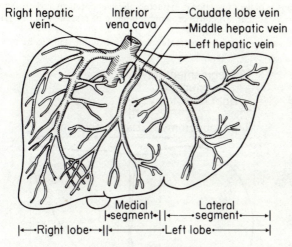

Right hepatic vein — Inferior vena cava — Caudate lobe vein — Middle hepatic vein — Left hepatic vein

Medial segment — Lateral segment — Right lobe — Left lobe

Fig. 80. The hepatic veins.

planes in the liver. The middle hepatic vein enters the inferior vena cava separately or more commonly joins the left hepatic vein to form a short common trunk.

Several smaller veins drain directly from the liver into the inferior vena cava. The important cause of death in hepatic vein injuries, apart from haemorrhage, is air embolism which may occur at the time of laparotomy.

Hepatic resections

Liver tissue has remarkable powers of regenerations and major resection are well tolerated. Hepatic resections may be either segmental or non-segmental.

Non-segmental resections are wedge resections or débridement of liver tissue.

Major lobar resections are planned in accordance with segmental anatomy. The portal venous, hepatic arterial and hepatic bile duct branches conform to the four-segment organization. The hepatic veins are an exception (*see above*).

In major lobar resections, the structures in the porta hepatis supplying that portion of the liver to be excised should be isolated first, when possible. The hepatic veins are short and large. In only about 60 per cent of cases can the right hepatic vein be ligated easily outside the liver. Usually it is safer to control the hepatic veins from within the substance of the liver. One of the techniques of liver resection is to fracture the liver parenchyma between one's fingers. Vascular structures crossing the plane of resection can be felt and ligated.

The various types of segmental resections are outlined in *Fig*. 81.

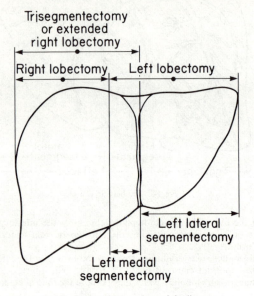

Fig. 81. Segmental resections of the liver.

BILE DUCTS

Hepatic ducts

The confluence of the right and left hepatic ducts almost always occurs outside the liver. In dissections in this area it may be necessary to push liver substance away to display the confluence completely. The common hepatic duct arises from the confluence of the ducts and, by definition, becomes the common bile duct where it is joined by the cystic duct.

The common bile duct

The length varies inversely with the length of the common hepatic duct and it is usually from 5 to 15 cm long. It runs down first in the right extremity of the lesser omentum to the right of the common hepatic artery and anterior to the portal vein. It passes behind the first part of the duodenum and then through or behind the head of the pancreas, to be joined by the main duct of the pancreas. The common channel so formed pierces the wall of the second part of the duodenum to open onto the duodenal papilla which is on the posteromedial part of the duodenum at the junction of the upper two-thirds with the lower third. The supraduodenal portion of the common bile duct has been shown to contain scattered bundles of smooth muscle arranged in a longitudinal direction. The muscle is very weak and contraction of the muscle is an unlikely cause of biliary colic.

When visualized by means of cholangiography (a radio-opaque substance in the biliary system) the upper limit of the normal diameter of the duct is 8 mm. Obstruction to the flow of bile into the duodenum causes dilatation of the duct. There is no evidence that the common bile duct becomes dilated after cholecystectomy.

ULTRASONOGRAPHY: The main application of ultrasound in biliary tract disease is to distinguish dilated from non-dilated biliary ducts in a jaundiced patient. Because of overlying gas, the common bile duct is often not well visualized. This does not apply to the common hepatic duct. The normal internal diameter of the common hepatic duct is 4 mm, where the right branch of the portal vein runs posterior to it. The normal internal diameter of the common bile duct on ultrasonography is 6 mm. The normal common bile duct is therefore smaller on ultrasonography than on intravenous cholangiography. This may be due to the choleretic effect of the contrast material causing distension of the duct and the X-ray magnification factor.

Ampulla of Vater

The union of the common bile duct and the pancreatic duct forms the ampulla of Vater; however, an actual widening of the lumen as suggested by the term 'ampulla' occurs in only about 5 per cent of cases. The distance between the point of junction of the pancreatic and common bile duct with the duodenal papilla is also variable. In some instances these ducts open independently on the papilla. A normal papilla will permit the passage of a dilator 3 mm in diameter.

Sphincters

The circular smooth muscle around the pancreatic and common bile duct is known as the sphincter of Oddi; however, a sphincter of the common bile duct, which begins just above the entrance of the duct into the duodenal wall, a pancreatic sphincter and an ampullary sphincter, are also described

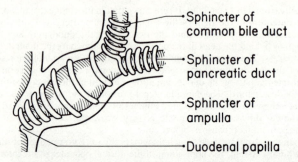

Fig. 82. Sphincters of the common bile, pancreatic duct and ampulla.

(*Fig.* 82). Of these the sphincter around the lower end of the common bile duct is the most constant and best developed.

Reflux of bile up the pancreatic duct has been postulated as a cause of biliary pancreatitis. Based on anatomical studies, it has been shown that the length of the ampulla is seldom long enough for a large stone lodged in the ampulla to cause reflux of bile up the pancreatic duct. Spasm of the sphincter of the ampulla may also be a cause of reflux.

Variations in the bile ducts

See Fig. 83.

1. The cystic duct usually joins the common hepatic duct to form the common bile duct within 2–5 cm of the upper border of the duodenum.
2. Frequently the common hepatic and cystic ducts lie parallel, being joined by connective tissue for some distance before becoming one duct.
3. The union of the cystic and common hepatic ducts is frequently behind the duodenum or the pancreas, and may only occur just before the duct pierces the wall of the duodenum.
4. Usually the cystic duct joins the common hepatic duct on its right side. It may, however, join the front, back, or even the left side of the common hepatic by taking a spiral course behind it.
5. An accessory bile duct is not uncommon. It is sometimes an accessory right hepatic duct which leaves the right extremity of the porta hepatis, runs down parallel to the cystic duct and behind it, in front of the right hepatic artery, and joins the common hepatic duct anywhere between the site of its formation and the entrance of the cystic duct into the common duct. It is more common to find ducts of varying size going directly from the liver into the gallbladder.

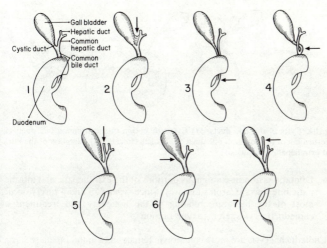

Fig. 83. Variations in the bile ducts. (1) The ducts as usually described; (2) the common hepatic and cystic ducts lie parallel, being joined by connective tissue; (3) the common hepatic duct and cystic ducts join just before the duct enters the duodenum; (4) the cystic joins the common hepatic duct on its *left*; (5) accessory right hepatic duct; (6) absence of cystic duct—the common hepatic duct enters the gallbladder and the common bile duct leaves it. (7) The right hepatic duct joins the neck of the gallbladder. (After Flint.)

6. The cystic duct may be absent, the common hepatic duct entering the gallbladder and the common bile duct leaving it. It is, perhaps, more accurate to describe the gallbladder in these cases as being sessile. The condition is important, as gall stones can readily enter the common duct.

7. A rare anomaly shows the right hepatic duct entering the gallbladder near its junction with the cystic duct. Its surgical importance is considerable. Should it be ligatured, jaundice would result as there is little communication of bile channels between the two parts of the liver drained by right and left hepatic ducts.

CONGENITAL DILATATION OF THE BILIARY TREE: Cystic dilatation of the common bile duct (choledochal cyst) (*Fig.* 84) is an uncommon abnormality. Cysts are divided into four types:

1. Congenital cystic dilatation of the common bile duct.
2. Congenital diverticulum of the common bile duct.
3. Congenital choledochocele.

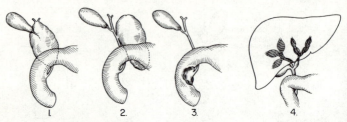

Fig. 84. Cysts of the bile ducts. (1) Cystic dilatation of the common bile duct; (2) diverticulum of the common bile duct; (3) choledochocele; (4) dilatation of the intra- and extrahepatic bile ducts.

4. Dilatations of non-contiguous portions of the extrahepatic and intrahepatic bile ducts (Caroli's disease). Since types 2, 3 and 4 rarely occur, most of the literature relating to the aetiology and treatment of choledochal cysts refers to type 1 lesions.

Choledochal cysts are more common in females and in the Japanese.

The clinical features include a classic triad of symptoms and signs, i.e. pain, a right upper quadrant abdominal mass and jaundice.

In at least 80 per cent of normal individuals, the common bile duct and main pancreatic duct terminate as a single channel at the ampulla of Vater. This unification occurs within the duodenal wall and the common channel is short in length. In cases with choledochal cysts this union occurs outside the duodenal wall, forming a long common channel which allows the reflux of pancreatic juice into the biliary tree, with damage and dilatation of the bile ducts.

Relations of the bile ducts to the arteries of the liver

Normally the hepatic artery lies to the left of the bile duct and divides near the liver into right and left branches, the right branch passing behind the common hepatic duct. The cystic artery is a branch of the right hepatic and lies most commonly between the cystic duct and liver, i.e. above and medial to the duct.

The cystic artery tethers the gallbladder. It can be felt as a taut string when the proximal part of the gallbladder is pulled laterally and can thus be identified. When the artery is divided the inner part of the gallbladder becomes much more mobile.

Arterial anomalies are very common (*Fig.* 85):

1. The right hepatic artery may pass in front of the common hepatic duct.
2. The right hepatic artery may lie parallel to and very near the cystic duct and is often behind it.

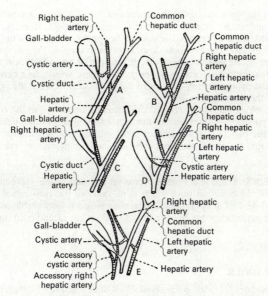

Fig. 85. Abnormalities in the arteries to the liver. **A**, The blood vessels as usually described—i.e. the normal. **B** The right hepatic artery passes in front of the common hepatic duct. **C**, The right hepatic artery parallel to and very near the cystic duct. **D**, The cystic artery passes in front of the common hepatic duct. **E**, An accessory right hepatic artery arising from the superior mesenteric artery and giving off an accessory cystic artery.

3. The cystic artery may pass in front of the common hepatic duct.
4. The right hepatic artery may arise from the superior mesenteric artery. An accessory cystic artery may exist, and arises from the right hepatic, the left hepatic, or some other branch of the hepatic trunk.

Vascular arrangements of the common bile duct

ARTERIAL SUPPLY: The blood supply to the extrahepatic bile ducts is generous, the main contributor being the posterior–superior pancreatico-duodenal artery assisted by the hepatic and cystic arteries. The blood supply to the common bile duct may be relevant in stricture formation of the duct which may occur following apparently minimal trauma to the duct and following liver transplantation.

Recent studies have shown that there is a vascular plexus around, in the wall of, and in the submucosa of the common bile duct. Branches of the gastroduodenal artery run on the sides of the common bile duct at the 3 and 9 o'clock positions. The gastroduodenal artery also supplies the retropancreatic portion of the common bile duct. A retroportal artery, which may arise from either the coeliac axis or superior mesenteric artery, runs behind the head of the pancreas and posterior to the portal vein to reach the posterior aspect of the common bile duct.

It is recommended that minimal dissection be done around the common bile duct particularly at the sides of the duct. In mobilizing the duodenum and head of the pancreas a thin fibrous layer on the back of the head of the pancreas and the portal vein should be left intact to protect the retroportal artery.

THE VEINS: There is a venous plexus on the wall of the supraduodenal portion of the common duct which is of value in the recognition of the common bile duct at operation. This venous plexus is only visible when the overlying peritoneum has been removed. It does not extend onto the cystic duct.

GALLBLADDER

The gallbladder (*Fig.* 86) holds about 45 ml of bile and is 7·5–10 cm long. It consists of fundus, body, infundibulum, neck, and cystic duct.

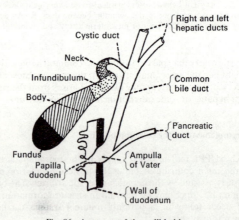

Fig. 86. Anatomy of the gallbladder.

The fundus projects beyond the liver. The body lies in a fossa on the inferior surface of the liver. The infundibulum is the part of the organ between the body and neck; it sags down as a pouch (pouch of Hartmann) towards the duodenum, and is the first part usually to form adhesions to this part of the gut. The neck leaves the upper part of the infundibulum and soon narrows to form the cystic duct.

Developmental anomalies of the gallbladder

Congenital absence of the gallbladder is extremely rare. Other congenital abnormalities are seen in *Fig.* 87.

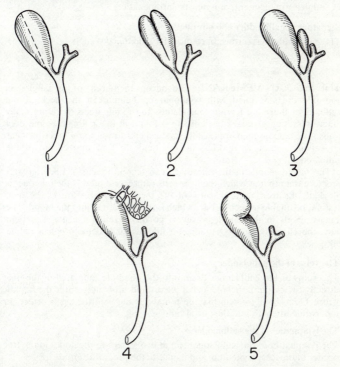

Fig. 87. (1) Longitudinal septate gallbladder. The communication between the two halves is not shown. (2) Double gallbladder with common serosa and cystic duct; (3) double gallbladder with separate serosa and cystic ducts; (4) persistent communications between gallbladder and bile ducts in liver; (5) Phrygian cap deformity.

1. The gallbladder may be septate, transversely or longitudinally.
2. The gallbladder may be double with a single cystic duct.
3. The gallbladder may be double with separate ducts opening into hepatic or common or both ducts. The serosa may be separate or common.
4. Small ducts may connect gallbladder with liver. Usually these become obliterated. They may persist, which is one of the reasons why drainage is advisable after cholecystectomy.
5. The folded fundus (Phrygian cap) deformity is the commonest congenital abnormality of the gallbladder. It has no pathological significance, but when present it can be seen on cholecystography.
6. The gallbladder may have a mesentery: it may be on the left of the falciform ligament, or it may be intrahepatic.

Structure of gallbladder and bile ducts

The gallbladder has serous, fibromuscular, and mucous coats.

THE MUCOUS MEMBRANE: The mucous membrane of the gallbladder and bile ducts is lined with columnar epithelium. In the neck of the gallbladder there are few mucous glands. In the bile ducts there are many mucus-secreting glands. Elastic tissue is found in the gallbladder and duct walls. The mucous membrane of the cystic duct forms a spiral fold which has no valvular action as it offers no resistance to flow into or out of the gallbladder.

The mucus glands in the bile ducts can secrete mucus at much greater pressure than that at which the liver cells can secrete bile. If the bile duct is blocked, the liver may, because of the increase of pressure in the duct system, be unable to secrete bile, which is then absorbed into the blood. The mucus glands in the ducts, however, go on secreting mucus. A patient may, therefore, be deeply jaundiced while his ducts contain mucus (white bile).

The veins of the gallbladder

The veins of the gallbladder drain into the quadrate lobe area of the liver directly or via the pericholedochal plexus and ultimately enter the hepatic veins. Occasionally a vein may be found passing with the cystic artery, or independently of it, into the portal vein.

The lymphatics of the gallbladder

The lymphatics of the gallbladder run in two groups to the nodes in the free border of the lesser omentum and thence to the pre-aortic group.

Shoulder tip pain in acute cholecystitis

In acute cholecystitis pain may be referred to the skin overlying the acromion. The phrenic nerve arises from the same segments of the spinal cord (C3, 4 and

5) as the supraclavicular nerve (C3, 4). Irritation of that portion of the diaphragmatic peritoneum supplied by the phrenic nerve accounts for the pain referred to the distribution of the supraclavicular nerve.

Cholecystectomy

The incision may be a upper paramedian or midline incision (Chapter 9), but some surgeons may prefer a transrectus approach (*see below*).

When performing a cholecystectomy, the surgeon must remember that there are many variations from the normal anatomy of the vessels and bile ducts in the hepatoduodenal ligament. The dissection of these structures can commence in the triangle of Calot which is formed by the common hepatic duct on the left, the cystic duct on the right and the liver above. The cystic artery is first ligated and divided after which the cystic duct and its junction with the common bile duct is defined. At this stage an operative cholangiogram is performed by passing a fine catheter down the cystic duct and injecting a radio-opaque fluid into the bile ducts. Apart from demonstrating the presence of stones and drainage of contrast material or drainage of dye into the duodenum, it may demonstrate congenital anomalies of the biliary system.

An alternative method of removing the gallbladder is to start the dissection at the fundus of the gallbladder and to continue the dissection down to the cystic duct by remaining in a plane close to the gallbladder. Although the dissection is somewhat haemorrhagic (the cystic artery is ligated only during the course of the dissection), there is practically no danger of damaging the common bile duct. This method of cholecystectomy should be used if any difficulty is experienced in defining the anatomy in Calot's triangle. To do so is good judgement and not an admission of defeat.

PRINGLE'S MANOEUVRE: The vessels in the free border of the lesser omentum may be controlled by compression between the thumb and index finger of the left hand. The measure is an emergency one which may be useful in cases of injury to one of the large vessels in the area or in hepatic injuries. It is safe for 30 minutes if the blood pressure is normal, but in the presence of shock the pressure should be released each 15 minutes.

SUPERIOR TRANSRECTUS INCISION: This is Kocher's incision for approach to the liver, gallbladder, and bile ducts. The incision commences at the tip of the xiphoid process and passes down, and to the right, parallel to the costal margin and two finger-breadths below it. The rectus is cut across in the line of the incision (*Fig.* 88). Deep to it is the 9th thoracic nerve which passes downwards and inwards.

It is preserved by being drawn carefully aside. (This advice may fail in practice, as the nerves are so easily damaged by the manipulations necessary to the operation.)

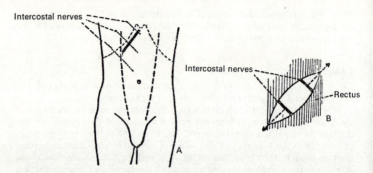

Fig. 88. A, Kocher's incision for gaining access to biliary passages. B, The nerves going to supply the rectus, exposed after the muscle has been divided. They are retracted in the line of the arrows.

The intercostal nerves to the upper rectus pass beneath the costal cartilages to gain the abdominal wall, insinuating themselves between the digitations of the diaphragm and the transversus abdominis. These nerves, having reached the abdominal wall, loop upwards in a manner reminiscent of costal cartilages. The 9th nerve is encountered in this incision; the 7th and 8th lie above the incision.

This incision divides: (*a*) skin; (*b*) anterior rectus sheath; (*c*) rectus; (*d*) posterior rectus sheath; (*e*) fascia transversalis; (*f*) extraperitoneal fat; (*g*) peritoneum.

Needle biopsy of the liver

An isotope scan or ultrasonography may be used to select the site for puncture of the liver.

INTERCOSTAL ROUTE: The patient must be cooperative and able to hold his breath. The needle is inserted in the midaxillary line. It may be entered in the 10th, 9th, or 8th right intercostal space (*Fig.* 89). Above this it will injure the lung. In any of these three spaces the needle traverses the intercostal muscles, the parietal pleura, the pleural recess below the lung (costophrenic sinus), the pleura covering the diaphragm, and then the diaphragm. It then pierces the peritoneum over the undersurface of the diaphragm and passes through the peritoneal recess between the liver and the diaphragm, the peritoneum on the liver, to reach the liver.

SUBCOSTAL ROUTE: This route is confined to liver biopsy in patients with

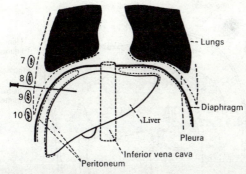

Fig. 89. Liver biopsy by the intercostal route: the needle transverses both pleural and peritoneal cavities.

livers enlarged below the right costal margin. The needle is usually inserted below the costal margin in the midclavicular line.

SUBPHRENIC ABSCESS

Six spaces may be defined in relation to the periphery of the liver. They are of surgical importance because pus may collect in them, forming abscesses. Such abscesses are termed 'subphrenic' because they are all related to the diaphragm. The ligaments of the liver take a large part in delimiting these spaces. Of these six spaces, three are on the right and three are on the left. They are named: (*a*) right anterior intraperitoneal compartment; (*b*) right posterior intraperitoneal compartment; (*c*) right extraperitoneal compartment; (*d*) left anterior intraperitoneal compartment; (*e*) left posterior intraperitoneal compartment; (*f*) left extraperitoneal compartment (*Fig.* 90).

Right anterior intraperitoneal compartment

BOUNDARIES:
  Anterior: Diaphragm and anterior abdominal wall.
  Posterior: Liver (anterior surface).
  Superior: Coronary ligament (anterior layer).
  Left: Right side of the falciform ligament.
  Right: The fossa communicates with the right posterior intraperitoneal compartment by the potential space between the diaphragm and the right lateral surface of the liver.
  Below: The fossa is open.

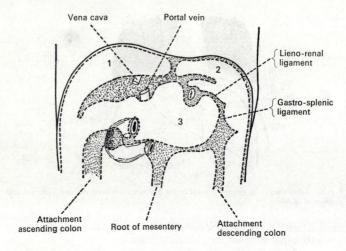

Fig. 90. Anatomy of the subphrenic spaces, the viscera having been removed. (1) Right anterior intraperitoneal compartment; (2) left anterior intraperitoneal compartment; (3) lesser sac. (After Strode, by courtesy of the Editor of *Surgery*.)

Observe that the right anterior intraperitoneal compartment is continuous with the right posterior intraperitoneal compartment round the anterior sharp margin of the liver. In cases where an abscess forms in one of the compartments, it is usually prevented from extending round this sharp margin by the formation of adhesions between the transverse colon and greater omentum to the anterior border of the liver, which serves to limit the abscess to one compartment (*Fig.* 91).

Right posterior intraperitoneal compartment (Morison's or the hepatorenal pouch)

BOUNDARIES:
  Anterior: Inferior surface of the liver.
  Posterior: Peritoneum covering the diaphragm and the upper pole of the right kidney.
  Above: Coronary ligament (posterior layer).
  Below: The pouch is open into the general peritoneal cavity.

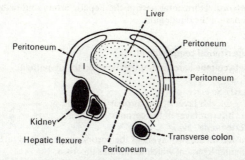

Fig. 91. Anatomy of subphrenic abscess. **X** denotes situation where adhesions form between anterior border of liver and transverse colon, thus separating the right posterior intraperitoneal compartment (I) from the right anterior intraperitoneal compartment (II).

Left anterior intraperitoneal compartment

BOUNDARIES:
   Anterior: Abdominal wall.
   Posterior: Liver.
   Above: Left triangular ligament.
   Right: Falciform ligament.
   Left: The fossa is open. The spleen is some distance away.
   Below: The fossa is open.
   The left and right anterior compartments are separated from each other, therefore, by the falciform ligament.

Left posterior intraperitoneal compartment

This is the lesser sac of the peritoneum and is open into the main peritoneal cavity through the epiploic foramen (Winslow). This foramen is 3 cm in size and is situated opposite the 12th thoracic vertebra.

BOUNDARIES OF THE FORAMEN OF WINSLOW:
   Anterior: Right free border of the lesser omentum containing the bile duct, the vertical part of the hepatic artery, and the portal vein. The duct is dexter (to the right).
   Posterior: Vena cava and the right adrenal gland.
   Superior: Caudate process of the liver.

Inferior: Horizontal part of the hepatic artery and below that the first part of the duodenum.

Right extraperitoneal compartment

The area between the bare area of the liver and the diaphragm.

BOUNDARIES:
  Anterior: Superior layer of the coronary ligament.
  Posterior: Inferior layer of the coronary ligament.
  Left: Inferior vena cava.
  Right: Fusion of the two layers of the coronary ligament to form the right triangular ligament which terminates the fossa.
  Above: Diaphragm, which is in actual contact with the lower boundary.
  Below: Posterior surface of the liver.
  This area is entirely shut in, and if it is distended by fluid, the liver tends to be pushed down and the diaphragm up.

Left extraperitoneal compartment

The space is merely the connective tissue around the upper pole of the left kidney. It is seldom infected and is the least important of the six spaces.

The accuracy of diagnosis of subphrenic abscess has been improved by computerized body tomography and ultrasound. Radiologists are now able to drain subphrenic abscesses by percutaneous catheters under the guidance of ultrasound.

Chapter 7

THE PANCREAS

EMBRYOLOGY

The liver and pancreas arise as dorsal and a ventral outpouching of the duodenum (*Fig. 92a*). The dorsal pouch is the rudiment of the pancreatic duct from which the neck, body and tail of the pancreas develops. The ventral pouch arises from the duodenum at a lower level and is the rudiment of the bile passages from which a pancreatic duct arises to form the head and the uncinate process.

Due to differential growth of the wall of the second part of the duodenum, the dorsal duct is carried to the front to form the primitive dorsal duct. The lower ventral duct is carried posteriorly thus bringing the common bile duct behind the primitive dorsal duct and the first part of the duodenum (*Fig. 92b*).

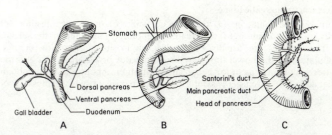

Fig. 92. Development of the pancreas. (A) Dorsal and ventral outpouchings of the duodenum; (B) rotation of the ventral pancreas; (C) the usual mature state.

After fusion of these component parts of the pancreas, the main pancreatic duct is formed from the ventral duct and distal part of the dorsal duct (*Fig*. 92c). The proximal part of the dorsal duct usually persists as the accessory pancreatic duct (Santorini) which opens into the duodenum about 2 cm proximal to the main duct (Wirsung). These two ducts usually communicate, but in about 9 per cent of people the two ducts persist without any communication.

CONGENITAL ANOMALIES OF THE PANCREATIC DUCTS

Pancreas divisum

In this condition (*Fig*. 93) there is failure of fusion of the dorsal and ventral ducts and the dorsal duct becomes the major ductal system of the pancreas.

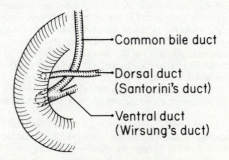

Fig. 93. Pancreas divisum.

Accessory pancreatic tissue

This may be found in: (*a*) the stomach wall; (*b*) the small intestine; (*c*) Meckel's diverticulum; (*d*) the greater omentum; (*e*) the hilum of the spleen.

The nodules are usually single, 1–6 cm in diameter, yellowish, and lobulated. In the bowel they may be submucous or intramuscular and the latter may be mistaken for neoplastic infiltration. About one-third contain islet cells. They are usually symptomless but may give rise to an intussusception.

Annular pancreas

Due to maldevelopment of the primitive pancreatic ducts, a ring of pancreatic tissue may surround the descending portion of the duodenum. It usually produces no symptoms but it may occur in association with duodenal stenosis in which case duodenal obstruction occurs.

In the presence of duodenal obstruction, a duodenojejunostomy is performed and no attempt is made to resect the pancreatic tissue which would result in a pancreatic fistula.

RELATIONS OF SURGICAL IMPORTANCE

The head of the pancreas lies within the concavity of the duodenum in front of the 2nd lumbar vertebra; the body lies in front of the 1st lumbar vertebra and the upwardly sloping tail is at the level of the 12th thoracic vertebra.

The common bile duct passes through the head of the pancreas and the portal vein is incompletely surrounded by the neck, head and uncinate process on its anterior, right lateral and posterior aspects.

The stomach and spleen are separated from the anterior surface of the body of the pancreas by the lesser sac. The tail of the pancreas projects a variable distance into the lienorenal ligament and may come into contact with the hilum of the spleen where it can be damaged during splenectomy.

The retroperitoneal position of the pancreas contributes to the severe epigastric pain radiating to the back in patients with acute pancreatitis.

In acute pancreatitis, collections of fluid with a high amylase content may form in the lesser sac or in the retroperitoneal tissue behind the lesser sac. These fluid collections are pseudopancreatic cysts which have no epithelial lining.

The main pancreatic duct courses the length of the gland and lies close to the upper surface of the gland. It joins the common bile duct at the ampulla of Vater (*see* p. 89) and passes through the duodenal wall. The duct of Santorini usually empties into the duodenum 2–3 cm proximal to the ampulla.

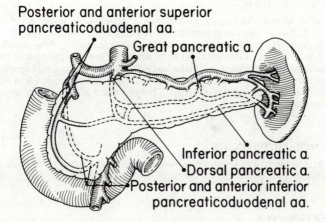

Posterior and anterior superior pancreaticoduodenal aa.

Great pancreatic a.

Inferior pancreatic a.
Dorsal pancreatic a.
Posterior and anterior inferior pancreaticoduodenal aa.

Fig. 94. The arterial supply to the pancreas.

ARTERIAL SUPPLY

The arterial supply (*Fig.* 94) consists of a vertically directed system of arteries (from the gastroduodenal and superior mesenteric arteries) around the head of the pancreas and a horizontally directed system (from the splenic or coeliac arteries), around the body and tail of the pancreas. There is a rich anastomosis between the two systems.

The anastomoses between the coeliac artery and the superior mesenteric artery form an important collateral pathway if either of these vessels is occluded. The dorsal pancreatic artery, which arises from the coeliac artery or one of its branches, may replace the middle colic artery and form part of the marginal artery.

In the operation of subtotal pancreatectomy, either the superior or inferior pancreaticoduodenal artery may be divided: division of both arteries causes necrosis of the duodenum.

When the main pancreatic duct has to be drained, it may be opened anteriorly to within 15 mm of the duodenum without serious haemorrhage or duodenal ischaemia occurring. If the incision extends closer to the duodenal wall the anterior superior pancreaticoduodenal artery will be damaged.

Occasionally the hepatic artery arises from the superior mesenteric artery in which case a pancreaticoduodenectomy might endanger the blood supply to the liver.

VENOUS DRAINAGE

Most of the veins draining the pancreas are tributaries of the splenic vein (*see Fig*. 74). Other veins empty into the superior mesenteric and portal veins.

In performing a pancreaticoduodenectomy for a carcinoma of the ampulla of Vater, a plane of dissection has to be developed between the neck of the pancreas and the portal vein. This has to be done strictly anterior to the portal vein because veins draining the head of the pancreas enter the right side of the portal vein and dissection to the right of the portal vein will, therefore, result in tearing of the vein.

LYMPHATIC DRAINAGE

This is to the root of the superior mesenteric artery and then to the coeliac nodes.

NERVE SUPPLY

The sympathetic nerve supply is from the splanchnic nerves and the parasympathetic supply is from the vagus. Afferent pain fibres are carried by the sympathetic nervous system but bilateral sympathectomy is not effective in alleviating pain of chronic pancreatitis or pancreatic carcinoma because intercostal nerves and retroperitoneal tissue also become involved. Motor fibres are carried by both sympathetic and parasympathetic systems.

Chapter 8

THE SPLEEN

The surge of enthusiasm for preserving the damaged spleen came about because of the fear of overwhelming postsplenectomy infection (OPSI) and has highlighted the immunological role of the spleen. The splenic macrophages are the most active of the body's macrophages in phagocytosing living and inert particles. The spleen also initiates cellular (T lymphocytes) and humoral (B lymphocytes) responses.

EMBRYOLOGY

The spleen develops on the left side of the dorsal mesogastrium. It is mesodermal in origin and later incorporates vascular and lymphatic elements.

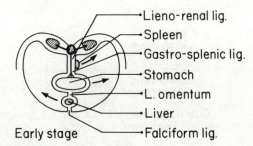

Fig. 95. Transverse section of the abdomen of the embryo: the stomach and spleen move to the left and the liver moves to the right.

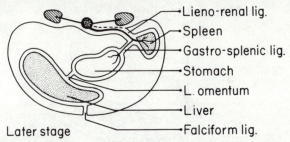

Fig. 96. There has been a partial re-absorption of the dorsal mesogastrium: the unabsorbed part is the lienorenal ligament.

As the stomach rotates, the left surface of the mesogastrium fuses with the peritoneum over the left kidney. This fusion explains the dorsal attachment of the lienorenal ligament and why the splenic artery runs posterior to the omental bursa (lesser sac) and anterior to the left kidney. (*See Figs* 95, 96.)

The spleen is rarely absent, but accessory spleens have been reported to occur in 10–35 per cent of individuals (*Fig.* 97). The majority of accessory spleens occur at the hilum, in the greater omentum or along the splenic vessels and pancreas. They are up to 3 cm in diameter and may undergo torsion. If the spleen is removed for haemolytic anaemia, a diligent search must be made for an accessory spleen, which can cause recurrent symptoms if not removed.

RELATIONS

The spleen is an intraperitoneal structure with a characteristically notched anterior border. The convex parietal surface of the spleen is in contact with

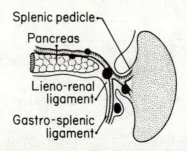

Splenic pedicle

Pancreas

Lieno-renal
ligament

Gastro-splenic
ligament

Fig. 97. More common locations of accessory spleens.

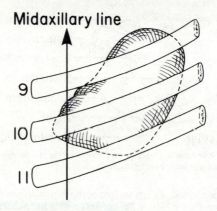

Midaxillary line

9

10

11

Fig. 98. The diaphragmatic surface of the spleen showing its relation to the 9th, 10th and 11th ribs.

the diaphragm deep to the 9th, 10th and 11th ribs. Its long axis follows the 10th rib up to the midaxillary line (*Fig.* 98). Through the diaphragm, the spleen is related to the pleural recess and to the thin inferior border of the left lung (*Fig.* 99).

In an adult, a fracture of the 9th, 10th or 11th ribs, where they overlie the spleen, alerts the surgeon to a possible splenic injury. In children the ribs are more pliable and a splenic injury following blunt trauma frequently occurs without a fractured rib.

The visceral surface of the spleen is shared by the stomach, kidney and colon (*Fig.* 100).

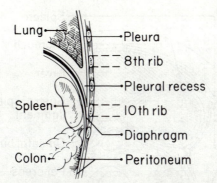

Fig. 99. Coronal section of the spleen to show its relation to the pleural recess.

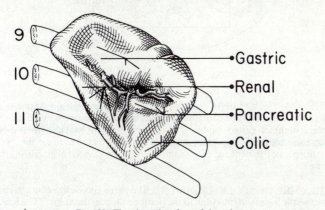

Fig. 100. The visceral surface of the spleen.

Splenic ligaments

The spleen is suspended at its hilum by two peritoneal folds, the lienorenal and gastrosplenic ligaments (*Fig.* 101). These folds form the lateral limit of the omental bursa.

THE LIENORENAL LIGAMENT: The lienorenal ligament is short and transmits the blood vessels to the spleen. The tail of the pancreas lies in this ligament but it does not always reach the hilum of the spleen. The tail of the pancreas can be damaged at the time of splenectomy.

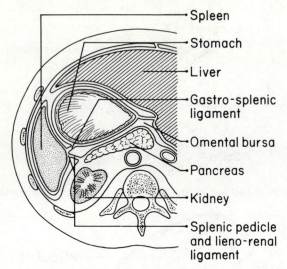

Fig. 101. The splenic ligaments.

THE GASTROSPLENIC LIGAMENT: The gastrosplenic ligament is directed anteriorly and contains the short gastric arteries (branches of the splenic or the left gastro-epiploic artery) which supply the left half of the greater curvature and fundic area of the stomach. In a subtotal gastrectomy, the lower gastrosplenic ligament and its contained arteries are divided in mobilizing the stomach.

THE PHRENICOCOLIC LIGAMENT: The phrenicocolic ligament attaches the splenic flexure of the colon to the peritoneum over the kidney. The lower pole of the spleen is in contact with this ligament which is thought to be one of the main supports of the spleen. The spleen may be accidentally damaged when the ligament is cut in the process of surgical mobilization of the splenic flexure.

BLOOD SUPPLY

Splenic artery

This is usually a branch of the coeliac artery, but it may arise from the aorta or superior mesenteric artery. It usually runs along the upper border of the

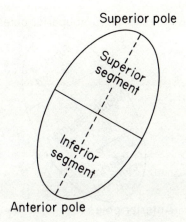

Fig. 102. Vascular segments of the spleen.

pancreas. At the tail of the pancreas it passes to the front of the pancreas and divides into its superior and inferior terminal branches.

The intrasplenic branches of the splenic artery do not usually anastomose: each supplies its own segment. There is a superior and inferior segment of the spleen separated by a relatively avascular plane perpendicular to the long axis of the organ (*Fig.* 102). These vascular territories correspond to the superior and inferior divisions of the splenic artery. In less than 20 per cent of patients three primary arterial branches supply a superior, middle and inferior segment (*Fig.* 103). This segmental blood supply makes segmental resection possible; this could be important where preservation of splenic tissue is necessary.

Potential sources of collateral circulation are available through the pancreatic, gastro-epiploic and short gastric branches of the splenic artery. The spleen may also receive a branch from the inferior pancreatic artery which itself may arise from the pancreaticoduodenal arteries.

Splenic veins

The splenic vein regularly runs on the posterior surface of the pancreas below the level of the splenic artery. It receives the inferior mesenteric vein and joins the superior mesenteric vein at a right-angle behind the neck of the pancreas to form the portal vein.

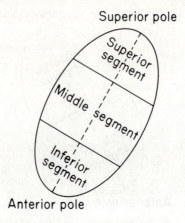

Fig. 103. Vascular segments of the spleen in 20 per cent of patients.

SPLENIC RUPTURE

Whenever possible the surgeon should attempt to conserve a ruptured spleen in children because of the danger of OPSI. If the splenic injury is not severe, the diagnosis can be confirmed by doing a radioactive technetium scan of the spleen. Delayed rupture of a subcapsular haematoma is very uncommon in children and resolution of the injury can be monitored by repeating the technetium scan.

A ruptured spleen found at laparotomy should be conserved if at all possible. Segmental resection may be done when either the upper or lower pole has been traumatized. The spleen is fully mobilized by dividing the lienorenal and gastrosplenic ligaments. The splenic artery and veins are gripped in the tail of the pancreas to control the bleeding and the appropriate polar artery is ligated.

If a splenectomy has to be performed, slithers of splenic tissue can be transplanted by burying the tissue in the retroperitoneum or greater omentum (autotransplantation).

Splenosis (implantation of splenic tissue) may occur when fragments of the spleen are spilled during rupture of the spleen. Multiple areas of splenic tissue are found disseminated over the peritoneum.

SPLENECTOMY

The usual incision is either a midline or a left subcostal incision. If the spleen is enormously enlarged, an incision can be made in the line of the 9th rib from the costal margin to the right iliac fossa. If necessary, the incision is extended into the chest along the line of the 9th rib and the diaphragm is also divided.

Due to stretching of the ligaments it is often easier to remove a grossly enlarged spleen than a spleen of normal size. If there are many adhesions between the spleen and diaphragm, the splenic artery should be exposed in the lesser sac by dividing the gastrocolic ligament. The splenic artery is ligated in continuity after which the splenic adhesions are divided.

DISTAL SPLENORENAL SHUNT

This is one of the favoured operations in the treatment of portal hypertension because it selectively decompresses the oesophageal varices via the short gastric veins into the splenic venous system. The splenic vein is disconnected from its junction with the superior mesenteric vein and anastomosed to the left renal vein.

The lesser sac is opened by dividing the gastrocolic omentum. The peritoneum over the inferior border of the pancreas is incised and the pancreas is gently mobilized, lifted from its bed and rotated cephalad. The splenic vein is identified attached to the posterior surface of the pancreas. The inferoposterior aspect of the splenic vein has the fewest collaterals which require ligation.

Chapter 9

THE ANATOMY OF ABDOMINAL INCISIONS

Incisions through the abdominal wall are based on anatomical principles. The intra-abdominal pressure is considerable, and the surgeon aims at leaving the abdominal wall as strong as possible after operation, otherwise there exists a very real fear that portions of the abdominal contents may leave the abdominal cavity through the weak area which is caused by a badly placed incision, resulting in a condition known as scar, incisional, or ventral hernia.

THE PRINCIPLES GOVERNING ABDOMINAL INCISIONS

1. The incision must give ready access to the part to be investigated, and must allow extension if required.
2. The muscles must be split in the direction of their fibres, rather than cut across.
3. The incisions must not divide nerves.

4. The rectus muscles may be cut transversely without seriously weakening the abdominal wall, as such a cut passes between two adjacent nerves without injuring them. The rectus has a segmental nerve supply, so that there is no risk of a transverse incision cutting off the distal part of the muscle from its nerve supply, as would be the situation if a muscle which depended on a single nerve were to be divided (*Fig.* 104).

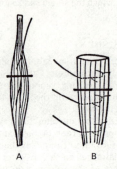

A   B

Fig. 104. Demonstrating that division of a muscle (A), with a single nerve supply causes paralysis distal to the section, whereas division of a muscle (B), such as the rectus, with a segmental supply produces no paralysis, as the nerves are uninjured.

Above the umbilicus, the tendinous intersections prevent retraction of the rectus muscle after it has been divided.

5. Drainage tubes should be inserted through separate small incisions, as their presence in the main wound may seriously prejudice the strength of the ultimate scar. For the same reason, a colostomy should be made through a separate incision and not through the main wound.
6. Closure of abdominal incisions has been more readily understood since it has been realized that they heal by forming a block of fibrous tissue, and that disruption is a mechanical problem, often due to ischaemia. Thus wound closure without tension is necessary for a secure closure.

GENERAL LAPAROTOMY INCISIONS

Specific incisions for particular purposes have been included in the consideration of individual organs. More flexible incisions may be required where wider or multipurpose exposure is desired.

Midline incisions

Midline incisions (*Fig.* 105) traverse the abdominal wall in a vertical direction

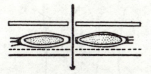

Fig. 105. Midline incision.

above or below the umbilicus. They are extensively used. The incision divides: (*a*) skin; (*b*) linea alba; (*c*) fascia transversalis; (*d*) extraperitoneal fat; (*e*) peritoneum.

The linea alba above the umbilicus is a dense, strong structure 1 cm wide, formed by the interlacing fibres of the rectus sheaths. It holds sutures well and it is relatively avascular.

The incision may be extended downwards by cutting around the side of the umbilicus. The side chosen is determined by the falciform ligament which travels from the umbilicus upwards and to the right.

A midline incision may be extended upwards by cutting or excising the xiphoid process of the sternum and, if necessary, splitting the sternum.

In exposing the bladder, the incision may stop short of the peritoneum so that the bladder is dealt with through its anterior surface which is devoid of peritoneum in the region of the space of Retzius (prevesical).

The midline lower abdominal incision is occasionally followed by an incisional hernia, particularly at the lower end just above the pubis. A major reason for this is that, at the time of closure of the incision, the surgeon sutures the external oblique fascia (Gallaudet's fascia) instead of the linea alba. The external oblique fascia lies on the outside of the external oblique aponeurosis, to which it is adherent. It is given off over the cord as the external spermatic fascia at the external ring, and extends over the pubis, into the perineum. It is not as strong as the linea alba and, unless the linea alba is sutured, a hernia will develop immediately above the pubis.

Where a supra-umbilical midline incision gives insufficient access, it may be combined with a second incision carried laterally at right-angles to the first (*Fig*. 106).

When more exposure is necessary, an oblique upward extension can be used. This will cut the rectus and the muscles of the lateral abdominal wall in the line of the intercostal nerves, which will therefore be preserved, and it will be possible to extend the wound further into an intercostal space (*Fig*. 107).

Paramedian incisions

A paramedian incision (*Fig*. 108A) is made vertical, parallel to the midline, and about 2·5 cm away from it to one or other side. It may be made of any

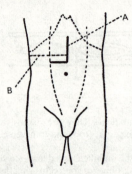

Fig. 106. **A**, Method of enlarging a supra-umbilical incision by a right-angle extension through the rectus. **B**, The dotted line shows Rutherford Morison's incision for difficult operations on the bile ducts.

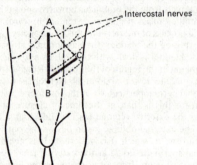

Fig. 107. Angular incision used for gaining access to a very large spleen or kidney. **AB**, Median supra-umbilical incision; **BC**, incision joining the umbilicus to the tip of the 10th costal cartilage; **C**, observe that no nerves are injured in the incision.

length, and, even if extended from costal margin to pubis, the scar does not greatly weaken the abdominal wall.

The incision traverses: (*a*) skin; (*b*) anterior rectus sheath; (*c*) rectus (*see below*); (*d*) posterior rectus sheath above the arcuate line; (*e*) fascia transversalis; (*f*) extraperitoneal fat.

The incision may be extended upwards to the xiphoid process of the sternum (Mayo-Robson incision). In this manoeuvre, troublesome haemorrhage from the superior epigastric artery is frequently encountered (*Fig.* 109).

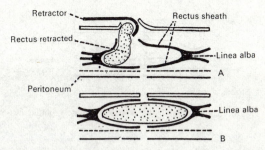

Fig. 108. A, Structures encountered in approaching peritoneal cavity by paramedian route with retraction of rectus; B, shows how incision line in the aponeuroses is protected by rectus muscle on closing the wound.

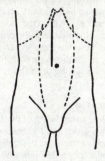

Fig. 109. Mayo-Robson incision: a paramedian incision, the upper end of which may be extended, if necessary, to the xiphisternum.

In this incision there are different ways of dealing with the rectus:

1. The muscle may be displaced outwards intact without any further interference with it. When the wound is closed the muscle returns to its bed and forms the most efficient protection possible to the line of the incision, which it directly covers (*Fig.* 108B). This is a sound incision extensively used on the right or left of the midline. When used to deal with the terminal part of the pelvic colon or for excision of the rectum, the incision extends low down so that the rectus may be mobilized down to its insertion to the pubis.

2. The muscle may be divided in the line of the incision (*Fig.* 110). The nerves to the rectus enter it from the side or back about its middle. Should the incision through the rectus be made too far laterally, the nerves will be divided and the muscle paralysed.

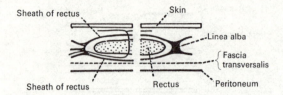

Fig. 110. Structures divided by the paramedian muscle-splitting incision.

Security in closure is based on the same principles as closure of a midline incision, but at this site the fibres of the anterior and posterior sheath are transverse and may not hold sutures well. Special care is therefore necessary in suturing. In addition, since the blood supply enters with the nerve, an extensive split, combined with a tight closure, may result in ischaemia to the medial part of the muscle enclosed within the incision.

However, if the muscle is split well medially, only the small medial segment of muscle will be affected and this has been shown by experience to have no ill effects. Splitting the muscle in the direction of its fibres is quicker, and closure is as effective as the muscle displacing procedure.

Incisions dividing the flat muscles

An oblique incision in the line from the tip of the 12th rib to halfway between the umbilicus and the pubis gives good exposure. The posterior limit will depend on requirements and, anteriorly, it usually ends at the lateral border of the rectus. It gives good exposure of laterally situated tumours, such as those of kidney or peripheral colon. The flat muscles are cut across and no nerves are divided. If necessary the rectus sheath may be opened and the muscles retracted medially or the muscle may be cut across. In the case of retroperitoneal structures, the peritoneum is not entered, but is displaced medially, and the dissection carried around the periphery of the peritoneum.

Chapter 10

THE GROIN AND SCROTUM

The anatomy and surgical conditions of the groin and scrotum can best be understood if the development of the testis is described first.

DEVELOPMENT OF THE TESTIS

The organ is developed between the 10th and 12th dorsal segments of the embryo. Its nerve supply is from the 10th dorsal or thoracic segment of the cord. This accounts for the fact that in cases of injury or inflammation of the testis the patient frequently complains of pain at the level of and lateral to the umbilicus, which receives its nerve supply from the same segment.

The testis develops on the posterior abdominal wall from the genital ridge situated on the medial side of the mesonephros. In its development it is constituted by the primordial sex cells, coelomic epithelium (seminiferous tubules) and mesenchyme (connective tissue).

Descent of the testis

The testis, lying in the lumbar region in front of the kidney, reaches the scrotum as a result of several factors, one of which is the gubernaculum testis. The gubernaculum is attached to the caudal end of the testis in a continuous column of mesenchyme extending through the inguinal region to the genital swelling. By the third month of fetal life the testis has reached the deep inguinal ring as a result of differential growth of the posterior abdominal wall while the gubernaculum fails to elongate.

A diverticulum of the coelomic epithelium, called the processus vaginalis, follows the path of the gubernaculum and invades the anterior abdominal wall. It carries with it a covering from each of the layers of the abdominal wall and in this way the inguinal canal is formed, with:

1. The fascia transversalis forming the internal spermatic fascia.
2. The internal oblique and transversalis muscles forming the cremasteric fascia.
3. The external oblique forming the external spermatic fascia.

The final descent of the testis through the inguinal canal to the scrotum is controlled by testosterone and maternal gonadotrophins. The gubernaculum keeps open the path of descent.

The testis descends:

1. From loin to iliac fossa in the third month of intra-uterine life.
2. From the fourth to the seventh month it rests at the site of the internal or abdominal inguinal ring.
3. During the seventh month it is travelling through the inguinal canal.
4. In the eighth month it lies at the external or subcutaneous inguinal ring.
5. In the ninth month it enters the scrotum, reaching its base at or after birth.

Three per cent of full-term infants and 21 per cent of premature infants do not have both testes in the scrotum: most of these reach the scrotum but a small percentage remains undescended. Descent does not occur after the infant is 1 year old.

FATE OF THE PROCESSUS VAGINALIS: This peritoneal diverticulum becomes occluded at two points soon after birth: first, at the internal abdominal ring, and second, just above the testis, cutting off the part of the sac in relation to the testis, which is henceforward known as the tunica vaginalis testis. The part of the sac between the two occlusions is the funicular process, which becomes obliterated forming a fibrous cord, the rudiment of the processus vaginalis.

IMPERFECT DESCENT OF THE TESTIS

Imperfect descent of the testis may be divided into incomplete descent of the testis and ectopia testis.

Incomplete descent of the testis

Cryptorchidism, i.e. absence of one testis from the scrotum, occurs in 0·1–0·2 per cent of all young adults. If left undescended the testis will not develop normally.

TYPES OF INCOMPLETE DESCENT: The testis may become arrested at any point along its long journey from lumbar region to the base of the scrotum. The incompletely descended testis may be:
1. *Lumbar:* Entire failure of descent.
2. *Iliac:* Partial descent in which the testis is situated at the entrance to the inguinal canal.
3. *Inguinal:* The testis is in the canal. Pressure on the inguinal canal may make the testis emerge from the external ring. A testis situated in the inguinal canal is impalpable.
4. *At the External Ring:* The testis frequently comes to rest just outside the external inguinal ring.
5. *Scrotal:* The testis is in the upper part of the scrotum. This is the so-called high retractile testis which will descend spontaneously at the time of puberty.

ECTOPIA TESTIS: Ectopia testis implies that the organ has deviated from the normal line of its descent. The ectopic testis is always one which has successfully completed its intra-abdominal descent and has negotiated the inguinal canal and external ring. It is usually fully developed.

An ectopic testis may be found at the following sites:
1. Superficial inguinal ectopic where it lies beneath Scarpa's fascia and on the external oblique aponeurosis usually at the external ring.
2. At the root of the penis.
3. In the perineum.
4. In the femoral triangle.

Imperfect descent of the testis is frequently misdiagnosed as a retractile testis. In a retractile testis the cremasteric reflex draws the testis back. If the testis can be coaxed into the scrotum it is not an imperfectly descended testis. If the child is asked to squat, this flexion manoeuvre relaxes the cremasteric reflex, and if the testis is only retractile it will descend spontaneously into the scrotum.

Orchidopexy

The basis for successful orchidopexy is the systematic mobilization of the cord and the placement of the testis in the scrotum without tension on the cord. At operation the cremaster and the hernial sac of the processus vaginalis, if present, are identified and separated from the cord. The internal spermatic fascia is freed from the vessels and vas. The testis is then suspended by the vas with its vessels and the testicular artery with the related pampiniform plexus of veins. Mobilization can be carried out proximal to the internal ring by dividing the muscles of the abdominal wall and mobilizing the testicular vessels up to the lower pole of the kidney. If the testis still does not reach the scrotum, it should be fixed outside the external ring and the second stage of the operation is done one year later.

Although there is an anastomosis between the cremasteric artery, the artery of the ductus deferens and the testicular artery, the latter should not be divided to lengthen the cord.

One of the methods of holding the testis in the scrotum is to create a pouch for the testis between the skin and dartos muscle.

INVERSION OF THE TESTIS

The organ is normally suspended in the scrotum, attached above, below and behind, to the epididymis, which in turn is blended with the ductus deferens and the vessels and nerves going to the testis and epididymis. It is thus held in a relatively fixed position, its vertical axis inclining obliquely from above down and from before back. The term 'inversion of the testis' implies an alteration of its normal position in the scrotum. Inversion is usually unilateral.

Types of inversion of the testis

There are four types (*Fig.* 111):

1. *Superior Inversion:* The long axis of the testis is tipped forwards, so that the posterior border of the testis looks upwards and the epididymis lies horizontally on this border.
2. *Anterior Inversion:* The epididymis is attached to the anterior border of the testis.
3. *Lateral Inversion:* The epididymis is attached to the lateral surface of the testicle.

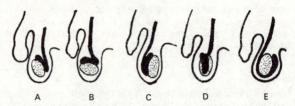

Fig. 111. Inversion of testis. A, Testis normally orientated; B, superior inversion; C, anterior inversion; D, lateral inversion; E, loop inversion. (After Campbell.)

4. *Loop inversion:* The epididymis and ductus deferens encircle the testicle like a sling.

The first condition is not uncommon; the second is quite common if anyone troubles to find it; the remaining two conditions are rare.

Anterior inversion is of practical importance in the operation of 'tapping' or withdrawing the fluid from a hydrocele. The testis is normally posterior to the fluid and the needle is entered in front. In anterior inversion, the testis is in front of the fluid and a needle entered anteriorly may damage the organ.

TORSION OF THE TESTIS

The term is synonymous with torsion of the spermatic cord. In this condition the testis undergoes rotation round a vertical axis, and its blood supply is partly or wholly cut off. In the latter event gangrene of the organ occurs.

The following facts are noteworthy:

1. Torsion frequently affects an incompletely descended testis as the organ is improperly fixed.
2. Torsion is sometimes found associated with lengthening of the peritoneal fold (mesorchium) attaching the testis to the epididymis, a condition predisposing to twisting. In such cases, the testis is completely surrounded by the tunica vaginalis and the torsion is intravaginal.
3. Torsion of the testis is usually associated with imperfect fixation of the organ, e.g. the epididymis is attached posteriorly to the ductus only and not to the mesoblastic structures.
4. Superior inversion predisposes to rotation. In such cases the torsion is usually extravaginal, the twist involving the whole cord which is shortened, so elevating the testis higher in the scrotum. This elevation is a useful diagnostic point in torsion of the testis.
5. Torsion of the testis is associated with dimpling of the skin of the scrotum because of shortening of the coverings of the cord (external, cremasteric, and internal spermatic fasciae) which blend with the scrotal septum and raphe. This scrotal dimpling may be of diagnostic value in testicular torsion.

VESTIGIAL STRUCTURES IN CONNECTION WITH THE TESTIS

There are four testicular appendages which may undergo torsion and present as a painful testicular swelling (*Fig*. 112).

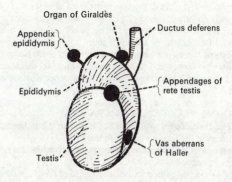

Fig. 112. Vestigial structures in connection with the testis.

1. The appendix testis, or hydatid of Morgagni, is found in more than 90 per cent of men and is a remnant of the Müllerian duct (paramesonephric duct).
2. The appendix of the epididymis which is a mesonephric remnant attached to the globus major of the epididymis.
3. The paradidymis or organ of Giraldès is attached to the lower spermatic cord and is a mesonephric remnant.
4. The vas aberrans or organ of Haller originates at the junction of the body and tail of the epididymis and is also a mesonephric remnant.

Of these, torsion of the appendix of the testis is the most common. Torsions of testicular appendages are very uncommon in adults and occur most frequently in patients 10–13 years old.

FASCIAE OF CAMPER, SCARPA AND COLLES

These are names applied to the superficial fasciae of the lower part of the anterior abdominal wall and perineum.

Fasciae of Scarpa and Camper

Midway between the umbilicus and pubis, the superficial fascia is condensed on its deep surface to form a membranous layer (the fascia of Scarpa).

Sandwiched between the skin and this fascial condensation is a layer of fat which corresponds to and is continuous with the subcutaneous fat of the body generally. This layer is Camper's fascia.

Just below the subcutaneous abdominal ring (external ring), Camper's and Scarpa's fasciae are replaced by the muscle of the scrotum (the dartos muscle). There is no subcutaneous fat in the penis or scrotum.

The dartos gives a muscle sheath to the penis and to each testicle. The muscle is much more extensive than is usually thought and is responsible for the corrugations of the scrotal skin, especially when cold. Normal spermato-genesis requires a controlled temperature which is maintained by the contraction of the dartos in cold environmental temperatures and relaxation when it is hot.

THE ATTACHMENTS OF SCARPA'S FASCIA:

Superior: The fascia fades away midway between the pubis and umbilicus above, and in the lumbar region at the sides.

Inferior: Just below the subcutaneous or external abdominal ring the fascia changes its name to fascia of Colles.

Lateral: The fascia is attached to the deep fascia of the thigh (the fascia lata) just below the inguinal ligament at the groin crease. Because of this attachment to the fascia lata, fluid tracking down from above under the superficial fascia cannot extend further into the thigh than the line of this attachment.

Fascia of Colles

Just below the subcutaneous inguinal ring, Scarpa's fascia changes its name to Colles' fascia or the superficial perineal fascia. This extends over the penis and scrotum, giving a fascial covering to each; it then covers the muscles in the superficial compartment of the perineum.

ATTACHMENTS:

Lateral: It is attached to the conjoined ramus of the ischium and pubis, as far back as the tuberosity of the ischium.

Posterior: It curves round the superficial transverse perineal muscles to join the posterior margins of the fascia of the urogenital diaphragm.

Anterior: It is continuous with the fascia of Scarpa.

Medial: It is continuous with its fellow of the opposite side. The fascia sends a median septum to be attached to the perineal muscles. This septum is not complete, and fluid may pass through it from one side to the other.

If a ruptured urethra results in extravasation of urine (*Fig.* 113) into the space deep to Colles' fascia (superficial perineal space), the attachments of Colles' fascia determine the direction of flow of the extravasated urine. The urine may pass into the areolar tissue in the scrotum, around the penis and upwards into the anterior abdominal wall. It cannot pass into the thighs

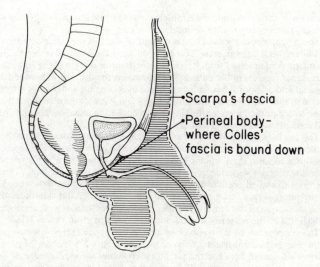

*Scarpa's fascia

*Perineal body-
where Colles'
fascia is bound down

Fig. 113. Extravasation of urine into the superficial perineal space.

because Scarpa's fascia is attached to the fascia enveloping the thigh muscles, nor can it pass posteriorly around the anus, because of Colles' fascia which is attached to the posterior border of the urogenital diaphragm.

ANATOMY OF THE INGUINAL REGION AND OF INGUINAL AND FEMORAL HERNIA

Inguinal canal

This is a triangular slit 4 cm long, almost horizontal in direction, which lies just above the inner half of the inguinal ligament. At its lateral end is the abdominal inguinal ring (internal inguinal ring), and at the medial end is the subcutaneous (external) inguinal ring.

The internal inguinal ring is an opening in the fascia transversalis midway between the anterior superior iliac spine and the symphysis pubis, just lateral to the inferior epigastric artery. The ring is shaped like the letter V with the open end pointing laterally and superiorly. The arms are called the crura. The superior crus is attached to the transversus muscle by fascial slips so that, when the transversus abdominis muscle contracts, the internal ring is drawn laterally, thus increasing the obliquity of the exit.

The subcutaneous inguinal ring is triangular, and lies very obliquely above and lateral to the pubic crest. It is an opening in the external oblique. The spermatic cord emerges from it, lying on the inferior margin of the ring, and lateral (not medial) to the pubic spine. However, the distinction between an inguinal and a femoral hernia is best made by sliding the index finger, from lateral to medial, down an imaginary line joining the anterior superior iliac spine to the pubic tubercle: the finger displaces an inguinal hernia upwards and medially and a femoral hernia downwards and laterally.

The fascia transversalis is part of the endo-abdominal fascia, deriving its name from the overlying transversus muscle. The lower part of this fascia is thickened to form the iliopubic tract (Thomson's ligament) which stretches from the anterior superior iliac spine laterally to the pubis medially. It lies posterior to and adjacent to the inguinal ligament, forms the inferior border of the internal ring, bridges across the femoral vessels, and reinforces the anterior margin of the femoral sheath. The iliopubic tract, if well developed (which it is in the majority of cases), can be used in groin hernia repair.

The aponeurosis of the transversus abdominis muscle extends downwards from the arched muscle to become attached into a variable length of Cooper's ligament between the pubic tubercle and the medial edge of the femoral vein. It is intimately adherent to the underlying fascia transversalis. The strength of the posterior wall of the inguinal canal will vary with the extent of this aponeurosis.

The boundaries of the canal are:

Anterior: External oblique in its whole length. Internal oblique in its lateral third.

Posterior: Fascia transversalis and the aponeurosis of the transversus abdominis muscle in its whole length with falx inguinalis (conjoint tendon) in its inner half. Reflex inguinal ligament in its inner third.

Floor: The upper surface of the inguinal ligament (external oblique), which forms a furrow (Poupart's ligament).

Inguinal hernia

An indirect inguinal hernia is congenital as a result of failure of obliteration of the processus vaginalis. If the processus vaginalis fails to close at the internal abdominal ring, a passage is left through which the abdominal contents may pass. Such an event may occur soon after birth or not for many years, though it is important to realize, even in the latter case, that the sac into which the hernia occurs may have existed since birth. The processus vaginalis closes a little sooner on the left than on the right, therefore hernia is commoner on the right.

An indirect inguinal hernia traverses the canal. It is invested by the coverings of the spermatic cord (from outside in): (*a*) external spermatic

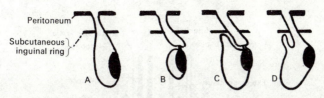

Peritoneum

Subcutaneous
inguinal ring

A   B   C   D

Fig. 114. Types of indirect inguinal hernia. A, Vaginal; B, funicular; C, infantile;
D, encysted.

fascia from external oblique; (*b*) cremasteric fascia from internal oblique;
(*c*) internal spermatic fascia from fascia transversalis.

TYPES OF INDIRECT HERNIAE: *See Fig*. 114.

1. *Vaginal:* The processus vaginalis has failed to become occluded in any
   part of its course. The hernia therefore descends to the base of the
   scrotum and the testis is behind it and may be difficult to locate.
2. *Funicular:* The processus is obliterated above the testis. The testis can
   be felt separately from the hernia, below it.
3. *Infantile:* As (2), but a process of peritoneum of the processus vaginalis
   is found in front of the hernia as high up as the external ring.
   Therefore, at operation, a peritoneal sac is found in front of the hernial
   sac.
4. *Encysted:* As (1), but a process of peritoneum lies in front of the sac up
   to the external ring.

    Types (3) and (4) are due to a diverticulum of the processus vaginalis
being caught up at the external ring during development.

5. *Interstitial:* In this type a diverticulum of the processus vaginalis has
   been caught between the layers of the developing abdominal wall. The
   sac may be (*Fig*. 115):

    Proparietal or extraparietal (superficial) between the superficial
    fascia and external oblique.
    Interparietal (intramuscular) between the internal and external
    oblique muscles.
    Retroparietal or intraparietal (properitoneal) between the fascia
    transversalis and peritoneum.

    This type of hernia is rare, and is usually found in association with an
    imperfectly descended testis.

The constriction in strangulated inguinal hernia is in 50 per cent of cases at
the internal ring, and in the remaining 50 per cent at the external ring. The
constriction at the internal ring must be divided in a lateral direction because
the inferior epigastric artery is medial to the ring.

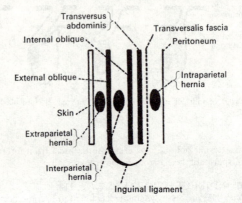

Fig. 115. Varieties of interstitial hernia.

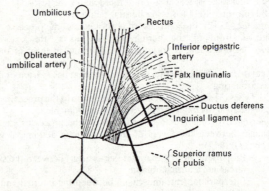

Fig. 116. Posterior surface of lower part of anterior abdominal wall showing the triangle of Hesselbach.

DIRECT INGUINAL HERNIA: Direct inguinal hernia is acquired as a result of weakening of the posterior wall of the inguinal canal. Direct hernia leaves the abdominal cavity medial to the inferior epigastric artery through the triangle of Hesselbach (*Fig.* 116). The triangle is seen on looking at the inner surface of the anterior abdominal wall and its borders are: lateral boundary—inferior epigastric artery; medial boundary—outer border of the rectus; lower boundary—inguinal ligament.

Hesselbach's triangle is divided into medial and lateral halves by the obliterated umbilical artery (lateral umbilical ligament). A direct hernia leaves this triangle through its outer or inner part, and is therefore: (*a*) a lateral direct hernia or (*b*) a medial direct hernia.

Coverings of Direct Hernia:

Lateral direct hernia: The same coverings as the indirect type, except that the covering it receives from the fascia transversalis is not that part of the fascia prolonged from the margins of the internal ring. The inferior epigastric artery is lateral to the hernia opening.

Medial direct hernia: (*a*) External spermatic fascia; (*b*) falx inguinalis or conjoint tendon; (*c*) fascia transversalis.

Direct hernia is generally less oblique in direction than indirect, though this is not always true. In direct hernia the opening in the fascia transversalis lies directly opposite the external ring, and the examining finger passes straight back through the openings and not in an oblique direction as in indirect hernia.

Femoral region

A femoral hernia passes through two orifices: (*a*) the femoral canal, which is the inner compartment of the femoral sheath; (*b*) the fossa ovalis (saphenous opening)—an opening in the fascia lata of the thigh, 4 cm below and 4 cm lateral to the pubic tubercle.

The femoral sheath is a funnel-shaped fascial channel which invests the femoral vessels and passes down behind the inner half of the inguinal ligament. It is formed by two fascial layers (*Fig.* 117). Its anterior wall is formed by the fascia transversalis continued down behind the inguinal ligament in front of the femoral vessels. Its posterior wall is formed by the fascia iliaca passing down behind the vessels.

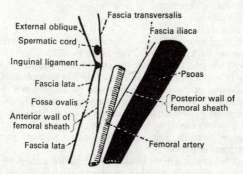

Fig. 117. Longitudinal section of femoral sheath.

Anterior wall: Covered by fascia lata in which is the fossa ovalis.
Posterior Wall: Lies on the psoas and pectineus.
Outer Wall: Straight.
Inner Wall: Oblique and shorter than outer wall.
Compartments: Three, a lateral for the femoral artery, an intermediate for the vein, and a medial called the 'femoral canal'. The femoral nerve lies behind and lateral to the fascia iliaca; it is not included in the sheath (*Fig.* 118).

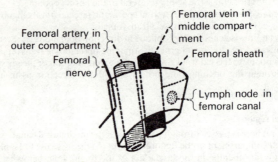

Fig. 118. Compartments of femoral sheath.

FEMORAL CANAL: This is 1·2 cm long and 1·2 cm wide. It lies under cover of the fascia cribrosa, which covers over the saphenous opening. It contains fat and a lymph node belonging to the deep subinguinal group. The femoral ring is the mouth of the canal.

The boundaries of the femoral ring are:
Anterior: Inguinal ligament.
Posterior: Pectineus.
Lateral: Femoral vein.
Medial: Lateral sharp edge of the lacunar ligament. This edge gives a fascial extension backwards for 12 mm along the iliopectineal line (brim of pelvis) where it blends with the periosteum. This fascial extension is called Cooper's ligament. It is now held that aponeurotic fibres of the transversus or the transversalis fascia itself insert into the pectineal ligament 4–8 mm, lateral to the lacunar ligament. Only when the ring is enlarged is it bordered by the lacunar ligament. The surgeon closes up the femoral canal by sewing Cooper's ligament to the inguinal ligament or to the falx inguinalis (conjoint tendon), to prevent the recurrence of hernia.
Abnormal Obturator Artery: Usually the obturator and inferior epigastric vessels each gives a pubic branch which is small, and these anastomose

at the back of the pubis. In 30 per cent of cases the pubic branch of the inferior epigastric is very large, taking the place of the obturator artery, and is known as the abnormal obturator artery. It passes down in relation to the femoral ring to reach the obturator foramen (*Fig.* 119).

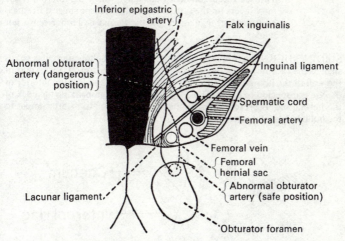

Fig. 119. Posterior surface of lower part of anterior abdominal wall showing the course of the abnormal obturator artery.

In its descent it may stick to the side of the femoral vein lateral to the femoral ring (the safe position). In 10 per cent of persons with an abnormal artery, the vessel passes down along the edge of the lacunar ligament, which is the medial boundary of the femoral ring (the dangerous position). In strangulated femoral hernia the constricting agent is sometimes the outer edge of the lacunar ligament, and it must be divided to relieve the pressure. It is necessary, therefore, to exercise great care in dealing with this ligament, as serious haemorrhage follows division of the vessel.

Coverings of Femoral Hernia: A hernia passing down the femoral canal emerges through the saphenous opening. It has, therefore, as covering: (*a*) fat—forming the femoral septum; (*b*) anterior wall of femoral sheath; (*c*) fascia cribrosa.

Having become subcutaneous, the hernia, if it continues to enlarge, often takes a recurrent course across the inguinal ligament, following the line of the superficial inferior epigastric vessels.

The neck of the femoral hernial sac is narrow which is important because it results in:

1. A cough impulse often being absent on palpation over the hernial sac.
2. Strangulation of bowel in the hernial sac occurs commonly.
3. The sac often contains fluid only, which together with the fatty layers on the outside of the hernial sac suggest irreducibility and strangulation but the hernia is neither tense nor tender.

SLIDING HERNIA: In this condition (*Fig.* 120), a hollow muscular viscus such as the caecum or bladder, which is partly extraperitoneal, forms part of the wall of the hernial sac. These structures are at risk unless the interior of the sac is inspected to exclude this possibility prior to transfixing the neck of the hernial sac. If present the sac must be closed distal to its attachment to the hollow muscular viscus.

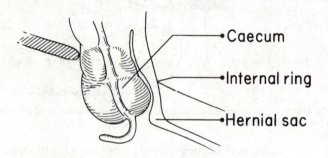

Fig. 120. Sliding hernia: the caecum forms part of the hernial sac.

GROIN HERNIA REPAIR

Inguinal hernia

An incision one finger-breadth above the inner half of the inguinal ligament is the classic incision for dealing with an inguinal hernia (*Fig.* 121). In infants a skin crease incision is used. The incision divides the skin and two layers of superficial fascia (Camper and Scarpa). It exposes the external oblique aponeurosis, the external abdominal ring, and the cord at the inner end of the inguinal ligament. The external oblique aponeurosis is cut in the line of its fibres and the cord is exposed lying in the inguinal canal.

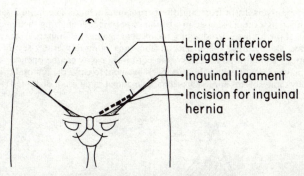

Fig. 121. Incision for an inguinal hernia.

In the case of an indirect hernia, the sac is amputated at its junction with the parietal peritoneum, as is indicated by the presence of extraperitoneal fat (herniotomy). If considered necessary the internal ring is narrowed and the posterior wall of the canal is strengthened by suturing local structures (herniorrhaphy) or by the introduction of extraneous material (hernioplasty). The external oblique is sutured to restore the normal position.

In the case of a direct hernia, the sac may have a very wide neck and then simple inversion may be preferable. Repair of the posterior wall of the canal is always necessary.

Femoral hernia

LOTHEISSEN OPERATION: The same incision as for inguinal hernia repair is widely used in the Lotheissen operation for the cure of femoral hernia. The steps of the operation are the same as those for inguinal hernia up to the exposure of the cord in the canal. The cord or round ligament is then drawn aside to expose the posterior wall of the canal. This fascia is divided, exposing the femoral canal lying behind the inguinal ligament. The sac of the femoral hernia is found in this canal. The major drawback of this approach is that it disrupts the inguinal canal mechanism.

McEVEDY OPERATION: A vertical incision is made from just over the femoral hernia to a point about 8 cm above the inguinal ligament. The medial skin flap is elevated and the anterior rectus sheath exposed. In this situation the aponeuroses of the flat muscles of the abdomen are all anterior to the rectus. The sheath is incised 1 cm medial to the lower fourth of the linea semilunaris, and the rectus retracted inwards, which exposes the fascia transversalis. When this is incised the dissection is carried down between the fascia transversalis in front and the peritoneum behind. The hernial sac is identified as a funnel-shaped protrusion of peritoneum entering the femoral canal. If the hernia is irreducible, the lacunar ligament (Gimbernat) may be divided under direct vision and an abnormal obturator artery secured if required. Should it be necessary, the peritoneal cavity can be opened. The inguinal ligament is sutured to Cooper's ligament to close the femoral canal. An advantage of this approach is that the inguinal canal is not disrupted (*Fig.* 122).

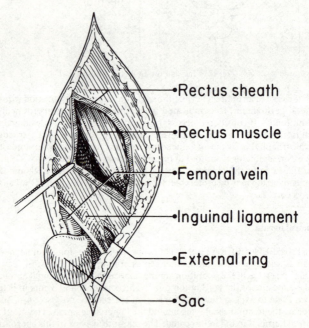

Fig. 122. The McEvedy approach for femoral hernia.

INFRA-INGUINAL APPROACH: This is also referred to as the low or crural approach. The skin incision is made over the hernia and about 2 cm below and parallel to the inguinal ligament. The subcutaneous fat is easily separated from the thick extraperitoneal coverings of the sac. Once the neck of the sac has been closed and the sac excised, the inguinal ligament is sutured to the pectineal ligament on the superior ramus of the pubis. The femoral vein must not be compromised by placing a suture too far laterally as this may precipitate a thrombosis of the femoral vein. If strangulation of bowel is present, the occasional surgeon should resect the bowel through a lower paramedian incision with which he is more familiar.

HYDROCELE

In this condition there is a collection of fluid in some part of the processus vaginalis. There are various types of hydrocele (*Fig.* 123):

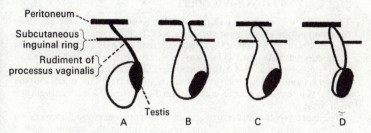

Peritoneum

Subcutaneous }
inguinal ring }

Rudiment of }
processus vaginalis }

Testis

A   B   C   D

Fig. 123. A, Vaginal hydrocele; B, congenital hydrocele; C, infantile hydrocele; D, hydrocele of cord.

1. VAGINAL: This is a collection of fluid in the tunica vaginalis testis. It is not due to any fault of development. It is always necessary in this type to determine whether it is of the common idiopathic (or primary) variety, or whether it is secondary to some disease of the testis or epididymis.

2. CONGENITAL: This is also known as intermittent hydrocele. It is in fact a congenital hernial sac but with a tiny communication between the processus vaginalis and the peritoneal cavity, which permits the escape of fluid into the abdominal cavity, but not of the entrance of intestine into the sac. It lessens in size on lying down. It may be confused with a congenital hernia. The latter, however, reduces much more readily than the hydrocele and its reduction may be associated with a gurgle.

3. INFANTILE: The processus vaginalis is occluded at the internal abdominal ring only, and the hydrocele therefore extends into the canal.

4. HYDROCELE OF THE CORD: The funicular process fails to shrink into a fibrous cord, so that a tubular cavity results, shut off from peritoneum above and tunica vaginalis below. It becomes distended with fluid, forming one or more swellings separate from the testis.

SPERMATOCELE

This is a cystic enlargement occurring behind the testicle in close relationship with the epididymis. Since it is connected with the sperm-conducting apparatus it contains a milky fluid. When this connection is not present the fluid is crystal clear and it is then more appropriately called a cyst of the epididymis. Clinically, a spermatocele can be felt apart from the testis while a hydrocele envelops the testis.

THE ANATOMY OF A VARICOCELE

The testicular veins on each side arise in the testis and epididymis and form the pampiniform plexus in the spermatic cord. It consists of from 8 to 10 veins most of which lie in front of the ductus deferens and may communicate with the ductus deferens veins. The plexus ends near the deep inguinal ring in two main trunks which ascend with the corresponding testicular artery. The two veins soon unite to form a single vein which, on the right side, opens into the inferior vena cava at an acute angle and, on the left, into the left renal vein at a right-angle.

There are valves in the testicular veins which prevent blood flowing down the veins and so protect the unsupported veins in the scrotum against increased intra-abdominal pressure. A varicocele is a dilatation of the veins of the pampiniform plexus.

Varicoceles are usually considered to result from absence of competent valves in the proximal portion of the testicular vein as demonstrated on venography. Varicoceles are more common on the left side. This has been attributed to:
1. The left testicular vein enters the renal vein at a right-angle.
2. The left testicular vein is overlaid by the descending colon.
3. A renal carcinoma extending along the left renal vein may occlude the testicular vein.
4. The left renal vein passes anterior to the aorta and posterior to the superior mesenteric artery. The angle between these two arteries, which form the 'nutcracker', may be too narrow and causes compression of the left renal vein as it passes between them.
5. The left common iliac vein is crossed by the right common iliac artery and the increased pressure in the iliac vein is transmitted to the pampiniform plexus through the ductus deferens veins which drain into the internal iliac vein.

OPERATION FOR VARICOCELE: The veins draining the pampiniform plexus may be ligated in the inguinal canal near the internal ring. Inadvertent damage to the testicular artery at this point may, however, result in testicular atrophy. An alternative approach is a supra-inguinal incision and an extraperitoneal approach to the testicular vein which is then ligated as high as possible. Patients in whom a varicocele persists or recurs may require ligation of the veins of the ductus deferens to overcome the effects described in (5) above.

A varicocele is the commonest correctable cause of male infertility. The low sperm count found in association with a varicocele may be due to increased scrotal temperature resulting from the increased vascularity of the region.

Chapter 11

THE CHEST WALL, LUNGS AND MEDIASTINUM

THE CHEST WALL

Parts of the sternum can be used to determine with accuracy the situation of deeper structures. The sternal notch corresponds to the lower border of the 2nd thoracic vertebra. In the child, the top of the aortic arch may reach the upper border of the manubrium, whereas, in the adult, it is above the level of the centre of the bone.

The angle of Louis, a slight transverse prominence formed by the junction of the manubrium with the body of the sternum, is an important landmark. Here the 2nd costal cartilage articulates with both of these bones. Although the 1st rib is mainly concealed by the calvicle, the 1st costal cartilage can be palpated below it. The 2nd rib is the one most easily identified in counting the ribs. The angle of Louis corresponds to:

The lower border of the 4th thoracic vertebra.

The bifurcation of the trachea (this is one vertebra higher in the infant).

The site where the pleural sacs meet.

The arch of the aorta begins its ascent at this level and ends its descent at the same level posteriorly as it arches back. The highest point of the arch reaches the midpoint of the manubrium in the adult.

This vital anatomical level is illustrated in the CT scan-cut in *Fig*. 124.

The intercostal spaces are widest between the inner ends of the 2nd and 3rd costal cartilages. They become narrower between the lower ones. The internal mammary vessels are best ligated in the 2nd or 3rd space where they are 1 cm from the side of the sternum. The vessels lie on the pleura above the 3rd costal cartilage. Below this level they are separated from it by slips of the transversus thoracis muscle. The 3rd intercostal space is thus the site of choice for internal mammary ligation. The course of this artery should be remembered when evaluating penetrating wounds of the thorax. It gives two anterior branches to each of the upper five spaces, and perforating branches pass through the great pectoral muscle, supplying it and the breast. Those emerging from the 2nd, 3rd and 4th spaces are of considerable size.

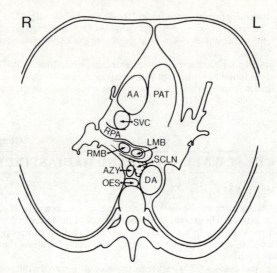

Fig. 124. Diagram of CT scan-cut: AA, ascending aorta; AZY, azygos vein; DA, descending aorta; PAT, pulmonary artery trunk; LMB, left main bronchus; RMB, right main bronchus; OES, oesophagus; RPA, right pulmonary artery; SVC, superior vena cava; SCLN, subcarinal lymph nodes.

The ribs and costal cartilages, by virtue of their attachments to the sternum and vertebrae, form a series of hoops. Conditions which affect one part of the circle alter the shape of the rest. Any prominence or depression of the skeletal thorax must be considered in relation to the thoracic cage as a whole. A notable example is the prominence sometimes seen at the costochondral junction and often mistaken for a tumour; it is in fact a buckling due to unequal rib growth.

THE LUNGS AND BRONCHIAL TREE

Fissures

Each lung is divided into lobes by the oblique or the horizontal fissure. The surface marking begins at the 6th costochondral junction and follows the line of the 6th rib to meet the tip of the 3rd thoracic spinous process. The upper end of the fissure is somewhat higher on the left than on the right and generally lower than usually stated in anatomy texts, being at the 5th rib or interspace or even the 6th rib.

The horizontal fissure occurs on the right side only. It is marked out by a line extending from the 4th costal cartilage to strike the oblique fissure in the midaxillary line at the level of the 5th rib. This fissure is frequently absent or incomplete.

Segments of the lungs

The significance of the segmental structure of the lungs is apparent when it is realized that:

1. The segmental architecture of the lungs is fairly uniform.
2. Infections and neoplastic processes are often localized to one or more adjacent segments.
3. Conservation of lung tissue is thus often possible in removal of diseased areas.

Each lung consists of 10 segments which, although they appear to be in continuity, are separate entities (*Fig.* 125). The parenchymal substance of adjacent segments is distinct. They fill with air proximodistally like the opening of a fan. Each has its own bronchus, artery and veins. There is little anastomosis between adjacent segments and thus individual segments can be excised with little loss of blood or air leakage if strict adherence to intersegmental planes is practised.

The lung segments have a constant disposition and relationship to the overlying ribs. Each extends to the pleural surface and, but for the fact that the lingular bronchus comes from the left upper lobe bronchus, the arrangements on the two sides would be similar. On both sides the superior segment of the lower lobe is often fused with the upper lobe. The apparent complexity of the segmental anatomy is simplified in the diagram (*Fig.* 125).

Each bronchopulmonary segment is a unit in the architecture of the lung. Its parenchyma is distinct from that of its neighbours. It is supplied by one or more branches of the pulmonary artery and is drained by its own veins. In general the bronchus and its main branches to the segments are central in position. The arteries tend to occupy a position nearer the centre of the segments than the veins, which tend to lie mainly along the intersegmental planes and are thus useful guides in delineating the intersegmental divisions.

Lung abscess commonly follows aspiration. The site of the abscess or suppurative pneumonitis is dependent on posture and bronchial anatomy. The right lung is more commonly affected than the left.

Right lung

UPPER LOBE: This lobe comprises three segments: apical, anterior and posterior. The dome of the lung is formed by the apical segment which has

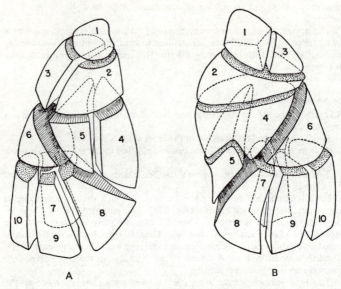

Fig. 125. A, The segments of the right lung. Upper lobe: 1, apical; 2, anterior; 3, posterior. Middle lobe: 4, medial; 5, lateral. Lower lobe: 6, superior; 7, medial basal; 8, anterior basal; 9, lateral basal; 10, posterior basal. B, The segments of the left lung. Upper lobe: 1, apical; 2, anterior; 3, posterior; 4, superficial lingular; 5, inferior lingular. Lower lobe: 6, superior; 7, medial basal; 8, anterior basal; 9, lateral basal; 10, posterior basal. (By courtesy of Sweet—modified by Thomas.)

anterior, posterior, medial and lateral surfaces. The anterior segment has anterior and medial surfaces, while the posterior segment presents laterally and posteriorly. The inferior surfaces of the anterior and posterior segments form the base of the upper lobe. The inferior aspect of the anterior segment is separated from the middle lobe by the horizontal fissure, whereas the posterior part of the longitudinal fissure intervenes between the posterior segment of the upper and the superior segments of the lower lobe. The posterior segment of the right upper lobe is frequently the primary site of tuberculosis, septic pneumonitis or aspiration abscesses. Lesions in the anterior segment of the upper lobe tend to be cancerous.

MIDDLE LOBE: This lobe is vertically demarcated into the lateral segment which is anterolateral and the medial segment which is anteromedial. The middle lobe does not reach the chest wall behind. Its anterior surface is largest, while triangular surfaces lie against the 4th and 5th ribs laterally and the pericardium medially.

The inferior surface of the medial lobe lies on the diaphragm. The middle lobe bronchus is long and lies in the lymphatic pathway from the right lower lobe. It is surrounded by lymph nodes and is vulnerable to external compression by node enlargement. Thus bronchiectasis, tuberculosis or viral conditions may cause middle-lobe collapse.

Lymph nodes are present in the acute angles formed by the branching of the bronchi. The presence of calcified nodes, so often seen near the lung hilum on X-ray plates, is a consequence of severe lymphadenitis.

LOWER LOBE: This lobe, the largest of the three, is made up of superior and inferior segments. The superior segment (often called apical) is related by its posterior surface to the 4th and 8th ribs. The medial and lateral aspects extend around to the fissure and come into contact with the posterior segment of the upper lobe. This segment, therefore, has one surface abutting on the mediastinum and another against the lateral chest wall. It is prone to aspiration and its sequelae.

The inferior portion of the lower lobe comprises four basal segments and lies on the diaphragm. The posterior segment contributes to the mediastinal surface of the lobe, the lateral segment is also partially posterior, and the anterior segment is also lateral. The medial aspect (cardiac) is entirely medial and diaphragmatic.

AZYGOS LOBES: These are accessory lobes which may appear in any three situations:
1. The lobe of the azygos vein (due to abnormality of the azygos vein).
2. The upper azygos lobe, not associated with abnormality of the azygos vein.
3. The lower azygos lobe.

The second and third types are of no practical importance; they are accessory lobules of lung tissue and are rarely found.

The Lobe of the Azygos Vein: This is important because it may cause unusual appearances on chest X-rays and it may be the site of disease in the lung.

Part of the upper, inner surface of the right lung is cut off from the rest by a double pleural septum, the meso-azygos, which contains at its apex the upper part of the azygos vein (*Fig.* 126). The meso-azygos therefore divides the pleural cavity into an upper compartment, containing the accessory lobe, and a lower one for the rest of the lung. The lobe may vary in size. The fissure formed by the pleural septum cuts the lung at any level from an oblique plane, cutting the outer surface of the lung 5 cm below the apex, to a vertical plane cutting off a small tongue-shaped lobe from the mediastinal surface.

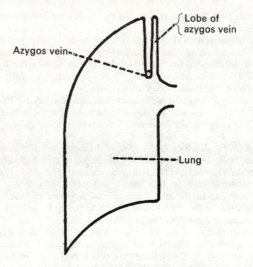

Fig. 126. The lobe of the azygos vein.

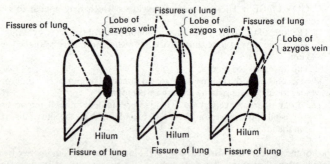

Fig. 127. Various forms which lobe of azygos vein may assume. Mediastinal surface of lung is depicted.

The fissure containing the meso-azygos and the vein extends almost to the root of the lung, resembling a normal lung fissure (*Fig.* 127). It is visible on radiography as a line coursing from the apex of the lung towards the hilum. The line itself is the meso-azygos, and the dense shadow at its end is the azygos vein.

Left lung

UPPER LOBE: This lobe consists of five segments. The lower two comprise the superior and inferior lingular segments. The lower part of the inferior lingular segment extends to lie on the diaphragm adjacent to the pericardium. The upper lobe division of this lobe is arranged very much as on the right, having anterior, apical and posterior segments. The apical and posterior segments often have a single bronchus which subdivides causing them to be described as a single apicoposterior segment. As each receives an independent bronchus, artery and vein they are fittingly described separately.

LOWER LOBE: The left lower lobe is smaller than the right one. It comprises five segments with an arrangement similar to that on the right. Thus there are one superior and four basal segments.

Bronchial tree

RIGHT LUNG: The right main bronchus is more vertical, wider and shorter than the left. The bronchus to the upper lobe passes laterally and slightly upwards for just over 1 cm and then branches rapidly into three divisions: apical, anterior and posterior.

On the front of the main bronchus, just beyond the origin of the upper lobe branches, there is a groove in which the pulmonary artery lies. Just distal to this the middle lobe bronchus arises from the anterolateral aspect and divides into the medial and lateral segments. Distal to the origin of the middle lobe bronchus, all bronchi are destined for the segments of the lower lobe. The bronchus to its superior segment comes off posteriorly and runs horizontally backwards. The relationship of the origin of this bronchus to that of the middle lobe is surgically important. Though it usually comes off distal to the middle lobe bronchus, it may arise exactly opposite or even proximally. The implications of this close anatomical contiguity between middle and lower lobes is that removal of the middle lobe is often necessary when surgery for inflammatory or neoplastic disease of the lower lobe is undertaken.

LEFT LUNG: The left main bronchus is longer than the right and less vertical. About 5 cm from the trachea it divides into the left upper-lobe stem bronchus and a branch to the lower lobe. After this bifurcation the upper stem bronchus curves laterally. The bronchus to the lingular segment occurs as a bifurcation of this tube a little more than 1 cm from its origin; it divides into superior and inferior segmental bronchi. The stem bronchus to the upper lobe, having divided to form the lingular bronchus, soon subdivides into one branch to the anterior segment and another to the apical and posterior segments which again subdivides into a bronchial division for each segment.

The left lower lobe first gives off the bronchus to the superior segment which comes from its posterior aspect. There are usually three bronchi to the basal segments: one for the posterior, one for the lateral and one that subdivides into anterior and medial basal segmental bronchi. This description of the bronchial tree is the common one but anomalies are frequent (*Fig.* 128).

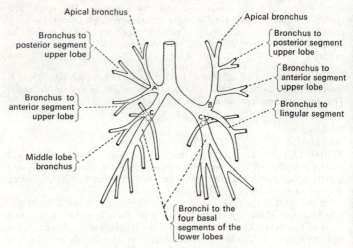

Fig. 128. The anatomy of the bronchial tree. A, Right upper lobe stem of bronchus, B, left upper lobe stem of bronchus; C, the dotted circle shows the origin of the bronchus to the superior segment of the lower lobe. It arises from the posterior aspect of the stem bronchus. (Redrawn from Shanks and Kerley.)

A supernumerary bronchus is apparent on about 30 per cent of radiographs. It arises just distal to the origin of the superior segmental bronchus to the lower lobe. It may occur in either lung and is sometimes called the subsuperior bronchus. It assumes importance in the interpretation of bronchograms.

PULMONARY VESSELS

Right pulmonary artery

This artery runs transversely for a short distance in front of the right main bronchus and reaches the anterior aspect of the upper lobe bronchus where it supplies its first branch to the upper lobe. This branch soon divides into an apical and an anterior vessel. The main pulmonary artery continues downwards, lying in a groove on the anterior surface of the bronchus below its upper-lobe branch. In this situation, the artery gives off the posterior segmental branch to the upper lobe. The vessel can be found only by dissection in the depths of the fissure as it enters the lobe beneath the fissure.

The middle lobe is supplied as a rule by two branches of the pulmonary artery which arise at the base of the confluence of the fissures distal to the posterior segmental branch to the upper lobe. They enter the middle lobe closely related to the bronchus. The pulmonary artery ends by supplying the lower lobe segments. The vessel to the superior segment arises by first passing downwards and backwards. A spray of vessels then supplies the remaining four basal segments.

Left pulmonary artery

The main trunk is longer than on the right. The artery curves upwards and over the main bronchus then gives off the first branch which supplies the apical and posterior segments. The vessel then arches behind the upper lobe bronchus giving off branches to the upper three segments of the lobe. In the interlobar fissure the main vessel gives off a single lingular artery which divides into a vessel to each segment of the lingula. There may, however, be only one vessel to the lingula. The left lower-lobe arteries come from the interlobar part of the main vessel, much as on the right. They come off more distally, arising close to the bronchi of their segments of supply (*Fig.* 129).

Venous system

This is similar on the two sides. The veins draining the segments converge to form large trunks and end as the superior and inferior pulmonary veins at the hilum of the lung. The superior pulmonary vein receives the apical, posterior and anterior segmental veins and two or more veins from the middle lobe. The inferior pulmonary vein receives the veins from the lower lobe segments. At the hilum of the lung the veins are the most anterior structures.

Bronchial vessels

The bronchial arteries are small vessels which supply nutrition to the lungs. There is usually one main artery to each lung. They arise from the aorta just beyond the origin of the left subclavian or they may come from one of the upper aortic intercostals. One or more smaller arteries may arise from the thoracic aorta.

Bronchopulmonary circulation

The bronchial and pulmonary circulations intercommunicate freely on both the arterial and venous sides. These are not, therefore, closed circuits as was

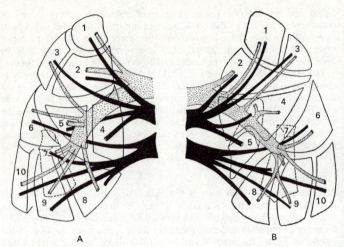

Fig. 129. Diagrams of the blood supply to (A), the right lung, (B), the left lung; arteries, stippled; veins, black. (By courtesy of Richard Sweet.) See *Fig.* 125 for segment names.

at one time believed. The bronchial circulation is unique in that the artery arises from the systemic circulation, whereas its venous component enters the pulmonary system. It thus constitutes an AV shunt.

Numerous anastomoses between the bronchial and pulmonary arterial systems are of significance in inflammatory lung disease. Early in the course of inflammatory disease thrombosis of the bronchial artery branches occurs. Progressive enlargement of the bronchial arterial system follows. Massive haemoptysis is always from enlarged bronchial vessels. The recent development of bronchial artery embolization techniques to control catastrophic tracheobronchial haemorrhage demands a thorough knowledge of the bronchial arterial supply to each lung and its variations. It is of moment that the intercostal bronchial–vascular interplay supplies reticular branches to the midthoracic section of the spinal cord. Paraplegia has occurred following embolization of important spinal branches from the bronchial system.

LYMPH NODES OF THE THORAX

These fall into two main groups: parietal and visceral.

Parietal nodes

These consists of: (*a*) anterior, or internal mammary nodes; (*b*) posterior, or posterior mediastinal nodes; (c) lateral, or intercostal nodes; (d) inferior, or diaphragmatic nodes.

INTERNAL MAMMARY NODES: They lie along the internal mammary vessels. Two nodes are found in each of the first two intercostal spaces; they are not found lower than the 3rd space. They receive lymph from the skin over the breast, the deep structures forming the abdominal wall above the level of the umbilicus, and the upper surface of the liver on the right. Their lymph passes by a single trunk on each side into the junction of the subclavian and jugular veins.

POSTERIOR MEDIASTINAL NODES: They lie behind the pericardium in relation to the oesophagus and aorta. They drain: (a) the oesophagus; (b) the diaphragm; (c) the upper surface of the liver. Their lymph enters the thoracic duct.

LATERAL OR INTERCOSTAL NODES: They lie in front of the rib necks in the posterior ends of the intercostal spaces. They drain the deep structures forming the side and back of the chest. The lymph from the lower four or five spaces drains into the thoracic duct on the left and into the main lymph duct on the right.

DIAPHRAGMATIC NODES: They are arranged in four groups: anterior, posterior, right lateral, and left lateral. They all rest on the upper surface of the diaphragm.

Visceral nodes

These consist of: (1) superior mediastinal nodes and (2) peritracheobronchial nodes.

1. SUPERIOR MEDIASTINAL NODES: They lie in front of the trachea behind the aortic arch. They drain: (a) the trachea and oesophagus; (b) the heart. A single efferent from these nodes unites with the efferent from the peritracheobronchial nodes to form the bronchomediastinal trunk.

2. PERITRACHEOBRONCHIAL NODES: This group (*Fig.* 130) comprises many nodes among which are some of the largest in the body. It is made up of: (a) pretracheobronchial nodes which lie in front and lateral to the trachea and bronchi; (b) intertracheobronchial (subcarinal) nodes which lie between the two main bronchi; (c) interbronchial nodes which lie between the divisions of each bronchus at the hilum of and actually in the substance of the lung. These nodes drain the lungs and bronchi. A single efferent joins the efferent of the superior mediastinal group to form the bronchomediastinal trunk. The trunk usually opens both on the right and left into the junction of

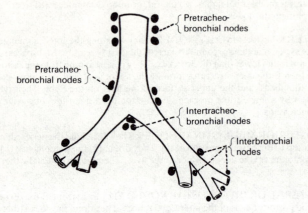

Fig. 130. The peritracheobronchial nodes.

the subclavian and internal jugular veins. It may join the right lymph duct on the right or the thoracic duct on the left.

Lymphatic drainage of the lungs

Lymph converging on the hila of the lungs is not drained in a strictly lobar manner. From the right lung, lymph passes directly or indirectly to node groups related to the bifurcation of the trachea, i.e. the intertracheobronchial and pretracheobronchial nodes.

On the left there are three regions of lymph drainage. The superior part of the upper lobe drains to the left pretracheobronchial nodes. Lymph from the lower part of the upper lobe and upper part of the lower lobe drains to the same node group, but also to the subcarinal nodes, passing through them to the right group of pretracheobronchial nodes. The remaining part of the lower lobe drains to the nodes at the tracheal bifurcation and thence to the right pretracheobronchial nodes. Some lymph from the nodes in relation to the sides of the trachea passes to the inferior deep cervical nodes and so to the jugular lymph trunk.

The tracheobronchial nodes give rise on each side to a lymph trunk which receives the efferent vessel draining the superior mediastinal group, the bronchomediastinal trunk. Usually it enters the related jugular–subclavian junction; it may, however, enter the right lymph duct or the thoracic duct according to the side.

PROCEDURES USED TO INVESTIGATE THORACIC DISEASE

Prescalene node biopsy

The most accessible nodes are those of the inferior deep cervical group lying lateral to the internal jugular vein. These nodes can be felt only in advanced disease. They may be biopsied to determine the operability of the bronchogenic carcinoma or to determine the aetiology of the more obscure pulmonary diseases such as sarcoidosis. The procedure is usually carried out in the absence of lymphadenopathy. The finding of cancer in a deep cervical lymph node indicates an inoperable bronchogenic tumour. Usually the ipsilateral scalene fat pad and contained node are removed. Care should be taken to avoid injury to the phrenic nerve which lies on the scalenus anterior muscle. It is apparent from the lymphatic drainage of the lower two-thirds of the left lung field that scalene-node biopsy would need to be bilateral.

Cervical mediastinoscopy

This procedure is carried out through a tracheostomy type incision above the suprasternal notch. The pretracheal fascia is opened and, by blunt finger dissection, a plane is carried down along the trachea deep into the thorax. A mediastinoscope introduced along this plane can visualize and biopsy paratracheal nodes, the superior tracheobronchial nodes and the inferior tracheobronchial (carinal) group. This valuable procedure allows staging of the lymphatic spread of lung cancer and has spared many patients from fruitless exploratory thoracotomy.

Anterior mediastinotomy

The drainage of upper lobes to the anterior mediastinal lymph node groups has been responsible for this procedure. The right or left second costal cartilage is removed, the internal mammary lymph nodes of the second space are biopsied *en passant*, and the pleura is stripped with a swab off the mediastinal structures. This allows biopsy of the anterior mediastinal lymph node chains without formal thoracotomy. If upper-lobe cancer has spread to these nodes it is inoperable. The mediastinal structures and hilum can likewise be assessed through this approach.

SURGICAL ACCESS TO THE THORAX

Three operative approaches are in common use: median sternotomy, posterolateral thoracotomy and thoraco-abdominal transthoracic approach.

Median sternotomy

The skin incision is from the sternal notch to the xiphisternum. The suprasternal tissues and the periosteum of the sternum are divided in the midline with a diathermy. The xiphoid process is excised and a finger is inserted substernally, pushing away the pleural and pericardial sacs. Superiorly, a right-angled instrument is inserted close to the sternum around the notch and opened, allowing the insertion of the digit behind the sternal notch. The sternum is lifted by a hooked retractor inserted at its notch above and at the xiphoid stump below and the lungs are deflated, while the sternum is divided in the midline with a saw. This gives surgical access to the thymus, the heart and great vessels, and to both pleural sacs.

Posterolateral thoracotomy

A skin incision commencing 5 cm below the nipple is made in a curving motion posterosuperiorly, skirting the inferior angle of the scapula by at least 2 cm. The large muscles of the chest wall are encountered: the first is the latissimus dorsi, which is divided from medial to lateral and the second is the serratus anterior, which is detached from its costal origins.

Wide access is obtained by removing a rib, usually the 6th, and entrance to the pleural space gained through the rib bed. Rib removal is unnecessary in young to middle-aged persons as a fair degree of mobility of the ribs is present. In such cases the intercostal muscles can be detached with a diathermy along the upper border of the rib until the pleura is reached. This avascular plane allows safe access. The pleura is opened and a rib spreader inserted. The rib spreader is opened by degrees and some forward stripping of the intercostal muscle attachment of the rib can be completed by the use of a notched periosteal elevator pushed along the upper border of the rib. A similar manoeuvre can be repeated posteriorly.

This entrance to the pleural space puts one exactly on the fissures of the lungs, in a central position for surgery of any of the lobes and segments, or for pneumonectomy on either side.

Thoraco-abdominal incision

The thoracotomy part of the thoraco-abdominal incision is carried out as described above, but entrance into the pleural space is effected above or through the bed of the 8th rib. The aortic hiatus and the lower oesophagus can be well visualized and mobilized after division of the mediastinal pleura overlying them. If surgery has been undertaken for malignant disease of the oesophagogastric junction, operability can be assessed from above by detaching the diaphragm at its periphery and slipping a hand intra-abdominally, allowing bimanual assessment of the tumour.

Once operability has been determined, the definitive procedure can be carried out either through the diaphragmatic incision or by extension of the thoracotomy incision across the costal margin towards the umbilicus. The rectus muscle is retracted medially, the peritoneum and lateral flat muscles are divided in the line of the fibres of the external oblique and the diaphragm is opened. The costal cartilage, which was divided during the extension of the thoracotomy towards the abdomen, is generally excised.

Incision of the diaphragm should take into account the distribution of the major branches of the phrenic nerve. Damage to the nerve will interfere with diaphragmatic function postoperatively. Circumferential diaphragmatic detachment totally avoids the phrenic innervation and, once access to the undersurface of the diaphragm has been achieved, the major subdivisions of the phrenic nerve and accompanying blood vessels can be visualized and avoided (*Fig.* 131).

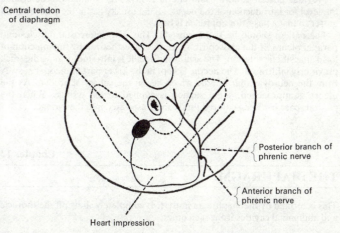

Central tendon of diaphragm

Posterior branch of phrenic nerve

Anterior branch of phrenic nerve

Heart impression

Fig. 131. The usual type of distribution of the left phrenic nerve. Any extensive division of the diaphragm would damage the nerve. (After Perera and Edwards in the *Lancet*.)

The diaphragm is repaired with figure-of-eight, non-absorbable stitches. The abdomen is closed and a single intercostal drain is laid across the base of the appropriate pleural space. The thoracotomy is closed following the insertion of two or three pericostal sutures. The pericostal suture should be placed through a hole in the inferior rib to avoid compression of the intercostal neurovascular bundle when it is tightened.

INTERCOSTAL NERVE BLOCK

This is a very effective way of relieving the pain caused by a fractured rib.

Apart from blocking the intercostal nerve of the fractured rib, two intercostal nerves above and below the fractured rib should also be blocked, because of an overlap of the segmental nerve supply. The needle is advanced until a rib is struck, withdrawn a little, then slid under the inferior margin of the rib an additional 0·5–1 cm. Aspiration is attempted and if no blood is aspirated, 1–5 ml of local anaesthetic solution is injected.

ASPIRATION OF THE CHEST

Fluid in the pleural cavity may be aspirated for diagnostic and/or therapeutic purposes. A diagnostic biopsy of the parietal pleura may be performed at the time of aspiration.

Previous postero-anterior and lateral X-rays are examined to determine the level for introduction of the needle. Fluid usually lies in the paravertebral gutter so that a posterior approach is best.

The patient should be sitting upright. The skin, intercostal muscles and parietal pleura of the chosen rib space are anaesthetized by the injection of local anaesthetic solution. The aspirating needle is introduced along the track previously infiltrated. The needle is kept in the lower part of the space, away from the neurovascular bundle which lies in the subcostal groove. As the pleura is approached, slight suction is applied to the syringe. When the pleural space has been entered fluid can be aspirated into the syringe.

Chapter 12

THE DIAPHRAGM

This is formed by the diaphragm muscle. It completely shuts off the thoracic and abdominal cavities from each other.

DEVELOPMENT OF THE DIAPHRAGM

The diaphragm, pericardium, and heart are formed in the neck and obtain their innervation there (C3, 4, 5). They migrate to their ultimate destinations carrying their nerve supply with them. The diaphragm develops from four structures (*see Fig.* 132).

The septum transversum

The septum transversum is composed of mesoderm which forms the central tendon of the diaphragm. The septum transversum grows from the ventral body wall, and separates the pleuropericardial cavities from the peritoneal

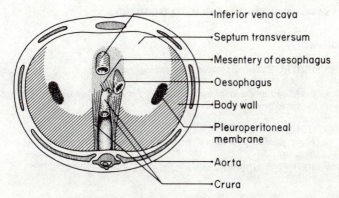

Inferior vena cava

Septum transversum

Mesentery of oesophagus

Oesophagus

Body wall

Pleuroperitoneal membrane

Aorta

Crura

Fig. 132. The development of the diaphragm.

cavity. Dorsally it fuses with the mesenchyme ventral to the oesophagus and the pleuroperitoneal membranes.

The pleuroperitoneal membranes

Pleuroperitoneal membranes are partitions separating the pleural from the peritoneal cavities and they fuse with the dorsal mesentery of the oesophagus and with the septum transversum. Only small areas in the fully developed diaphragm are derived from this precursor.

The dorsal mesentery

Dorsal mesentery of the oesophagus constitutes the median portion of the diaphragm. The crura of the diaphragm develop from muscle fibres which grow into the dorsal mesentery of the oesophagus; because they form an arch which overlies the aorta, the crura are sometimes referred to as the aortic component of the diaphragm.

The body wall

The lungs and pleural cavities enlarge and burrow into the lateral body wall which is split into two layers: an outer layer which will form part of the definitive body wall, and an inner layer that contributes to the peripheral portions of the diaphragm.

With fusion of the component parts of the diaphragm, the mesenchyme of the septum transversum extends into these areas and forms myoblasts that differentiate into the muscle of the diaphragm.

ANATOMY OF THE DIAPHRAGMATIC MUSCLE

Origin

ANTERIOR: By two slips from the xiphoid process.

LATERAL: From the inner surface of the lower six cartilages, interdigitating with the transversus abdominis.

POSTERIOR:
1. From medial and lateral lumbocostal arches and median arcuate ligament.
2. By two crura from the bodies of the upper three lumbar vertebrae.

Insertion

The fibres converge on a central tendon shaped like a trefoil leaf.

Nerve supply of the diaphragm
1. The phrenic nerve is the motor nerve to the diaphragm and is also sensory to the central region. This explains referred pain from the diaphragm to the shoulder.
2. The peripheral region of the diaphragm which develops from the body wall receives sensory nerves from the lower six or seven intercostal nerves.

The distribution of the phrenic nerve on the diaphragm is best seen on the inferior surface (*Fig.* 131, Chapter 11).

Action

It is the chief (involuntary) muscle of respiration but can also be used voluntarily to increase pressure in the abdomen.

Relations

UPPER SURFACE: Pleura and lung on each side, and pericardium and heart between these.

CIRCUMFERENTIALLY: Costal cartilages, ribs and internal intercostal muscles, quadratus lumborum and psoas muscles.

LOWER SURFACE: Liver and stomach, spleen and kidney. The adrenals, the kidneys, and the pancreas lie on the crura. Much of the superior surface of the muscle is covered by pleura, and most of the inferior surface by peritoneum. A part of the posterior surface of the kidneys and the bare area of the liver are in direct contact with the muscle, no serous membrane intervening. Disease of the kidney or liver may spread through to the chest at these unprotected areas.

Openings in the diaphragm

The three large openings (*Fig.* 133) in the diaphragm are shown in *Table* 2.

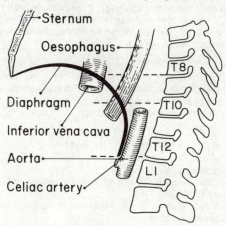

Fig. 133. The openings in the diaphragm.

Table 2   The three openings in the diaphragm

Name of opening	Level	Shape	Position
Inferior vena caval	8T	Square	Slightly to right of median plane
Oesophageal	10T	Oval	Slightly to left of median plane
Aortic	12T	Round	Central

CAVAL OPENING: Transmits the inferior vena cava and half of the right phrenic nerve (the nerve first pierces the muscle and then supplies it from below).

OESOPHAGEAL OPENING: This opening is strengthened by the crura interlacing around it. In addition to the oesophagus it transmits the right and left vagi and the oesophageal branches of the left gastric artery with the accompanying veins. These vessels communicate here with the oesophageal branches of the aorta. This is one of the sites where portal and systemic circulations communicate. Therefore, in obstruction to the veins in the liver (cirrhosis), these veins at the lower end of the oesophagus become very dilated and frequently rupture.

The left vagus passes through the anterior angle of the oval, to supply the anterosuperior surface of the stomach and the right vagus goes through the posterior angle to the postero-inferior surface of the stomach. The alimentary canal is, at an early developmental stage, a median tube with right and left sides. The right vagus supplies the right side, the left supplies the left side; with the outgrowth of the liver the stomach rotates so that its left side becomes anterior, carrying its nerve supply with it.

AORTIC OPENING: This lies between the crura; the aortic orifice is completed by the median arcuate ligament which connects the crura. Three unpaired structures pass through it. From right to left these are the vena azygos major, the thoracic duct, and the aorta.

SMALLER ORIFICES IN THE DIAPHRAGM:

Between Xiphoid Slip and that from the 7th Costal Cartilage: Superior epigastric vessels pass.

Between the Slips from the 7th and 8th Costal Cartilages: Musculophrenic vessels pass.

Between each Pair of the remaining Slips: One of the lower five intercostal vessels and nerves pass.

Behind the Lateral Lumbocostal Arch: Last thoracic nerve and subcostal vessels pass.

Behind the Medial Lumbocostal Arch: The sympathetic trunk passes.

Each Crus is pierced by: The great, lesser, and least splanchnic nerves.

The Left Crus is pierced in addition by: The vena hemi-azygos.

Suprapleural membrane (Sibson's fascia)

The cervical pleura rises to the neck of the 1st rib which is almost 4 cm above the level of the sternal end of the 1st costal cartilage. It is protected externally by the scalene muscles which are lined internally by a dense fascia, the suprapleural membrane (Sibson's fascia) (*Fig.* 134).

The fascia, spreading out like a fan from the transverse process of the 7th cervical vertebra, is attached to the inner border of the 1st rib.

It thins out medially and fades into the pleura. The fascia gives rigidity to the thoracic inlet and prevents it ballooning in and out during respiration.

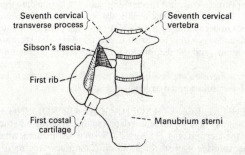

Seventh cervical transverse process

Seventh cervical vertebra

Sibson's fascia

First rib

First costal cartilage

Manubrium sterni

Fig. 134. The diaphragm of the upper aperture of the thorax—Sibson's fascia.

CONGENITAL DIAPHRAGMATIC HERNIA

There are different types depending on the nature of the congenital defect.

1. POSTEROLATERAL HERNIA: It occurs about once in 2000 births and leads to herniation of abdominal contents into the thoracic cavity which compresses the lung and displaces the heart. The hernia results from defective formation and fusion of the pleuroperitoneal membrane which closes the pleuroperitoneal canal in the fetus. There is a large defect in the posterolateral portion of the diaphragm. The hernia occurs most commonly through the left hemidiaphragm. Bochdalek's name is commonly associated with this hernia, although it is not a hernia through the 'foramen' described by him. Apart from causing confusion it is of no practical importance.

A posterolateral hernia is an important neonatal emergency. Infants present with a clinical triad of dyspnoea, cyanosis and apparent dextrocardia. An endotracheal tube should be passed as soon as the condition is diagnosed, and the infant subjected to surgery.

A thin hernial sac may or may not be present. A rim of diaphragmatic muscle is often present at the edge of the defect posteriorly. The lung on the affected side is small and hypoplastic due to compression by the bowel in the chest.

2. RETROSTERNAL HERNIA: The foramina of Morgagni (1769) are the names given to the openings which originally exist between the ventral (xiphisternal) and the lateral (costal) slips of origin. When the diaphragm is fully formed there is a small natural space between these slips. It contains a little areolar tissue and transmits the superior epigastric vessels. Thus a hernia in this situation may occur on either side. It is more common on the right, the reason being that the pericardial attachment is more extensive on the left and

offers more protection against the development of a hernia than the liver does on the right. Thus such a hernia usually lies between the pericardium and the right pleura. On occasions the hernia may enter the pericardial sac.

A hernial sac may or may not exist. Costal cartilages and sternum form the anterior boundary and the diaphragm forms the rest of the circumference of the defect.

Retrosternal herniae are less likely to present in the neonate but patients complain of discomfort and dysphagia at a later age.

3. CONGENITAL PARA-OESOPHAGEAL OR ROLLING HERNIA:

In this condition (*Fig.* 135) there is a defect in the diaphragm to the right and anterior to the oesophagus. There is a hernial sac present which usually contains the anterior wall of the stomach rolling upwards until it may be upside down in the posterior mediastinum. An important feature of this hernia is that the normal relationship of the cardio-oesophageal junction to the diaphragm is undisturbed.

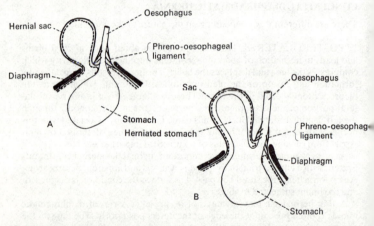

Fig. 135. A, Congenital oesophageal hiatal hernia; B, portion of stomach in hernial sac.

There is a difference of opinion about the origin of this hernia. The one theory proposes that there is a peritoneal process left in the posterior mediastinum when the developing stomach invaginates the peritoneum from behind. The other theory is that there is a congenital defect in the right crus of the diaphragm allowing the stomach to herniate into a sac-like space to the right of the oesophagus and the pressure of the herniating stomach results in the disappearance of the crural muscle separating the congenital defect from the oesophageal hiatus.

This is an extremely rare type of hernia and the only way it can disturb the mechanics of the oesophagus is if by its bulk it compresses the oesophagus against the vertebral column.

Comment:

    a. Congenital herniae are often associated with other maldevelopment, more especially malrotation of the midgut loop, which may be the cause of obstruction.

    b. Eventration of the diaphragm is not a true hernia as the gut is below the diaphragm. Half of the diaphragm has defective musculature due to failure of muscular tissue to extend into the pleuroperitoneal membrane on the affected side. As a result there is upward displacement of abdominal contents into an outpouching of the diaphragm.

    c. The herniation of bowel through the right diaphragm is relatively uncommon because of the protection afforded by the liver.

ACQUIRED DIAPHRAGMATIC HERNIAE

These may be either:
1. Traumatic.
2. Hiatal (sliding).

1. Traumatic hernia

This may follow an open injury to the diaphragm as the result of a penetrating wound of the chest or a closed injury to the diaphragm associated with a sudden increase in intra-abdominal pressure following a road traffic accident. The hernia is usually through the left side of the diaphragm as the right side is protected by the liver.

The injury to the diaphragm often goes undetected initially. The negative intrathoracic pressure is responsible for sucking the stomach, small bowel or colon into the chest. The gut in the chest may undergo strangulation months or years after the injury. The defect in the diaphragm is repaired through the abdomen or the chest. The latter route is generally preferred if the herniated gut is thought to be densely adherent to the pleura.

2. Acquired hiatal (sliding) hernia

This is commonest of all internal herniae (*Fig.* 136). The gastro-oesophageal junction is displaced into the chest, but only the anterolateral portion of the herniated stomach is covered by peritoneum, so the stomach itself is not within a hernial sac. The stomach forms part of the wall of the hernial sac and

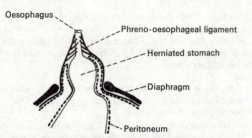

Fig. 136. Sliding hernia. (Redrawn from Allison.)

is comparable to the large bowel or bladder in a sliding inguinal or femoral hernia (*see* p. 132). A sliding hiatal hernia is commonly diagnosed on barium meal examination of the oesophagus.

A sliding hiatal hernia has little clinical significance unless accompanied by abnormal gastro-oesophageal reflux.

FACTORS PREVENTING GASTRO-OESOPHAGEAL REFLUX:

a. Gastro-oesophageal sphincter is a functional sphincter at the gastro-oesophageal junction which represents a barrier to reflux. The sphincter cannot be identified anatomically but demonstrates a resting pressure of 10–15 cm of water.

b. The intra-abdominal segment of the oesophagus. Internally the gastro-oesophageal mucosal junction lies just below the diaphragm, but externally the oesophagus and stomach join more distally. There is a definite intra-abdominal segment of the oesophagus measuring at least 2 cm. It is flaccid and is compressed on all sides, like a flutter valve, by an increase in intra-abdominal pressure.

c. The phreno-oesophageal membrane (*Fig.* 137) holds the cardio-oesophageal junction in its normal position. It is formed by a reflection of the fascia transversalis (endo-abdominal fascia) on the undersurface of the diaphragm onto the lower end of the oesophagus. The membrane is elastic and allows a fair degree of mobility of the cardia which is necessary in vomiting. A hernia will result from a weakness of the phreno-oesophageal membrane (e.g. after operations on this area) or an increase in intra-abdominal pressure (e.g. obesity). The cardia will then slide up through the hiatus.

An abnormally low insertion of the phreno-oesophageal membrane has been incriminated as an indirect cause of reflux, by eliminating the intra-abdominal segment of the oesophagus.

d. A mucosal rosette is formed by the bunched-up gastric mucosa at the

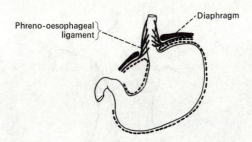

Fig. 137. The phreno-oesophageal ligament.

non-distended cardiac orifice. It may act as a watertight plug in preventing reflux.

e. The oesophageal hiatus in the diaphragm probably supports the sphincter. It lies anterior to the aorta and is in the right crus in 55 per cent of cases, while in the remainder the left crus of the diaphragm plays a variable part in the formation of the hiatus. The width of the hiatus varies between 1·8 and 2·5 cm.

f. The gastro-oesophageal angle may be important. An acute angle of entry of the oesophagus into the stomach is said to act as a flap valve in preventing reflux.

REPAIR OF THE SLIDING HERNIA: As for all other sliding herniae this requires removal of the sac, reduction of the contents, closure of the hernial orifice and fixation of the mobile organ. In this case, closure of the hiatal orifice cannot be complete and care must be exercised to avoid oesophageal compression by excessive approximation of the crura around the oesophagus. Reduction alone does not guarantee competence of the oesophageal sphincter and an antireflux procedure, such as the Nissen fundoplication, is practised in addition to hernia reduction. The principle of this procedure is to completely encircle the abdominal portion of the oesophagus with the cardiac portion of the stomach which has a flutter-valve effect on the oesophagogastric junction.

Chapter 13

THE BREAST

DEVELOPMENT OF THE BREAST

The epithelial lining of the ducts and acini of the breast is developed from ectoderm and the supporting tissue is derived from the mesenchyme. On each

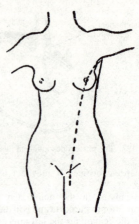

Fig. 138. The milk line.

side of the ventral surface of young embryos, a thickened band of ectoderm develops (the milk ridge). It extends obliquely from the axilla to the inguinal region (*Fig.* 138). In the human, the whole of this ridge atrophies, excepting only a small portion in each pectoral region from which the breasts arise. Accessory breast tissue will form along the course of the milk ridge, if it does not disappear outside the area where the breast normally develops. Normally, a tiny portion of the ridge which is going to form the breast enlarges, projecting slightly on the skin and extending deeply in the shape of buds which form long slender tubes from which the ducts and secreting tissue of the breast are formed. The nipple is either flat or depressed at birth, but later it projects beyond the surrounding skin.

CONGENITAL ABNORMALITIES OF THE BREAST

Amastia

Bilateral absence of breast tissue and nipple is exceedingly rare. When breast tissue is absent unilaterally, the pectoral muscles are often absent.

Polymastia

There is more than one breast on one or both sides. The accessory breast tissue may occur anywhere along the milk ridge but is usually 7–10 cm below and medial to the normal nipple. Usually all that is seen is a rudimentary nipple, but deep to the nipple there is breast tissue. Accessory breast tissue may exist without ducts projecting onto the skin and swelling of breast tissue which cannot discharge its contents may lead to difficulties in diagnosis. It may be confused with a lipoma especially when there is no nipple visible.

Polythelia

There is imperfect development of the mammary rudiment so that supernumerary nipples are situated irregularly over the breast and not on the milk ridge.

ANATOMY

Extent

VERTICAL: 2nd to 6th ribs inclusive.

HORIZONTAL: The side of the sternum to the midaxillary line. About two-thirds of the breast rests upon the pectoralis major, one-third on the serratus anterior. At its lower medial quadrant the gland rests on the aponeurosis of the external oblique, which separates it from the rectus abdominis.

The breast lies in the subcutaneous tissue and is separated from the underlying muscles by the deep fascia.

AXILLARY TAIL OF SPENCE: This is a prolongation from the outer part of the gland which passes up to the level of the 3rd rib in the axilla, where it is in direct contact with the main lymph nodes of the breast (anterior axillary nodes). This process of breast tissue gets into the axilla through an opening in the axillary fascia, known as the foramen of Langer. It follows that the axillary tail is under the deep fascia, and not, like the rest of the breast, superficial to this layer.

When it enlarges it may be mistaken for a lipoma.

Architecture of the gland

The breast is composed of acini which make up lobules, aggregations of which form the lobes of the gland. The lobes are arranged in a radiating fashion like the spokes of a wheel and converge on the nipple, where each lobe is drained by a duct. Ten to fifteen collecting ducts open onto the nipple, each duct draining a segmental system of smaller ducts and lobules. The ducts are surrounded by connective tissue which is characteristically loose and vascular in the distal ductules.

Different portions of the duct system are associated with different diseases. The larger ducts are the site of duct papilloma and duct ectasia; the distal smaller ducts are the site of fibro-adenoma during development of the breast, and cyst formation and sclerosing adenosis during the involutional period. The majority of cancers of the breast arise from the intralobular portions of the terminal ducts.

The roundness of the organ is due to fat which fills the gaps between the portions of the parenchyma.

LIGAMENTS OF COOPER: The breast is anchored to the overlying skin and to the underlying pectoral fascia by bands of connective tissue called 'ligaments of Cooper' (*Fig.* 139).

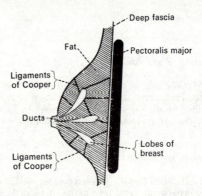

Fig. 139. Vertical section of the breast showing the ligaments of Cooper.

In cancer of the breast, the malignant cells may invade these ligaments and consequent contraction of these strands may cause dimpling of the skin or attachment of the underlying growth to the skin which then cannot be pinched up from the lump.

If cancer cells grow along the ligaments of Cooper binding the breast to the pectoral fascia, the breast becomes fixed to the pectoralis major. It cannot then (as normally) be moved in the long axis of the muscle.

Blood supply of the breast

This is derived from:

1. The lateral thoracic artery, from the 2nd part of the axillary.

2. The perforating cutaneous branches of the internal mammary to the 2nd, 3rd and 4th spaces.
3. The lateral branches of the 2nd, 3rd and 4th intercostal arteries.

Venous drainage

The superficial veins radiate from the breast and are characterized by their proximity to the skin. They are accompanied by lymphatics and drain to axillary, internal mammary and intercostal vessels.

Phlebitis of one of these superficial veins feels like a cord immediately beneath the skin. The condition produces no discoloration and may be tensed like a bowstring by putting traction on it (Mondor's disease).

Nerve supply

The secreting tissue is supplied by sympathetic nerves which reach it via the 2nd to the 6th intercostal nerves. The overlying skin is supplied by the anterior and lateral branches of the 4th, 5th and 6th intercostal nerves.

Axillary lymph nodes

The breast drains mainly to the axillary nodes, of which there are five sets (*Fig.* 140).

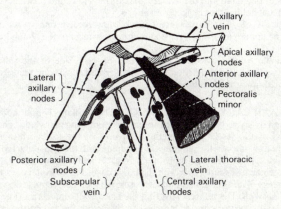

Fig. 140. Lymph nodes of the axilla.

ANTERIOR SET: Situated along the lateral thoracic vein under the anterior axillary fold. They lie mainly on the 3rd rib. The axillary tail of Spence is in actual contact with these nodes and, therefore, cancer involving this process may be misdiagnosed as an enlarged node with an apparently healthy breast and the anterior axillary nodes may be involved, by direct continuity of tissue.

POSTERIOR SET: These lie along the posterior axillary fold in relation to the subscapular vessels.

LATERAL SET: Along the upper part of the humerus in relation to the axillary vein.

CENTRAL SET: Situated in the fat of the upper part of the axilla. The intercostobrachial nerve passes outwards amongst these nodes. Enlargement of these nodes, such as occurs in cancer, may, by pressure on the nerve, cause pain in the distribution of the nerve along the inner border of the arm.

APICAL SET: These are also called the 'infraclavicular nodes'. They are very important and constant in position being bounded below by the 1st intercostal space, behind by the axillary vein, in front by the costocoracoid membrane. These nodes lie very deeply, but can be palpated by pushing the fingers of one hand into the axillary apex from below, and the fingers of the other hand behind the clavicle from above.

They are of great importance because they receive one vessel directly from the upper part of the breast and ultimately most of the lymph from the breast.

A single trunk leaves the apical group on each side of the subclavian trunk, and enters the junction of the jugular and subclavian veins, or may join the thoracic duct on the left.

THE AXILLARY FASCIAL 'TENT': The axillary lymph nodes are enclosed by layers of fascia which resemble a tent lying on its side. The 'tent' consists of the fascia covering the structures of the axilla which can be described as follows (the patient is lying supine with the arm abducted):

Anterior Wall: The pectoralis minor muscle and the clavipectoral fascia which fuses superiorly with the fascia covering the axillary vessels.

Posterior Wall: The subscapularis muscle lying on the scapula.

Medial Wall: Deep fascia covering the chest wall, upper ribs, intercostal and serratus anterior muscles. In dissecting the fascia, the nerve to serratus anterior, which runs just deep to the fascia, is lifted off the chest wall.

Apex: Points upwards and medially where the layers of fascia come into contact with each other.

Base: Points downwards and laterally and is open.

The lymph nodes are enclosed in this tent. A block dissection of the axillary lymph nodes should excise the 'tent' intact.

Lymphatic drainage

The breast is drained by two sets of lymphatics:

1. The lymphatics of the skin over the breast.
2. The lymphatics of the parenchyma of the breast.

LYMPHATICS OF THE OVERLYING SKIN: These drain the integuments over the breast, but not the skin of the areola and nipple. They pass in a radial direction and end in the surrounding nodes. Those from the outer side go to the axillary nodes. The skin of the upper part drains by vessels which go to the supraclavicular nodes (members of the lower deep cervical nodes). Certain of these vessels may end in the cephalic node which lies in relation to the vein of the same name in the deltopectoral triangle. The vessels from the skin over the inner part of the breast go to the internal mammary nodes which lie in relation to the veins of that name. These nodes lie in the upper four or five intercostal spaces or behind the related costal cartilages.

The lymphatics of the skin over the breast communicate across the middle line, and a unilateral disease may become bilateral by this route.

Mammary cancer may spread along these superficial lymphatic vessels to produce nodules in the skin.

LYMPHATICS OF THE PARENCHYMA OF THE BREAST: The subareolar lymph plexus of Sappey is a collection of large lymph vessels situated under the areola. Though the subareolar plexus communicates with the lymphatics of the breast tissue, it is not a collecting zone for the breast lymph.

The axillary nodes receive about 75 per cent of lymph draining the breast tissue (*Fig.* 141). Lymphatics arising in the lobules pass directly outwards in the substance of the breast, receive tributaries on the way, and pass through the axillary tail to the axilla. Most go to the anterior group of nodes; a few pass to the posterior group, and from there they run to central and apical groups, coming to lie on the inferomedial and anterior aspects of the axillary vein.

Lymphatics from the deep surface of the breast pass through the great pectoral muscle on their way to the axillary or internal mammary nodes (*Fig.* 142).

The lymphatic plexus of the deep fascia consists of fine vessels which do not act as a normal pathway for lymph from the breast to the regional nodes.

The internal mammary nodes receive lymph from both the medial and lateral portions of the breast. Lymph enters the thorax along the anterior perforating branches of the internal mammary artery and along the lateral perforating branches of the intercostal vessels. Most of this lymph goes to the

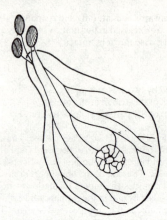

Fig. 141. The main lympathic pathways from the breast passing through the axillary tail to the anterior node group.

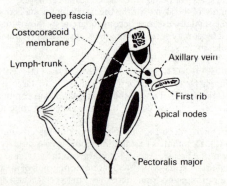

Fig. 142. Showing the direct pathway of deep lymphatics of the breast through the great pectoral muscle to the axillary nodes.

internal mammary chain, but a small amount may pass to the posterior intercostal nodes lying near the heads of the ribs (*Fig.* 143).

At the level of the first interspace, fine lymphatics connect the right and left internal mammary chains behind the manubrium sterni, and nodes may be found there. Even in apparently early breast cancer, tumours of the outer half of the breast may metastasize to the internal mammary nodes without involvement of the axillary nodes.

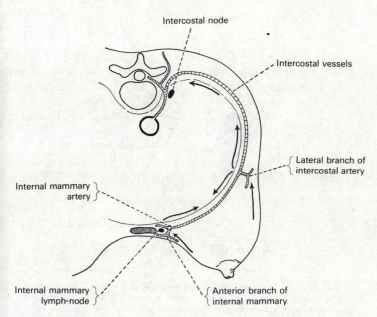

Fig. 143. The routes into the chest of lymph from the breast. The arrows show the direction of lymph flow.

'RETRACTION' IN BREAST PATHOLOGY

The physical sign of 'retraction' (*Fig.* 144) may occur under the following circumstances:

Congenital retraction of the nipple

In the development of the breast there is first a downgrowth of epithelium from the future site of the nipple, forming a pocket or invagination of the skin. Only shortly before birth is this depression pushed up to become an evagination or nipple. This evagination may never occur and a depression exists throughout life.

Inflammatory retraction of the nipple

The duct may fill with secretion. If infection occurs, the resultant abscess may

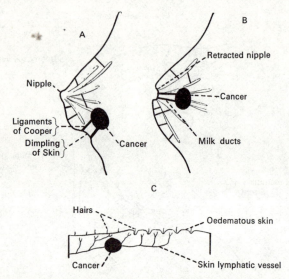

Fig. 144. Illustrating the pathology of breast retraction. A, Dimpling of the skin due to the pull exerted by the ligaments of Cooper; B, retraction of the nipple due to retraction of the milk ducts, C, peau d'orange due to lymphatic obstruction.

burst through the skin near the edge of the areola. The resultant fistula may close and later the process will be repeated or a persistent lactiferous duct fistula may form. The persistent or recurrent inflammation will result in fibrosis and nipple retraction.

Retraction in relation to cancer of the breast
There are three varieties of retraction which may occur, each due to a different cause:

1. RETRACTION OF THE SKIN: Due to invasion of the ligaments of Cooper, as explained above.

2. RETRACTION OF THE NIPPLE: Due to extension of growth along the main milk ducts and subsequent retraction as fibrosis occurs, leading to indrawing of the nipple.

3. PEAU D'ORANGE: In this condition the pits of the hair follicles appear to be retracted beneath the level of the surrounding skin. The condition is due

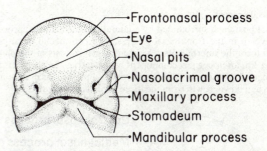

Frontonasal process
Eye
Nasal pits
Nasolacrimal groove
Maxillary process
Stomadeum
Mandibular process

Fig. 145. Frontal aspect of face in a 5-week-old embryo.

to blockage of the lymphatics draining the skin, leading to a stagnation of lymph and oedema of the skin.

SURGERY FOR BREAST CANCER

The classic operation of radical mastectomy attempts to excise the whole organ and its lymphatic field which includes the skin overlying the tumour, the cutting of thin skin flaps, total removal of the breast with its axillary contents and the pectoralis major and most of the pectoralis minor muscles. However, the concept of total surgical excision of mammary cancer is receiving reconsideration and the modern trend is a more limited extirpation and reliance on adjuvant treatment to eliminate more distant cancer cells. This change in surgical approach is based on the concept that all lymph eventually drains into the venous system and that lymphovenous anastomoses abound. It is, therefore, considered that extension of the cancer cannot usually be extirpated by surgery alone.

Chapter 14

DEVELOPMENTAL ANOMALIES OF THE FACE AND BRANCHIAL ARCHES

DEVELOPMENT OF THE FACE

The face is formed from five processes which surround an opening (the stomadeum) at the anterior end of the embryo (*Fig.* 145). These are: (*a*) frontonasal—a single process; (*b*) maxillary—one on each side; (*c*) mandibular—one on each side.

Frontonasal process

Two nasal pits, each surrounded by a lateral and medial nasal process (*Fig.* 146), develop in the frontonasal process. The two medial nasal processes merge to form the intermaxillary segment which consists of the philtrum of the upper lip, an upper jaw component which carries the four incisor teeth, the triangular primary palate (premaxilla), and the nasal septum which develops as a downgrowth from the fused medial nasal processes.

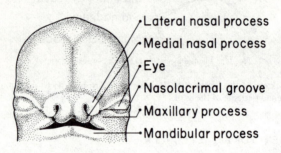

Fig. 146. Frontal aspect of face in a 10-week-old embryo.

The lateral nasal process forms the side of the nose. It takes no part in the formation of the upper lip.

The maxillary process

The maxillary processes fuse with the lateral nasal process at the nasolacrimal groove (the future nasolacrimal duct) and with the medial nasal processes to form the lateral part of the upper lip. Two lateral palatine processes, which fuse in the midline to form the secondary palate, develop from the inner aspect of the maxillary processes. The palate is formed by the fusion of secondary palate to the primary palate. The incisive foramen marks the junction of the two components of the palate (*Fig.* 147).

The mandibular process

The mandibular processes give rise to the lower lip and jaw. The lines of fusion of these processes are depicted in *Fig.* 148.

When these epithelial structures have fused, a mesodermal mass flows in between the two layers of the fused epithelium, to provide the supporting structures of the face.

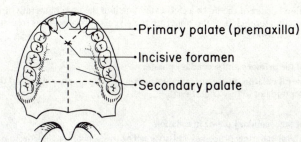

Fig. 147. The normal palate.

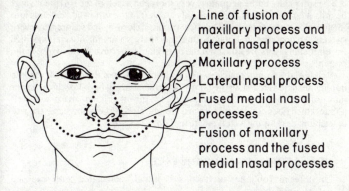

Fig. 148. The facial fusion lines.

HARE-LIP AND CLEFT PALATE

Hare-lip and cleft palate are the most common congenital anomalies of the head and neck occurring in 1 per 750 live births. It is now thought that these anomalies result from a failure of the separate mesodermal masses to flow between the various processes which are already joined by two layers of epithelial cells. The epithelial layers become stretched until the cells are so attenuated that they give way, resulting in a cleft.

Hare-lip and cleft palate may be classified as follows:

Cleft of the primary palate

The cleft (*Fig*. 149A, B, C) may vary from a barely perceptible cleft in the vermilion border of the lip to a cleft extending into the nose bilaterally. In a complete bilateral cleft of the upper lip the alveolar process hangs free and projects anteriorly.

Cleft of the primary and secondary palates

The lateral palatine processes, the mesoderm of the primary palate and the nasal septum fail to fuse (*Fig*. 149D).

Cleft of the secondary palate in isolation

The lateral palatine processes fail to meet with each other and the nasal septum. The extent of the cleft (*Fig*. 149E) may vary from a cleft of uvula only to a complete cleft of the hard and soft palates as far as the incisive foramen.

The soft palate in the neonate is very short and a cleft of the soft palate may be mistaken as a cleft of the uvula only. A cleft of the soft palate extends into the muscles of the palate, which effect oronasal closure, and so interferes with speech. An uncommon, but important, anomaly is a submucous cleft in which the epithelial layers are intact but the muscular layers have failed to fuse in the midline.

A cleft of the primary palate with or without a cleft of the secondary palate implies an increased risk in the family of further cases of hare-lip which may or may not be associated with a cleft palate. On the other hand, an isolated cleft palate which does not extend forward into the alveolus only increases the risk of a sibling developing a cleft palate and not a hare-lip.

RARE MALFORMATIONS OF THE FACE

1. Orbitofacial (oblique) cleft: this is usually associated with exposed nasolacrimal duct.
2. Macrostomia: a lateral or transverse cleft which runs from the mouth to the ear.
3. Microstomia due to excessive merging of the mesodermal masses of the maxillary and mandibular processes.
4. Bifid nose which results from an incomplete fusion of the medial nasal processes.
5. Median cleft of the upper lip which results from a mesodermal deficiency and failure of the medial nasal processes to merge.
6. Median cleft of the lower lip is caused by failure of the mesenchymal masses of the mandibular processes to merge completely.

BRANCHIAL CYSTS AND FISTULAE

The neck and pharynx are formed from five branchial arches of which the

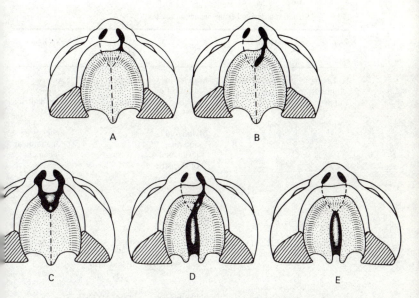

Fig. 149. A, Unilateral hare-lip extending into the nose; B, unilateral hare-lip involving lip and premaxilla; C, bilateral hare-lip involving lip and premaxilla; D, cleft of primary and secondary palate; E, isolated cleft palate.

most caudal is poorly defined (*Fig.* 150). Between the arches are depressions both internally and externally. Those internally are called 'pharyngeal pouches', those externally are the 'branchial grooves' or 'clefts'. Between the two is a membrane, which is lined externally with squamous epithelium and internally with columnar epithelium. A typical branchial arch contains a plate of cartilage, a muscle mass, a nerve, and an artery. The branchial arch derivations are listed in *Table* 3 and the outcome of the branchial arteries is considered further in Chapter 22.

The growth of the second arch is much faster than that of the arches below, so that it soon overhangs them, forming a deep groove—the cervical sinus (*Fig.* 150).

Ultimately, the overgrown 2nd arch meets the 5th and the two fuse. Now the cervical sinus is a buried space lined by squamous epithelium. It disappears entirely. Should a part of the space persist, it will form a branchial cyst. Should the 2nd arch fail to fuse with the 5th, an opening will be found

Table 3. Structures derived from branchial arches

Arch	Nerve	Muscles	Skeletal structures	Ligaments
1st (man-dibular arch)	Mandibular nerves (Vth)	Muscles of mastication	Malleus Incus	Anterior ligament of malleus
		Mylohyoid and an-terior belly of digastric		Spheno-mandibular ligament
		Tensor tym-pani		
		Tensor palati		
2nd (hyoid arch)	Facial (VIIth)	Muscles of facial expression	Stapes Styloid pro-cess	Stylohyoid ligament
		Stapedius	Lesser cornu of hyoid	
		Stylohyoid	Upper part of body of hyoid bone	
		Posterior belly of digastric		
3rd	Glosso-pharyngeal (IXth)	Stylo-pharyngeus	Greater cornu of hyoid	
			Lower part of body of the hyoid bone	
4th and 6th	Superior laryngeal branch of vagus (Xth)	Cricothyroid	Thyroid cartilage	

Arch	Nerve	Muscles	Skeletal structures	Ligaments
	Recurrent laryngeal branch of vagus (Xth)	Levator palati Constrictors of pharynx Intrinsic muscles of larynx	Cricoid cartilage Arytenoid cartilage Corniculate cartilage Cuneiform cartilage	
5th	This arch is rudimentary only			

on the neck at birth—a lateral cervical (branchial) sinus. Such an orifice will be found along the line of the anterior border of the sternomastoid muscle, at the junction between the upper three-quarters with the lower one-quarter of the muscle. This opening is connected to a tract which will always be separated from the pharynx by a septum which represents the remains of the cleft membrane. This membrane, due to its tenuous nature, as it contains no mesodermal structure, usually breaks down establishing a fistula which extends from the skin to an internal opening in the tonsillar fossa. This is known as a branchial fistula.

Branchial fistula
As the fistula is the remains of the cervical sinus it is below the 2nd arch and, as it usually arises in connection with the 2nd cleft, it is above the 3rd arch.

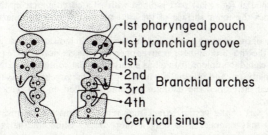

Fig. 150. Branchial arches and the cervical sinus.

The nerve of the 2nd arch is the facial, its artery the external carotid and the nerve of the 3rd arch is the 9th, its artery the internal carotid. The fistula would therefore run between these structures (*Fig*. 151).

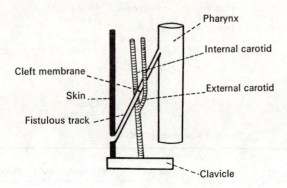

Fig. 151. Course of a branchial fistula.

From its opening on the skin, the fistula passes subcutaneously through the platysma to the level of the upper border of the thryoid cartilage where it pierces the deep fascia. The fistula then passes beneath the posterior belly of the digastric muscle and the stylohyoid, crosses the hypoglossal nerve and internal jugular vein, to traverse the fork of the carotid bifurcation, the external carotid being superficial and the internal carotid deep.

It then crosses the glossopharyngeal nerve and the stylopharyngeus muscle to pierce the superior constrictor and open on the posterior pillar of the fauces behind the tonsil.

The lateral (external) part of the fistula is lined with squamous epithelium and the medial (internal) part is lined with ciliated columnar epithelium (which lines the inner surface of the cleft membrane and the pharyngeal pouch).

The site of the opening on the skin surface is not an indication of its groove origin, as the 2nd, 3rd, and 4th grooves open into the cervical sinus.

The so-called 'complete' fistula has a muscular coat continuous externally with the platysma and internally with the palatopharyngeus. If this muscle coat is well developed the fistulous opening is pulled on and puckers on swallowing.

Only a part of the vestigial track may remain. Thus a sinus presenting externally may connect with only a short track. Blind internal sinuses resulting from persistence of the pharyngeal pouch rarely cause symptoms and are probably commoner than reported.

Fistulae are bilateral in at least 30 per cent of cases. Cysts are usually unilateral.

There is a definite familial tendency, and other congenital abnormalities may coexist, such as pre-auricular sinuses, or subcutaneous cartilaginous nodules on one side corresponding in situation to a fistulous opening on the other.

Branchial cysts

These occur along the line of the anterior border of the sternomastoid, usually in the region of the angle of the jaw. Their relations are similar to those of the fistula. The cyst is lined with squamous epithelium (like the cervical sinus).

ANOMALIES OF THE FIRST BRANCHIAL GROOVE

The ectodermal portion of the 1st branchial groove takes part in the formation of the adult external auditory meatus. The corresponding entodermal portion of the first pharyngeal pouch becomes the tympanic cavity of the middle ear and the Eustachian tube.

Anomalies of the 1st branchial groove are very rare. The line of obliteration of the 1st branchial groove runs parallel with the mandible and extends from the external auditory meatus to just below the midpoint of the mandible. If only the skin edges of the 1st ectodermal groove fuse without obliteration of the branchial groove, a tunnel is formed which is lined throughout by squamous epithelium. The external opening of this channel is situated between the lower border of the mandible and the hyoid bone.

The fistulous track passes inward and upward superficial to the posterior belly of the digastric muscle, through the parotid gland, and extends to the junction of the bony and cartilaginous portions of the external auditory canal (*Fig.* 152). Its relationship to the facial nerve varies, being either superficial or deep to the branches of the facial nerve. It would be expected that the track would be superficial to the facial nerve (which is the nerve of the 2nd arch), but the branches of that nerve are taken by their muscles as they migrate to the superficial region of the face over the surface of the first arch, hence the variable relationship of the first cleft to the branches of the facial nerve.

Any portion of the track may persist to form a branchial cyst (of the first groove) anywhere along its course. Such squamous-lined cysts may thus be found in the parotid gland or in the submandibular region.

PRE-AURICULAR SKIN TAGS AND SINUSES

The pinna is formed from a merger of six tubercles which arise from the 1st and 2nd branchial arches. Pre-auricular sinuses result from abnormal

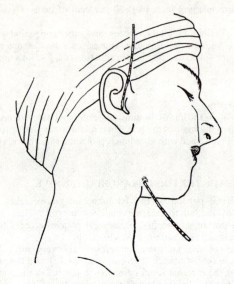

Fig. 152. Complete aurocervical fistula.

infolding and entrapment of epithelium during merger of these tubercles and pre-auricular skin tags may result from accessory auditory tubercles.

Pre-auricular sinus

A sinus may occur in the skin in front of the tragus, on the helix of the ear above the tragus or rarely in other sites on the ear. These sinuses occur bilaterally in about a quarter of cases. The sinuses are short and never connect internally with the external auditory canal. There is a strong tendency to familial recurrence.

The patient may present with an abscess in the cheek which initially requires drainage. The sinus and its small cyst-like extensions should be totally excised to prevent a recurrence.

Pre-auricular skin tags

Small skin tags (auricular appendages) may occur anterior to the ear as a result of the development of accessory auditory tubercles. They are usually unilateral and consist of skin only, but may contain cartilage.

THE MANDIBLE AND MAXILLA

THE BLOOD SUPPLY OF THE MANDIBLE

The mandible has a rich blood supply from the following sources:

1. The inferior alveolar artery is the only arterial vessel which enters the mandible, and it supplies the medullary bone of the mandible and the alveolus.
2. The blood supply to the cortical plates of the mandible is via the muscles of mastication.
3. There is a significant blood supply to the condylar processes and parts of the ramus from the capsule of the temporomandibular joint.
4. There is also a significant vascular component which arises from the muscles of facial expression, namely the buccinator and mentalis muscles. An additional supply to the lingual aspect of the body of the mandible is derived from the mylohyoid muscle as well as the geniohyoid and genioglossus muscles.
5. There is an extensive anastomosis between the inferior alveolar arteries, periosteal vessels and vessels derived from the muscles of mastication. With increasing age, the blood supply to the mandible from the inferior alveolar artery decreases progressively and is compensated for by the vessels arising from muscles of mastication and the periosteum.

This rich blood supply makes it possible to section the mandible in three or more places in order to reposition it for aesthetic or functional reasons. It should be noted, however, that extensive stripping of the periosteum and muscles of mastication should be avoided because, if this is done, avascular necrosis of the bone occurs.

THE BLOOD SUPPLY OF THE MAXILLA

Blood supply to the maxillary bone is derived from a network of anastomosing vessels formed by branches of the maxillary artery:

1. THE SUPERIOR ALVEOLAR ARTERIES: The supply to the maxillary incisor and canine teeth, as well as the labial mucosa covering the alveolus, is derived from the anterior superior alveolar artery which has its origin within the infra-orbital canal. The maxillary premolars and associated buccal soft tissues derive their blood supply from the middle superior alveolar artery which arises from the infra-orbital artery, within the infra-orbital canal. The blood supply to the maxillary molar teeth and associated soft tissues is derived from the posterior superior alveolar artery.

2. LONG SPHENOPALATINE ARTERY: The palatal mucosa related to

the hard palate and soft tissues associated with the palatal aspect of the maxillary incisors and canines derives its blood supply from the long sphenopalatine artery.

3. GREATER PALATINE ARTERIES: The remainder of the bony hard palate and the associated soft tissues are supplied by the two greater palatine arteries. They exit from the hard palate through the two greater palatine foramina which are situated anteromedially to the pterygoid hamulus.

4. LESSER PALATINE ARTERIES: The blood supply to the soft palate is via a number of lesser palatine arteries which exit from the hard palate distal to the greater palatine arteries. A significant supply to the soft palate is derived from the muscles of the soft palate, namely, palatoglossus, tensor palati, levator palati, palatopharyngeus and the uvular muscle.

Unlike the mandible there are few muscles attached to the maxilla from which it can obtain a blood supply, although a significant blood supply to the cortex is derived from a periosteal network of vessels derived mainly from the palatal vasculature.

In recent years, maxillary osteotomies for correction of facial deformities in the middle third of the facial skeleton have been used extensively. The blood supply via the palatine vessels in the maxilla accounts for a significant proportion of the blood supply to the bone and great care must be taken not to compromise the blood supply via greater and lesser palatine vessels, by unnecessary reflection of palatal soft tissues.

SENSORY NERVE SUPPLY TO THE JAWS

Sensory supply to the lower jaw

Total sensory supply to the lower jaw (*Fig.* 153) is derived from the mandibular branch of the trigeminal nerve.

1. The long buccal nerve arises from the anterior division of the mandibular nerve, passes between the two heads of lateral pterygoid and runs down, deep to temporalis muscle whilst lying on the lateral pterygoid. It continues laterally to reach the buccinator muscle (which it does not supply) and gives off a small branch to supply the skin below the zygomatic bone. The nerve pierces buccinator and terminates by supplying sensation to the mucosa opposite the last three molar mandibular teeth on their buccal aspect. It also conveys secretomotor fibres to the molar and buccal salivary glands from the otic ganglion.

2. The inferior alveolar nerve which arises from the posterior division of the mandibular nerve and passes down deep to the lateral ptergyoid

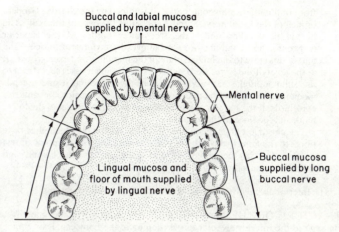

Buccal and labial mucosa
supplied by mental nerve

Mental nerve

Buccal mucosa
supplied by long
buccal nerve

Lingual mucosa and
floor of mouth supplied
by lingual nerve

All teeth supplied by inferior alveolar nerve

Fig. 153. Sensory innervation of the mandible.

muscle whilst lying on the medial pterygoid muscle. It passes forward between the mandible and the sphenomandibular ligament towards the medial surface of the mandible. Just before it enters the mandibular foramen below the lingula, it gives off the nerve to mylohyoid and the anterior belly of digastric. This nerve is the only motor nerve in the posterior division of the mandibular nerve.

The inferior alveolar nerve enters the mandibular foramen under cover of the lingula. It continues inside the mandible in the mandibular (inferior alveolar) canal, and supplies the molars and premolars of the lower jaw. At a point between the lower premolars, the bulk of the nerve leaves the mandible through the mental foramen to become the sensory supply to the lower lip, the buccal mucosa from the incisor to the premolars and the skin over the chin. This is known as the mental nerve. It carries a few secretomotor fibres from the chordae tympani to labial minor salivary glands. The lower incisor and canine teeth are supplied by the incisive nerve, which is the continuation of the inferior alveolar nerve anterior to the mental foramen within the substance of the mandible. It is commonly found that the lower first incisor has a dual nerve supply, from the incisive nerve on its own side, and from the terminal twigs of the incisive nerve of the other side.

3. The lingual nerve, which arises from the posterior division of the mandibular nerve, courses downwards on the medial pterygoid muscle in

front of the inferior alveolar nerve. It is joined by the chordae tympani branch of the facial nerve about 2 cm below the base of the skull. The lingual nerve slips under the free lower border of the superior constrictor and continues forward above the mylohyoid muscle. The nerve runs close to the lingual plate of the mandible and even grooves it at the level of the lower third molar tooth. It then crosses superficial to the submandibular salivary gland duct, hooks round it and ascends medial to the duct on the hyoglossus to supply sensation to the anterior two-thirds of the tongue, the mucosa on the lingual aspect of the lower teeth and the floor of the mouth.

The chordae tympani component of the lingual nerve supplies taste fibres to the anterior two-thirds of the tongue and secretomotor fibres, which relay in the submandibular ganglion, to the lingual and submandibular salivary glands.

The inferior alveolar nerve may be involved in various conditions:

FRACTURE OF THE MANDIBLE: In any fracture of the mandible, damage to the inferior alveolar nerve running in the bony canal can occur. This can be neurapraxia with spontaneous recovery within days or weeks if displacement of the segments is minimal, or a fully developed neurotmesis if gross displacement or a comminuted fracture has occurred. Initially, presenting features are similar, viz. numbness of the distribution zone of the mental nerve, especially lower lip and chin.

INFECTIONS: The same numbness of the lower lip is found in cases of osteomyelitis of the mandible when the inferior alveolar nerve is affected.

SURGICAL PROCEDURES: The removal of an impacted lower third molar tooth can damage the inferior alveolar nerve if the tooth lies on the inferior alveolar canal, or if the nerve lies between the roots of the impacted tooth. The lingual nerve can also be traumatized as the nerve runs on the lingual aspect of the mandible at the level of the lower third molar. An elevator or guard should be slipped in on the lingual aspect of the mandible under the periosteum prior to the elevation of the root or bone removal, to protect the lingual nerve.

ORTHOGNATHIC SURGERY: Injury of the inferior alveolar nerve may follow sagittal mandibular osteotomy where the buccal and lingual plates of the ramus are separated from one another to allow advancement or retrusion of the tooth-bearing segment of the mandible.

INTRA-ORAL BLOCK OF THE INFERIOR ALVEOLAR NERVE: The procedure (*Fig.* 154) has three steps:
Position 1: With the mouth open, the index finger can palpate the sharp

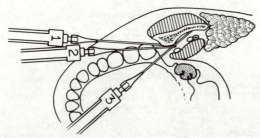

Fig. 154. The three positions of the needle in a mandibular injection. Position (1) insertion of needle striking bone. Position (2) injection of lingual nerve. Position (3) injection for inferior alveolar nerve.

anterior border of the ramus of the mandible. The needle is inserted just medial to this anterior border 1 cm above the occlusal surfaces of the lower molar teeth. With the syringe held parallel to the occlusive surfaces of the lower molar teeth, the needle is advanced for a short distance until it strikes bone.

Position 2: The needle is disengaged from periosteum, redirected medial to the ramus of the mandible and advanced about 6 mm. The needle is now in the space between the lingual nerve and the ramus. At this point 0·5 ml of local anaesthetic is injected to block the lingual nerve.

Position 3: The syringe is now rotated to lie over the premolar teeth of the opposite side of the jaw and the needle is advanced posteriorly and outwards until it strikes the ramus of the mandible. The needle is slightly withdrawn and the remainder of the local anaesthetic is injected in the region of the inferior alveolar nerve.

The buccal nerve arises from the mandibular nerve above the inferior alveolar nerve and to anaesthetize the buccal side of the mucosa, local anaesthetic is injected into the cheek from the inside of the mouth, immediately above its junction with the gum of the third molar tooth.

Sensory supply to the upper jaw

The upper jaw is supplied by the maxillary nerve (*Fig.* 155). The teeth are supplied by outer and inner nerve loops.

1. The outer nerve loop supplies the pulps of the teeth, the outer (buccal and labial) alveolar plate, the periosteum and mucous membrane covering the alveolar plate. It is formed from the posterior superior alveolar and infra-orbital branches of the maxillary nerve.

2. The inner nerve loop innervates only the inner (lingual or palatal) alveolar plate, and the overlying periosteum and mucous membrane. The nerves forming the inner nerve loop are the nasopalatine, the

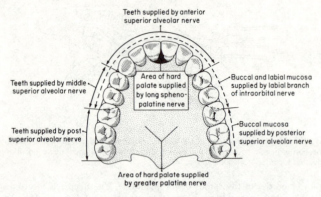

Fig. 155. Sensory innervation of maxilla.

greater palatine and the lesser palatine nerves which pass through the pterygopalatine ganglion.

This nerve supply is of importance in the following conditions:

LOCAL ANAESTHETIC TECHNIQUE: In operations on the upper teeth only the outer nerve loop need be anaesthetized provided the inner alveolar plate is not involved. In extractions both nerve loops must be anaesthetized.

The buccal cortical plate surrounding the upper dentition is thin, unlike the thick alveolar plate of the mandible. Hence, it is practical to obtain anaesthesia of the upper teeth by infiltration of local anaesthetic in the deepest point of the buccal sulcus next to the tooth that one wishes to anaesthetize. The solution diffuses through the thin bony wall to the nerve ending supplying that particular tooth through its apex.

ORTHOGNATHIC SURGERY TO THE MAXILLA: In total maxillary osteotomy in which the whole of the tooth-bearing area of the maxilla is freed from its attachment to the base of the skull, the position of the bony cuts is such that the posterior, middle and anterior superior alveolar nerves are usually severed. Stabilization of the fragment using infra-orbital rim suspension usually results in a neurapraxia of the infra-orbital nerve. The palatal mucosa is left undisturbed and sensation to the palate is uninterrupted.

FRACTURES OF THE ZYGOMATIC BONE: The bony attachments of the zygomatic bone and its arch are frequently fractured.

A fracture of the zygomatic bone may be associated with damage to the infra-orbital nerve (anaesthesia of the upper lip, also of the nose and lower eyelid) or the zygomaticofacial nerve (anaesthesia over the malar prominence). When the zygomatic arch is fractured the zygomaticotemporal nerve may be damaged (anaesthesia of the skin of the temporal region).

When the temporal process of the zygomatic bone is depressed, the patient is unable to open his mouth fully because of impingement of the coronoid process on the zygomatic bone.

THE TEMPOROMANDIBULAR JOINT

Anatomy

The temporomandibular joint is a synovial joint between the convex condyle of the mandible, the concave glenoid (mandibular) fossa and the articular eminence on the undersurface of the squamous part of the temporal bone (*Fig.* 156).

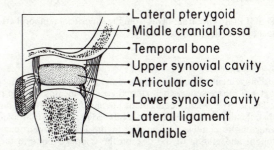

- Lateral pterygoid
- Middle cranial fossa
- Temporal bone
- Upper synovial cavity
- Articular disc
- Lower synovial cavity
- Lateral ligament
- Mandible

Fig. 156. The temporomandibular joint in a frontal section.

The temporomandibular joint is divided into two compartments by a deformable meniscus of dense fibrous tissue with elastic fibres predominating in the posterior portion. The disc is much thinner in its central portion than along the periphery, where it is attached to the joint capsule and to the upper fibres of the lateral pterygoid muscle anteriorly.

The synovial-lined articular capsule is attached to the temporal bone around the edges of the glenoid fossa and to the neck of the mandible. It is thin and loose between the temporal bone and articular disc, but between the disc and mandible it is thicker and stronger.

On the lateral side, the capsule is reinforced by the lateral (temporomandibular) ligament which extends from the zygomatic arch downward and backward to the lateral and posterior aspect of the neck of the mandible.

The sphenomandibular ligament, inserted into the lingula, and the stylomandibular ligament, inserted into the angle of the mandible, do not support the capsule and are regarded as accessory ligaments. These ligaments are thought to act as pivots during protrusion and opening of the jaw.

MUSCLES RESPONSIBLE FOR MOVEMENT OF THE JAW:
Protrusion: Both lateral pterygoid muscles.
Retraction: Posterior fibres of the temporalis muscle.
Lateral excursion: Unilateral contraction of lateral and medial pterygoid muscles.
Opening: Lateral pterygoid and digastric muscles.
Closing: Masseters, medial pterygoid and temporalis muscles.

NERVE SUPPLY: The auriculotemporal nerve which runs below and behind the joint. The nerve to the masseter sends a twig to the joint.

LYMPH DRAINAGE: Lymph drainage is to the pre-auricular, intraparotid and upper deep cervical nodes.

BLOOD SUPPLY: Blood supply is from the superficial temporal artery and fine branches from the maxillary artery.

Opening of the jaw

Backward movement of the ramus of the mandible is restricted by the parotid salivary gland, buttressed by the external acoustic meatus and the mastoid process. This restricts wide opening of the jaw and protrusion of the jaw has to occur when the mouth is opened. This combined movement is brought about by hinging of the condyle on the disc in the lower temporomandibular compartment and gliding of the disc on the temporal bone in the upper compartment. The disc is moved forward by its attachment to the lateral pterygoid muscle which contracts when the jaw is opened.

The elastic fibres in the posterior aspect of the disc restrain forward movement of the disc and return it to its resting position when the mouth is closed.

Dislocation of the jaw

The temporomandibular joint is stable in occlusion. The impact of a blow to the jaw is absorbed by contact between the upper and lower molar teeth.

Dislocation occurs when the capsule and the lateral ligament are sufficiently relaxed to allow the condyle to move to a point anterior to the articular eminence when opening the mouth. Muscle spasm locks the jaw in this position making it impossible for the patient to close the jaw.

The dislocation is reduced by downward pressure on the posterior teeth and upward pressure on the chin accompanied by posterior displacement of the entire mandible.

Chapter 16

LYMPH TISSUE OF THE HEAD AND NECK

WALDEYER'S LYMPHATIC RING

At the entrance to the pharynx there is a considerable amount of lymphoid tissue which is grouped in a circular fashion round this part of the gut (*Fig.* 157), and is constituted as follows:

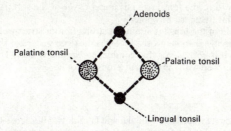

Fig. 157. Waldeyer's lymphatic ring.

Superior: The pharyngeal tonsils or adenoids—a central collection of lymphoid tissue in the roof of the pharynx.

Inferior: The lingual tonsil—situated on the posterior part of the dorsum of the tongue.

Lateral: The palatine tonsils, usually referred to as 'the tonsils', are situated at the isthmus of the fauces, one on each side.

THE TONSILS

Development

The tonsil lies in a fossa, the tonsillar fossa, which is the inner extremity of the second pharyngeal pouch. From the endoderm in the neighbourhood of the pouch, outgrowths invade the surrounding mesenchyme. These become canalized later, forming the crypts of the tonsil. Around these epithelial evaginations lymphoid tissue collects to form the lymphoid follicles of the organ. Part of this pouch remains as the intratonsillar cleft which penetrates the tonsil and may pass into the soft palate.

Situation

The tonsils are situated one on each side in the oropharynx, lying in the tonsillar fossa, between the palatoglossal and the palatopharyngeal folds (anterior and posterior pillars of the fauces). They are visible through the mouth when the tongue is depressed.

The tonsil is about 2 cm in its greatest dimension. When the tonsil enlarges, the area of tonsil exposed between arches depends on the direction in which enlargement has occurred. When expansion of the tonsil has occurred in an outward direction, much of the tonsil lies buried. In children, the upper third of the tonsil extends under cover of the soft palate, but by middle age this tissue has atrophied.

The capsule of the tonsil is a thin but strong fibrous structure, continuous with the pharyngeal aponeurosis. It covers the deep surface of the tonsil and extends into it to form septa that conduct nerves and vessels. The capsule is therefore removed with the tonsil in a tonsillectomy.

Relations

The organ has: two surfaces—medial and lateral; two borders—anterior and posterior; two poles—superior and inferior; two developmental folds related to it—the plica triangularis and plica semilunaris.

SURFACES:

Medial Surface: This faces inwards, bounding the passage from mouth to pharynx on each side. It is covered with squamous epithelium. On the surface are seen the opening of the 12–20 crypts of the organ. Plugs of pus or debris are often seen filling these openings.

Lateral Surface: This is separated by lax connective tissue from the superior constrictor muscle of the pharynx. The superior constrictor separates the tonsil from the following:

  1. The ascending palatine and tonsillar arteries.
  2. The glossopharyngeal nerve which may be temporarily affected by oedema following tonsillectomy, producing loss of taste over the posterior third of the tongue.
  3. The stylohyoid ligament.

Relation of the Tonsil to the Internal Carotid: This vessel lies 2·5 cm behind and lateral to the tonsil, separated from the pharynx by lax areolar tissue and fat, so that when the organ is pulled inwards with forceps prior to its removal, it is separated still further from the carotid.

BORDERS: The anterior border is in contact with the palatoglossus muscle. The posterior border is in contact with the palatopharyngeus muscle.

DEVELOPMENTAL FOLDS:
Plica Triangularis: This is a fold of mucous membrane passing from the lower part of the tonsil to the palatoglossal fold. It is constant in the fetus, but often disappears in the adult.
Plica Semilunaris: This is an occasional fold crossing the upper part of the tonsillar fossa.

BLOOD SUPPLY: This is very profuse, being obtained through the following arteries (*Fig.* 158):

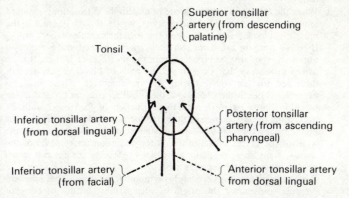

Fig. 158. The posterolateral surface of the left tonsil to show the blood supply. (After Morris.)

1. Anterior tonsillar—from dorsal lingual.
2. Posterior tonsillar—from ascending pharyngeal.
3. Superior tonsillar—from descending palatine.
4. Inferior tonsillar—from facial.

VENOUS DRAINAGE: The veins form a plexus around the capsule, draining into the pharyngeal plexus.

NERVES: The glossopharyngeal, having reached the base of the tongue, sends twigs upwards to supply the tonsil.

SPECIAL FEATURES OF PRACTICAL IMPORTANCE:

1. The tonsil capsule is separated by lax tissue from the superior constrictor, so that when the tonsil is pulled forward the wall of the pharynx is not pulled with it. While this fact is true for the normal or merely enlarged tonsil, it is not always the case.

2. Quinsy is a peritonsillar collection of pus, though the infection begins within the tonsil. After repeated attacks of quinsy the gland capsule is so densely adherent to the constrictor that only considerable force can separate the two. Under these circumstances the pulling forward of the tonsil displaces the pharyngeal wall inward also. It is obvious, therefore, that, having divided the attachments of the mucous membrane of the surroundings to that of the tonsil, the organ will, in the absence of previous inflammatory attacks, separate easily from the constrictor; should previous attacks of quinsy have occurred, no plane of cleavage exists and separation is difficult, i.e. the so-called 'adherent tonsil'.

3. When the tonsil and its capsule are removed, the constrictor is exposed and not the aponeurosis of the pharynx, which, though internal to the muscle, is blended with and is removed with the capsule of the tonsil.

4. Bleeding from the tonsillar fossa after removal of the tonsil presents an important similarity to bleeding from the uterus after labour. It is an axiom in surgery that clots round the ends of blood vessels are not disturbed for fear of restarting the haemorrhage. There are two exceptions, i.e. in the uterus and the tonsillar fossa, in both of which situations clots interfere with the retraction of the vessel walls by preventing the contraction of the surrounding muscles, i.e. the muscles bounding the tonsillar fossa in the one instance and those forming the walls of the uterus in the other. After operation for removal of the tonsils, many surgeons make a practice of clearing out any clot which may be present in the tonsillar fossa.

5. Bone or cartilage may very rarely be found in the tonsil. There are two possible sources for the origin of such tissue: spicules of bone or cartilage may be derived from embryonic 'rests' of the branchial arches, or ossification in the stylohyoid ligament may cause a very long styloid process to project into the tonsil.

LYMPHATIC DRAINAGE OF WALDEYER'S RING: This lymphoid tissue drains into:

1. The main lymph node of the tonsil; situated in the angle between the internal jugular and common facial veins just below the angle of the jaw. Other nodes in this region assist in the drainage.

2. Inframastoid (adenoid) nodes, which lie below the tip of the mastoid process under cover of the sternomastoid muscle, receive lymph from the adenoids (pharyngeal tonsils). These nodes lie in close relation to

the spinal accessory nerve which may be injured during biopsy of the nodes.

Both the tonsillar lymph node and the inframastoid nodes are members of the upper deep cervical lymph nodes.

LYMPH NODES OF THE NECK

Circular chain of nodes

This (*Fig.* 159) consists of the following node groups: (*a*) occipital; (*b*) posterior auricular; (*c*) pre-auricular; (*d*) parotid; (*e*) facial; (*f*) submandibular; (*g*) submental; (*h*) superficial cervical; (*i*) anterior cervical.

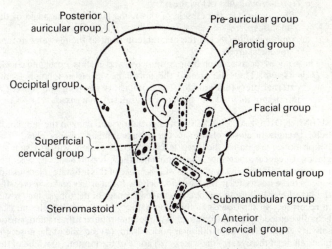

Fig. 159. The nodes of the circular chain.

OCCIPITAL NODES: One or two nodes situated midway between the mastoid process and the external occipital protuberance. They drain the back of the scalp.

POSTERIOR AURICULAR NODES: Situated on the mastoid process behind the pinna. They drain the temporal region of the scalp, back of the pinna, and external auditory meatus.

PRE-AURICULAR NODES: Situated immediately in front of the tragus; the situation is so definite that a swelling not exactly in front of the tragus cannot arise from this node. The node lies superficial to the parotid fascia. It drains the outer surface of the pinna and side of the scalp.

PAROTID NODES: These nodes are situated both in the substance of the parotid salivary gland and deep to it, i.e. between it and the side wall of the pharynx.

The deeper nodes drain: (a) the nasopharynx and (b) the back of the nose. The more superficial receive lymph from: (a) the eyelids; (b) front of the scalp; (c) external auditory meatus; (d) tympanic cavity.

FACIAL NODES: Consist of superficial and deep groups.
  Superficial Group: Consist of:
    a. *Infra-orbital:* Just below the orbit.
    b. *Buccinator:* On the muscle of this name lateral to the angle of the mouth.
    c. *Supramandibular:* On the mandible in front of the masseter around the facial artery.
  These nodes receive lymph from conjunctiva and eyelids, nose, and cheek.
  Deep Group: These lie around the maxillary vessels in relation to the external pterygoid muscle. They drain: (a) the temporal fossa; (b) infratemporal fossa; (c) back of the nose; (d) pharynx.

SUBMANDIBULAR NODES: An important group lying in the submandibular triangle in close relation to the submandibular salivary gland. The lymph nodes are under the deep fascia in actual contact with the salivary glands. In cancer, therefore, the removal of these lymph nodes necessitates the removal of the salivary gland as well because of this intimate relationship. One of these nodes lies in the S bend which the facial artery makes in crossing the mandible. Failure to remove this node in cancer of the tongue may result in recurrence of the disease in this lymph node. Small lymph nodes may be actually embedded in the substance of the submandibular salivary and parotid salivary glands. The submandibular nodes drain: (a) the side of the nose; (b) inner angle of the eye; (c) the cheek; (d) angle of the mouth; (e) whole of the upper lip; (f) outer part of the lower lip; (g) the gums; (h) some lymph from the side of the tongue.

SUBMENTAL NODES: These lie in the submental triangle. They drain the central part of the lower lip and the floor of the mouth. They receive some lymph from the apex of the tongue.

SUPERFICIAL CERVICAL NODES: These lie on the outer surface of the sternomastoid around the external jugular vein. They drain the parotid region and lower part of the ear.

ANTERIOR CERVICAL NODES: These lie near the middle line of the neck in front of the larynx and trachea. They consist of superficial and deep sets of nodes.

Superficial Set: Lie in relation to the anterior jugular vein and drain the skin of the neck. They are unimportant.

Deep Set: Consists of:

   a. The infrahyoid nodes: These lie on the thyrohyoid membrane and drain the front of the larynx.

   b. The prelaryngeal nodes: These lie on the cricothyroid ligament and drain the larynx. Their afferents pass through a small foramen in the middle of the cricothyroid ligament. These nodes are often the first to become enlarged in cancer of the larynx. The nodes assist in the drainage of the thyroid.

   c. The pretracheal nodes: These lie in relation to the inferior thyroid veins in front of the trachea and drain the thyroid and trachea.

EFFERENTS OF THE CIRCULAR CHAIN: The deep cervical chain receives ultimately all the lymph from the nodes enumerated above. It receives the efferents directly from all these node groups except the facial and submental. The efferents from these two groups pass first to the submandibular nodes.

Vertical chain of deep cervical nodes

This consists of a number of large nodes lying in relation to the carotid sheath. A few members of this group occupy an outlying position behind the pharynx and are called the 'retropharyngeal nodes'. They drain the back of the nose and pharynx and the auditory tube.

The vertical chain of deep cervical nodes lies alongside the pharynx, trachea, and oesophagus, and extends from the base of the skull to the root of the neck. They are arbitrarily divided into superior deep cervical and inferior deep cervical groups by the point of bifurcation of the common carotid (or, alternatively, by the omohyoid). The nodes of both groups are in very intimate relationship with the internal jugular vein. Some of the nodes of the inferior group project beyond the posterior border of the sternomastoid into the posterior triangle of the neck. There are a few small nodes of this group which lie in the groove between the trachea and oesophagus alongside the recurrent nerve. They are called paratracheal nodes and assist in the drainage of the thyroid. Two of the deep cervical group are named.

MAIN NODE OF THE TONSIL (JUGULODIAGASTRIC): *See above*.

JUGULO-OMOHYOID NODE: A node situated on the common carotid just above the point where the anterior belly of the omohyoid crosses this vessel. It plays a very important part in the lymph drainage of the tongue, receiving some vessels from the apex which take a circuitous route to reach the node.

The deep cervical nodes receive the lymph from the entire head and neck, either directly or indirectly from the nodes of the circular chain.

The lymph from the deep cervical chain, i.e. all the lymph from that half of the head and neck, is collected into one trunk, the jugular lymph trunk, which leaves the inferior deep cervical nodes. On the right side this trunk enters the junction of the subclavian vein and internal jugular vein. On the left side the trunk enters the thoracic duct.

Lymph drainage of the lips

The lower lip drains to the submental and submandibular nodes, thence to the deep cervical nodes.

There is communication of lymphatics across the midline in the upper and lower lips, therefore cancer near the midline of the lips may spread to the nodes on both sides of the neck. Some lymph from the outer third of the lip enters the mandible through the mental foramen which allows direct spread into the mandible in cancer of the lip. The upper lip and the junctions of the upper and lower lips have a more extensive lymph drainage than the lower lip. Some lymph passes directly to the upper deep cervical lymph nodes.

Lymph drainage of the tongue

The tongue is drained by lymph vessels which may be divided into four groups: (1) apical vessels; (2) marginal vessels; (3) central vessels; (4) basal vessels.

1. APICAL VESSELS: Vessels from the tip of the tongue pass in two directions: (*a*) to the submental nodes; (*b*) to the jugulo-omohyoid node.

2. MARGINAL VESSELS: These drain the side of the tongue and pass to the mandibular nodes and to the nodes of the deep cervical chain. Many of these trunks pass down on the outer surface of the hyoglossus muscle. There may be lymph nodules lying on the hyoglossus in relation to these lymph vessels. They are sometimes called 'lingual nodes'. They are palpated by one finger in the floor of the mouth, the fingers of the other hand being beneath the mandible.

3. CENTRAL VESSELS: These are vessels which drain the area of the tongue on either side of the median raphe (*Fig*. 160). They pass vertically downwards in the midline of the tongue between the genioglossi muscles and then pass, some to the left and some to the right, to the deep cervical nodes.

4. BASAL VESSELS: These trunks drain the posterior part of the tongue.

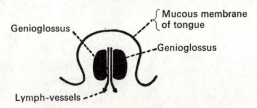

Fig. 160. Median group of lymphatic vessels of tongue.

Many of them pass freely from one side of the tongue to the other. They enter the deep cervical nodes.

From this description it will be seen that in cancer of the tongue, cancer cells may pass freely to lymphatic nodes on both sides of the neck.

In 50 per cent of normal individuals, the lymphatics of the tongue and floor of the mouth pass through the periosteum of the mandible on their way to the lymph nodes in the submandibular triangle, thus accounting for the frequency of early attachment of the metastases to the jaw. It is apparent that when cancer of the floor of the mouth approaches the jaw, removal of part or all of the body of the mandible is necessary. The mental foramen on the outer surface of the mandible is about equidistant from its upper and lower borders, and the foramen is, therefore, some distance from the intra-oral cavity. In older people who are edentulous, the alveolus is absorbed and the mental foramen may be only 1 mm from the upper border of the mandible instead of 15 mm. It is then an intra-oral structure being separated from the mouth by the mucoperiosteum only and offers a ready route for cancer of the floor of the mouth to invade the mandibular canal. Thus the situation of this foramen is an important factor in enabling the surgeon to plan the extent of bone removal in cancer of the floor of the mouth encroaching on the jaw. Once the mandibular canal is invaded, extensive resection of the mandible is necessary (*Fig.* 161).

RADICAL NECK DISSECTION

In this procedure all of the lymphatics and nodal tissue is removed between the platysma and the deep cervical fascia from the level of the mandible superiorly, the lateral border of the strap muscles medially, the anterior border of the trapezius posteriorly and the clavicle inferiorly. The following structures are preserved: the carotid artery, the mandibular branch of the facial nerve, the vagus, phrenic and hypoglossal nerves and the cervical sympathetic chain. The spinal accessory nerve is usually sacrificed but this produces a shoulder drop.

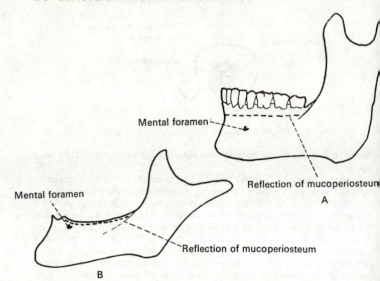

Fig. 161. A, The relation of the mental foramen to the mucoperiosteum when the teeth are in situ. B, The relation of the mental foramen to the mucoperiosteum in the edentulous jaw.

Note that the internal jugular vein is removed because of the close association of the deep cervical lymph nodes to this vessel.

When a radical neck dissection is combined with an incontinuity resection of lesions of the oral cavity and/or mandible, it is termed a composite or 'commando' resection.

Chapter 17

THE THYROID, THYMUS AND THE PARATHYROID GLANDS

THE THYROID GLAND

Development
The thyroid gland develops as a median downgrowth of a column of cells from the pharyngeal floor between the first and second pharyngeal pouches

(subsequently marked by the foramen caecum of the tongue). The canalized column becomes the thyroglossal duct which is displaced forwards by the developing hyoid bone and then, below the hyoid, lies slightly to one side, more commonly the left. The duct bifurcates to form the thyroid lobes and a portion of the duct forms the pyramidal lobe (*Fig.* 162).

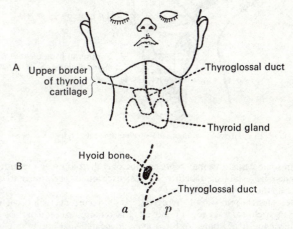

Fig. 162. A, Course of thyroglossal duct, anterior view; note divergence to left below upper border of thyroid cartilage. B, Lateral view, showing relationship between duct and hyoid bone, *a,* Anterior; *b* posterior.

Congenital anomalies

A few clinically relevant developmental errors may occur.

ECTOPIC THYROID TISSUE: Ectopic thyroid tissue may lie anywhere along the line of descent and may, in rare instances, be the only thyroid tissue present. An occasional site for this anomaly is in the base of the tongue. Ectopic thyroid tissue can be identified by isotope scanning.

THYROGLOSSAL CYST: A thyroglossal cyst results from persistence of a portion of the thyroglossal duct. It is the commonest congenital error and presents as an asymptomatic swelling somewhere along the course of the duct, but usually below the level of the hyoid bone (*Fig.* 163). These cysts usually become clinically evident in the late teens, presumably because the lining becomes secretory. There is often thyroid tissue associated with the cyst

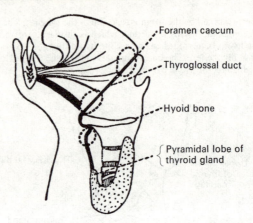

Fig. 163. Thyroglossal duct, and sites occupied by thyroglossal cysts.

and, in some cases, this may represent the only thyroid tissue present. This fact must be established before surgical excision is performed to avoid rendering the patient hypothyroid.

After surgical removal of thyroglossal cysts, recurrence will occur if the whole thyroglossal track is not removed. This requires excision of the central section of the hyoid bone and it is even advocated that coring out of the suprahyoid portion of the duct remnant is necessary. Surgical practice often ignores this advice and its importance is in doubt.

AGENESIS: Total agenesis of one thyroid lobe may occur. This is rare but can be clinically important, leading to confusion in diagnosis, especially in toxic glands, when it could be diagnosed as a secreting nodule.

Anatomy

The thyroid gland occupies an important position in the centre of the visceral compartment of the neck, lying astride the trachea just above the thoracic inlet. Normally weighing about 25 g, the anatomy of this vital endocrine gland is relevant both to the non-operating clinician and in operative surgery.

The gland has two lobes, shaped roughly like slender pears, hugging the anterolateral aspect of the cervical trachea from the level of the thyroid cartilage to the 5th or 6th tracheal ring. The right lobe is often larger than the left and the lobes are joined together across the midline by a thin isthmus plastered quite firmly to the anterior surface of the trachea, at the level of the 2nd and 3rd tracheal rings. A variable-sized, but usually small, pyramidal lobe arises from the isthmus somewhere along its upper border near the midline. The thyroid gland is covered by fascia and the strap muscles and, more laterally, it is tucked under the diverging anterior borders of the sternomastoid muscles.

Clinical beginners often search for the gland too high in the neck. It should be palpated from behind the subject with the middle and index fingers lying just above the sternoclavicular joint across the trachea, as though spreading the converging sternomastoid muscles. Because of its fascial attachments, the gland moves upwards with swallowing and, therefore, it slides under the examining fingers. The normal gland can be felt in thin necks. It is soft and supple and the tracheal rings can be palpated through it.

The important anatomical features with surgical relevance are:

1. THE MUSCULOFASCIAL COVERINGS: The strap muscles are ensheathed by the general investing layer of cervical fascia and this unites them in the midline. These muscles are applied to the anterior surface of the gland, but separated from it by a loose condensation of fascia derived from the pretracheal fascia. This false capsule covers the gland which is enclosed by its diaphanous true capsule with its very rich blood supply, clearly visible just beneath its surface. (*See Fig.* 164.)

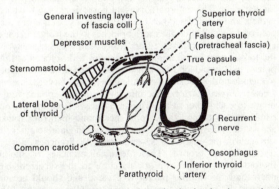

Fig. 164. The relations of the thryoid arteries to the gland and to the capsules. Observe that, whereas the superior thyroid artery enters the superficial aspect of the gland, the inferior thyroid enters its deep aspect.

In the surgical approach to the thyroid gland, the musculofascial envelope is incised down the midline, which is relatively avascular, and the 'space' between the two capsules of the gland is entered. This loose plane is easily developed and the gland exposed by retracting the strap muscles. The nerve supply of these muscles, the sternohyoid and its deeper neighbour, the sternothyroid, comes from cervical roots 1, 2 and 3 via branches from the ansa cervicalis. These branches enter the muscle at its lateral border and on the deep surface and, though it is not often necessary, the muscles may be divided transversely to facilitate access to the gland. Provided they are resutured, there does not appear to be any impairment of function.

The other important implication of the musculofascial covering of the gland is that at the end of thyroid operations the divided fascial envelope is resutured in the midline and this again closes the visceral space. If there is postoperative haemorrhage into this closed space, respiratory embarrassment from tracheal compression results and requires immediate release of the sutures to restore the airway.

2. THE VASCULAR SUPPLY: As would be expected from its endocrine function, the blood supply of the thyroid gland (*Fig*. 164) is very rich in the hyperthyroid state, and there may be an enormous increase in the volume of blood circulating through the gland. Each thyroid lobe is supplied by a superior and an inferior thyroid artery and drained by three veins.

The Superior Vascular Pedicle: The superior vascular pedicle contains the superior thyroid artery, which is the first branch of the external carotid, and its accompanying vein, which drains into the internal jugular vein. The external laryngeal nerve is closely related to this pedicle and is discussed below. The superior vessels enter the upper pole of the gland at its apex with branches to the front and back of the gland. These superior vessels are easily dealt with surgically, because the loose space between the two capsules is developed at the upper pole of the thyroid lobe and a ligature is placed close to the upper pole, to include both vessels and exclude the external laryngeal nerve.

The Inferior Thyroid Artery: The inferior thyroid artery and vein do not relate to each other at all. The artery arises from the thyrocervical trunk, passes behind the carotid sheath and then runs transversely across the space between this and the thyroid gland to enter the deep surface of the gland as several separate branches close to the tracheothyroid groove. These terminal branches of the inferior thyroid artery are uncomfortably close to the recurrent laryngeal nerve and the inferior parathyroid gland and should be surgically shunned. If the inferior thyroid artery is to be ligated, it should be done in its transverse portion medial to the carotid sheath.

The Inferior Thyroid Veins: The inferior thyroid veins, of which there are always a few on each side, leave the lower border of the gland and pass through the loose fascial space to join the left brachiocephalic vein. They are fragile and require to be ligated singly (*Fig*. 165).

The Middle Thyroid Vein: The applied anatomy of the middle thyroid vein is important because it is a short, thin-walled vessel, leaving the middle of the gland and directly coursing laterally to pass in front of or behind

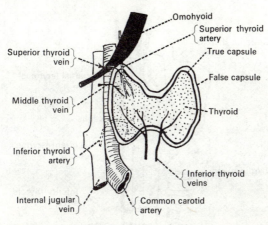

Fig. 165. The blood vessels of the thyroid. The veins do not accompany the arteries.

the carotid artery and enter the internal jugular vein. It is the first vessel encountered in thyroidectomy and merits careful ligation when it is met early on during the development of the intercapsular space mentioned above.

The Thyroidea Ima Artery: The thyroidea ima artery from the brachiocephalic trunk extending in front of the trachea is small and surgically irrelevant.

3. THE IMPORTANT CLOSE SURGICAL RELATIONS OF THE THYROID GLAND: These are the recurrent laryngeal nerves, the external laryngeal nerves and the parathyroid glands. Like all important relations they should be recognized immediately and cared for respectfully.

The External Laryngeal Nerve: The external laryngeal nerve (*Fig.* 166), a branch of the superior laryngeal nerve, descends on the fascia of the inferior pharyngeal constrictor, relates closely to the superior vascular pedicle of the thyroid and then leaves this at a variable height above the gland to travel medially to its destination in the cricothyroid muscle. It is functionally important to the pitch of the voice because the cricothyroid muscle is a tensor of the vocal cord. Damage to this nerve alters the voice quite significantly, and is especially noticeable in singers. Its surgical avoidance has been mentioned.

The Recurrent Laryngeal Nerve: The recurrent laryngeal nerve (*Fig.* 167) is a branch of the vagus arising embryologically in relation to the 4th aortic arch vessels. Because of the descent of these vessels forming the subclavian artery on the right and the aortic arch on the left, the

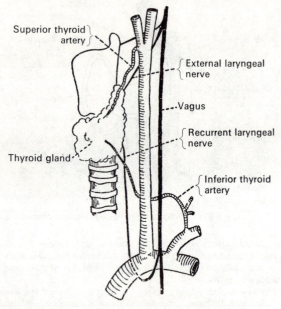

Fig. 166. Shows the intimate relationship of the external laryngeal branch of the vagus to the superior thyroid artery. (After Lennox Gordon.)

recurrent nerves are taken caudally and thus run an upward course to reach their vocal cord destination. The nerves usually lie in the tracheo-oesophageal groove and then bear a variable relationship to the branches of the inferior thyroid artery before entering the larynx. In the majority of cases, the nerve is found easily in the tracheo-oesophageal groove just below the thyroid gland, but its course may be anomalous and it may be much more lateral. In very rare instances, because of failure of development of the 4th arch vessel and a resultant anomalous right subclavian artery, the nerve on that side will be non-recurrent and then passes directly medially at a much higher level from the vagus to the larynx. In this position it could be in danger at the time of ligation of the middle thyroid vein, though the difference between these two structures should be easily apparent.

The Parathyroid Glands: The anatomy of the parathyroid glands is described below and from a consideration of this it will be obvious that they will be at risk during operations on the thyroid gland.

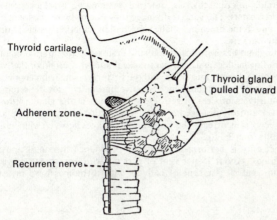

Fig. 167. The recurrent laryngeal nerve is well posterior to the gland, lying in the tracheo-oesophageal sulcus.

LYMPH DRAINAGE: Numerous lymphatic vessels leave the gland and drain to lymph nodes situated:
1. In the midline on the front surface of the larynx and trachea.
2. In the tracheo-oesophageal groove extending downwards into the superior mediastinum.
3. Upwards and laterally to the deep cervical chain and nodes lateral to this.

A consideration of the complexity of this lymphatic drainage and the anatomical distribution of the regional nodes becomes important in management of metastatic papillary thyroid cancer. Because of the wide distribution of the nodes, standard radical neck dissection has been abandoned in favour of 'regional' node removal.

Nodular retrosternal enlargements of the thyroid occur by downward extension. It is important to note that the blood supply of such retrosternal thyroid tissue comes from the neck and this means that its operative removal can always be conducted by the normal cervical approach.

THE THYMUS

The thymus gland lies behind the manubrium, anterior to the great vessels of the superior mediastinum. It is noteworthy that:
1. The organ is always connected to the thyroid by a strand of tissue known as the thyrothymic ligament.
2. It receives a good arterial supply from the vessels in the neighbour-

hood: inferior thyroid, internal mammary, brachiocephalic and intercostals. The venous drainage is by one or two large lobular veins going to the brachiocephalic veins and by superior vessels joining the thyroid veins.

3. The gland has a profuse lymphatic drainage (into internal mammary, anterior mediastinal, and paratracheal nodes). Certain of the lymphatics open directly into veins, without first traversing lymph nodes.

4. The gland is an organ which is active during the growth period. After maturity, a process of retrogression occurs in the gland, although it never entirely disappears. The old idea that the gland disappears at puberty is incorrect. The size varies at all ages between wide limits—in adults from 2·7 to 32 g.

Thymectomy is performed for thymic tumours (thymoma) and myasthenia gravis. About 15 per cent of patients with myasthenia gravis have thymomas and 30 per cent of patients with thymomas have myasthenia gravis.

THE PARATHYROID GLANDS

The number of parathyroids vary from 2 to 6, but, in 80 per cent of cases, there are 4 (2 on each side). The total weight of 4 normal glands is about 140 mg.

Embryology

The upper parathyroids arise from the 4th branchial pouch and come to lie in close association with the upper part of the lateral lobes of the thyroid. This position is constant.

The lower parathyroids arise from the 3rd branchial pouch in association with the thymus, and descend with the thymus. Because of this embryological migration they may be found anywhere from the upper pole of the thyroid to the anterior mediastinum.

Anatomy

The glands are the size of a split pea. They are pink or brown in colour, but are frequently covered by fat, making them difficult to recognize.

The superior glands lie on the posterior surface of the middle third of the thyroid, usually above the inferior thyroid artery, but well posterior to this plane. If enlarged they may descend into the posterior mediastinum.

The inferior glands are mostly found on the posterior surface of the lower pole of the thyroid or within 1 cm below the lower pole. They may be higher or lower, occasionally as far down as in the thymus in the anterior mediastinum. They lie in a more anterior plane than the upper glands.

A parathyroid gland located within the surgical false capsule of the thyroid, when diseased, remains in place locally. A gland outside the capsule is often displaced into the posterior mediastinum. Sometimes the parathyroids may be embedded in the thyroid gland.

Blood supply

A special small parathyroid artery supplies each gland. The lower parathyroid artery comes from the inferior thyroid artery and is a guide to the gland if it lies below the lower margin of the thyroid.

The upper parathyroid artery arises from the inferior artery or from an anastomosing artery joining the superior and inferior thyroid arteries and only very occasionally from the superior thyroid artery.

There is a good collateral arterial supply from the tracheal vessels and adequate parathyroid function persists even if all four major thyroid arteries are ligated.

Surgical significance

During thyroidectomy, the parathyroids may be damaged or removed, resulting in postthyroidectomy hypoparathyroidism. This must be avoided by exposing and protecting the glands.

Due to the use of the auto-analyser, asymptomatic hypercalcaemia is being increasingly diagnosed in patients with hyperparathyroidism. The hypercalcaemia is usually due to an adenoma or hyperplasia of the parathyroids. This is treated by excision of the affected glands. It can almost always be achieved through a cervical incision, but in about 1 per cent of cases a mediastinotomy is required.

Chapter 18

THE AUTONOMIC NERVOUS SYSTEM

The autonomic nervous system is concerned with the innervation of viscera, glands, blood vessels and non-striated muscle (*Fig.* 168). The peripheral autonomic nervous system, which is comprised of the sympathetic system (thoracolumbar outflow) and the parasympathetic system (craniosacral outflow), is under the control of central autonomic centres in the brain stem, hypothalamus and the cerebral cortex.

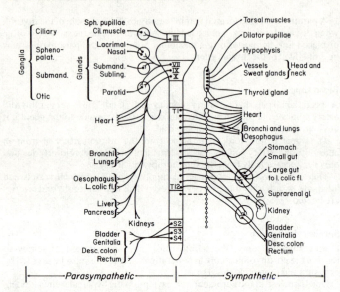

Fig. 168. The autonomic nervous system.

GENERAL ARRANGEMENT OF THE AUTONOMIC NERVOUS SYSTEM

Efferent autonomic nerve fibres

All efferent fibres of the sympathetic and parasympathetic nervous systems are interrupted in their course by a synapse in a peripheral ganglion. The preganglionic fibres which arise in the central nervous system are medullated while the postganglionic fibres are non-medullated.

In the sympathetic nervous system, the preganglionic fibres are the axons of nerve cells in the lateral column of grey matter of all the thoracic and upper two lumbar segments of the spinal cord. The preganglionic fibres synapse with nerve cells in

  a. The paravertebral sympathetic trunk.
  b. Prevertebral nerve plexuses (collateral ganglia).
  c. The adrenal medulla.

In the parasympathetic nervous system, the preganglionic cranial fibres arise from Edinger–Westphal (IIIrd nerve), salivary (VIIth and IXth nerves), ambiguus and dorsal motor (Xth nerve) nuclei in the brain stem. The sacral fibres arise in the grey matter of the spinal cord from the 2nd to 4th sacral segments. The preganglionic fibres synapse with ganglia nearer to the structures innervated than to the central nervous system or with ganglia dispersed in the walls of the viscera themselves.

Preganglionic sympathetic fibres are usually short and synapse with many postganglionic nerves which gives sympathetic discharges a widespread effect. This is in contrast with preganglionic parasympathetic fibres which are long and synapse with only a few postganglionic neurones, giving parasympathetic discharges a more limited effect.

Afferent autonomic nerve fibres

Afferent sensory fibres from viscera and the walls of blood vessels are distributed with the pre- and postganglionic fibres of the autonomic nervous system. These sensory fibres are not interrupted in autonomic ganglia, but have their cell bodies in some of the cranial and the dorsal spinal nerve ganglia.

These fibres subserve the following functions:

1. Visceral reflexes which usually do not reach the level of consciousness, e.g. in breathing.
2. Vascular reflexes such as the carotid sinus reflex in response to arterial pressure.
3. Organic visceral sensations such as hunger or visceral distension.
4. Visceral pain which is poorly localized and described as dull, but can be severe and varying in intensity. The pain may be referred to the skin or some other somatic structure, of which the sensory fibres are associated with the same segment of the spinal cord as the afferent fibres of the viscus causing the pain.

   This is in contrast with somatic pain which occurs when a serous lining, e.g. peritoneum, becomes inflamed. Pain sensation is then transmitted in the somatic nervous system and is accurately localized to the region of the body wall overlying the viscus.

Transmitter substances in autonomic nerve synapses

SYMPATHETIC NERVOUS SYSTEM:
   Preganglionic Nerve Endings: Acetylcholine is the transmitter substance (this includes preganglionic nerve endings in the adrenal medulla).
   Postganglionic Nerve Endings: Noradrenaline is the transmitter substance except in the case of the postganglionic nerve fibres to sweat glands where acetylcholine is the transmitter substance.

PARASYMPATHETIC NERVOUS SYSTEM: Acetylcholine is the transmitter substance at all parasympathetic nerve endings both pre- and postganglionic.

THE SYMPATHETIC NERVOUS SYSTEM

Preganglionic nerve fibres arise from the lateral column of grey matter in T1–L2 segments of the cord. They leave the cord in the anterior roots of the corresponding spinal nerves, run a short course in the mixed spinal nerve and beyond the junction of the posterior primary rami leave the spinal nerves as white rami communicantes (myelinated) to join the sympathetic trunk. A white ramus joins the sympathetic trunk (*Fig.* 169) from each spinal nerve from T1 to L2.

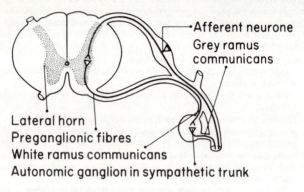

Fig. 169. Sympathetic reflex arc.

The sympathetic trunks

These trunks present as paired paravertebral sympathetic trunks which consist of ganglia joined by nerve fibres. The trunks extend from the base of the skull to the front of the coccyx where they join to form the ganglion impar. There are 3 cervical, 11 thoracic, 4 lumbar and 4 sacral ganglia. Developmentally there are ganglia for each spinal nerve but fusion of adjacent ganglia has reduced the number.

It should be noted that only the ganglia from T1 to L2 receive white rami communicantes and that the trunk above and below these levels is formed by the continuation of white rami.

Intermediate sympathetic ganglia may be found in spinal nerve roots or rami communicantes. Preganglionic fibres destined for these ganglia bypass the sympathetic trunk which is one of the explanations of failure after surgical removal of part of the sympathetic trunk.

From the sympathetic trunk the fibres may follow one of the following paths:

1. SOMATIC FIBRES: These enter the paravertebral sympathetic trunk to synapse in ganglia corresponding to their spinal segment of origin or with a ganglion higher or lower in the sympathetic trunk and are then distributed as grey rami communicantes (non-myelinated postganglionic fibres) to every one of the 31 paired spinal nerves. These postganglionic fibres supply vasoconstrictor fibres to arterioles, secretory fibres to sweat glands and pilomotor fibres to the somatic distribution of the skin. Grey fibres do not run up or down in the sympathetic trunk. Where fusion of ganglia has occurred, the fused ganglion will give rise to the same number of grey rami, as the number of ganglia from which it was constituted. The three cervical ganglia give rise to somatic branches which accompany the cervical nerves, but the superior cervical ganglion also gives rise to somatic branches which are distributed to the skin area of the trigeminal nerve through the internal and external carotid arteries.

2. VISCERAL FIBRES:
   a. To the thoracic viscera synapse in the cervical and upper thoracic ganglia and the grey (postganglionic) fibres reach the viscera through the cardiac, oesophageal and pulmonary plexuses.
   b. To the abdominal viscera traverse the ganglia in the paravertebral chain without synapse, enter one of the splanchnic nerves and synapse in the ganglia of one of the abdominal prevertebral plexuses.
   c. To the adrenal medulla run through the paravertebral trunk without synapsing and proceed in the greater splanchnic nerve through the coeliac plexus to the adrenal medulla, where they synapse with ganglion cells which have the same embryonic origin as sympathetic ganglia.
   d. To the cranial structures, such as the dilator pupillae, superior tarsal muscle, the nasal and salivary glands, are conducted by grey rami which accompany the carotid vessels, like their somatic counterparts. The lower larynx, trachea, hypopharynx and upper oesophagus receive grey (postganglionic) fibres from the middle cervical ganglion, which accompany the inferior thyroid artery.

The cervical sympathetic trunk

This nerve trunk (*Fig.* 170) lies in the prevertebral fascia between the carotid sheath in front and the prevertebral muscles (longus colli and capitis) behind. At its lower part it is continuous with the sympathetic trunk in the thorax; above it is continued into the skull as the internal carotid nerve which forms a plexus of nerves around the internal carotid artery.

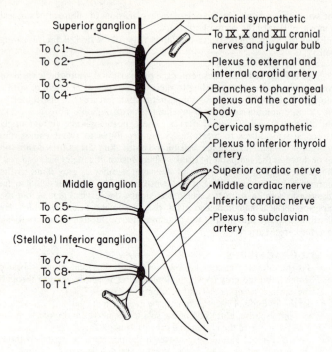

Fig. 170. The cervical sympathetic trunk.

There are three ganglia on the cervical sympathetic trunk. The upper and lower are large, the middle small. Each of the three ganglia gives: (i) grey rami communicantes to the cervical nerves, (ii) a cardiac nerve, and (iii) a plexus to an artery.

THE SUPERIOR CERVICAL SYMPATHETIC GANGLION: The largest ganglion in the neck. It lies in front of the transverse processes of the 2nd and 3rd cervical vertebrae on the longus capitis, behind the carotid sheath.

It gives rise to:

1. Lateral Branches:
    a. Grey rami communicantes to the upper four cervical nerves.
    b. Twigs to the glossopharyngeal, hypoglossal and vagus nerves.
    c. The jugular bulb.

2. Medial Branches:
   a. Laryngopharyngeal to the carotid body and the pharyngeal plexus.
   b. Cardiac branches to the cardiac plexus.
   c. Anterior branches to the internal and external carotid arteries.
      These branches are both somatic to the skin area of the
      trigeminal nerve and visceral to the dilator pupillae, the
      superior tarsal muscle and the nasal and salivary glands.

THE MIDDLE CERVICAL GANGLION: The smallest of the three, and
lies on the 6th cervical vertebra, in front of or behind the inferior thyroid
artery at about the level of the cricoid cartilage and the transverse process of
C6. The ganglion sometimes occupies a lower position, near the inferior
ganglion, of which it is considered a part.
   It gives rise to:
   1. Grey rami communicantes to the 5th and 6th cervical nerves.
   2. Cardiac nerve which is the largest of the sympathetic cardiac branches.
   3. A vascular branch which runs with the inferior thyroid artery to the
      thyroid and parathyroid glands.

CERVICOTHORACIC (STELLATE) GANGLION: This is a large
ganglion formed by the fusion of the lower two cervical segmental ganglia
with the first thoracic ganglion. When not fused with the first thoracic
ganglion the upper mass is known as the inferior cervical ganglion.
   It lies behind the vertebral artery between the neck of the 1st rib and the
transverse process of the 7th cervical vertebra. It is separated from the
posterior aspect of the cervical pleura by the suprapleural membrane.
   It gives rise to:
   1. Grey rami communicantes to the 7th, 8th cervical and 1st thoracic spinal
      nerves.
   2. A plexus to the subclavian artery and its branches. There is a separate
      vascular branch to the vertebral artery which is purely vasomotor.
   Sympathetic Supply to the Head and Neck: The preganglionic fibres to the
      head and neck are derived from T1 to T5 segments of the spinal cord.
      Fibres ascend in the sympathetic trunk and synapse in the cervical
      ganglia from where they are distributed to the head and neck.
         It is of surgical importance that the sympathetic nerve supply to the
      pupil and the smooth muscle of the eyelids (oculopupillary fibres)
      joins the sympathetic trunk at the cervicothoracic ganglion from the
      1st thoracic segment of the cord.
Kuntz described a communicating branch between the 1st and 2nd
thoracic nerves in the chest. This branch receives grey rami from the stellate
and 2nd thoracic ganglia. When the communicating branch joins the 1st
thoracic nerve (not the 1st intercostal nerve), it constitutes a pathway through

which sympathetic fibres can leave the sympathetic trunk below the stellate ganglion and reach the upper limb through the 1st thoracic nerve contribution to the brachial plexus.

Less commonly the 3rd thoracic ganglion supplies a similar pathway to the upper limb via the 2nd thoracic nerve (nerve of Kirgis and Kuntz) (*Fig.* 171).

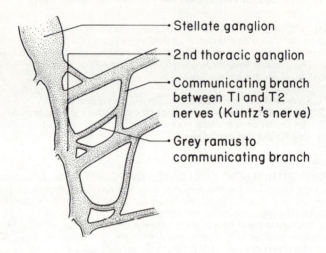

- Stellate ganglion
- 2nd thoracic ganglion
- Communicating branch between T1 and T2 nerves (Kuntz's nerve)
- Grey ramus to communicating branch

Fig. 171. The nerve of Kuntz.

The thoracic sympathetic trunk

This portion of the trunk is usually comprised of 11 ganglia of which the first is fused to the inferior cervical ganglion in 80 per cent of dissections.

The upper 10 ganglia lie outside the parietal pleura against the heads of the ribs and the lower 2 ganglia lie on the sides of the bodies of the corresponding vertebrae. The sympathetic trunk becomes continuous with the lumbar sympathetic trunk when it passes into the abdomen dorsal to the medial arcuate ligament.

Branches:

1. Grey rami communicantes to all the spinal nerves.
2. Visceral branches from the upper 6 ganglia to the pulmonary and cardiac plexus.

3. The splanchnic nerves:
   a. The greater splanchnic nerve consists of myelinated preganglionic fibres from the 5th to the 10th thoracic ganglia. It descends obliquely on the bodies of the vertebrae, perforates the crus of the diaphragm and the majority of fibres end in the coeliac ganglion in the coeliac plexus.
   b. The lesser splanchnic nerve arises from the 9th and 10th thoracic ganglia and also pierces the crus of the diaphragm. It joins an aorticorenal ganglion.
   c. The lowest splanchnic nerve arises from the last thoracic ganglion. It enters the abdomen with the sympathetic trunk and ends in the renal plexus.

The coeliac plexus

This plexus is formed largely by contributions from the greater splanchnic and 1st lumbar splanchnic nerves.

The plexus is situated around the origin of the coeliac artery, there being a large nerve mass on each side of this vessel known as the coeliac ganglion.

This plexus is continuous with a network of sympathetic nerves in relation to the aorta—the aortic plexus.

Numerous branches accompany the blood vessels arising from the aorta and are known by the same names, e.g. phrenic, adrenal, renal plexuses etc.

Nerves from these plexuses run to the abdominal viscera via the blood vessels.

The lumbar sympathetic trunk

There is a lumbar sympathetic trunk on each side. The trunk lies retroperitoneally on the anterolateral surface of the bodies of the lumbar vertebrae along the medial margin of the psoas major muscle. The trunk lies anterior to the lumbar arteries and veins but some veins may pass anterior to it. On the right side the trunk is overlapped by the inferior vena cava and on the left side it is partially covered by the aorta. The lateral aortic lymph nodes lie in close association with the trunk. The genitofemoral nerve passes through the fibres of the psoas major muscle and then lies on the anterior surface of the muscle lateral to the sympathetic trunk. The ureter also lies lateral to the sympathetic trunk.

The 1st and 2nd lumbar ventral rami send white rami communicantes to the corresponding lumbar ganglia. There are usually 4 ganglia on each side, but they are variable in number, size and position. The 1st lumbar ganglia may lie above the fascia of the medial arcuate ligament or under the insertion of the crus. It is impossible to assign a constant position to the various ganglia in relation to the lumbar vertebrae.

The sympathetic trunk below the last lumbar ganglion divides into 2 or 3 fine branches which pass posterior to the common iliac artery and continues as the pelvic part of the sympathetic trunk.

Branches:
1. Splanchnic nerves pass from the ganglia to join the coeliac, intermesenteric and superior hypogastric plexuses.
2. Grey rami communicantes from all the ganglia to the lumbar spinal nerves.

The hypogastric plexuses

The nerves from these plexuses run to the abdominal viscera via the blood vessels.

The superior hypogastric (or presacral) plexus lies in front of the sacral promontory. It is formed by strands from the lower end of the aortic plexus, receiving also branches from the ganglionated trunk on each side. The plexus divides into two nerves which run down on either side of the rectum to form the inferior hypogastric plexus behind the base of the bladder. This plexus supplies the bladder, rectum, and internal and external genitalia along the branches of the internal iliac artery (*Fig.* 172).

The hypogastric plexuses receive autonomic sensory fibres from the pelvic viscera, e.g. sympathetic pain fibres and parasympathetic fibres transmitting the sensation of bladder distension.

The inferior hypogastric plexus also receives parasympathetic contributions from the pelvic splanchnic nerves (nervi erigentes) from segments S2, S3 and S4.

Pelvic part of the sympathetic system

This part of the sympathetic trunk is situated in the extraperitoneal tissue in front of the sacrum medial to the anterior sacral foramina. The trunks converge caudally to form the ganglion impar on the anterior aspect of the coccyx. There are normally 4 or 5 sacral ganglia. The sympathetic trunk gives rise to grey rami to the sacral and coccygeal nerves. Medial branches join the inferior hypogastric plexus.

THE PARASYMPATHETIC NERVOUS SYSTEM

The parasympathetic nervous system is smaller than the sympathetic nervous system and has only visceral branches. It consists of a cranial and a sacral component.

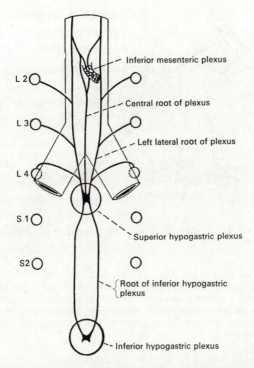

Fig. 172. Showing the superior and inferior hypogastric plexuses and the method of their formation. The small circles are part of the lateral chain of sympathetic ganglia.

Cranial

1. Four cranial ganglia: ciliary (p. 358), pterygopalatine (p. 360), submandibular (p. 362) and otic (p. 361). Only the parasympathetic fibres synapse in these ganglia which are also traversed by a sympathetic and a sensory root (*Fig.* 173).
2. The vagus nerve contains efferent parasympathetic fibres which arise in its dorsal nucleus and the nucleus ambiguus, and which are destined for the thoracic and abdominal viscera via the cardiac, pulmonary oesophageal and coeliac plexuses. These fibres are relayed in small ganglia which lie in the walls of the individual viscera.

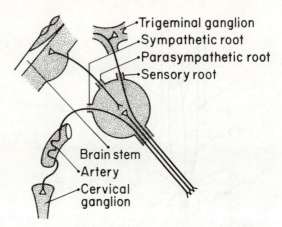

Fig. 173. Connections of the cranial parasympathetic ganglia.

Sacral

The anterior rami of the 2nd, 3rd and, frequently, the 4th sacral spinal nerves give rise to preganglionic fibres which form the pelvic splanchnic nerves (nervi erigentes). These nerves join the inferior hypogastric plexus and supply the pelvic viscera either directly or by accompanying the branches of the external iliac artery. Damage to these nerves during pelvic surgery may result in impotence.

SURGICAL SYMPATHECTOMY

Indications

Sympathectomy is used in peripheral vascular disease, to abolish excessive sweating and to relieve pain.

1. PERIPHERAL VASCULAR DISEASE:
   a. Sympathectomy may be used in organic occlusion of arteries in which direct vascular surgery will not relieve the obstruction. Sympathectomy often produces at least temporary vasodilatation and may accelerate the development of collaterals.
   b. Sympathectomy has also been used in certain vasospastic conditions. Raynaud's disease is a condition in which there is intermittent closure of

small arteries supplying the digits when the hands or feet are exposed to cold. This may be exacerbated or precipitated by sympathetic over-activity.

2. HYPERHIDROSIS: Gross sweating of the hands, axillae and feet is a severe disability. Sympathectomy is certain to give permanent relief and this constitutes the most cogent indication for sympathectomy.

3. RELIEF OF PAIN:
   a. *Visceral Pain:* Excision of the coeliac ganglion or its destruction by the injection of absolute alcohol or phenol has been used to relieve pain of pancreatic cancer or chronic pancreatitis.
   b. *Causalgia:* This condition is characterized by intense pain at the site of previous injury or operation. In some patients sympathectomy may produce relief but in general this is an unrewarding procedure.

Upper thoracic and cervical (cervicothoracic) sympathectomy

The aim of this operation is to obtain sympathetic denervation of the upper limb without dividing the oculopupillary fibres. Division of the latter fibres results in Horner's syndrome (p. 385).

The sympathetic supply to the upper limb comes from the upper thoracic segments of the spinal cord T2–T6 as white rami which leave the spinal nerves and ascend in the thoracic sympathetic trunk to the stellate (cervicothoracic) ganglion and sometimes to the 2nd and 3rd thoracic sympathetic ganglia. Postganglionic (grey rami) are supplied to the brachial plexus.

To achieve complete denervation of the upper extremity either a ganglionectomy or division of the rami to the relevant ganglia may be performed.

GANGLIONECTOMY: The stellate ganglion is best left undisturbed to prevent damage to the oculopupillary fibres from the 1st thoracic nerve, but the 2nd and 3rd ganglia are freed of all rami and the trunk is divided above the 2nd and below the 3rd ganglion and both ganglia are excised.

Following ganglionectomy of the 2nd thoracic ganglion but with preservation of the stellate ganglion there is, however, a reported incidence of Horner's syndrome, which has been attributed to disruption of oculopupil-lary fibres from T1, initially descending in the sympathetic trunk as far as the 2nd ganglion before coursing upwards to synapse in the superior cervical ganglion.

DIVISION OF THE RAMI TO THE 2ND AND 3RD GANGLIA: The trunk is divided below the 3rd ganglion and the rami of the 2nd and 3rd ganglia are sectioned. This procedure has the lowest incidence of Horner's syndrome. The mobilized ganglia are displaced into the sternomastoid muscle which is said to prevent the regeneration of sympathetic fibres.

OPERATIVE TECHNIQUE: There are three surgical approaches in common use for ablation of the sympathetic nerve supply of the upper limb: (1) supraclavicular; (2) transaxillary; (3) anterior thoracotomy through the 3rd intercostal space.

1. *Supraclavicular:* A horizontal skin incision is made a finger-breadth above the medial half of the clavicle. The platysma and external jugular veins are divided and at least the lateral two supraclavicular cutaneous nerves are preserved. The clavicular head of the sternomastoid is divided and also the inferior belly of the omohyoid. The phrenic nerve is identified lying deep to fascia on the scalenus anterior. The nerve and the internal jugular vein are displaced medially and the muscle is divided. The lower margin of the brachial plexus is identified and the subclavian artery is exposed and retracted downwards. The costocervical branch of the subclavian artery may need to be divided. The suprapleural membrane (Sibson's fascia) must now be divided to expose the dome of the pleura which lies beneath it.

   The parietal pleura is then peeled off the vertebral column and the posterior portions of the ribs to the level of the 4th rib. The pleura is kept intact during this process. The sympathetic trunk is identified by palpation as a thick cord with the nodular enlargements of the ganglia along its length.

   The sympathectomy can now be performed, keeping in mind the anatomical considerations mentioned above.

2. *Transaxillary:* With the patient in the lateral position and the upper arm raised, an incision, about 15 cm long, is made between the anterior and posterior axillary folds along the line of the 3rd rib. The pectoralis major and latissimus dorsi muscles are retracted and the nerves to serratus anterior and latissimus dorsi are protected. The serratus anterior is detached from the 3rd rib and the pleural cavity is entered through the bed of the rib. The lung is retracted downwards. The sympathetic trunk can be seen where it lies deep to the mediastinal pleura which is incised. The sympathectomy can now be performed. Meticulous haemostasis is necessary and the lung is expanded before closing the chest.

3. *Anterior Thoracotomy:* The incision overlies the 3rd interspace and extends from the lateral margin of the sternum to the midaxillary line. The pectoralis major muscle is incised in the line of its fibres and the chest is opened through an incision in the 3rd intercostal space. The lung is retracted downwards and the sympathetic trunk is identified where it lies deep to the mediastinal pleura.

Lumbar sympathectomy

Preganglionic fibres to the lower limb are derived from the lower 3 thoracic and upper 2 or 3 lumbar segments of the spinal cord. They reach the lower thoracic and upper 2 lumbar ganglia through white rami, some of which pass down the trunk to synapse about cells in the lumbar ganglia. Grey rami pass from the 1st and 2nd ganglia to the femoral and obturator nerves which supply the anterior part of the thigh. Other white rami extend farther down the trunk and synapse with the upper 2 or 3 sacral ganglia from where grey rami are distributed with the sciatic nerve to supply the posterior thigh and the limb below the knee.

Sympathetic denervation of the leg below the knee can, therefore, be obtained by removing the 3rd and 4th lumbar ganglia. Removal of the 1st lumbar ganglion is not usually necessary and is also potentially harmful by interfering with ejaculation. This complication is the result of impaired closure of the internal vesical sphincter allowing seminal fluid to flow retrogradely into the bladder. Removal of the first lumbar ganglion may also do harm by creating a 'steal' phenomenon which diverts blood to the thigh.

However, removal of L1 may be required in rare cases where improvement of circulation in the thigh is required to permit an above-knee amputation to heal.

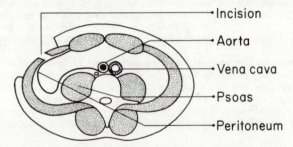

Fig. 174. Extraperitoneal approach to the lumbar sympathetic chain.

THE ANTERIOR APPROACH: With the patient supine, the incision extends from just below the umbilicus to just below the 10th rib (*Fig.* 174). The abdominal muscles are dealt with by splitting external oblique in the line of its fibres and cutting internal oblique and transversus in the line of the skin incision. The peritoneum is left intact and the dissection is carried retroperitoneally by mobilizing the peritoneal contents and extraperitoneal fat medially and anteriorly until the vertebral column is encountered. The genitofemoral nerve is identified over the medial third of the psoas muscle and preserved. Care must be taken to identify and protect the ureter which usually remains attached to the peritoneum. The sympathetic trunk is found by palpating it on the anterolateral aspect of the bodies of the vertebrae. On the right side, care must be taken to avoid injuring the vena cava immediately anterior to the sympathetic chain.

The sympathectomy is effected by removing L3 and L4 ganglia. The exact ganglia cannot be determined by their relationship to specific lumbar vertebrae. L1 ganglion lies above, in or behind the crus of the diaphragm and the sympathetic chain is, therefore, divided below the crus.

L4 ganglion lies at a level just above the sacral promontory and should be removed together with the interposed sympathetic chain which will include the L3 ganglion.

During the dissection, an atheromatous plaque may be dislodged and embolize from the aorta or the iliac artery to create serious distal ischaemia. The surgeon should avoid this complication by gentle technique.

SYMPATHETIC GANGLION BLOCK

Sympathetic ganglion block with local anaesthetic solution is performed to determine whether any benefit can be expected from surgical sympathectomy. The stellate, upper thoracic and lumbar ganglia and the splanchnic nerves and their adjacent ganglia are the most usual ganglia blocked. In the limbs a peripheral sympathetic block can be achieved with intravenous guanethidine.

It should be kept in mind that sympathetic fibres are conducted to the periphery along peripheral nerves and local anaesthetics when applied to peripheral nerves therefore interrupt the sympathetic outflow. In a regional block, e.g. brachial plexus block, dilatation of peripheral vessels occurs. A spinal or epidural anaesthetic produces more widespread sympathetic blockage and may cause a dangerous fall in blood pressure.

Stellate ganglion block

See Fig. 175. The anterior approach is the preferred approach. The patient lies supine with the head and neck extended. A 6-cm needle is inserted at a point 1·5 cm lateral and 1·5 cm superior to the suprasternal notch and directed posteriorly between the trachea and the carotid bundle to the lateral aspect of the vertebral body of C7.

The needle is then withdrawn slightly and redirected laterally to miss the vertebral body and advanced until it strikes its transverse process. At this point the needle is withdrawn 0·5 cm to place it in the correct fascial plane and 10 ml of a 1 per cent local anaesthetic solution is injected. A successful injection will produce a temporary Horner's syndrome.

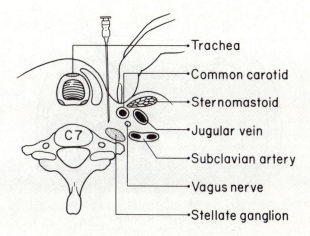

Trachea

Common carotid

Sternomastoid

Jugular vein

Subclavian artery

Vagus nerve

Stellate ganglion

Fig. 175. Stellate ganglion block.

Upper thoracic ganglion block

The patient lies on his side with the head supported by a pillow. The needle is inserted 4 cm from the midline of the back at right-angles to the skin, in line with the appropriate thoracic spinous process. When the needle strikes the transverse process it is remanipulated until it lies at the lower edge of the bone. It is now redirected 20 degrees to the sagittal plane and advanced 3 cm until the point strikes the body of the vertebrae. If aspiration produces no blood, cerebrospinal fluid or air, 5 ml of 0·5 per cent local anaesthetic solution is injected. The upper 4 thoracic ganglia can be injected serially using this technique with a separate injection site for each ganglion.

Lumbar ganglion block

The needle is inserted 3 cm from the midline of the back at a level halfway between the 2nd and 3rd lumbar spinous processes. The needle is directed towards the midline between the transverse processes of the lumbar vertebrae. When the needle strikes the body of the lumbar vertebrae, it is aspirated and if no blood or cerebrospinal fluid is withdrawn 30 ml of 0·5 per cent local anaesthetic solution is injected. A semipermanent block is obtained by injecting 10 per cent phenol in water.

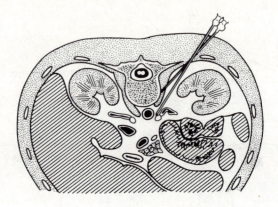

Fig. 176. Posterior splanchnic block.

Posterior splanchnic block

This procedure (*Fig.* 176) will produce a block of the nerves and ganglia anterior to the 1st lumbar vertebra and therefore a block of the visceral autonomic nerve fibres. The injection is made about 8 cm from the midline of the back at the level of the 1st lumbar spinous process. The needle is inserted at an angle of 30 degrees to the sagittal plane through the erector spinae muscle to strike the body of the 1st lumbar vertebra. The needle is withdrawn 3 cm and advanced at about 20 degrees to the sagittal plane past the lumbar vertebra into the retroperitoneal space. If no blood or cerebrospinal fluid is withdrawn, 40 ml of 0·5 per cent local anaesthetic solution is injected which diffuses across the midline and anaesthetizes both sides from one injection.

Chapter 19

COLLATERAL CIRCULATION

When a major artery is occluded, the viability of the parts supplied by that artery depends on the efficacy of the collateral circulation. The latter is an accessory circuit which consists of pre-existing branches of the main artery above and below the site of the occlusion (*Fig.* 177).

The branches anastomose with each other through their smaller branches (midzone vessels) which normally have a resistance to flow preventing

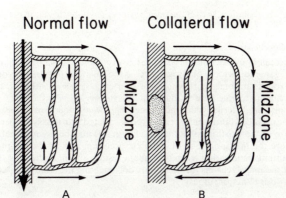

Fig. 177. A, Normal flow; B, collateral flow.

significant forward flow. However, in the event of an occlusion in the main vessel, the pressure distal to the occlusion drops and this allows reversed flow into the branches arising below the obstruction. The end result is physical enlargement of these collaterals which allow increased forward flow to nourish the area distal to the obstruction.

If the collateral flow is inadequate to meet the metabolic demands of the tissue at rest, acute ischaemia, manifested by rest pain and/or gangrene, results. If the blood flow is adequate for the metabolic demands at rest but not on effort, chronic ischaemia results. Intermittent claudication (ischaemic pain in the muscles being exercised) is a characteristic symptom of chronic ischaemia. If the metabolic demands are met both at rest and on exercise the patient is asymptomatic.

FACTORS AFFECTING COLLATERAL FLOW

Pressure gradient across the site of occlusion
Blood flow through the collateral circulation is heightened by increasing the pressure gradient across the site of occlusion.

Anatomic site of block
Occlusion of an artery with adequate side branches, such as the brachial artery, is less likely to cause severe ischaemia than occlusion of an artery with relatively few side branches, such as the popliteal. An 'end' artery with no

collateral circulation, such as the retinal artery, inevitably results in ischaemia.

Rate of occlusion

If the circulation is suddenly interrupted, as in embolic disease or ligation of an artery, gangrene is more likely to ensue, as the collateral pathway has not had time to develop. A gradual occlusion of an artery, as is seen in atherosclerosis, allows adequate time for existing collaterals to develop.

Major limb arteries which have been narrowed by atherosclerosis may become occluded during enforced bedrest associated with illness or operation. Because of the existing collateral circulation this may be asymptomatic and therefore the first indication of complete occlusion may be the symptom of intermittent claudication when the patient resumes normal activities. This is one of the many reasons for accurately documenting the state of a patient's pulses prior to major surgery.

Extent of occlusion

If a long segment of an artery is occluded, important side branches arising within the area of occlusion are not available for the collateral circulation and the outcome is therefore less favourable.

Sympathetic activity

Sympathetic denervation by either chemical or surgical means may hasten the speed with which collaterals develop.

MESENTERIC COLLATERALS

The coeliac, superior mesenteric and inferior mesenteric arteries are three unpaired branches of the abdominal aorta that supply the gastrointestinal tract (*Fig.* 178).

The coeliac artery

The coeliac axis arises from the anterior portion of the abdominal aorta opposite the thoracolumbar junction, as a single trunk 3–4 cm long and 6–8 mm in diameter. In about 20 per cent of people, part of the origin of the coeliac axis is compressed by the median arcuate ligament, which may result in a median arcuate ligament syndrome. This syndrome, which is almost confined to women, results in chronic ischaemia of the abdominal viscera with cramp-like postprandial epigastric pain and an epigastric bruit on auscultation of the abdomen. An aortogram shows compression of the coeliac artery by the median arcuate ligament.

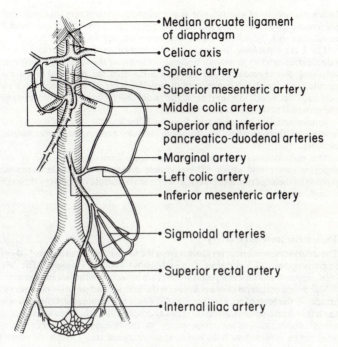

- Median arcuate ligament of diaphragm
- Celiac axis
- Splenic artery
- Superior mesenteric artery
- Middle colic artery
- Superior and inferior pancreatico-duodenal arteries
- Marginal artery
- Left colic artery
- Inferior mesenteric artery
- Sigmoidal arteries
- Superior rectal artery
- Internal iliac artery

Fig. 178. Mesenteric collaterals.

The superior mesenteric artery arises from the aorta not more than 1·5 cm caudal to the coeliac artery and may sometimes also be affected by median arcuate ligament compression.

This syndrome may occur either because the arteries arise at a higher level than usual or because the ligament crosses the aorta at a lower level.

Superior mesenteric artery

The superior mesenteric artery arises at a 20–30 degree angle from the abdominal aorta, opposite the middle of the 1st lumbar vertebra. The acute angle of origin explains why this artery is most commonly occluded by an aortic embolus. The diameter of the artery is 8–10 mm and it has an unbifurcated course for 3–6 cm before giving origin to the inferior pancreaticoduodenal artery which establishes a collateral circulation with the coeliac axis through the superior pancreaticoduodenal artery. About 1 cm below the origin of the inferior pancreaticoduodenal artery, the superior mesenteric gives rise to the middle colic artery which establishes a collateral circulation with the inferior mesenteric artery through its left colic branch.

The 1 cm separating the origins of the inferior pancreaticoduodenal and middle colic arteries is crucial, because occlusion of the superior mesenteric involving this segment of the artery will obstruct the potential collateral circulation through the coeliac and the inferior mesenteric systems. Such an occlusion will result in gangrene of the entire midgut from the duodenum to the proximal half of the transverse colon.

Jejunal and ileal branches arise from the left side of the superior mesenteric artery and through their anastomosing arcades form a profuse collateral network.

The right colic and ileocolic branches arise from the right side of the superior mesenteric artery. These vessels anastomose with the terminal portion of the superior mesenteric artery and the middle colic artery through a single arcade.

The inferior mesenteric artery

The inferior mesenteric artery arises from the aorta at about an angle of 70–90 degrees opposite L3 vertebra. It is only about 4 mm in diameter. The left colic, sigmoid and superior rectal arteries are branches of the left colic artery.

The major collateral channel between the inferior and superior mesenteric arteries is the arch of Riolan (*see Fig.* 43) which is a communication between the left and middle colic arteries. It has also been called the 'mesomesenteric artery', the 'central anastomotic artery' or the 'meandering artery', but it must not be confused with the less tortuous marginal artery which lies nearer the colon. The arch of Riolan is sometimes seen as a major collateral in cases of occlusion of the aorta.

In ligation of the inferior mesenteric artery at its origin from the aorta, as may be necessary in colonic resection or during aneurysmectomy, colonic infarction occurs in 1–2 per cent of patients. This incidence of colonic infarction is related to the variation in collateral blood supply because: (*a*) the middle colic artery is absent in 20 per cent of patients, (*b*) the marginal artery may be discontinuous, and (*c*) when the inferior mesenteric artery is ligated some distance from the aorta, the arch of Riolan may be included in the ligature.

The superior rectal artery forms a collateral network with the middle rectal arteries (internal iliac) and inferior rectal arteries (internal pudendal).

The collateral potential between the arteries supplying the gastrointestinal tract is so great that a gradual occlusion of all three unpaired arteries may occur without infarction of the gut. In these cases blood reaches the gut through the internal iliac, rectal arteries and the arch of Riolan.

AORTO-ILIAC DISEASE

The aorta and iliac vessels are common sites of partial or total occlusion in vascular disease. Because the occlusion usually occurs insidiously, it produces characteristic symptoms and signs of vascular disease described by Le Riche, with claudication in the thighs and buttocks, absent pulses in the lower limbs, muscular atrophy of both lower limbs and impotence in male patients.

Localized aorto-iliac occlusion may extend proximally to the inferior mesenteric artery which acts as an outflow tract proximal to the occluding thrombus. If the inferior mesenteric artery is already occluded, the thrombus will extend more proximally to the renal arteries which function as the next major outflow tract of the aorta. Rarely, both renal arteries become occluded which results in acute renal failure.

The viability of the lower limbs is maintained by bridging collateral systems:

Somatic collateral system

This consists of the internal mammary, superior epigastric and lower intercostal arteries which produce reversed flow through their anastomoses with the inferior epigastric and circumflex iliac arteries into the femoral and profunda femoris arteries. This collateral flow may be interrupted by lumbar sympathectomy which could precipitate gangrene.

Visceral collateral system

This occurs through the superior mesenteric, left colic, superior rectal, middle and inferior rectal, internal iliac, and inferior gluteal which anastomoses with the perforating vessels of the profunda femoris in the back of the thigh.

SUPERFICIAL FEMORAL ARTERY OCCLUSION

Occlusion of the superficial femoral artery is a common cause of intermittent claudication. The profunda femoris artery is an important collateral pathway through its anastomoses with the geniculate branches of the popliteal artery and the recurrent tibial arteries.

In the operation of profundoplasty, the origin of the artery from the common femoral artery is made wider where narrowing due to atherosclerosis is present. This comparatively simple procedure often relieves symptoms of chronic ischaemia.

POPLITEAL ARTERY

In occlusion of the popliteal artery the collateral circulation consists of:

The articular anastomosis

This occurs around the knee which has a rich network made up by the descending genicular branch of the femoral artery and the genicular branches of the popliteal artery which anastomose with the recurrent fibular and tibial arteries.

The muscular anastomosis

This takes place between the vessels to the muscles of the thigh (the hamstrings) and the muscles of the calf.

In gradual occlusion of the popliteal artery due to atherosclerosis, these genicular anastomoses develop sufficiently to maintain patency of the lower part of the popliteal artery which is then available for bypass grafting.

BRACHIOCEPHALIC ARTERY

After occlusion of this vessel the collateral circulation is abundant. The blood reaches:

Head and neck

The blood reaches the head and neck by the common carotid and vertebral of the opposite side. The external carotids communicate freely and the two vertebrals and internal carotids anastomose freely in the circle of Willis.

In some patients with occlusion of the brachiocephalic artery, flow in the right vertebral and right carotid arteries is reversed which results in a 'steal' phenomenon from the circle of Willis.

Arm

The blood reaches the arm by two alternative collateral systems:
1. The intercostal anastomoses, both anterior (from internal mammary) and posterior (from the aorta), communicating with the costocervical trunk (second part of the subclavian) and with the lateral thoracic, thoraco-acromial, and subscapular branches of the axillary.
2. The internal mammary (first part of the subclavian) communicates by its superior epigastric branch with the inferior epigastric (external iliac).

SUBCLAVIAN ARTERY

Origin of the subclavian artery

Obstruction of the subclavian artery proximal to the origin of the vertebral, results in the vertebral acting as a collateral to the arm and 'stealing' flow from the basilar. This may result in ischaemic neurological symptoms, associated with ischaemia in the affected arm (subclavian 'steal' syndrome; *see Fig*. 179).

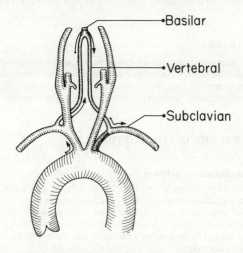

Fig. 179. The subclavian 'steal' phenomenon.

Third part of the subclavian artery

In occlusion of this artery collaterals are formed with (*a*) the intercostal anastomosis as described under occlusion of the brachiocephalic artery; (*b*) in addition there is a scapular anastomosis between the suprascapular and the descending branch of the transverse cervical artery (which are branches of the thyrocervical trunk from the first part of the subclavian artery) and the subscapular and circumflex humeral branches of the axillary artery.

BRACHIAL ARTERY OCCLUSION

In the upper arm there is a good collateral system made up by numerous muscular and articular branches.

At the elbow joint level, the rich collateral flow is dependent on the anterior and posterior branches of profunda brachii laterally and superior and inferior ulnar collaterals medially anastomosing below with the interosseous and ulnar recurrent arteries.

As a result of this rich collateral system, occlusion of the brachial artery does not usually cause gangrene unless the collaterals have been damaged by injury or surgery. However, labourers may experience forearm claudication during strenuous work.

This artery is not infrequently injured following cardiac catheterization.

SPLENIC ARTERY

This vessel is unique inasmuch as it may be mobilized and anastomosed to renal, superior mesenteric, or hepatic arteries, when the indications exist. It is unnecessary to remove the spleen because of the collateral supply it receives through its short gastric vessels via the left and right gastro-epiploic arteries.

COLLATERAL CIRCULATION TO THE BRAIN

Common carotid artery occlusion

The internal carotid artery has no branches in the neck and, consequently, in occlusion of the common carotid artery the collateral circulation to the brain is dependent upon an anastomosis between the branches of the subclavian and external carotid arteries, which will allow flow to run retrogradely down the external carotid to the carotid bifurcation into the internal carotid artery. This is achieved through:

1. Free communication between the branches of the left and right external carotid arteries.
2. Good communication between the left and right internal carotid arteries via the circle of Willis.
3. The superior thyroid artery, which is a branch of the external carotid artery, anastomoses with the inferior thyroid artery which is a branch of the thyrocervical trunk (first part of subclavian).
4. The descending branch of the occipital artery (external carotid artery) anastomoses with the deep cervical and ascending branch of the transverse cervical arteries below.
5. The vertebral arteries may take over the entire supply of the carotids within the skull.

The circle of Willis

This anastomosis lies in the subarachnoid space at the base of the brain (*Fig*.

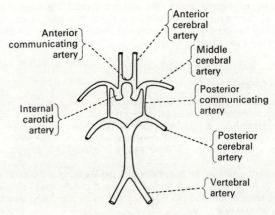

Fig. 180. The circle of Willis.

180). This arterial circle provides a potentially rich collateral circulation to the brain. The circle is fed by the two vertebral arteries and the two internal carotid arteries. Posteriorly, the two vertebrals fuse to form the single basilar artery. This divides into the paired posterior cerebral arteries, each of which is connected to the internal carotid by the posterior communicating artery. Anteriorly, the intracranial carotid artery gives rise to the paired anterior and middle cerebral arteries. The two anterior cerebral arteries anastomose with each other through the anterior communicating artery. Normally little mixing of the blood from opposing streams occurs in the communicating arteries because the pressures of the two streams are equal. Should either vertebral or carotid system be occluded, redistribution of blood occurs through the circle of Willis. The circle of Willis is incomplete to a greater or lesser degree in 5–20 per cent of cases. Congenital absence of the posterior communicating artery explains the 7 per cent incidence of hemiplegia following carotid artery ligation even in young patients. A rare anomaly is the persistence of the early embryonic channel connecting the cavernous part of the internal carotid artery with the upper third of the basilar artery. It is termed the 'trigeminal artery' and may be as large as the internal carotid. When present, it passes lateral to the posterior clinoid process or through the dorsum sellae, being in close proximity to the semilunar ganglion or 5th nerve.

Although on the surface of the brain there are rich anastomoses between vessels, once an artery enters the brain no anastomosis occurs.

A rich anastomosis is possible between the branches of the external and internal carotid on each side. The superficial temporal and facial arteries anastomose with the supra-orbital and ophthalmic arteries and, in occlusion of the internal carotid artery, the external carotid can supply a major portion of the internal carotid territory. Other branches of the external carotid may establish collateral pathways via the meningeal vessels and through the foramina of the skull.

BYPASS GRAFT

A bypass grafting procedure using the patient's own vessel, or prosthetic material, to bridge an arterial obstruction, is a commonly performed vascular procedure. The principle of the procedure is to create a new collateral pathway with a lower resistance to flow than the patient's own collateral system and at the same time not damaging existing collateral vessels.

In aorto-iliac disease an aortobifemoral bypass using a synthetic graft is commonly performed. Occlusions of the superficial femoral artery can be bypassed using a reversed (so that the valve cusps allow flow proximodistally) saphenous vein graft.

VENOUS COLLATERAL MECHANISMS

The venous collateral mechanisms are on the whole more generous than the arterial ones, but the integrity of certain veins is essential because of the absence or paucity of collaterals, such as the retinal, the superior vena cava, and the inferior vena cava above the renals, the portal and the superior mesenteric veins.

As a rule, either brachiocephalic vein may be tied off with safety, as can the subclavian. The removal of a single internal jugular vein is a safe procedure. If it is necessary to remove the remaining internal jugular, it is usually done as a staged procedure to allow the collateral to become established.

The venous collateral after ligation of the internal jugulars

In bilateral radical clearance of lymph nodes of the neck, not only the internal jugulars but the anterior and external jugular veins will also be sacrificed. The intracranial venous sinuses which drain the brain communicate extensively with the system of emissary veins, with the veins of the orbit, and with the prevertebral venous plexuses. The intracranial venous drainage is thus assured to the exterior of the skull from where it will reach the heart by three main routes:

1. Along the visceral compartment of the neck via pterygoid and pharyngeal plexuses, tracheal, thyroid, and oesophageal veins to the vertebral and brachiocephalic veins.

2. Through the occipital and the deep cervical plexuses to the first and superior intercostal veins, the vertebral, subclavian, and uppermost intercostal veins.

3. Through the vertebral venous plexuses via their communications with the intracranial sinuses above and their drainage into vertebral, brachiocephalic, and intercostals below.

Brachiocephalic vein occlusion

When one of the brachiocephalic veins is obstructed the other is usually spared. It supplies a ready collateral pathway to the superior vena cava through the cross communications of the numerous veins in the anterior part of the neck (*Fig.* 181).

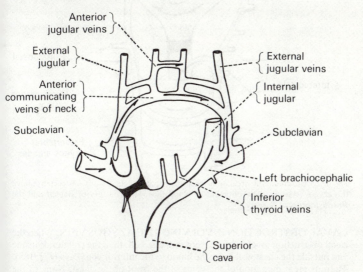

Fig. 181. Obstruction of the right brachiocephalic vein. The arrow shows the direction of the blood flow. (By courtesy of Barrett and the *British Journal of Surgery*.)

Superior vena caval obstruction

OBSTRUCTION OF THE SUPERIOR VENA CAVA ABOVE THE ENTRANCE OF THE AZYGOS: The main collateral pathways are the superior intercostal veins, which carry the blood to the azygos and hemi-azygos systems and so to the heart. The more superficial veins, such as chest wall veins and the internal mammary, which anastomose with the inguinal veins, do not carry sufficient of the load to cause prominence of the veins on the front of the chest. (*See Fig.* 182.)

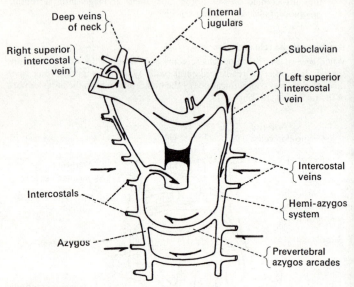

Fig. 182. The collateral circulation when the superior vena cava is obstructed, above the azygos. Arrows show direction of blood flow. (By courtesy of Barrett and the *British Journal of Surgery.*)

CAVAL OBSTRUCTION INVOLVING THE AZYGOS VEIN: When the caval obstruction involves the azygos entry as well, then the collaterals inside and outside the chest wall carry the blood to the inferior vena cava (*Fig.* 183). There is great dilatation of the veins of the front of the chest. None of the great veins mentioned has valves.

THE COMPARTMENTAL SYNDROME

Certain muscular compartments of the limbs are totally enclosed by unyielding deep fascia on the superficial aspect of the limb, and equally unyielding bone and interosseous membrane on the deep aspect. The

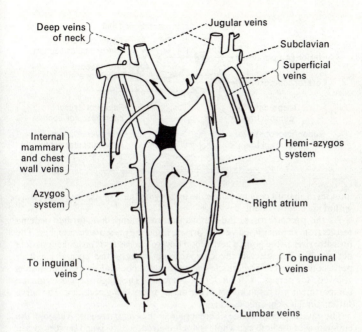

Deep veins of neck

Jugular veins

Subclavian

Superficial veins

Internal mammary and chest wall veins

Hemi-azygos system

Azygos system

Right atrium

To inguinal veins

To inguinal veins

Lumbar veins

Fig. 183. When the azygos and superior vena cava are both blocked, all blood is carried to the inferior vena cava by collaterals within and without the chest. The arrows show the rerouting of blood. The long lateral arrows denote the passage of blood from upper limbs etc. to the veins in the inguinal region. (By courtesy of Barrett and the *British Journal of Surgery*.)

relatively fixed space in the muscular compartment is occupied by muscles and tendons. In each case the nutrition of the soft tissues and innervation of the compartment are dependent upon vessels and nerves which traverse the compartment. In many instances the tissues distal to the compartment are also dependent on the nerve supply and blood supply of the neurovascular bundle that traverses the muscular compartment. The four compartments of the leg are illustrated in *Fig.* 184.

Any process which results in additional mass or fluid being introduced into this restricted osteofascial space cannot readily be accommodated, and the pressure rapidly rises. Bleeding due to trauma or a fracture, oedema following on a period of ischaemia to the muscles, or even excessive use of the

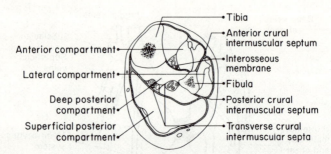

Fig. 184. The compartments of the leg.

muscles in an unfit person, can be the underlying cause of such rise in pressure within the compartment.

As the pressure rises, the venous outflow is impeded, further oedema results from the increased venous pressure and the pressure rises higher. The pressure rises to the point where blood flow to the tissues is no longer possible because the pressure in the compartment exceeds the normal capillary perfusion pressure. The muscles become ischaemic and, if the condition is allowed to persist, will undergo necrosis. The high pressure in the compartment will result in flow in the major artery being occluded. The nerve suffers similar ischacmic damage.

The clinical picture is one of great pain in the compartment. Although the circulation of the limb as a whole is not impaired, paralysis and sensory loss in the distribution of the nerve passing through the compartment may be a feature. In the anterior compartment of the leg the pain is over this compartment, and is associated with a foot drop at an early stage. The distal pulse will only disappear when the pressure in the compartment almost equals arterial pressure. If not treated promptly permanent muscle loss occurs rapidly. Distal tissue loss as a result of reduced blood flow can be seen in cases where several compartments have been affected simultaneously and arterial flow to the distal limb has suffered as a consequence.

Treatment consists of urgent decompression of the compartment by surgical opening of the fascial space involved to allow the muscles and other contents of the compartment additional space into which they may decompress.

Although the anterior compartment of the leg is most commonly involved in the compartmental syndrome, this phenomenon is seen in the deep posterior compartment of the leg, the anterior compartment of the forearm, the lateral compartment of the leg and the superficial posterior compartment of the leg. It is rarely seen in the quadriceps, the gluteal muscles and the posterior compartment of the forearm.

Chapter 20

VASCULAR APPROACH

Operations on blood vessels may be required for vascular disease or vascular trauma. In the case of vascular trauma, haemorrhage from a compressible vessel must be controlled by local pressure where possible and not by tourniquets, which may occlude important collaterals and produce venous thrombosis.

ASCENDING AORTA AND AORTIC ARCH

These are approached through a median sternotomy incision.

DESCENDING AORTA

These are usually approached through an incision in the appropriate rib bed or intercostal space on the left side.

CERVICOMEDIASTINAL VESSELS

These include the brachiocephalic, carotid, subclavian and vertebral arteries which may be diseased or damaged by a penetrating wound in the root of the neck. As a rule, penetrating wounds medial to the sternal head of the sternomastoid are approached by a median sternotomy, whereas lateral wounds are approached initially by a cervical incision which can be extended by a median sternotomy (*Fig.* 185).

Position of the patient

Exposure is facilitated by a sandbag placed between the scapulae and the neck is extended and rotated away from the side of the lesion. The arm on the side of the stab wound is abducted to 90 degrees.

Median sternotomy

A full-length median sternotomy gives adequate exposure. The left brachiocephalic vein and thymus may obscure the origin of the arteries from the aortic arch. The vein can be displaced upwards.

The left subclavian artery at its origin from the aortic arch lies on a more posterior plane. Exposure is improved by the surgeon standing on the side opposite to the injury and rotating the table to his side.

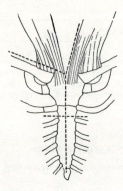

Fig. 185. The surgical approach to the great vessels of the upper mediastinum (dotted lines).

Left anterior thoracotomy

Left anterior thoracotomy through the 3rd or 4th intercostal space can be used for exposure of the intrathoracic portion of the left subclavian and left common carotid arteries.

EXPOSURE OF THE CERVICAL SEGMENT OF THE SUBCLAVIAN ARTERY AND THE VERTEBRAL ARTERY AT ITS ORIGIN FROM THE SUBCLAVIAN ARTERY

The skin incision is made 1 cm above the clavicle extending from the suprasternal notch about 10 cm laterally. The platysma and sternomastoid muscles are divided. The adipose tissue in front of the scalenus anterior is identified and the subclavian vein which crosses in front of the muscle is carefully mobilized. On the left side, the thoracic duct enters the junction between the subclavian and internal jugular veins. The phrenic nerve which crosses the scalenus anterior muscle from its lateral to its medial side is seen and preserved, after which the muscle is divided to expose the subclavian artery.

EXPOSURE OF THE BRACHIOCEPHALIC ARTERY

The periosteum of the medial two-thirds of the right clavicle is incised and stripped. The clavicle is transected with a Gigli saw and the medial portion is removed subperiosteally. The suprascapular vessels run close to the posterior surface of the periosteum and may be torn. The sternal end of the incision allows exposure of the brachiocephalic and carotid vessels.

EXPOSURE OF THE CAROTID ARTERY AND THE VERTEBRAL ARTERY IN ITS BONY CANAL

The median sternotomy incision is continued along the anterior border of the sternomastoid muscle to the tip of the mastoid process or it is commenced in the neck. The incision is carried down through the subcutaneous tissue and the platysma. After the division of the external jugular vein, the cervical fascia is opened along the anterior border of the sternomastoid which is retracted laterally to expose the carotid artery.

The vertebral artery is exposed by dividing the sternomastoid muscle near its insertion. The trachea, oesophagus, thyroid gland and carotid bundle are retracted anteriorly. A finger can be placed in an easily identifiable groove between the body of the cervical vertebra and the anterior tubercle of its transverse process. The longus colli muscle which lies in this groove is elevated out of the groove with an osteotome, revealing the thin anterior plate of the costotransverse bar. This plate is easily removed with bone nibblers thus exposing the vertebral canal and allowing direct ligature of the artery and the application of bone wax plugs to the vertebral venous plexus.

EXPOSURE OF THE AXILLARY ARTERY

The axillary artery extends from the outer border of the first rib to the lower border of the teres major muscle beyond which it is known as the brachial artery. The axillary artery is divided into three segments corresponding to the part of the vessel situated proximal, behind and inferior to the pectoralis minor muscle. The nerves of the brachial plexus surround the inferior segment of the axillary artery.

Deltopectoral approach

The skin incision extends from the clavicle to the distal edge of the pectoralis major muscle along the deltopectoral groove. The cephalic vein is preserved. The pectoralis major muscle is retracted medially to expose the clavipectoral fascia and the pectoralis minor muscle which are divided thus exposing the axillary artery lying between the cords of the brachial plexus laterally and the axillary vein medially.

The incision used to expose the subclavian artery in the neck can be extended across the clavicle into the deltopectoral groove.

Axillofemoral bypass

The proximal anastomosis is made to the first part of the axillary artery. A subclavicular incision 1 cm below the clavicle is commenced at the junction of the medial quarter with the outer three-quarters of the clavicle and extended laterally for 6 cm. The fibres of the pectoralis major are split in the direction of its fibres and the clavipectoral fascia is incised. The axillary artery lying superior to the vein is exposed between the 1st rib and the pectoralis minor.

EXPOSURE OF THE BRACHIAL ARTERY

A medial longitudinal incision is made along a groove which separates the medial border of the biceps anteriorly from the triceps posteriorly. The incision must be made anterior to the basilic vein. The biceps muscle is retracted laterally which exposes the median nerve lying over the brachial artery.

Exposure of the bifurcation of the brachial artery

A Z-shaped incision is made over the cubital fossa and the bicipital aponeurosis is divided to expose the artery. The median nerve lies medial to the artery.

EXPOSURE OF THE RADIAL ARTERY

Upper third

The incision is in the groove between the brachioradialis and pronator teres muscles.

Lower third

The artery is superficial but subfascial and situated lateral to the flexor carpi radialis longus tendon.

EXPOSURE OF THE ULNAR ARTERY

The ulnar artery reaches the medial side of the forearm at a point midway between the elbow and the wrist. The skin incision commences 6 cm below the medial epicondyle on a line which extends from the latter to the pisiform bone. The deep fascia is incised to expose the flexor carpi ulnaris which overlaps the artery. The ulnar nerve lies on its medial side.

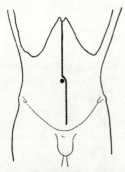

Fig. 186. The incision for a resection of an abdominal aneurysm.

EXPOSURE OF THE ABDOMINAL AORTA AND ITS BRANCHES

The abdominal aorta is exposed by a long midline incision extending from the xiphoid process to pubis (*Fig*. 186). The most common indication for exposure of the abdominal aorta is for aneurysm which lies below the level of the renal arteries in 95 per cent of cases. Should the aneurysm involve the upper abdominal aorta (suprarenal aneurysm) or extend into the thoracic aorta, adequate access and proximal control of the aorta can be obtained by extending the long midline abdominal incision into an appropriate left rib space, as a thoraco-abdominal incision with peripheral detachment of the diaphragm. The peritoneum in the left paracolic gutter is incised lateral to the left colon and extended above to the diaphragm and below to the brim of the pelvis. The left colon, left kidney, spleen, body and tail of the pancreas, and fundus of the stomach are retracted upwards and to the right in the relatively avascular retroperitoneal plane.

AORTO-ILIAC EXPOSURE

These vessels are commonly the site of atherosclerosis and are frequently the site for arterial surgery. The aorto-iliac bifurcation, as far distally as the origin of the external iliacs, may be approached through a transperitoneal route via a long midline incision as for the abdominal aortic aneurysm.

These vessels can also be approached extraperitoneally by an oblique incision such as is used for the ureter (*Fig*. 187). The incision runs obliquely forward from the loin in the direction of the symphysis pubis up to the lateral border of the rectus abdominis. The external oblique is split in the direction of

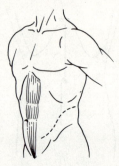

Fig. 187. The incision for extraperitoneal exposure of the aorto-iliac vessels.

its fibres, and the internal oblique and transversus fibres are cut. In this way minimal section of nerves is possible. This incision exposes the whole length of the iliac vessels, including the aortic bifurcation, but the exposure afforded to the opposite iliac vessels is poor. It is ideal for such procedures as unilateral iliac surgery or the placing of a heterotopic transplanted kidney on the iliac vessels.

FEMORAL VESSELS

The femoral vessels are best exposed by a vertical incision 15 cm long and centred over the midfemoral point. If dissection of the profunda femoris vessels is intended, the incision is extended inferiorly. The deep fascia of the leg is incised, and the artery is found lying lateral to the common femoral vein. The profunda femoris artery arises from the posterolateral aspect of the common femoral artery 2–4 cm distal to the inguinal ligament. Exposure to the proximal common femoral artery and distal external iliac artery can be facilitated by section of the inguinal ligament. The contents of the inguinal canal are protected by upward retraction.

POPLITEAL ARTERY

This vessel is 20 cm long. It begins at the hiatus in the adductor magnus as the continuation of the superficial femoral artery, and ends at the lower border of the popliteus muscle by dividing into anterior tibial artery and tibioperoneal trunk. This corresponds in level to the lower border of the tubercle of the tibia. Because of its anatomical features, the artery is prone to a number of specific disorders.

The site of the passage of this artery through the adductor hiatus is a common area for atherosclerotic stenosis and occlusion, possibly as a result of repeated injury to the vessel in the hiatus.

The fixity of the distal popliteal vessels at the lower border of the popliteal fossa results in frequent injury to this vessel when fracture and dislocation occur around the knee joint.

The popliteal artery may deviate medially from its normal course and pass deep to the femoral origin of the medial head of the gastrocnemius which may arise from a more lateral situation than usual (*Fig.* 188). This causes constriction of the artery which can lead to secondary thrombosis. The condition results in disappearance of ankle pulses when the knee is forcibly extended and, on arteriography, the vessel is deviated medially. It may be bilateral.

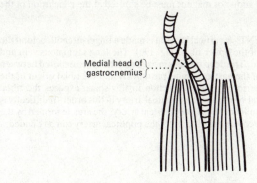

Medial head of gastrocnemius

Fig. 188. Popliteal artery passing deep to the medial head of the gastrocnemius muscle.

Medial approach

When extensive exposure of the popliteal artery is required and particularly when a femoropopliteal graft is contemplated, the medial approach is used. It also allows access to the saphenous vein which may be required as the graft, so that particular care must be taken to preserve the vein when making the skin incision. The patient lies supine with the thigh externally rotated and the knee in 30 degrees of flexion, supported with a rolled sheet placed underneath it.

UPPER SEGMENT: The incision is made longitudinally along the lower third of the medial aspect of the thigh crossing the adductor tubercle (*Fig.* 189). The deep fascia is divided in front of the sartorius muscle which is retracted posteriorly. The tendon of the adductor magnus, which hides most of the proximal portion of the popliteal artery after it has passed through the

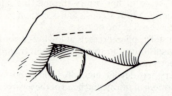

Fig. 189. Incision for exposure of the upper segment of the popliteal artery.

adductor canal, may have to be divided. Two veins are encountered, lateral and posterior to the artery with communicating veins which require division. The tendon of the adductor magnus must be sutured at the conclusion of the procedure.

LOWER SEGMENT: A vertical incision is made a finger-breadth behind the posterior border of the upper tibia (*Fig.* 190). The long saphenous vein and nerve are protected. The deep fascia is incised and the space exposed between the medial head of the gastrocnemius posteriorly and the tibial origin of the soleus muscle anteriorly. Blunt dissection in this space exposes the tibial nerve, two popliteal veins, and the popliteal artery in this order. If difficulty is experienced in mobilizing the distal popliteal artery, the arcade formed by the soleus muscle as it covers the division of the popliteal artery can be divided.

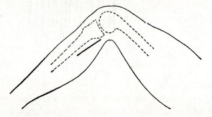

Fig. 190. The incision for exposing the lower segment of the popliteal artery.

ENTIRE POPLITEAL ARTERY: The skin incision is a combination of that used for exposure of the upper and lower segments of the artery. The sartorius, semimembranosus, gracilis and semitendinosus muscles are divided near their insertion into the tibia. Next the origin of the medial head of the gastrocnemius muscle is divided near the medial femoral condyle. Exposure of the entire length of the popliteal artery is now obtained. The tendons are resutured at the conclusion of the procedure.

Posterior approach

With the patient lying prone, the popliteal artery is readily approached by a vertical incision in the popliteal space. This incision should never be straight as a retractile scar readily develops in this area. It may consist of several gentle alternating curves (the lazy S) or a Z incision may be made.

The first structure encountered on dividing the strong deep fascia is the tibial nerve. The popliteal vein covers the artery which is the deepest structure in the neurovascular bundle.

EXPOSURE OF THE POSTERIOR TIBIAL ARTERY

Proximal segment

A 10-cm skin incision is made at midcalf level behind the posteromedial border of the tibia. The deep fascia is incised and the gastrocnemius muscle is retracted posteriorly. To expose the vessel either the soleus muscle is divided longitudinally or the muscle is detached from its tibial attachment.

Distal segment

A vertical incision is made above the medial malleolus, parallel to the posteromedial border of the tibia. The Achilles tendon is retracted posteriorly and the deep fascia is incised anteriorly, which exposes the posterior tibial vessels.

EXPOSURE OF THE ANTERIOR TIBIAL ARTERY

A longitudinal incision is made overlying the groove between the tibialis anterior and extensor digitorum longus. The muscles are separated by blunt dissection until the neurovascular bundle is located on the anterior surface of the interosseous membrane.

MYOCUTANEOUS FLAPS

Many muscles and their overlying skin receive their blood supply primarily from a single pedicle of vessels. The skin overlying such muscles together with the muscle and its major vascular pedicle can be mobilized. Provided the vascular pedicle is not compromised, this myocutaneous flap can be moved a considerable distance from the original site to provide a well-vascularized island of skin and muscle to cover a tissue defect.

Muscles with such an axial vascular supply and which are frequently used for myocutaneous flaps are:

1. The latissimus dorsi flap is based on the thoracodorsal vessels and can be used in chest wall reconstruction.
2. The pectoralis major flap is based upon the thoraco-acromial axis and can be used to cover defects over the sternum, neck and lower face.
3. The trapezius flap is based on the transverse cervical artery and can be used to cover defects of neck, face and scalp.
4. The gluteus maximus flap can be based upon either the superior or the inferior gluteal vessels. This flap is ideal for coverage of skin loss in deep bedsores and covering skin defects around the sacrum and ischium.
5. The gracilis flap is based on the medial femoral circumflex artery and can be swung to cover perineal defects.
6. The gastrocnemius flap is based on the medial or lateral head of the gastrocnemius, with the appropriate branch of the popliteal artery, and is useful to cover defects of the knee and anterior tibial areas.

FREE FLAPS

The ability to construct a flap and isolate an axial vessel allows the surgeon to transect the vascular pedicle of the flap, transport the flap to a totally remote site, and there to restore blood flow to the flap by microvascular anastomoses to local vessels of approximately the same size at the host location. In this way, a large vascularized flap can be placed at any point on the body that has host vessels to which the graft can be sutured. Toe-to-finger transplants are an example of this technique.

Chapter 21

THE VEINS AND GREAT LYMPH DUCTS

There are many reasons why the veins and their anatomy have become increasingly important to the practising surgeon.

Dilatation and tortuosity of the veins of the legs (varicose veins) are exceedingly common; autogenous vein grafts are used to bypass arterial obstructions in the coronary arteries and the arteries distal to the inguinal ligament; cannulation of veins is important for total parenteral nutrition and invasive monitoring of the patient; vascular access, which is necessary for haemodialysis in patients in chronic renal failure, has become a surgical discipline in its own right.

All veins except those enclosed by bones or by the cranium have smooth muscle in their walls. Because of hydrostatic pressure, the dependent veins in the standing posture have a thicker wall in relation to the diameter of the lumen than the more proximally situated veins. The density of sympathetic innervation by sympathetic constrictor fibres of the veins is proportional to the smooth muscle content in their walls.

All veins have valves except very small veins, the venae cavae, and the veins from the brain and viscera. The valves tend to be immediately distal to the point of entry of a major tributary. The valves direct the blood flow from distal to proximal and from superficial to deep veins, except in the perforating veins of the hands, feet and forearm in which flow is from deep to superficial.

THE ANATOMY OF VASCULAR ACCESS

Whenever possible the upper limb veins are used for intravenous infusions. When lower limb veins are used for this purpose there is an increased risk of deep vein thrombosis.

The venous blood of the arms drains through two intercommunicating main veins, the basilic and the cephalic. The median cubital vein in the cubital fossa (*Fig.* 191) is a common site for venepuncture.

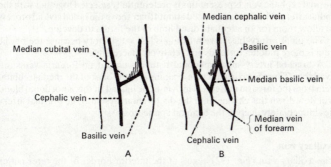

Fig. 191. Veins at bend of elbow. A, Arranged H fashion; B, arranged M fashion.

Cephalic vein

Runs up on the outer side of the forearm and arm. In the arm its position is very constant, first along the outer border of the biceps, then in the groove between the deltoid and pectoralis major where it pierces the deep fascia. In the deltopectoral triangle it dips deeply, pierces the costocoracoid membrane, and ends in the axillary vein. The virtual right-angle at which the cephalic vein joins the axillary vein is responsible for the obstruction frequently encountered at this point when attempting to pass a central venous catheter through the cephalic vein. The cephalic vein may communicate with the anterior jugular vein by a vessel which crosses the clavicle.

Basilic vein

Commences from the inner side of the dorsal venous plexus and runs up along the inner border of the forearm and arm, as far as the middle of the arm at the level of the insertion of the coracobrachialis. Here two structures pierce the deep fascia: the basilic vein going from superficial to deep and the medial cutaneous nerve of the forearm going from deep to superficial. Having pierced the deep fascia, the basilic becomes a vena comitans of the brachial artery which already has two accompanying veins. These three vessels join to form the axillary vein. Cannulation via the basilic vein is more liable to be successful than cannulation via the cephalic vein because the basilic vein becomes the axillary vein without angulation (*see* Cephalic vein *above*).

Internal arteriovenous fistulae

In chronic renal failure, fistulae are established between a forearm artery and vein to permit repeated venepuncture access to the blood stream. When a normal cephalic vein is present this is preferentially selected together with the radial artery. The fistula is created about 10 cm above the radial styloid process to allow room for an adequate distal limb of the fistula to develop.

The ulnar artery–basilic vein fistula is less satisfactory because the basilic vein is more mobile, tortuous and relatively inaccessible.

A brachial artery–median cubital fistula is used if no forearm veins are available. There is a constant vein draining into the back of the median cubital vein from the forearm muscles, which must be ligated. If this is not done, blood will flow down this channel into the deep venous system. The brachial artery lies immediately deep to the bicipital aponeurosis.

Axillary vein

The axillary vein (*Fig.* 192) begins at the inferior border of the teres major muscle as a continuation of the basilic vein. It ends at the outer border of the 1st rib. The axillary vein lies on the medial side of the axillary artery and partly overlaps it. It completely overlaps the artery anteriorly when the arm is abducted as in an axillary lymph node dissection.

The part of the vein in front of the first part of the axillary artery has a valve and is grooved by the subclavius muscle when the arm is abducted. The latter may be one of the factors responsible for axillary vein thrombosis which may follow prolonged abduction of the arm above the head, as in painting a ceiling.

The first part of the axillary vein is relatively superficial, being separated from the skin by fascia and fatty tissue. The medial cutaneous nerve of the arm lies on its surface and separates it from the axillary artery. The first part of the

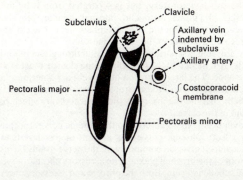

Fig. 192. Way in which subclavius muscle indents axillary vein in full abduction of arm. This is one of the factors in primary thrombosis of this vein.

axillary vein may be used for venepuncture. The axillary artery is palpated with the arm abducted; the axillary vein lies medial to it.

The subclavian vein

The subclavian vein (*Fig.* 193) lies in the lower part of the supraclavicular triangle. This triangle is bounded medially by the posterior border of the sternomastoid muscle, caudally by the middle third of the clavicle and laterally by the anterior border of the trapezius.

The subclavian vein is the continuation of the axillary vein and begins at the lateral border of the 1st rib. The subclavian vein passes over the 1st rib

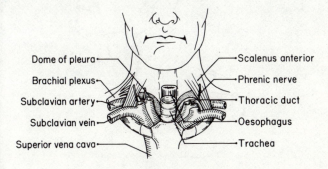

Fig. 193. The subclavian vein.

parallel to the subclavian artery, but is separated from it by the scalenus anterior muscle. It unites with the internal jugular vein behind the sternoclavicular joint to form the brachiocephalic vein. The external jugular vein is the only real tributary of the subclavian vein.

Anteriorly, the vein is separated from the skin throughout its entire course by the clavicle. Just medial to the midpoint of the clavicle it rises to the upper border of the bone. The lateral portion of the vein lies anterior to and below the subclavian artery, as both these structures cross the upper surface of the 1st rib. Medially, behind the artery, is the cervical pleura which rises above the sternal end of the clavicle.

The subclavian vein passes anterior to the phrenic nerve. In a postmortem study, an accessory phrenic nerve was present in just less than half the cadavers dissected. It arises in common with the nerve to subclavius from the 5th cervical root of the brachial plexus. The accessory phrenic nerve may pass in front of the subclavian vein. Both the phrenic and accessory phrenic nerves may be paralysed by local anaesthetic solution injected around the vein.

The thoracic duct arches over the apex of the pleura on the left side to enter the angle made by the junction of the internal jugular and subclavian veins.

Cannulation of the subclavian vein is done either by the supra- or infraclavicular approach. In obese patients, the vein can be located by use of the ultrasound flow probe. In the infraclavicular approach, the needle is inserted below the midpoint of the clavicle (*Fig*. 194) and aimed at the suprasternal notch. It is important to keep the needle and syringe roughly

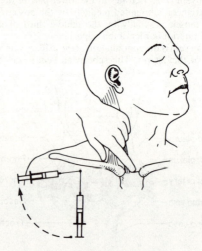

Fig. 194. Subclavian vein puncture.

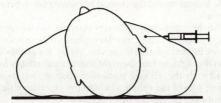

Fig. 195. The needle and syringe are parallel to the coronal plane.

parallel to the coronal plane to avoid producing a pneumothorax (*Fig*. 195). The subclavian artery may also be damaged during insertion of the needle.

Internal jugular vein

The internal jugular vein (*Fig*. 196) commences 1–2 cm below the base of the skull by the union of the transverse sinus with the inferior petrosal sinus. It

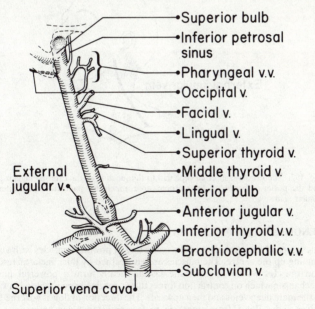

Fig. 196. The right internal jugular vein.

ends behind the sternal end of the clavicle by joining the subclavian to form the brachiocephalic.

It lies lateral to the internal carotid artery above and to the common carotid below. Its relations are, therefore, similar to those of these vessels. The deep cervical nodes are in close relation to the vein. At the lower ends both internal jugulars tend to the right, so that the right comes to lie farther from the right common carotid while the left vein tends to overlap the left common carotid artery. The lower part of the vein lies behind the junction of the sternal and clavicular insertions of the sternomastoid muscle.

Most techniques for cannulating the vein depend on identifying the sternomastoid muscle and its sternal and clavicular insertions. One technique is to insert a needle along the posterior border of the sternomastoid muscle cephalad to the point where the external jugular vein crosses the posterior border of the muscle (*Fig*. 197). The needle is directed towards the sternal notch and elevated 10 degrees above the coronal plane.

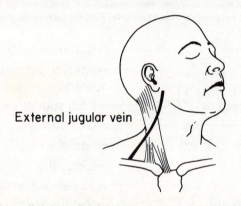

External jugular vein

Fig. 197. The needle is inserted cephalad to the junction of the external jugular vein and the posterior border of the sternomastoid muscle for puncture of the internal jugular vein.

VENOUS SYSTEM OF THE LEG

The leg can be regarded as a tube consisting of powerful muscles with veins running up the centre. The muscles are ensheathed by thick inelastic fascia. The muscles within the inelastic fascial sheath form a powerful pump mechanism which on contraction forces their contained venous blood inward to the main deep veins and then upwards. The direction of flow is governed by valves so that flow is from superficial to deep and from below upwards.

Each limb has three anatomically and functionally distinguishable sets of veins:

Superficial

The veins have relatively thick muscular walls. The major trunks are the long (great) and short (small) saphenous veins. These trunks run in tunnels created by a condensation of superficial fascia. This support from the condensation of fascia explains why the greater saphenous vein itself is very often not varicose while its tributaries are tortuous.

THE LONG SAPHENOUS VEIN: The long saphenous vein is the longest vein in the body. It commences from the inner part of the dorsal venous arch of the foot, passes in front of medial malleolus straight up to the posteromedial aspect of the knee joint, one hand-breadth posterior to the patella, and then up to the fossa ovalis or saphenous opening (4 cm below and lateral to pubic tubercle) where it enters the femoral vein. The saphenous nerve is closely associated with the long saphenous vein. The nerve is posterior to the vein at the knee, but at the ankle it lies anterior to the vein in 60 per cent of cases.

The saphenous vein at the ankle is a common site for a 'cut down' in emergencies. The saphenous nerve must not be included in a ligature around the vein.

Just below the knee the great saphenous vein receives a major tributary, the posterior arch vein (*Fig.* 198). This collects blood from a complex of veins overlying the posteromedial aspect of the calf and its main drainage is into the deep system via multiple veins perforating the deep fascia. The posterior arch vein may drain into a thin-walled accessory saphenous vein running parallel to the long saphenous vein. This vein also drains into the long saphenous vein.

The anterior veins of the leg ascend diagonally across the shin and join either the long saphenous or posterior arch veins. Other tributaries are from the short saphenous vein and veins around the knee.

In the thigh, near its junction with the femoral vein, the great saphenous receives the posteromedial and anterolateral veins, and the external pudendal, inferior epigastric and circumflex iliac veins enter the long saphenous vein at the fossa ovalis (*Fig.* 199). In the Trendelenburg or high ligature operation, these tributaries must be ligated and divided. If the long saphenous vein is divided distal to its junction with one of these tributaries, the patient will develop recurrent varicose veins (*Fig.* 200).

The junction of the long saphenous vein with the femoral vein is clearly visible as a white line.

The long saphenous vein may enter the femoral vein more distal to its usual termination or its tributaries may go directly to the femoral vein.

Vulval varicosities may occur during pregnancy. Most cases have incompetent long saphenous veins and their superficial tributaries. Other sources of such varicosities are:

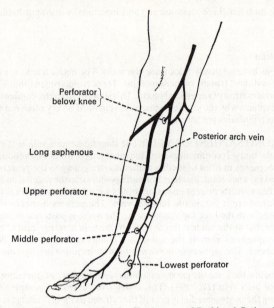

Fig. 198. The posterior arch vein. (By courtesy of Dodd and Cockett.)

1. Some veins from the labia majora pass with the round ligament through the inguinal canal. They may become varicose and cause a hernia-like swelling in the groin and may cause a considerable swelling of the labia majora.
2. Tributaries of the internal pudendal vein, when enlarged, cause swelling of the perineum and posterior part of the labia.

These conditions occur in the latter part of pregnancy and may be sufficiently severe to require operation.

When the long saphenous vein is removed for arterial grafting, it is important to place the incision over the vein. Undermining of the skin results in skin necrosis. Because of its valves, the vein has to be reversed when it is used to replace or bypass an arterial obstruction. In an *in situ* vein graft, the valves have to be destroyed to allow arterial blood to flow down the vein.

THE SHORT SAPHENOUS VEIN: The short saphenous vein begins by the fusion of a number of small veins below and behind the lateral malleolus, where it comes into relationship with the large sural nerve which lies just lateral to the vein in the lower third of the leg. The vein then runs along the

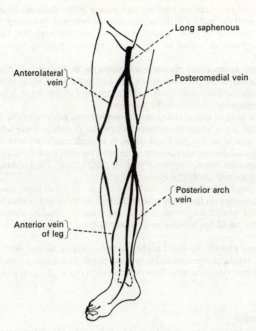

Fig. 199. The long saphenous vein and its tributaries. (By courtesy of Dodd and Cockett.)

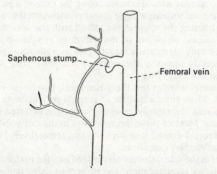

Fig. 200. Showing how a carelessly performed Trendelenburg operation will not prevent return of varicosity.

outer edge of the Achilles tendon, and passes to the midline; from here it continues until the middle of the popliteal space, where it dips sharply to enter the popliteal vein in most cases. Where it goes through the fascia, the posterior cutaneous nerve of the thigh emerges, passing from deep to superficial.

There are several less common terminations to the vessel. It may run non-stop through the popliteal space and end in the deep veins in the lower thigh, or join the long saphenous in the upper third of the thigh. It may enter the long saphenous just below the knee joint.

In 90 per cent of cases, the short saphenous vein perforates the investing fascia of the leg a variable distance below the popliteal fossa and runs a subfascial course to the popliteal fossa. If in such cases the vein is merely ligated in its subcutaneous position, recurrent varicosities will occur because the incompetent upper segment will be left intact. Exploration of the popliteal space will avoid this error.

Several small vessels connect the lower part of the small saphenous vein to the venous arches on the inner side of the leg. As these are connected to the medial ankle-perforating veins, venous hypertension may be transmitted to or from the small saphenous vein depending on which of the systems is incompetent.

The upper part of the short saphenous vein communicates with the long saphenous via the posteromedial vein of the thigh. This is also a possible route for the transmission of venous hypertension from one saphenous to the other.

The deep veins

The deep veins lie amongst and are supported by powerful muscles. These veins are the tibial, peroneal, popliteal, and femoral and their tributaries. The deep veins accompany named arteries taking the form of a plexus below the level of the knee and forming a single major vein towards the root of the limb.

The veins draining the muscles are valved with the notable exception of those in the soleus, which are of the nature of venous sinuses. They are unvalved and empty segmentally into the posterior tibial and peroneal veins, sometimes directly opposite the entry of the perforating veins into the posterior tibial vein (*Fig.* 201).

When the muscles are at rest there is sluggish movement of blood in the soleal sinuses. More than a quarter of surgical patients over the age of 40 develop deep vein thrombosis following surgery as detected by radioactive fibrinogen tests. Most of these thrombi form in the calf veins and undergo lysis. If the thrombi extend into popliteal and femoral veins there is a high incidence of pulmonary embolism.

Thrombosis in the soleal sinuses may extend into the perforating veins and, after spontaneous recanalization, the protective valve is destroyed which allows the blood to go from the deep to the superficial system. The resulting

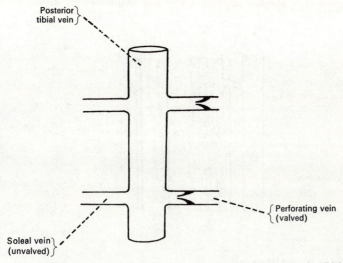

Fig. 201. The diagram shows soleal and perforating veins entering the posterior tibial vein exactly opposite each other.

venous congestion of the overlying skin can cause venous ulceration, usually above the medial malleolus.

Perforating veins

These are communicating vessels (*Fig.* 202) between the superficial and deep veins. They show a predilection for intermuscular septa occurring on either side of the sartorius, between the vastus lateralis and the hamstrings, on either side of the peroneal group and along the anterior border of the soleus.

1. INDIRECT: These consist of small superficial vessels which penetrate the deep fascia to connect with a vessel in a muscle, which in turn is connected to one of the deep veins. It is significant that in the ankle region there is little muscle and therefore few indirect perforators, and consequently the return of blood from the superficial tissues is dependent on the direct perforators. This is one of the most significant factors in the pathology of ankle ulceration.

2. DIRECT: These are the long and short saphenous veins, and smaller perforating veins.

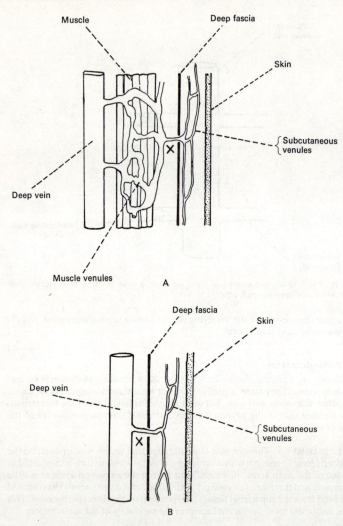

Fig. 202. A, Diagram of an indirect perforating vein (X); B, diagram of a direct perforating vein (X).

The Long and Short Spahenous Veins: The long and short saphenous veins are communicating veins between the superficial and deep venous systems of the leg. They are so valved as to prevent flow from deep to superficial systems. When valves become defective venous hypertension becomes evident as varicose veins.

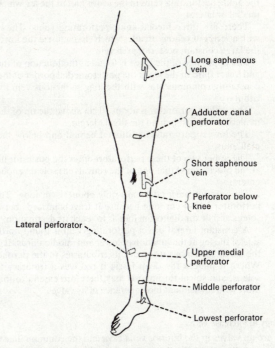

Long saphenous vein

Adductor canal perforator

Short saphenous vein

Perforator below knee

Lateral perforator

Upper medial perforator

Middle perforator

Lowest perforator

Fig. 203. The chief perforating veins of the lower limb.

The Smaller Perforating Vessels: The smaller perforating vessels are fairly constantly situated and are of great surgical significance (*Fig.* 203). They are intimately related to the posterior border of the tibia and fibula and are so valved that in health only an inward flow is possible. They commence from tributaries of the saphenous vessels and perforate the deep fascia to join the deep veins, being valved at each end, and being accompanied as a rule by a small artery. These small perforators are as follows:

In the thigh: A constant communicating vein between long saphenous, or a tributary in the lower half of the thigh, and the femoral vein in Hunter's canal.

In the leg: A communicating vein just distal to the knee connecting the long saphenous or posterior arch vein to the posterior tibial vein and the ankle perforating veins in the lower half of the leg which may be medial or lateral.

There are three medial ankle-perforating veins. They connect with a series of venous arcades which characterize the lower part of the large constant posterior arch vein.

The upper one of the three is found at the junction of the middle and lower third of the leg at the posteromedial border of the tibia. It constantly communicates with the long saphenous vein by a small tributary.

The middle perforator is about 10 cm above the tip of the medial malleolus and just behind the tibial margin.

The lowest perforator is situated behind and below the medial malleolus.

The upper two of these perforators enter the posterior tibial vein at the precise level that one of the (unvalved) soleal venous sinuses enters.

The inferior perforators are only about 1 cm long. The upper perforator is 3–4 cm long because it travels inwards between the soleus and flexor digitorum longus to reach its destination.

A constant lateral direct perforating vein is found on the outer side of the leg at the junction of lower and middle thirds. It connects the small saphenous or one of its tributaries to the peroneal vein. Where it pierces the deep fascia it receives a tributary from the soleus, and soleal thrombosis may therefore extend to the perforator, with subsequent incompetence of its valves.

Aetiology of varicose veins

There are no valves in the inferior vena cava and the common iliac veins. In about 80 per cent of people there is a valve in the external iliac vein which protects the saphenofemoral junction against high pressure. The remaining 20 per cent of people, with congenital absence of this valve in the external iliac vein, are prone to venous hypertension which may overcome the valve at the saphenofemoral junction with resultant varicose veins commencing at the saphenofemoral junction and proceeding down the vein. This accounts for some cases of varicose veins particularly in young people with a family history of varicose veins.

Another suggested cause for varicose veins is that the disease starts as thrombosis in soleal sinuses which extends to one of the calf-perforating veins. After recanalization the perforator becomes incompetent and venous hypertension can be transmitted from the deep to the superficial veins. Distension of the latter causes a secondary incompetence of the valves in the superficial veins.

The diagnosis

Two clinical tests are in common use and of great value.

THE TOURNIQUET TEST: A diagnosis of varicose veins having been made, the patient lies with the lower limbs exposed.

The limb is elevated above the level of the heart which empties the varicose veins. Rubber tubing is applied round the upper thigh sufficiently firmly to occlude the saphenous but not the femoral vein.

The patient now stands and exercises gently by intermittently raising the heels:

1. If the varicosities remain empty for 30 s, the communicating veins below the tubing are competent; if, however, they fill in this time the communicating veins below the tubing are incompetent.
2. If the veins remain collapsed as in (1) but fill at once on removal of the tubing, then a perforator above the tubing is incompetent (most probably the saphenofemoral junction).
3. If the varicosities fill in 30 s with the tourniquet in place, but distend even more when it is removed, then both the saphenofemoral and the valves of the lower perforating veins are incompetent.
4. Two tourniquets may be used at different levels in the lower limb to isolate and determine the exact position of incompetent perforators.

PERTHES' TEST: While the patient stands, a tourniquet is applied around the thigh tight enough to occlude the long saphenous vein but not the deep veins. The patient walks for 5 min.

If the fullness of the varicose veins disappears, then the valves of the perforating veins are competent and the deep veins are patent. If the fullness of the varicose veins remains unchanged or increases then the valves of the perforating veins are incompetent. Aggravation of the varicosities with significant calf pain suggests occluded deep veins.

EMBRYOLOGY OF THE INFERIOR AND SUPERIOR VENA CAVA

Numerous venous channels take part in the early formation of the primitive embryo. The surgeon is particularly concerned with anomalies of the inferior and the superior vena cava.

Inferior vena cava

The hepatic segment of the inferior vena cava (*Fig.* 204) is derived from the

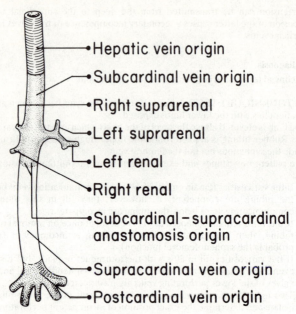

- •Hepatic vein origin
- •Subcardinal vein origin
- •Right suprarenal
- •Left suprarenal
- •Left renal
- •Right renal
- •Subcardinal – supracardinal anastomosis origin
- •Supracardinal vein origin
- •Postcardinal vein origin

Fig. 204. Development of the inferior vena cava.

hepatic veins (proximal part of the right vitelline vein) and hepatic sinusoids. The infrahepatic segment is derived from changes in three parallel sets of veins: the postcardinal, subcardinal and supracardinal.

1. The postcardinal vein is the primitive system and develops in association with the mesonephros. It anastomoses with the developing subcardinal system and persists only as the iliac bifurcation.
2. The right and left subcardinal veins, which are in a plane ventral to the aorta, communicate across the midline; blood is diverted to the right subcardinal system which forms the suprarenal portion of the inferior vena cava.
3. The supracardinal system appears as two parallel veins in a plane dorsal to the aorta; these veins anastomose with each other across the midline and also with the subcardinal system. This group of anastomoses forms a vascular ring around the aorta.

   The right supracardinal vein persists as the normal infrarenal right inferior vena cava and the ventral part of the cuff around the aorta persists as the normal left renal vein.

Should the left supracardinal vein persist, either a double inferior vena cava or a single left-sided vena cava results.

The entire venous cuff may persist to form a circumaortic renal vein.

The ventral portion may disappear leaving only a retro-aortic left renal vein.

RENAL VEIN ANOMALIES:

Retro-aortic Left Renal Vein: If the pre-aortic normal renal vein is not found during dissection of the abdominal aorta, one should suspect the presence of an isolated retro-aortic left renal vein, and perform a very cautious dissection. This vein takes an oblique course behind the aorta and is inserted more caudally into the inferior vena cava. It is often joined by lumbar and retroperitoneal veins. These veins are particularly susceptible to injury during aortic surgery.

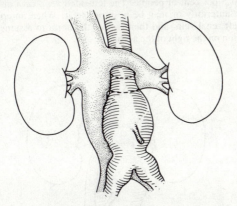

Fig. 205. Circumaortic renal venous cuff.

Circumaortic Renal Venous Cuff: In this condition (*Fig.* 205) the normal pre-aortic left renal vein is present, but in addition there are either small retro-aortic renal veins, or a single large retro-aortic left renal vein, which drains into the inferior vena cava. The former anomaly occurs in about 16 per cent of people, but a large retro-aortic renal vein component of the cuff is very uncommon.

During aortic surgery the small retro-aortic renal veins may not be noticed, but the presence of a large retro-aortic vein can result in serious haemorrhage if it is damaged. The vein drains into the inferior vena cava more caudally than the anterior vein and will be identified only if the surgeon dissects around the aorta under direct vision. If identified, special care must be taken to place the occluding clamp on the aorta at a higher level. Repair of a damaged vein may require division of the aorta to gain control.

Ligation of the Left Renal Vein: In a high abdominal aortic aneurysm, the left renal vein is sometimes ligated and divided to facilitate exposure of the aorta just below the renal arteries. The safe division of the vein depends on the efficiency of the collateral circulation through the adrenal and gonadal veins. This can be assessed by measuring the pressure of the left renal vein after it has been temporarily occluded with a vascular clamp. A pressure in excess of 40 mmHg suggests that the collaterals are inadequate.

INFERIOR VENA CAVA ANOMALIES:

Left-sided Vena Cava: A single left-sided vena cava (*Fig.* 206) occurs in 0.2–0.5 per cent of people. The left-sided vena cava may cross the aorta anteriorly or may be posterior to it. When anterior, it joins the left renal vein, and then crosses the aorta to assume its normal position on the right of the aorta.

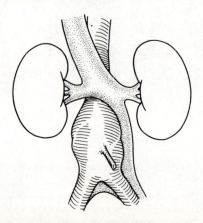

Fig. 206. Left-sided vena cava.

In the presence of such an anomaly the neck of an abdominal aneurysm can be dissected by dividing the right renal vein, provided the adrenal and genital veins join it to ensure a collateral path for the venous return from the right kidney.

Double Inferior Vena Cava: Duplication of the inferior vena cava may be anterior or postior to the aorta *Fig.* 207). Dissection of the neck of

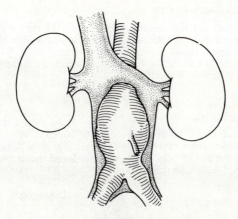

Fig. 207. Double inferior vena cava.

an abdominal aortic aneurysm may require division of the left renal vein or resection of the left portion of the inferior vena cava. The left portion of a double inferior vena cava may be quite small and easily overlooked, in which case it presents no difficulties to aortic resection.

Superior vena cava

In contrast to the inferior vena cava, development of the superior vena cava is comparatively simple. This vessel develops from two parallel anterior cardinal veins. During the second month of fetal development an oblique anastomosis shunts the blood from the left to the right cardinal vein and becomes the left brachiocephalic vein when the caudal part of the left anterior cardinal vein degenerates. The right anterior and the right common cardinal veins become the superior vena cava.

ANOMALIES OF THE SUPERIOR VENA CAVA:

Double Superior Vena Cava: This is due to persistence of the left anterior cardinal vein. The left-sided vena cava drains into the right atrium via the coronary sinus.

Left Superior Vena Cava: The right anterior and right common cardinal veins have degenerated. Blood from the right side drains via the brachiocephalic vein into the left superior vena cava which opens into the coronary sinus.

THE GREAT LYMPH DUCTS

These comprise: (a) the thoracic duct—single; (b) the right and left subclavian trunks; (c) the right and left bronchomediastinal trunks; (d) the right and left jugular trunks; (e) the right lymph duct.

These vessels, like all but the very smallest lymphatics, are supplied with bicuspid valves to prevent backflow.

Cisterna chyli

This lymph sac (*Fig*. 208) lies in front of the bodies of the 1st and 2nd lumbar vertebrae between the aorta and the right crus of the diaphragm. It is present in 50 per cent of cases. It receives three lymph trunks, the right and left lumbar and the intestinal.

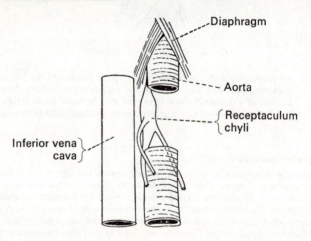

Fig. 208. The cisterna (receptaculum) chyli.

Each of the lumbar trunks is a short vessel which leaves the para-aortic glands to enter the cisterna. The lumbar trunks convey the lymph from the lower limbs, the pelvis including its viscera, kidneys and adrenals, and deep lymphatics of the abdominal walls. The left lumbar trunk reaches the cisterna by passing behind the aorta.

The intestinal trunk passes from the pre-aortic nodes to the cisterna. It conveys lymph from: (a) the stomach; (b) the pancreas; (c) the spleen; (d) most of liver; (e) the intestines.

Thoracic duct

This vessel commences from the upper end of the cisterna chyli. The duct conveys the entire lymph from the body excepting that from the: (i) right side of the head and neck; (ii) right upper limb; (iii) thoracic wall on the right; (iv) right lung; (v) right side of the heart; (vi) part of convex surface of the liver; (vii) lower part of the left lung.

The vessel in the adult is the same length as the spinal cord, viz. 45 cm.

The thoracic duct has a short abdominal course and continues up through the chest to terminate in the neck.

ABDOMINAL COURSE: Leaving the cisterna, the duct passes through the aortic orifice of the diaphragm, having the vena azygos on its right.

THORACIC COURSE: It runs up the posterior mediastinum, having the azygos vein on its right and the aorta on its left side. Behind it are the vertebrae, the right intercostal arteries, and the hemi-azygos and accessory hemi-azygos veins. In front are the oesophagus, diaphragm, and pericardium. The duct, on reaching the 7th thoracic vertebra, begins to cross to the left. It does so very obliquely, reaching the left side at the level of the 5th thoracic vertebra, having crossed behind the oesophagus. It now runs up along the left border of the oesophagus, medial to the pleura and behind the left subclavian artery into the neck.

CERVICAL COURSE: In the neck the duct forms an arch which reaches as high as the 7th cervical vertebra. The duct arches behind the 'carotid system' and in front of the 'vertebral system', i.e. it passes behind the common carotid artery, internal jugular vein, and the vagus nerve, and in front of the vertebral artery, vein and the sympathetic trunk. As the duct arches to the left it also crosses the scalenus anterior and phrenic nerve and the transverse cervical and suprascapular arteries (*Fig.* 209).

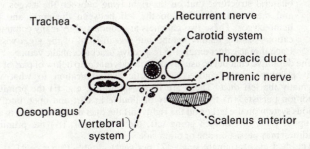

Fig. 209. Relationship of termination of thoracic duct.

TERMINATION: It usually ends as a single vessel by entering the junction of the left internal jugular and subclavian veins. The opening is guarded by valves to prevent regurgitation of blood into the duct. The duct sometimes divides into two, one vessel entering the veins on the right side of the head and neck. This is important in wounds of the duct. It used to be thought that if the duct were severed the injury would be fatal. This is not so, for after leaking lymph for a while the patient usually recovers. This indicates that there exist numerous communications with the venous system whereby the lymph in the thoracic duct may enter the circulation.

TRIBUTARIES:
In the Abdomen: The duct receives on either side a trunk from the lateral intercostal lymph nodes of the lower six spaces.
In the Thorax: It receives:
1. A trunk from either side draining the upper lumbar nodes which pierces the crus of the diaphragm to join the duct.
2. Efferents from the posterior mediastinal nodes.
3. Efferents from the lateral intercostal nodes of the upper six left spaces.
In the Neck: It receives:
1. The left jugular lymph trunk from the left side of the head and neck.
2. The left subclavian lymph trunk from the left upper limb.
It may receive:
3. The left bronchomediastinal trunk from the left side of the thorax.

ANOMALIES OF THE THORACIC DUCT: It requires protection and the appreciation of the possibility of, and practical implications of, the existence of anomalies.
Development: At the end of the second month the thoracic duct is a bilateral structure, that on the right lying between the azygos vein and the aorta, and that on the left between the aorta and the hemi-azygos. These two channels are connected by many communications passing mainly behind but also in front of the great vessel. Each thoracic duct enters the respective brachiocephalic vein.
The definitive channel as usually described is made up below of part of the right primitive vessel and a retro-aortic communication to what was originally the left duct. There are many variations, e.g. (i) the primitive condition persists; (ii) the duct may be double in part and open into the venous system on the left or on the right; (iii) the duct may divide into two in its upper part, one branch going left, the other right; (iv) the primitive condition may persist on one or other side.
The duct may terminate singly (77 per cent), doubly (9 per cent), triply (9 per cent), and quadruply (in 5 per cent).

Quite frequently the duct ends in other veins than in the left angulus venosus, e.g. on the left side in the subclavian, internal jugular, or vertebral; on the right in the angulus venosus, the internal jugular, or the subclavian.

INJURY TO THE THORACIC DUCT: The thoracic duct may be damaged as the result of penetrating injuries of the chest or neck. The patient may develop an accumulation of lymph in the chest (chylothorax) which collapses the lung on the affected side. A chylothorax very rarely becomes infected which has been attributed to the bacteriostatic effect of chyle.

A chylothorax is treated by aspirating the lymph from the pleural cavity. If the chylothorax recurs, chest tube drainage is instituted. Ligation of the thoracic duct is required only if the lymph leak persists after 2–3 weeks of conservative treatment.

During operations in the chest, the root of the neck and the upper abdomen, e.g. when mobilizing the upper end of an aortic aneurysm, the major lymphatic ducts may be damaged and chyle is seen to leak into the surrounding tissues. All that is then required is ligature of the duct. Smaller lymphatic leaks are presumably common but close spontaneously. Persistent chylous ascites does not occur.

Right lymph duct

This is a short vessel 1·25–2·5 cm long which runs down on the scalenus anterior to join the junction of the right internal jugular and subclavian veins. It is formed by the union of the right jugular, subclavian, and bronchomedias-

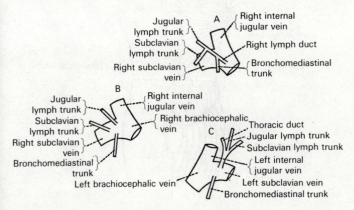

Fig. 210. Termination of the great lymph trunks. A and B, on the right side; C, on the left side.

tinal trunks (*Fig.* 210). These vessels may all open separately into the junction between the right subclavian and internal jugular veins.

The lymphatic watersheds of the skin

It is important to realize that the lymph from the skin and its appendages drains in the first instance to the plexus on the deep fascia. In cancer of the skin, or a skin appendage, radical operation implies the removal of that part of the plexus on the deep fascia.

The lymphatic drainage of the skin and its appendages falls naturally into six great territories. A vertical line through the sagittal plane of the body divides the lymphatic drainage of the skin into three areas on each side. There is some communication across the middle line, but it is not free (*Fig.* 211).

The three areas on each side of the body are demarcated from each other by two horizontal lines, one at the level of the clavicle, the other at the level of

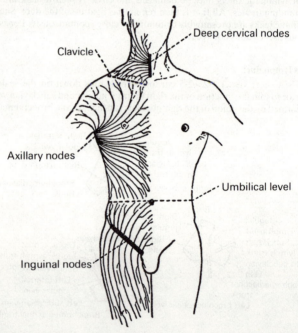

Fig. 211. To show the lymphatic watersheds of the skin. (Redrawn from Sampson Handley.)

the umbilicus. These lines are the lymphatic watersheds, and the skin lymph flows in a direction away from them. Each line also represents the meeting place of two adjacent territories, so that cancer situated on one of these lines may spread by two routes along the lymphatics running away from the watershed. Similarly, a cancer situated anywhere in the middle line of the surface of the body may spread in two directions because of the lymphatic communication across the midline. Cancer situated at the umbilicus may spread in four directions, viz. towards both axillae and both groins, as lymphatics draining to these glands come into communication at the umbilicus.

The importance of these facts is realized when it is remembered that the treatment of cancer is removal of the growth itself and also removal of the lymphatics and nodes which drain the area in which the cancer is situated.

Chapter 22

THE HEART AND GREAT VESSELS

THE HEART

Embryology
At an early stage of development (three weeks) the heart consists of a relatively straight tube in which five sacculations develop. Caudocranially they are the sinus venosus with its right and left horns, atrium, ventricle, bulbus cordis and truncus arteriosus. The cardiac tube undergoes looping and

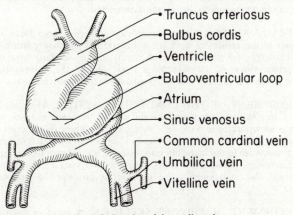

Fig. 212. Looping of the cardiac tube.

partitioning (septation) in the process of developing into a four-chambered heart.

LOOPING: The right ventricle develops from the bulbus cordis and the left ventricle from the primitive ventricle. A bulboventricular loop (*Fig.* 212) directed to the right and frontally is responsible for the position of the ventricles in the mature state. Differential growth results in the atrium lying anterior to the sinus venosus.

PARTITIONING: By a process of septation the cardiac tube is divided into right and left chambers and the truncus arteriosus into the aorta and pulmonary trunk. While these septa are dividing the atrium and ventricles, the common atrioventricular canal is being divided into right and left canals by the ingrowth of anterior and posterior endocardial cushions. The right and left atria come to drain into the right and left ventricles as the result of a shift of the atrioventricular canal to the right. Ridges which develop in the bulbus cordis fuse with the ventricular septum in such a manner that the aorta arises from the left ventricle and the pulmonary trunk from the right ventricle.

INCORPORATION OF THE SINUS VENOSUS INTO THE ATRIUM: During the process of partitioning, the right horn of the sinus venosus becomes incorporated in the right atrium, while the left horn of the sinus venosus forms the coronary sinus and the oblique vein (of Marshall).

PULMONARY VEINS AND LEFT ATRIUM: The common pulmonary vein and its tributaries are incorporated into the left atrium when septation of the cardiac chambers has been almost completed.

CARDIAC VALVES: The semilunar valves develop from three valve swellings at the orifices of both the aorta and the pulmonary trunk. The atrioventricular valves (tricuspid and mitral) develop similarly from localized proliferations of subendocardial tissue around the atrioventricular canals. These swellings become hollowed out on their ventricular sides.

DEVELOPMENT OF THE CONDUCTION SYSTEM: The sino-atrial node is originally situated in the right wall of the sinus venosus which becomes incorporated into the right atrium and lies where the superior vena cava enters the atrium. The primordial conductive cells of the left wall of the sinus venosus are found in the interatrial septum just anterior to the opening of the coronary sinus. These cells, together with similar cells from the atrioventricular canal region, make up the atrioventricular node and bundle of His.

DEVELOPMENT OF FIBROUS SKELETON: A band of connective

tissue grows in from the epicardium as the chambers of the heart develop and separates the muscle of the atria from that of the ventricles.

DEVELOPMENT OF CORONARY ARTERIES: These develop as endothelial sprouts from the left and right posterior quadrants of the bulbus cordis at the end of the sixth week. At this time the bulbus cordis is not yet divided into aortic and pulmonary trunks.

FETAL CIRCULATION: By the end of the eighth week the heart has assumed the features which it retains until birth. The right atrium in the fetal circulation receives blood from the superior vena cava and oxygenated blood from the placenta via the left umbilical vein, ductus venosus and right vitelline vein. The latter later becomes the hepatic part of the inferior vena cava. Some of the venous blood, especially that from the superior vena cava, flows into the right ventricle thence into the pulmonary artery and, by way of the ductus arteriosus, into the descending aorta. The oxygenated inferior vena caval blood is directed through the foramen ovale in the atrial septum into the left atrium from where it reaches the left ventricle and aorta. The ductus closes within hours of birth by contraction of its own smooth muscle, and the relatively high pressure in the left atrium closes the valve of the foramen ovale.

Position of the heart in the thorax

In its normal anatomical position, the long axis of the heart extends from the left hypochondrium towards the right shoulder. This axis is intersected at right-angles by that of the atrioventricular junction. The right atrium and right ventricle lie for the most part anterior to the left atrium and left ventricle. (*See Fig.* 213.)

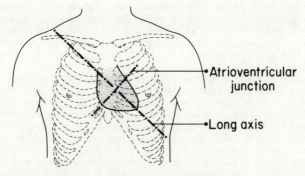

Fig. 213. Position of the heart in the thorax.

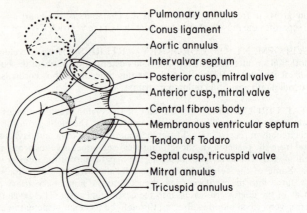

Fig. 214. The fibrous skeleton.

Structure

THE FIBROUS SKELETON OF THE HEART: The fibrous skeleton (*Fig.* 214) is formed by four fibrous annuli or rings and the extensions that arise from them. Two of the rings surround the atrioventricular orifices and two contribute to the roots of the aorta and pulmonary trunk. The pulmonary valve ring lies at a higher level than the aortic valve and is connected to the fibrous skeleton of the heart by the conus ligament.

The atrioventricular annuli give attachment to the muscle fibres of the atria and ventricles. The fibrous skeleton also provides attachment for the aortic, mitral, tricuspid and pulmonary valve leaflets. From the postero-medial wall of the aorta (between the right posterior and left posterior sinuses), a fibrous membrane (the intervalvar septum or subaortic curtain) becomes continuous with the anterior cusp of the mitral valve. This fibrous membrane acts as an aortic baffle placed between the inflow and outflow tracts of the left ventricle.

Between the posterior wall of the aortic root and the upper parts of the two atrioventricular orifices, a band of fibrous tissue extends to the right and left to form the right and left fibrous trigones. The right fibrous trigone, measuring 10 mm by 5 mm, is the larger and more important, and lies between the two atrioventricular rings behind the non-coronary cusp of the aortic valve. It is also called the 'central fibrous body'. The latter extends downwards in a triangular manner between the right and left atrioventricular annuli to become continuous with the membranous part of the interventricular septum which also forms part of the fibrous skeleton. The membranous septum separates the left ventricle from the right ventricle and also the right atrium because part of the septal cusp of the tricuspid valve is attached to the right side of the septum. The membranous septum is a strategic area of the heart because it links together both ventricles and the right atrium and also the aortic, tricuspid and mitral valves.

The Tendon of Todaro: This band of collagen is an extension of the right fibrous trigone which is palpable in the subendocardial tissue of the right atrium. It forms one side of the triangle of Koch. The other sides are formed by the septal leaflet of tricuspid valve and the antero-medial margin of the orifice of the coronary sinus.

If tension is placed on the remnants of the valve (Eustachian) of the inferior vena cava, the tendon of Todaro becomes prominent.

The tendon indicates the septal site of the atrioventricular node and its conducting tissue.

Clinical Significance:

1. The fibrous skeleton of the heart is capable of holding sutures under persistent tension.
2. In rheumatic heart disease the mitral annulus is often thickened due to the inflammatory process. This may result in an atrioventricular conduction defect.
3. In many types of congenital heart disease, such as some types of ventricular septal defects, the tetralogy of Fallot and tricuspid atresia, the central fibrous body is deformed and the course of the conduction system is altered.
4. Mönckeberg's sclerosis involving the aortic sinuses of Valsalva may extend to the membranous septum and injure or destroy the bundle of His.

THE CONDUCTION SYSTEM: *See Fig.* 215.

1. *Sino-atrial Node:* This is a small area measuring $15 \times 3 \times 1$ mm of specially differentiated muscle fibres in the wall of the right atrium to the right of the opening of the superior vena cava. the node lies in a dense matrix of fibrous tissue through which runs the nodal artery. Arrhythmias following atrial surgery are invariably due to damage to the sino-atrial node or its blood supply.
2. *Atrioventricular Node:* It measures about $7 \times 3 \times 1$ mm and lies subendocardially in the medial wall of the right atrium about 1 cm above the opening of the coronary sinus and immediately behind the basal attachment of the septal cusp of the tricuspid valve.
3. *Atrioventricular Bundle of His:* It is the only muscular connection between the atria and ventricles. It is 2–3 cm long and passes through the central fibrous body to reach the lower margin of the membranous part of the interventricular septum from which it passes upwards and forwards. In this position, the bundle is more or less directly related to the mitral, tricuspid and aortic valves and the membranous septum and is at risk during surgery on any of these structures. The

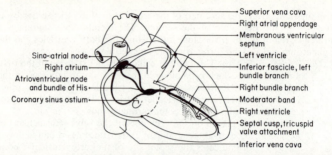

Fig. 215. The conducting system.

non-coronary sinus and cusp of the aortic valve lie behind and above the membranous part of the interventricular septum and the atrioventricular bundle may be affected by lesions that cause aortic valvulitis.

4. *Ventricular Conduction Tissue:* Having penetrated into the subaortic outflow tract, the atrioventricular bundle sits astride the muscular ventricular septum. It divides into (*a*) the right bundle-branch—a thin cord-like structure which passes through the posterior limb of the septomarginal trabeculum (moderator band) and extends towards the right ventricular apex, and (*b*) left bundle-branches. This branching occurs along the length of the bundle, the left bundle-branches tumbling down the smooth left side of the septum. Three major branches (anterior, septal and posterior) can be identified in the descending fan of left bundle-branch cells, but the three are intimately connected.

MORPHOLOGY OF THE CARDIAC CHAMBERS:

The Right Atrium: This chamber normally receives the systemic venous return. Both venae cavae and the coronary sinus enter the smooth-walled portion of the atrium which developmentally belongs to the sinus venosus. It is separated from a trabeculated portion of the atrium by a vertical ridge called the crista terminalis. The atrial appendage ends bluntly and projects to the left from the root of the superior vena cava and overlaps the right side of the root of the aorta.

The Left Atrium: This chamber forms the most posterior aspect or base of the heart. The four pulmonary veins enter a smooth-walled segment of atrium. There are only a few trabeculae (musculi pectinati) in the left atrial appendage which is a long finger-like projection from the left atrium.

The posterior septal surface of the right atrium is characterized by the fossa ovalis and the orifice of the coronary sinus. The fossa ovalis is the depression at the site of the fetal interatrial communication known as the foramen ovale. The true atrial septum is smaller than anticipated and incisions placed outside this area will penetrate the heart wall.

The characteristic shape of the right and left atrial appendages is the best way of distinguishing between the right and left atrium angiographically.

The Right Ventricle: This contains the smooth-walled infundibulum formed from incorporation of the bulbus cordis and it leads to the pulmonary valve. Although the leaflet pattern of the tricuspid valve is variable, it has a typical papillary muscle pattern consisting of a single anterior muscle, multiple posterior muscles and a medial (septal) papillary muscle. The supraventricular crest is a muscular arch placed between the right atrioventricular and pulmonary orifices so that blood from the right atrium must follow a U-shaped course to pass through the pulmonary orifice. The trabeculations of the right ventricle are coarse.

Angiocardiographic criteria of the right ventricle are the separation of the atrioventricular valve from the pulmonary valve by the infundibulum and the triangular shape of the ventricle on the anteroposterior projection.

The Left Ventricle: The cavity of the left ventricle is cone shaped and contains the two cusps of the mitral valve and two large papillary muscles. The aortic vestibule lies just below the aortic valve and is mainly fibrous. The interval between the right posterior (non-coronary) and left posterior (coronary) sinuses of the aortic valve is filled with a deformable subaortic curtain (intervalvar septum), which continues into the base of the central part of the anterior cusp of the mitral valve.

The left ventricle is identified angiocardiographically by the absence of an infundibulum which brings the aortic valve in line with the mitral valve. The ventricle has a cone shape on both lateral and frontal projections.

Congenital abnormalities of the heart

The incidence of congenital heart disease is approximately 9 per 1000 live births. The highest mortality from these anomalies occurs during the neonatal period. Advances in cardiac surgery have made surgical correction of many of these anomalies possible.

Congenital cardiac anomalies occur as a result of the following embryological mishaps: failure of septation and malalignment of septa, abnormal fusions, impeded growth and errors of looping.

1. FAILURE OF SEPTATION (PARTITIONING) AND MALALIGNMENT OF SEPTA

i. *The Cardiac Chambers:* There is a communication between the right and left atria (atrial septal defect) or the right and left ventricle (ventricular septal defect).

ii. *Atrioventricular Canal:* The normal development of the atrial or ventricular septum is dependent on the latter fusing with the endocardial cushions which divide the atrioventricular canal. The cushions also form the cusps of the atrioventricular valves. If the cushions fail to fuse or fuse incompletely a series of defects develop involving the atrioventricular canals, the atrioventricular valves (cleft valves) and the atrial and ventricular septa.

iii. *Truncus Arteriosus:* A persistent truncus arteriosus results from failure of an aorticopulmonary septum to develop. A single vessel gives rise to a pulmonary trunk and ascending aorta.

iv. *Great Vessels:* Malalignment of the great vessels occurs when the aorticopulmonary septum develops but fails to follow a spiral course. This malalignment results in complete transposition of the great vessels; the aorta arises from the right ventricle and the pulmonary trunk arises from the left ventricle.

2. ABNORMAL FUSIONS WHICH MAY OCCUR AT THE FOLLOWING SITES:

i. *Primitive Endocardial Valves:* Abnormal fusions of the endocardial swelling which will form the semilunar or atrioventricular valves give rise to pulmonary, aortic, tricuspid or mitral atresia or stenosis. The cardiac chamber situated downstream from an atretic valve is usually secondarily hypoplastic.

ii. *Foramen Ovale:* Premature closure results from adhesions of the valve of the foramen ovale to the wall of the atrial septum during fetal life. The right side cardiac chambers are enlarged and those of the left side hypoplastic.

3. IMPEDED GROWTH: There is a primary failure of the myocardium to develop which gives rise to a hypoplastic right or left ventricle. This abnormality is commonly associated with valvular atresia or stenosis.

4. ERRORS OF LOOPING: If the looping between the bulbus cordis and the ventricle is to the left instead of to the right, there is a mirror image development of the heart and its great vessels with displacement of the heart to the right (dextrocardia).

The coronary circulation

Coronary artery bypass grafting to revascularize an ischaemic myocardium and relieve angina pectoris is a commonly performed major surgical operation. An intimate knowledge of the coronary circulation has therefore become necessary. It is now also possible to dilate the orifice of obstructed coronary arteries with a balloon passed percutaneously (percutaneous transluminal angioplasty).

The heart is supplied by two coronary arteries, aptly named because they encircle the base of the ventricles like a crown (L. *corona:* crown).

The coronary arteries give rise to a capillary network in the myocardium. The capillary network drains into coronary veins which in turn empty into the coronary sinus of the right atrium.

The main coronary arteries are subepicardial and run in the atrioventricular and interventricular sulci. With age and ischaemic disease, the arteries are covered by an increasingly thick layer of fat, which makes it difficult to find the arteries at operation.

Minor branches from the subepicardial arteries in the atrioventricular sulcus ascend into the atria or descend into the ventricles round the circumference of the sulcus. Similar branches arising from the arteries in the interventricular sulcus penetrate to supply the ventricular septum.

THE RIGHT CORONARY ARTERY: This artery (*Fig.* 216) arises from the right anterior aortic coronary sinus. It runs forwards and to the right, between the right atrial appendage and the root of the pulmonary trunk, in the right atrioventricular sulcus. The artery runs round the acute (inferior) margin of the heart to reach the crux cordis. (At this point the posterior interventricular sulcus leaves the atrioventricular sulcus.)

It has the following branches:

1. *Infundibular:* In 50 per cent of cases this artery arises from a separate ostium in the coronary sinus. The artery ramifies over the right ventricular outflow tract. A small branch of the infundibular artery passes to the left around the right ventricular infundibulum and anastomoses with a branch of the left coronary artery to form the ring of Vieussens.

2. *Sinus Node Artery:* An important artrial branch of the sinus node artery arises from the right coronary near its origin and supplies the sino-atrial node. In 45 per cent of individuals, this artery arises from the circumflex branch of the left coronary. Occlusion of the artery to the sino-atrial node may result in atrial arrhythmias.

3. *Right Anterior Ventricular Branches:* As the right coronary artery descends in the atrioventricular sulcus it gives off 3 or 4 right anterior ventricular branches that run to the left parallel to the lower anterior margin of the heart. The lowest and largest of these vessels is the marginal artery which may extend to the apex and supply part of the ventricular septum.

The right coronary terminates by dividing into the following branches:

4. *The Posterior Descending Interventricular Artery:* In 90 per cent of individuals this vessel arises from the right coronary at the crux cordis (right dominance). It may also arise more proximally as a right ventricular branch and rarely it may encircle the apex of the left ventricle.

5. *Atrioventricular Nodal Artery:* This is a small vessel.

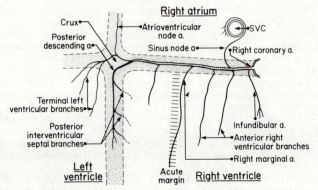

Fig. 216. The right coronary artery. [Redrawn from *Christopher's Textbook of Surgery*, ed D. C. Sabiston. Philadelphia, Saunders.]

6. *Posterior Left Ventricular Wall Arteries:* Occlusion of these arteries may result in posteromedial papillary muscle dysfunction. When arising from the right coronary artery, the posterior ventricular branches have a characteristic inverted, C-shaped appearance on angiography. Identification of their origin with retrograde collateral filling is important for the surgeon.

LEFT CORONARY ARTERY: This artery (*Fig.* 217) is very short. In the first part of its course it has a characteristic upward loop which lies free in the subepicardial tissue between the pulmonary trunk in front and the left atrial appendage behind. Just over 1 cm from its origin, it divides into the left anterior descending and circumflex arteries. In about 2 per cent of individuals, the vessels have a separate origin from the coronary sinus.

1. *Left Anterior Descending Artery:* This artery runs alongside the anterior interventricular vein in the interventricular sulcus. It then passes towards the apex which it encircles in 70 per cent of cases. The origin of the left anterior descending artery may be paired, yielding a bifid vessel frequently terminating proximal to the apex. Especially in its proximal and middle one-third, it may dip into the interventricular septum and occupy an intramuscular course (myocardial bridging), before returning to its epicardial position.

The left anterior descending artery has the following branches: (i) a series of perpendicular branches into the anterior interventricular septum. The first of these, originating 1 cm from the origin of the left anterior descending artery, is the largest, and gives off important

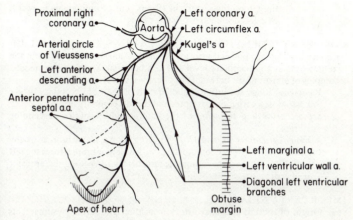

Fig. 217. The left coronary artery. [Redrawn from *Cristopher's Textbook of Surgery*, ed D. C. Sabiston. Philadelphia, Saunders.]

tributaries to the conduction system. (ii) One or more diagonal branches supplying the anterolateral left ventricular wall.

Angiographically, the left anterior descending artery may be recognized by: straight septal branches, lesser 'kinking' with myocardial contraction than the diagonal artery and it is usually the only vessel which runs round the apex and characteristically terminates in an inverted Y.

2. *Circumflex Coronary Artery:* This artery enters the atrioventricular sulcus close to the base of the left atrial appendage. Because of the proximity of the appendage, it may be injured in surgical procedures which amputate or ligate the left atrial appendage. The artery is in close proximity to that part of the fibrous annulus to which the posterior mitral valve leaflet is attached and may be damaged during mitral valve replacement or repair. It may also be obstructed by submitral aneurysms.

The artery has the following branches:

   i. Sino-atrial node artery (45 per cent of individuals).
   ii. A marginal branch originates from the proximal segment of the artery. This branch runs to the obtuse margin of the heart. In coronary artery bypass surgery, a vein graft is anastomosed to this artery and not the circumflex artery which is situated deeply in the atrioventricular sulcus.
   iii. A branch to the inferior left ventricular wall.
   iv. The posterior descending ventricular artery (it may arise from

the circumflex artery in 10 per cent of individuals in which case left dominance exists).

CORONARY COLLATERAL CIRCULATION: The right and left coronary arteries are not end arteries. There are anastomoses between the two networks at a precapillary level and also between larger calibre vessels. Examples of anastomoses between larger calibre vessels are:

1. *Vieussens' Ring:* An infundibular branch of the right coronary artery anastomoses with a similar branch of the left coronary artery.
2. *Septal Perforating Branches* of the anterior and posterior descending arteries.
3. *Arteria Auricularis Magna (Kugel's Artery):* An atrial branch of the right coronary artery communicates with a similar branch from the left circumflex artery. The communicating artery runs along the anterior atrial wall.

IMPORTANT VARIATIONS:

1. Origin of the left coronary artery from the right coronary sinus. This artery then courses anterior or posterior to the pulmonary artery before bifurcating. This anomaly is implicated in sudden death, presumably due to compression between the aorta and pulmonary artery. The circumflex branch might pass, separately, to the right and posterior to the aorta.
2. Origin of the left anterior descending or circumflex arteries from the right coronary artery. In this instance these arteries may be severed in operations designed to widen the right ventricular outflow tract, e.g. Fallot's tetralogy.

CORONARY ARTERY DISEASE: 'Three vessel disease' refers to the right coronary artery and circumflex and anterior descending branches of the left coronary artery. The proximal undivided segment of the left coronary artery is called the left main coronary artery.

Penetrating wound of the heart

Penetrating wounds of the heart are most commonly due to stab wounds which involve the right ventricle in more than half the patients, and then the left ventricle, the right atrium and the left atrium in decreasing order of frequency. The right ventricle is most commonly involved because this chamber forms the largest part of the sternocostal surface, and almost the entire inferior border of the heart.

Bleeding from the myocardial injury is usually contained by the pericardium, resulting in tamponade, which limits ventricular filling in diastole. Tamponade is more common in stab wounds of the right ventricle and the atria, because their relatively thin walls do not allow spontaneous arrest of bleeding to occur. Associated cardiac injuries, although uncommon, may involve the coronary arteries, the valves and the atrial or ventricular septa.

Operative management is best carried out through a full-length median sternotomy. This incision provides adequate exposure of the cardiac chambers.

An alternative approach is an anterolateral left thoracotomy through the 5th intercostal space. If wider exposure is required, the sternum may be divided transversely and extended into the corresponding intercostal space on the opposite side. This incision provides better exposure of the posterior mediastinal structures including the descending aorta and oesophagus.

Pericardiocentesis

In patients with cardiac tamponade, pericardiocentesis and aspiration of non-clotted blood from the pericardium may be life saving.

A large bore intravenous cannula is inserted beneath the costal margin at its angle with the xiphoid process and directed towards the left shoulder at an angle of 45 degrees to the horizontal.

THE GREAT VESSELS

Embryology

Six branchial arches develop during the fourth week of fetal development (*Fig.* 218). The ventrally placed truncus arteriosus supplies paired arteries (aortic arches) to the branchial arches. The junction of the aortic arches with the truncus arteriosus is somewhat dilated and is known as the aortic sac.

The aortic arches terminate in a dorsal aorta running on each side of the embryo.

The embryonic aortic-arch system develops as follows:

The truncus arteriosus forms the proximal portions of the ascending aorta and the pulmonary trunk.

The aortic sac forms the distal portion of the ascending aorta, the brachiocephalic trunk and the aortic arch up to the origin of the left common carotid artery.

The 1st aortic arch disappears and only a small remnant persists to form the maxillary artery.

The 2nd aortic arch also disappears but the dorsal portion persists as the stapedial artery.

The 3rd aortic arch forms the common carotid artery from its proximal portion and the distal portion joins the dorsal aorta to form the internal carotid artery. The external carotid artery develops as a vascular sprout from the 3rd arch.

The 4th aortic arch on the left side forms the aortic arch segment between the left common carotid and left subclavian arteries. The latter artery is the left 7th segmental artery which arises directly from the aorta. On the right side the 4th arch forms the proximal part of the right subclavian which is continuous with the right 7th segmental artery. The dorsal aorta between the 3rd and 4th arches disappears.

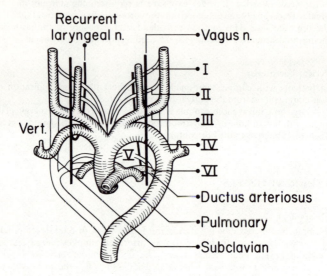

Fig. 218. The development of the branchial arch arteries.

The 5th aortic arch is transient and never well developed.

The 6th aortic arch differs on the two sides. The proximal portion of the left 6th arch persists as the proximal part of the left pulmonary artery and the distal part of this arch persists as the ductus arteriosus which passes from the pulmonary artery to the descending aorta. The proximal part of the right 6th arch forms the right pulmonary artery but the distal part disappears.

The recurrent laryngeal nerves supply the 6th pair of aortic arches and hook around the arches on their way to the larynx. On the right side, because the distal part of the right 6th arch and the 5th arch degenerate, the nerve passes round the right subclavian artery. On the left side the nerve hooks round the ductus arteriosus which develops from the distal half of the left 6th arch.

Malformations of the aortic-arch system

Anomalies of the aortic arch complex result from either disappearance of an embryonic vascular structure, which normally remains patent, or the maintenance of patency in a structure which normally disappears.

1. DOUBLE AORTIC ARCH: The ascending aorta bifurcates into two arches in front of the trachea which then pass posteriorly on either side of the trachea and oesophagus. The descending aorta is usually in the normal position. In the most common type, the right arch is larger than the left and a left ductus arteriosus joins the left-sided descending aorta.

2. RIGHT AORTIC ARCH: The entire right dorsal aorta persists and the distal segment of the left dorsal aorta involutes. The right arch arises from the ascending aorta and passes backwards to the right of the trachea and oesophagus to join the upper descending aorta. The branches of the arch are the mirror image of the left arch. The first branch is the brachiocephalic (left), followed by the right common carotid and right subclavian arteries. The most common type of right aortic arch is associated with an aberrant left subclavian artery and a left-sided ductus arteriosus. In this type there is a complete vascular ring around the trachea and oesophagus.

3. CERVICAL AORTA: In this very rare anomaly, there is an abnormal elongation of the aortic arch extending into the neck. The apex of the arch may reach as high as the hyoid bone usually on the right side. The descending aorta crosses from the right behind the oesophagus at the level of the tracheal bifurcation to continue its descent on the left side. A ductus arteriosus extending to the left subclavian artery completes the vascular ring.

4. ABERRANT RIGHT SUBCLAVIAN ARTERY: The right subclavian artery arises from the descending aorta and passes posterior to the trachea and oesophagus. The aberrant artery is usually asymptomatic but may cause dysphagia, in which case it is known as dysphagia lusoria. Radiologically the barium-filled oesophagus is indented by the artery at the level of the 3rd or 4th thoracic vertebra.

5. PATENT DUCTUS ARTERIOSUS: The ductus usually closes during the first week of postnatal life, but closure may be delayed in premature infants. It is one of the commonest congenital cardiovascular anomalies and is 30 times commoner in populations living at high altitudes. Patent ductus is more common in girls than in boys. The ductus is like an arteriovenous fistula and when large the infant presents with heart failure. However, 50 per cent of infants and children with this anomaly have no symptoms. If untreated, there is a risk of bacterial infection in the ductus. Division of the ductus is associated with a negligible mortality.

6. COARCTATION OF THE AORTA: This is the commonest primary cardiovascular cause of heart failure in an acyanotic infant in the first week of life. Boys are affected twice as often as girls.

Though this condition may affect any part of the aorta, 98 per cent of coarctations affect the first part of the descending aorta just beyond the arch. Two types of coarctation are recognized (*Fig.* 219).

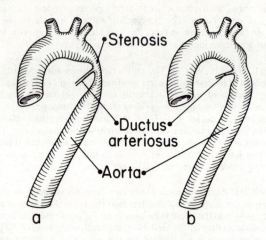

Fig. 219. Coarctation of the aorta. *a*, Isthmal or tubular. *b*, Juxtaductal.

Isthmal or Tubular: This is an exaggeration of the normal narrowing between the left subclavian artery and the ductus which results from poor blood flow in this segment, while the ductus remains patent.

Juxtaductal: This is an exaggeration of the normal indentation on the posterior wall of the aorta.

The outstanding clinical features of the condition are raised arterial pressure in the arm compared with the femoral pressure below this, grooving of the lower borders of the ribs by enlarging intercostal arteries and, often, visible arterial pulsation on the back. It is, therefore, necessary to determine the femoral or popliteal blood pressure in all cases of hypertension lest coarctation of the aorta be overlooked. In the neonate there is normally up to 20 mmHg systolic pressure difference between the upper and lower limbs because of isthmal narrowing.

Patients with coarctation should be operated on to relieve hypertension and its sequelae.

Rupture of the thoracic aorta

1. RUPTURE OF THE DESCENDING AORTA: In road traffic accidents, decelerating forces are engendered which can produce pressure waves in the aorta. The arch of the aorta is relatively fixed by the brachiocephalic, left common carotid and left subclavian arteries, but the more mobile descending aorta continues to travel forwards. Shearing forces between the relatively fixed and mobile portions of the aorta lead to rupture in the region of the attachment of the ligamentum arteriosum. If the adventitia of the aorta remains intact a false aneurysm forms which produces widening of the mediastinum on chest X-ray. These latter patients usually reach hospital alive and it is possible to repair the tear in the aorta.

2. RUPTURE OF THE ARCH BRANCHES: Rupture of the major aortic branches (usually the brachiocephalic artery) is due to aortopulmonary compression forces on the chest, combined with hyperextension of the cervical spine. The compressive forces displace the heart and ascending aorta towards the left, accentuating the curvature of the ascending aorta and therefore increasing tension on the origin of the brachiocephalic artery.

Operations on the descending aorta

The incidence of postoperative paraplegia following operations on the descending aorta is largely dependent on the blood supply of the spinal cord, which is derived from the neck vessels and the descending aorta, with a collateral circulation between them.

The calibre of the anterior spinal artery is narrowest in the midthoracic region. In this region (T8–L1), spinal cord blood supply may be largely dependent upon an artery arising directly from the descending aorta (artery of Adamkiewicz). (*See* Chapter 27.)

Chapter 23

THE KIDNEYS, URETERS AND ADRENALS

KIDNEYS

Position

The long axis of the kidney is parallel to, but not coincident with, the axis of the 12th rib. (The long axis of the spleen is parallel to and coincident with the long axis of the 10th rib.) Both kidneys normally lie entirely above the level of the umbilicus, the lower poles being about 2·5 cm above the highest point of the iliac crest. The right kidney reaches the upper border of the 12th rib, the left reaches the lower border of the 11th rib. The outer border of the organ lies 1·25 cm lateral to the outer border of the sacrospinalis muscle. The pelvis of the kidney is seen in pyelograms to lie opposite the 1st and 2nd lumbar transverse processes.

Relations

RELATIONS TO THE 12TH RIB: This rib is separated from the kidney by the pleura and the diaphragm. The diaphragm, therefore, intervenes between the kidney and the pleura. It sometimes happens that there is a small gap between the slips of the diaphragm arising from the lateral arcuate ligament and the 12th rib, in which case the kidney and the pleura are separated by a little connective tissue only (*Fig.* 223).

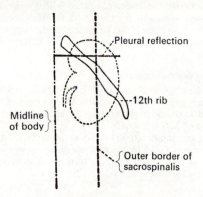

Fig. 220. Showing certain important posterior relationships of the kidney.

It is seen from *Fig.* 220 that the 12th rib is oblique while the lower border of the pleura is horizontal. The two cross like an X. The angle between the 12th rib and the outer border of the sacrospinalis is the kidney angle. Kidney pain is usually referred here, and pressure here may elicit pain in kidney lesions. The lumbar incision for exposure of the kidney commences here.

In cases where the 12th rib is very short it does not project beyond the outer border of the sacrospinalis. In such cases the pleura may be opened on exposing the kidney by this route, as the 11th rib is sometimes mistaken for the 12th.

HEPATORENAL (MORISON'S) POUCH: There is a deep recess above the upper pole of the right kidney. This is the hepatorenal pouch. It is lined by

Table 4 Relationship of kidneys

	Right	Left
Anterior (*Fig.* 221)	Below: hepatic flexure	Below: splenic flexure
	Medial: second part of duodenum	Crossing the middle: pancreas and splenic vessels Below pancreas is jejunum* Above pancreas is stomach* and spleen
	Above: adrenal, liver*	Above: adrenal
Medial	Inferior vena cava, ureter	Duodenojejunal flexure, inferior mesenteric vein, adrenal, ureter
Lateral	Below: ascending colon* Above: liver*	Below: descending colon* Above: spleen*
Posterior (*Figs* 222 and 223)	Same in both kidneys. Each kidney rests upon four muscles: psoas, transversus abdominis, quadratus, diaphragm. The lumbocostal arches, last thoracic, iliohypogastric and ilio-inguinal nerves, and subcostal vessels are between kidney and quadratus, the anterior layer of the lumbodorsal fascia intervening	

*Structures indicated thus are separated from the kidney by peritoneum.

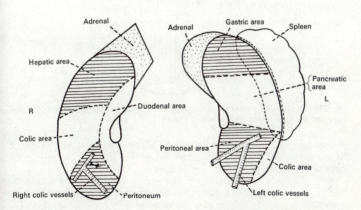

Fig. 221. Anterior relations of the kidneys. The hatched areas represent peritoneum.

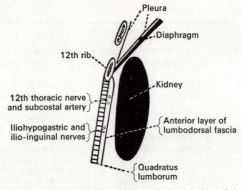

Fig. 222. Schematic representation of the posterior relations of the kidney.

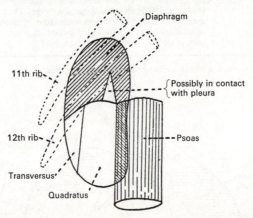

Fig. 223. The posterior relations of the kidney, showing its relation to diaphragm and ribs, and the area where it may lie in contact with the pleura.

peritoneum, and is bounded in front by the inferior surface of the liver, above by the posterior layer of the coronary ligament of the liver, behind by the peritoneum on the diaphragm (*Fig.* 224).

With the body lying horizontal, this recess is the lowest level of the peritoneal cavity, excluding the pelvis. Extravasations of fluid are likely to collect there, especially after operations on the liver and bile passages. The pouch is therefore usually drained after such operations if leakage is feared.

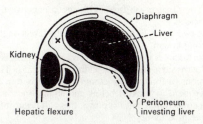

Fig. 224. The hapatorenal or Morison's pouch (X).

FASCIAL RELATIONS: The kidney has three capsules: (i) its proper capsule; (ii) fatty capsule; (iii) the renal fascia.

Proper Capsule: A fibrous membrane stripping easily from the organ. In inflammatory diseases it is frequently adherent and cannot be stripped without tearing the kidney tissue.

Fatty Capsule: The kidney is embedded in a peculiar type of fat. This fat is condensed at its periphery to form the renal fascia. It is likewise condensed where the kidney is in contact with it, because of the continuous impact due to the pulsation of the kidneys.

Renal Fascia: Is continuous with the extraperitoneal connective tissue (*Fig.* 225). It is arranged as follows:

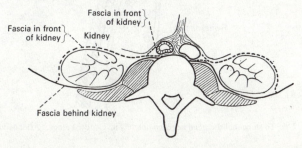

Fig. 225. The diagram shows that the renal fascia invests each kidney completely. (After Mitchell.)

Laterally: At the outer border of the kidney it splits to enclose the organ; lateral to this it is fused with fascia transversalis.

Posteriorly: It blends with the fascia on the psoas and quadratus. The attachments are feeble and the kidney and its capsules are readily separated from the underlying muscles.

Medially: The renal fascia fuses with the connective tissue round the great vessels.

Above: The two layers join, and fuse with the fascia on the under aspect of the diaphragm.

Below: The fascia is closed below. The renal fascia is an investment completely surrounding the kidney (*Fig.* 225). Thus perinephric collections of fluid will be completely enclosed in this fascia. The compartment is weakest below and should increasing pressure of such a collection lead to rupture, this will occur inferiorly into the pelvic cellular tissue.

The adrenal is enclosed in a separate loculus of this fascia; therefore in removal of the kidney, when it is shelled out from its fatty capsule, the adrenal remains *in situ*; furthermore, for the same reason in movable kidney the adrenal does not move with the kidney (*Fig.* 226). The integrity of the adrenal gland is not always secured by such a fascial arrangement.

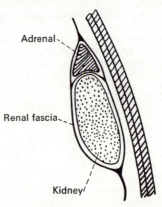

Fig. 226. To show that the renal fascia completely invests the kidney. (After Mitchell.)

Postmortem studies have shown that in less than 0·5 per cent of cases the adrenal is so intimately fused with the kidney that a nephrectomy would result in a coincident adrenalectomy. There is a small interspace filled with connective tissue between the inferomedial angle of the adrenal and the kidney where a separation of the two structures can be started in such cases.

The kidney is retained in place mainly by intra-abdominal pressure; the fatty capsule assists. In thin patients the lower pole of the right kidney is usually palpable in the lumbar region. The kidneys move about 3 cm in a vertical direction during deep breathing.

Blood supply

Renal arteries are large vessels that arise from the aorta at right-angles at the level of the intervertebral disc between L1 and L2 vertebrae. The renal artery origin is an important landmark in abdominal aortic aneurysm surgery. Over 95 per cent of such aneurysms arise below the level of origin of the renal arteries. In resecting an abdominal aortic aneurysm it is usually possible to place an occluding vascular clamp on the aorta distal to the renal arteries.

The kidney is anatomically divided into segments by its blood supply (*Fig.* 227). In the hilar area of the kidney, the main renal artery divides into anterior and posterior divisions. The anterior division supplies the apical, upper, middle and lower segments while the posterior division supplies the posterior segment of the kidney.

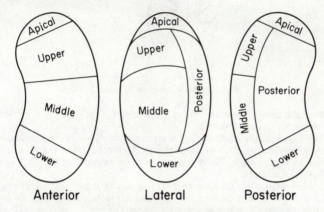

Fig. 227. Segments of kidney.

The junction of the area supplied by the anterior and posterior divisions of the renal artery is an important anatomical landmark. This junction encroaches on the posterior half of the kidney and is situated about two-thirds of the way from the hilum to the lateral margin of the kidney (*Fig.* 228). In the operation of anatrophic nephrolithotomy, a functionally avascular plane between the posterior segment and the upper and middle segments is entered. This technique enables stones lodged in the renal calices to be removed with minimal damage to the renal tissue.

The fact that the major calices also have some constancy of pattern makes it possible to carry out segmental resections of the kidney. The blood supply of the lower segment lends itself best to such a local resection, though the procedure is also carried out with other segments. Although there is no

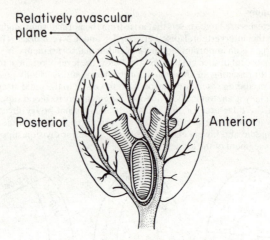

Fig. 228. Avascular plane of kidney.

collateral arterial circulation between the segments of the kidney, there is free intercommunication of all veins.

The blood supply to the kidney is interrupted temporarily in operations such as anastomosis of the splenic to the renal artery beyond a stenosis which is causing hypertension. The duration of ischaemia should not exceed 30 min at body temperature.

Studies on cadavers have shown that there is more than one renal artery in 15 and 20 per cent of cases on the right and left sides, respectively. As the renal arteries are end arteries, anastomoses must be made to all the arteries of the donor kidney in kidney transplantation operations. Accessory veins may be ligated as there are generous venovenous anastomoses throughout the kidney.

Nerve supply

Thoracic 10, 11, and 12 through the lesser and lowest splanchnic nerves. The nerve supply of the large intestine is the same. Renal lesions such as calculus, therefore, may, and often do, cause reflex interference with peristalsis. Such cases may simulate acute obstruction of the large gut.

Lymphatics of the kidney

The lymph vessels in the kidney run with the renal vessels, and reach the para-aortic lymph nodes. The intrarenal lymph vessels communicate freely with the plexus in the perinephric fat. Therefore in removal of the kidney for conditions which spread via lymphatics, it is essential to remove the perinephric fat.

Development of the urinary organs

The metanephros, which becomes the permanent kidney, develops from two

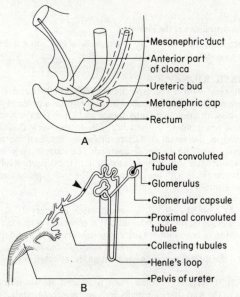

Fig. 229. A, The origin of the ureteric bud from the mesonephric duct; B, the point of union between derivatives of the ureteric bud and metanephric cap indicated by an arrow.

sources (*Fig.* 229): (1) the ureteric bud (metanephric diverticulum), from the mesonephric duct. The ureteric bud gives rise to the ureter, the renal pelvis, calyces and collecting tubules. (2) The intermediate mesoderm condenses around the ureteric bud to form the metanephric cap. The latter forms the glomerular capsule (Bowman's capsule), the proximal and distal convoluted tubules and the loops of Henle. The glomerular capsule becomes invaded by a cluster of capillaries that forms the glomerulus. Both primordia of the metanephros are of mesodermal origin.

The developing kidney is first a pelvic organ, but by differential growth of the embryo's body caudal to the kidney, it assumes progressively higher levels and eventually comes to lie on the posterior abdominal wall. As the kidneys 'ascend' they are vascularized by successively higher lateral splanchnic arteries which are branches of the aorta. Inferior branches undergo involution but variations in blood supply to the kidneys reflect changing patterns of supply in their 'ascent' from the pelvis.

Initially the hilum of the kidney faces ventrally, but as it 'ascends' it rotates almost 90 degrees so that its hilum is directed anteromedially.

Congenital abnormalities of the kidney

About 10 per cent of infants are born with some abnormality of the genito-urinary system.

1. POLYCYSTIC KIDNEYS:
   i. Infantile type with a recessive inheritance which occurs bilaterally. Some are present at birth but may present later as a juvenile form.
   ii. Adult type with a dominant inheritance and which is an important cause of chronic renal failure in the adult. The former view that these cysts developed as the result of failure of fusion between the meta- and mesonephros has now been discounted. The current view is that they are the result of an abnormal development of the collecting tubules. The cysts communicate with the glomerulus. The liver, spleen and pancreas may also contain cysts.

2. RENAL AGENESIS: It occurs about once in every 1000 births. A normal kidney is found on one side only. It is obviously important to assess the renal function of both kidneys prior to renal surgery to avoid the disaster of removing a patient's only functioning kidney. It can be suspected in the male patient if the ductus deferens is absent on the affected side.

3. HORSESHOE KIDNEY: As the renal rudiments are ascending from the pelvic region to the loin, they normally remain entirely separate. They may, however, come in contact and should they adhere, a horseshoe kidney may result, the two kidneys being joined by an isthmus.

Though this isthmus may connect the upper poles of the kidneys, in the vast majority of cases it connects their lower poles. This isthmus usually receives its blood supply directly from the aorta by a special vessel. The isthmus crosses in front of the aorta and vena cava. When the isthmus is large, the ureters have to ascend from the renal pelvis to cross it (*Fig.* 230), and this may cause some degree of obstruction to the outflow of urine. The inferior mesenteric artery may cross the isthmus when the latter is at the lower pole. As the fused kidney is heavy, it usually lies at a lower level than the normal kidney.

The condition is usually symptomless and unsuspected, but may in very

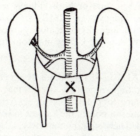

Fig. 230. Horseshoe kidney with isthmus below. Note that isthmus (X) necessitates curving of ureters in negotiating isthmic ridge.

exceptional cases produce pressure on the vena cava, which is evidenced by oedema of the lower limbs.

A horseshoe kidney is a problem in abdominal aortic aneurysm surgery. In only 20 per cent of these cases do the renal arteries arise normally. In the remaining cases there are 5 or more additional arteries arising from the aorta or iliac vessels. Division of these vessels may result in ischaemia of the kidney.

4. UNILATERAL FUSED KIDNEY: In this condition (*Fig*. 231A) the renal rudiments have become fused and the combined mass has passed to one side, the organ proper to that side being above, the other being below. The ureter of the displaced kidney crosses to its own side and opens into the bladder in its normal situation.

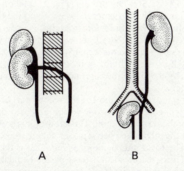

A   B

Fig. 231. Abnormalities in development of the kidneys. A, Unilateral fused kidney; ureteric orifices in bladder are normal. B, Left kidney normal; right has remained pelvic.

5. ECTOPIC KIDNEYS: One or both kidneys may be in an abnormal position. Most ectopic kidneys (*Fig.* 231B) are located in the pelvis, but some are low in the abdomen. Ectopic kidneys receive their blood supply from vessels near them. A pelvic kidney may sometimes be felt on rectal or vaginal examination.

6. MULTIPLE RENAL VESSELS: About 25 per cent of kidneys have two or more renal arteries. Supernumerary arteries may arise from the adrenal artery and pass to the superior pole of the kidney. Arteries may arise from the aorta and pass to the inferior pole of the kidney and obstruct the ureter at the ureteropelvic junction. These supernumerary vessels result from persistence of embryonic vessels that normally disappear when definitive renal arteries form.

URETERS

The ureters are muscular tubes 25–30 cm long depending on the height of the individual. They have an abdominal and a pelvic course. The ureters lie in a bed of loose areolar connective tissue in the retroperitoneal space, but when the peritoneum is reflected the ureters remain attached to the undersurface of the peritoneum. Such displacement could expose them to surgical injury. Because they are not fixed to surrounding structures, wormlike movements due to peristalsis can be seen under normal circumstances and the ureters can be displaced or obstructed by retroperitoneal masses such as aortic aneurysms and tumours.

ABDOMINAL COURSE: The ureters (*Fig.* 232) lie on the medial portion of the psoas major which intervenes between it and the tip of the transverse processes of the lumbar vertebrae. On an excretory urogram this relationship of the ureters to the tips of the transverse processes and where it crosses the pelvic brim at the sacro-iliac joints is clearly seen. It crosses the genitofemoral nerve and is itself crossed obliquely by the testicular (ovarian vessels). It enters the pelvis by crossing either the end of the common or beginning of the external iliac artery.

The right ureter is usually covered by the second part of the duodenum. It is crossed by the right colic and ileocolic vessels and near the pelvis lies behind the mesentery of the terminal ileum. The left ureter is crossed by the left colic vessels and near the inlet of the pelvis passes behind the pelvic mesocolon and its mesentery. The fossa intersigmoidea (*Fig.* 233) is the surgeon's guide to the left ureter. The pelvic mesocolon has a parietal attachment shaped like an inverted V. At the apex of the V is a fossa or a dimple. With a finger in the fossa or dimple the ureter can be rolled on the underlying common iliac artery.

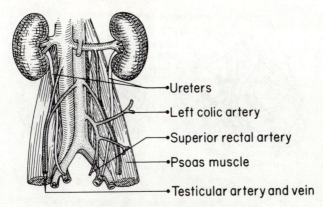

Fig. 232. Abdominal course of the ureters.

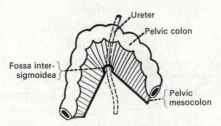

Fig. 233. To show the fossa intersigmoidea lying at the apex of the Λ attachment of the pelvic mesocolon. The ureter is shown passing down behind the fossa.

PELVIC COURSE: Each ureter runs retroperitoneally along the postero-lateral wall of the pelvis and passes in front of the internal iliac artery and its anterior division (*Fig.* 234). At the level of the spine of the ischium, it leaves the pelvic wall by turning slightly medially. During this part of its course it is less closely related to the peritoneum and in the male the ductus deferens crosses in front of it to gain its medial side (*Fig.* 235).

In the female, the pelvic part of the ureter forms the posterior boundary of a shallow depression named the ovarian fossa in which the ovary is situated. At the level of the ischial spine the ureter passes forwards and medially. In this part of its course, it is well hidden in a tunnel formed from loose cellular tissue in the base of the broad ligament and is adherent to the posterior leaf of the ligament. Here the uterine artery crosses over the ureter about 2 cm lateral to the cervix. The ureter passes above the lateral fornix of the vagina

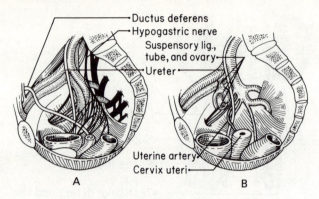

Fig. 234. Pelvic course of the ureter in the male, in the female.

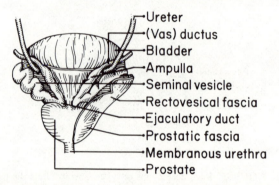

Fig. 235. The ductus passes anterior to the ureter to gain its medial side.

and lies in close proximity to the anterior wall of the vagina for a short distance before it pierces the bladder wall obliquely.

Nerve supply

Although the ureter has a sympathetic innervation from the renal, inferior mesenteric, testicular (ovarian), and pelvic plexuses, its urinary transport function is not dependent on this, as is well demonstrated in the transplanted kidney with its ureter attached.

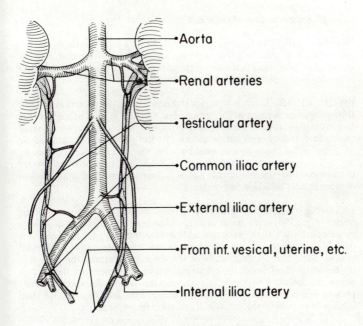

Aorta

Renal arteries

Testicular artery

Common iliac artery

External iliac artery

From inf. vesical, uterine, etc.

Internal iliac artery

Fig. 236. Blood supply of the ureter.

Arterial supply to the ureter

See Fig. 236.

1. The upper segment of the ureter is supplied by branches of the renal, gonadal or adrenal arteries.
2. In the pelvis the ureter obtains its blood supply from the common iliac artery or the internal iliac artery and its branches.
3. The middle portion receives only small peritoneal twigs and branches from the arteries of the posterior abdominal wall. These vessels run up and down the ureter to form an anastomotic plexus in the adventitial coat of the ureter, but in 10–15 per cent of individuals the anastomosis is deficient, in which case the cut end of the ureter is liable to necrose if it has been excessively mobilized. The surgeon should therefore inspect the cut end of the ureter for bleeding before performing an anastomosis.

Pelvic portions of the ureter must be mobilized by dividing the fascia on their medial side because vessels reach them from their lateral side; the reverse is true of the abdominal portion of the ureter.

Congenital abnormalities of the ureter

DOUBLE PELVIS: Double pelvis (*Fig.* 237a) of the ureter is usually unilateral. It is due to premature division of the ureteric bud near its termination. The upper pelvis drains the upper group of calyces and the lower pelvis drains the middle and lower group.

BIFID URETER: Double ureters and double pelves are present and result from premature division of the ureteric bud (*Fig.* 237b, c). The ureters may join in the lower third of their course and open through a common orifice into the bladder. If they open independently into the bladder the ureter draining the upper pelvis opens into the bladder below the orifice of the other ureter. In the latter case one ureter crosses its fellow and may produce urinary obstruction. Patients with double pelves or double ureters are more likely to develop urinary infection and calculi.

ECTOPIC URETERIC ORIFICE: The presence of an ectopic ureteric orifice (*Fig.* 237d) is the result of a second ureteric bud arising from a single mesonephric duct. In the male, the additional ureter may open into the lower part of the trigone, the prostatic urethra, the ejaculatory duct or seminal vesicle. Since the opening is above the sphincter urethrae the patient is continent. In the female, the additional ureter may open into the urethra below the sphincter urethrae or even into the vagina. Such patients may present with dribbling incontinence, especially during the day. When a child is lying down at night she remains dry (vertical incontinence).

RETROCAVAL URETER: The right ureter may 'ascend' posterior to the inferior vena cava and may be obstructed by it (*Fig.* 237e). This abnormality occurs when the posterior cardinal vein persists during the development of the inferior vena cava.

Surgical damage to the ureter

1. IN THE ABDOMEN:
    i. Right or left hemicolectomy may result in damage to the right and left ureters, respectively, when the colic vessels are ligated.
    ii. Ligation of the inferior mesenteric artery during excision of the rectum. The left ureter lies close to this artery.

2. IN THE PELVIS:
    i. Ovariectomy: the ureter runs behind and below the infundibulopelvic ligament of the ovary. The ureter must be identified by opening the peritoneum over the lateral wall of the pelvis between the round and infundibulopelvic ligaments.

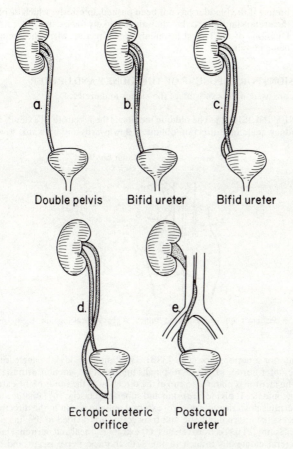

a. Double pelvis   b. Bifid ureter   c. Bifid ureter

d. Ectopic ureteric orifice   e. Postcaval ureter

Fig. 237. Congenital abnormalities of the ureter.

ii. Hysterectomy and ligation of the uterine arteries lateral to the cervix. The ureters are 2·5 cm lateral to the cervix and are crossed anteriorly by the uterine artery.

iii. Ligation of the lateral ligaments of the uterus.

iv. Application of clamps to the angles of the vagina may damage the ureters if the bladder has not been pushed anteriorly, which displaces the ureters laterally so that they are less likely to be damaged.

v. Divisions of the lateral ligaments of the rectum when the rectum is being mobilized.

INCISIONS FOR EXPOSURE OF THE KIDNEY AND URETER

These are used in the exposure of the kidney and ureter.

KIDNEY INCISIONS: The oblique incision is the favourite. It extends from the kidney angle in a direction obliquely downwards and outwards towards

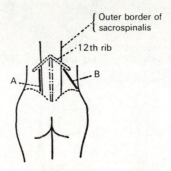

Fig. 238. Posterior approaches to the kidney; **A**, by vertical incision; **B**, by oblique incision.

the anterior superior spine (*Fig.* 238B). The kidney angle is the angle formed by the outer border of the sacrospinalis muscle at its junction with the 12th rib. The incision is planned to run in the direction of the fibres of the external oblique muscle. It divides: (*a*) skin and superficial fascia; (*b*) latissimus dorsi and serratus posterior inferior; (*c*) external oblique is split in the direction of its fibres; (*d*) internal oblique and transversus are divided in the line of the skin incision; (*e*) fascia transversalis; (*f*) extraperitoneal and perirenal fat; (*g*) the lateral cutaneous branch of the 12th thoracic nerve is cut and there results an area of anaesthesia the size of the palm of the hand over the gluteal region. The outer border of the quadratus is exposed at the upper part of the cut. Care must be exercised towards the lower part of the cut that the peritoneum is not injured, as it lies exposed when the fascia transversalis is divided.

The incision gives good exposure to the kidney and also to the upper half of the ureter. Its great advantage is that it may be extended forwards above and parallel to the outer half of the inguinal ligament to expose the lower half of the ureter and the base of the bladder. The incision and its continuation allow exposure of the whole length of the kidney and ureter.

At the kidney angle, the pleura crosses the inner half of the 12th rib. If the 12th rib is very short, as it not uncommonly is, then the kidney angle is formed by the sacrospinalis and the 11th rib and the pleura crosses this angle (*Fig.* 239). The pleura may be inadvertently opened.

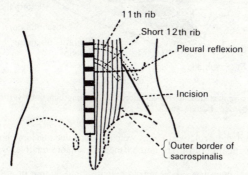

Fig. 239. To show danger of opening pleura by oblique kidney incision when the 12th rib does not project beyond outer border of sacrospinalis.

VERTICAL INCISION: This extends perpendicularly along the outer border of the sacrospinalis from the 12th rib to the iliac crest (*Fig.* 238A). The incision divides: (*a*) skin and fascia; (*b*) latissimus dorsi and serratus posterior inferior; (*c*) the three layers of lumbodorsal fascia; (*d*) the fascia transversalis and extraperitoneal fat (*Fig.* 240). The incision is planned to interfere as little as possible with the muscles. It has the disadvantage that it does not give exposure of the ureter, and cannot easily be extended to effect such exposure.

HORIZONTAL URETERIC INCISION: A transverse incision a little above the level of the iliac crest extending outwards from the lateral border of the sacrospinalis is sometimes used to expose the ureter when it is wished to implant its divided proximal end into the skin.

ADRENAL GLANDS

Embryology
The cortex develops from mesoderm and the medulla from neuro-ectoderm (neural crest cells). The adrenal gland of the human fetus is 20 times larger

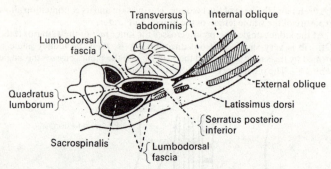

Fig. 240. Anatomical structures encountered in exposing kidney by vertical incision along outer border of sacrospinalis. The kidney capsules are not shown.

than the adult gland relative to body weight. This is due to a large fetal cortex which regresses after birth. The adrenal medulla remains relatively small until after birth.

Each gland measures 30–50 mm in height, about 30 mm in breadth and from 4 to 6 mm in thickness. Each gland weighs from 3 to 5 g.

Relations

The right adrenal is shaped like a top hat. The left adrenal is shaped like a cocked hat. Each has an anterior and a posterior surface. Each of these surfaces has two relations (*Fig.* 241).

The left adrenal has 'slipped' down the medial border of the kidney, being arrested by the renal vessels, its lower pole being in contact with these, whilst its upper pole is in contact with the upper pole of the spleen. Thus it comes about that the right adrenal is usually higher than the left, just the reverse of the relative positions of the kidneys.

Between the two adrenals are the crura, the aorta, the coeliac artery, the coeliac plexus, and the inferior vena cava.

Arteries

There are three to each: (*a*) superior adrenal from the inferior phrenic; (*b*) middle adrenal from the aorta; (*c*) inferior adrenal from the renal.

Veins

One only which drains, on the right, into the vena cava and, on the left, into the left renal.

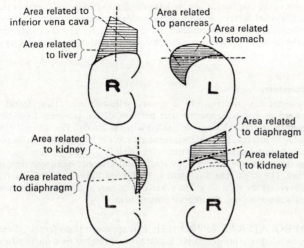

Fig. 241. The relations of the adrenals. R Right kidney; L, left kidney. The anterior surfaces are shown above, the posterior below.

Innervation

The coeliac plexus and splanchnic nerves supply branches. Most of the fibres are preganglionic sympathetic and go directly to the cells of the medulla. The hormones secreted by the medulla take the place of postganglionic fibres.

Table 5 Relationship of adrenal glands

	Right	Left
Anterior	Medial: inferior vena cava	Superior: stomach
	Lateral: part of bare area of liver	Inferior: pancreas
Posterior	Inferior: kidney	Medial: crus of diaphragm
	Superior: crus of diaphragm	Lateral: kidney
Hilum	Near upper end	Near lower end
Peritoneal relations	Not related to peritoneum, except a tiny area below	Separated from stomach by peritoneum

Lymphatic drainage

There is a lymphatic plexus under the capsule and in the medulla. From the right adrenal lymphatic drainage is to para-aortic nodes and nodes near the right crus of the diaphragm. On the left side, drainage is to nodes at the origin of the left renal artery and para-aortic nodes. Lymphatics may accompany any vessel reaching the adrenal and, for this reason, lymphatic drainage may reach the posterior mediastinum directly along the inferior phrenic artery.

Adrenalectomy

The adrenal has a characteristic canary yellow colour. This should be recognized as it has happened that portions of the pancreas have been removed by mistake during a left-sided adrenalectomy. The adrenal gland will not hold forceps. Parts of its investing fascia can be gripped by forceps to facilitate removal of the gland without tearing it.

The three adrenal arteries are small, and give off numerous tenuous branches. The single vein is as thick as a lead pencil and very short on the right where it enters the vena cava. The adrenal veins may be double and drain into unusual situations, e.g. the inferior phrenic vein.

POSTEROLATERAL APPROACH: This approach is preferable if there has been adequate pre-operative localization of disease to a single adrenal gland and if there is no need for exploration for ectopic tissue (as in phaeochromocytoma) or for wider dissection (as in adrenocortical carcinoma). This approach is especially useful on the right side, because the adrenal veins commonly enter the vena cava posteriorly.

An incision is made through the posterior layer of the lumbodorsal fascia. The sacrospinalis muscle is retracted medially, its attachment to the 12th rib divided and the rib is removed subperiosteally. Sometimes the 11th rib is removed or an incision can be made between the 11th and 12th ribs. The anterior layer of the lumbodorsal fascia is incised to expose the kidney. The inferior surface of the diaphragm is exposed by blunt dissection and the parietal pleura is separated from the superior surface. Downward retraction of the kidney allows the adrenal to be seen.

ANTERIOR APPROACH: This approach is preferable if the disease has not been localized to one adrenal or if wider abdominal exploration or dissection has to be done. Either a midline or long transverse upper abdominal incision ('chevron' or 'bucket-handle') is adequate (*Fig.* 242). A left adrenal tumour may be approached by reflecting the mobilized spleen and pancreatic tail medially and the splenic flexure inferiorly, or by dividing the gastrocolic omentum and retracting the tail of the pancreas, spleen and stomach upward. The right adrenal is approached by mobilizing the hepatic flexure of the colon, displacing it inferiorly, and dividing the lateral peritoneal attachments of the duodenum to permit the duodenum and inferior vena cava to be retracted medially.

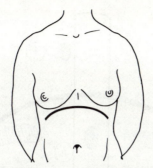

Fig. 242. The chevron or bucket-handle incision.

PARAGANGLION SYSTEM

Paraganglion cells are derived from the neural crest and migrate in proximity with autonomic ganglion cells which is why they are called 'paraganglion cells'. The largest collections of these cells come to rest in the adrenal medulla where they may also be called 'phaeochromocytes' (which stain a golden-brown colour when fixed with chromium salts). The remainder of the paraganglion system which consists of scattered minute masses of neural crest tissue is distributed symmetrically in the para-axial regions of the trunk (chromaffin paraganglia) (*Fig*. 243) and round the branchial grooves (non-chromaffin paraganglia) (*Fig*. 244).

NON-CHROMAFFIN PARAGANGLIA: These are chemoreceptors responding to alteration in pH and blood gases. They occur in relation to the following arches:

1st Arch: Orbital ciliary body.

2nd Arch: Glomus tympanicum (on the tympanic branch of the glosso-pharyngeal nerve in the temporal bone).

3rd Arch: Carotid body and glomus jugulare (on the jugular bulb).

4th Arch: Glomus intravagale (in the inferior ganglion of the vagus nerve).

6th Arch: Aortic and pulmonary glomus bodies (on the arch of the aorta and pulmonary vessels).

All paraganglia store catecholamines in their cells. Chromaffin staining correlates poorly with the catecholamine content of tumours arising from paraganglia.

Tumours arising from paraganglia

Tumours of paraganglia can be classified according to their secretory characteristics:

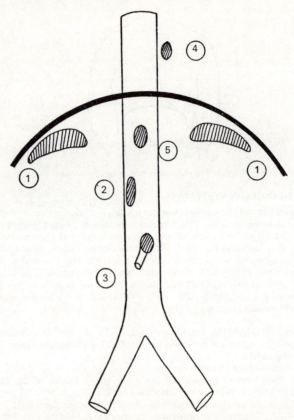

Fig. 243. Situations where chromaffin tissue may be found. (1) Normal position in adrenal; (2) lumbar paravertebral space; (3) organ of Zuckerkandl; (4) paravertebral space in left thorax; (5) in front of great vessels.

FUNCTIONALLY ACTIVE TUMOURS: These tumours produce hypertension which may be paroxysmal or sustained.

Tumours of the adrenal medulla are called 'phaeochromocytomata' and secrete noradrenaline and adrenaline. Approximately 10 per cent of such tumours are malignant, in 10 per cent more than one is present, and 10 per cent are extra-adrenal.

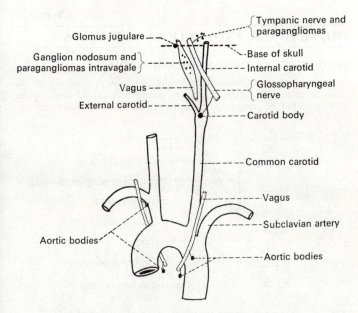

Fig. 244. The situations in which paragangliomas may be found. (Redrawn from Lattes, R. (1950), *Cancer*, vol. 3, p. 667.)

Extra-adrenal secretory tumours are usually called 'paragangliomas' and have been described in para-axial ganglia from the skull to the bladder. These tumours secrete primarily noradrenaline.

Tumours with more immature cells (neuroblastoma), secrete mainly dopamine which is an adrenaline precursor.

NON-SECRETORY TUMOURS: These arise from 'non-chromaffin' paraganglia and are called 'chemodectomata'. The commonest site for a chemodectoma is in the carotid body (carotid body tumour) which lies on the posterior surface of the carotid bifurcation. As it enlarges it splays out the internal and external carotid arteries which enables the arteriographic diagnosis to be made. The main artery of supply to a carotid body tumour is a branch from the external carotid artery.

Chapter 24

THE BLADDER, PROSTATE AND URETHRA

DEVELOPMENT OF THE BLADDER AND URETHRA

The terminal portion of the hindgut (cloaca) is subdivided posteriorly into the anorectal canal, and anteriorly into the primitive urogenital sinus, by the development of the urorectal septum which fuses with the cloacal membrane

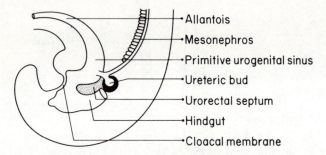

- Allantois
- Mesonephros
- Primitive urogenital sinus
- Ureteric bud
- Urorectal septum
- Hindgut
- Cloacal membrane

Fig. 245. Development of the bladder from the cloaca.

(*Fig.* 245). That portion of the primitive urogenital sinus which is continuous with the allantois and into which the mesonephric ducts drain becomes the urinary bladder. When the mesonephric ducts are incorporated into the dorsal bladder wall, the ureters come to lie cranial to the ejaculatory ducts in males.

That part of the dorsal bladder wall marked off by the openings of these four ducts forms the trigone of the bladder. When congenital diverticula of the bladder occur, they are formed somewhere along a line joining the two ureteric orifices and in close proximity to a ureteric orifice.

The allantois becomes a fibrous cord—the urachus—attached to the dome of the bladder. In the adult the urachus becomes the median umbilical ligament.

The definitive urogenital sinus is formed distal to the entrance of the mesonephric ducts. In the male (*Fig.* 246), it forms the urethra distal to the entrance of the ejaculatory ducts and, in the female (*Fig.* 247), it forms a small portion of the urethra, the lower one-fifth of the vagina and the vestibule.

The fate of the mesonephric duct in the male is discussed with the development of the testes (p. 123). In the female the mesonephric duct largely disappears, except for vestigial tubular remnants lying in the mesosalpinx between the uterine tube and ovary (*Fig.* 248). These are as follows:

1. The hydatid of Morgagni arising from the broad ligament next to the fimbrial end of the tube.

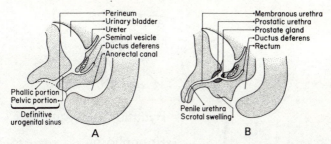

Fig. 246. Formation of the urethra in the male. The definitive urogenital sinus forms a pelvic and phallic portion, which, in turn, develop into the lower prostatic, membranous, and penile urethra, respectively. A and B show successive stages of development.

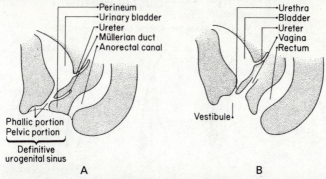

Fig. 247. Formation of the urethra in the female. The definitive urogenital sinus forms the lower portion of the urethra, a small portion of the vagina, and the vestibule. A and B show successive stages of development. The Müllerian duct gives rise to the uterus and part of the vagina.

2. The epoöphoron lying above the ovary.
3. The paroöphoron lying medial to the ovary.
4. The duct of Gartner which is that part of the mesonephric duct corresponding to the ductus deferens and ejaculatory ducts in the male. In the female, it runs in the broad ligament along the lateral wall of the uterus or vagina and gives rise to cysts.

Congenital abnormalities of the urachus

See Fig. 249. Defective development may be responsible for:

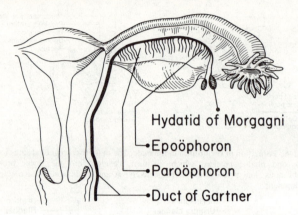

Fig. 248. Vestigial tubular remnants of the mesonephric ducts.

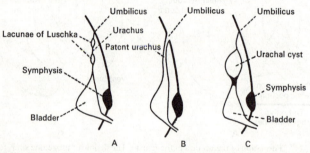

Fig. 249. Abnormalities of the urachus. A, Lacunae of Luschka; B, patent urachus; C, urachal cyst.

1. PATENT URACHUS: The ligament remains open in its whole length and, when the cord falls off, urine discharges at the umbilicus. It is said that this condition is always associated with an obstruction to the outflow of urine from the bladder.

2. LACUNAE OF LUSCHKA: Small cavities may remain in the urachus which are unsuspected during life and are only found postmortem. They are called 'lacunae of Luschka'.

3. CYSTS OF THE URACHUS: One of these lacunae enlarges to form a cyst which may be very large. It is below the umbilicus and central in position, though it may occur lateral to the midline where it has gravitated because of its weight.

THE BLADDER
Relations of the bladder

The urinary bladder lies in the pelvis posterior to the pubic bones from which it is separated by the retropubic space.

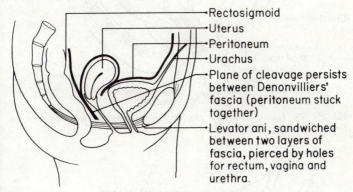

Rectosigmoid
Uterus
Peritoneum
Urachus
Plane of cleavage persists between Denonvilliers' fascia (peritoneum stuck together)
Levator ani, sandwiched between two layers of fascia, pierced by holes for rectum, vagina and urethra.

Fig. 250. The pelvic peritoneum in the female.

In the female (*Fig.* 250), the peritoneum is reflected from the superior surface of the bladder near its posterior border onto the anterior wall of the uterus close to the junction of the body of the uterus and the cervix. In the male (*Fig.* 251), the peritoneum is reflected from the superior surface of the bladder over the superior surface of the deferent ducts and seminal vesicles. The bladder can expand into the loose extraperitoneal tissue when full. The shape of the empty bladder is seen in *Fig.* 252.

The neck of the bladder in the male lies on the prostate below which the pelvic diaphragm (formed by the levator ani muscle, sandwiched between two layers of fascia), supports the contents of the pelvis. In females the bladder rests on the anterior vaginal wall which is also supported by the levator ani muscle.

Structure of the bladder

The smooth muscle of the bladder wall consists of interlacing fibres which criss-cross the bladder wall. Outside the bladder wall there is connective tissue and fat containing many veins. The urothelium consisting of transitional epithelium can easily be separated from the bladder wall except over the trigone.

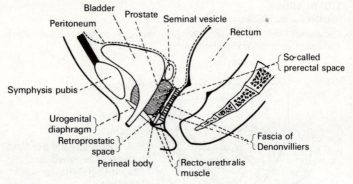

Fig. 251. The fasciae behind the prostate and the peritoneal reflection over the bladder.

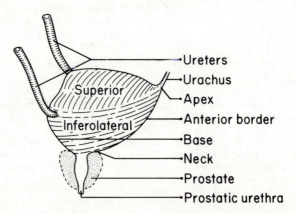

Fig. 252. The shape of the bladder.

Sphincters of the bladder

The bladder has two sphincters: the internal and external sphincters.

INTERNAL SPHINCTER: This consists of smooth muscle and is situated at the neck of the bladder. It is innervated by the autonomic nervous system and is an involuntary muscle. The normal tone of the muscle controls continence and micturition can only take place when this muscle relaxes.

The muscle lies proximal to the opening of the ejaculatory ducts into the urethra and therefore prevents reflux of ejaculatory fluid into the bladder.

This sphincter is disrupted during prostatectomy after which ejaculation cannot occur because the ejaculated fluid flows back into the bladder.

EXTERNAL SPHINCTER: This consists of striated muscle and arises from the rami of the pubis. It is situated distal to the internal sphincter and surrounds the urethra between the fascial layers of the urogenital diaphragm.

It is under voluntary control but can maintain urinary continence after the internal sphincter has been disrupted by prostatectomy.

The nerve supply is derived from the perineal branch of the pudendal nerve (S2 and 3).

Blood supply of the bladder

ARTERIAL: The bladder has a profuse arterial supply which enables the surgeon to fashion tubes from the bladder wall to replace portions of a damaged ureter. The superior vesical artery, which is a branch of the internal iliac artery, is the main artery of supply. The inferior vesical arteries supply the base of the bladder.

VENOUS DRAINAGE: The veins pass to the internal iliac veins but the vesical veins also connect the bladder and prostate directly with the veins of the hip bones, the heads of the femora and the vertebral bodies. Any increase in intra-abdominal pressure forces blood from the pelvis into the bony plexuses. This accounts for the site of occurrence of bony metastases in carcinoma of the bladder and prostate.

Lymphatic drainage

The lymphatics of the bladder drain to the internal iliac or obturator nodes, but also to the lymph spaces of the bones of the pelvis and the upper ends of the femora.

Nerve supply of the bladder

MOTOR: Sympathetic supply arises in the 1st and 2nd lumbar segments of the cord. From the cord the nerves pass to the lateral sympathetic chain and then form the hypogastric plexus (presacral nerve). Nerves from the hypogastric plexus form hypogastric ganglia on the lateral wall of the rectum. From here postganglionic fibres pass to the bladder and also the prostate, seminal vesicles, uterus and rectum. Sympathetic fibres are probably inhibitory to the bladder.

The parasympathetic fibres, derived from the 2nd, 3rd and 4th sacral segments of the cord, run in the pelvic splanchnic nerves (nervi erigentes) and synapse on the outer submucosal coats of the bladder wall. The parasympathetics are motor to the detrusor muscle and inhibitory to the internal sphincter.

SENSORY: The sensation of bladder distension is carried in the parasympathetic filaments of the pelvic splanchnic nerves (nervi erigentes) to the S2 and S3 segments of the cord.

Pain afferents are conducted in sympathetic nerves located in the presacral plexus and may reach levels as high as T6 in the cord.

Abdominal incision for exposure of the bladder and prostate

Transverse incision (Pfannenstiel's exposure) is generally used.

A curved incision concave upwards is made 2·5 cm above the symphysis pubis, through the skin, subcutaneous tissues, rectus sheath and, laterally, the aponeurosis of the external oblique. The rectus sheath is digitally dissected off the anterior aspect of the muscle on either side of the midline, there being no tendinous intersections attaching the sheath to muscle below the umbilicus. In the midline the sheath is detached from the linea alba by sharp dissection. The recti and pyramidalis muscles are separated in the midline to open the extraperitoneal prevesical and preprostatic space. The transversalis fascia is incised and the bladder is recognized by the tortuous veins running over its surface. The peritoneum should be identified on the upper surface of the bladder.

THE PROSTATE

The organ is composed of glandular tissue in a fibromuscular stroma. It is the size and shape of a chestnut. It surrounds the first 3 cm of the urethra. It is traversed by the ejaculatory ducts. It and the caecum are both broader than they are long: prostate 3 cm long, 3·8 cm broad; caecum 5·7 cm long, 6·4 cm broad. The organ consists of five lobes and has five surfaces.

Lobes

The five lobes (*Fig.* 253) are: anterior, posterior, two lateral, and middle.

ANTERIOR LOBE: Lies in front of the urethra and contains little or no glandular tissue. Benign hypertrophy ('adenomata') therefore seldom, if ever, occurs here.

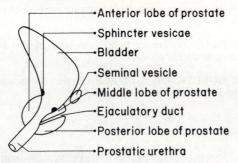

Fig. 253. Sagittal section of bladder and prostate showing normal projection of middle lobe of prostate into prostatic urethra.

POSTERIOR LOBE: Lies behind the middle lobe. 'Adenomata' never occur here but primary carcinoma of the prostate is said to begin here.

LATERAL LOBE: 'Adenomata' may occur here.

MIDDLE LOBE: This is the wedge of tissue situated behind the urethra and in front of the ejaculatory ducts. It is just below the neck of the bladder and contains much glandular tissue. Here also lie the subtrigonal glands and all the subcervical glands of Albarran. These are mucous glands, separate and distinct from the prostate, and are important because, owing to their intimate relation to the bladder neck, very slight degrees of enlargement of these glands may lead to obstruction to the outflow of urine.

The middle lobe projects normally into the urethra, raising a prominence on its floor—crista urethralis or verumontanum. The internal urethral meatus is indented below by a slight elevation (uvula vesicae) also due to the subjacent middle lobe.

Surfaces
These are: base or superior surface (above), apex (below), posterior surface, two inferolateral surfaces, and anterior surface. Their relations are:

BASE: Continuous with neck of bladder, a groove intervening in which are veins.

APEX: Rests on upper surface of superior layer of the urogenital diaphragm, therefore 'adenomata' of the prostate tend to grow upwards into the bladder, this being the path of least resistance.

POSTERIOR: Rests on anterior wall of rectum and can be felt by a finger in the rectum.

INFEROLATERAL (2): Related to and supported by that part of the levator ani called the levator prostatae.

ANTERIOR BORDER OR SURFACE: Behind the symphysis and connected with it by puboprostatic ligaments.

Fascial relations

CAPSULES: Two—true and false (*Fig*. 254). The false (surgical) capsule is formed around an area of adenomatous enlargement by a condensation of prostatic tissue which is pushed to the periphery of the gland and the 'adenomata' can be shelled out of this compressed gland tissue.

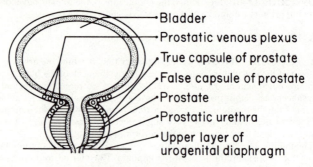

- Bladder
- Prostatic venous plexus
- True capsule of prostate
- False capsule of prostate
- Prostate
- Prostatic urethra
- Upper layer of urogenital diaphragm

Fig. 254. The capsules of the prostate.

The true (anatomical) capsule is formed by the visceral layers of pelvic fascia which gives a sheath common to bladder and prostate and is absent where the two organs are in contact.

The prostatic plexus of veins lies between the two capsules and receives in front the deep dorsal vein of the penis. In the operation of transvesical prostatectomy the surgeon 'enucleates' the 'adenoma' leaving the prostatic plexus of veins between the sheaths undisturbed. The prostatic urethra is removed with the gland and the ejaculatory ducts are torn across.

As the result of prostatectomy the patient will be sterile because the mechanism at the internal sphincter has been disturbed. Although the ejaculatory ducts discharge into the prostatic cavity, ejaculation will be retrograde into the bladder. Adrenergic-blocking agents have a similar effect.

FASCIA OF DENONVILLIERS: In the early fetus the peritoneum of the pelvic floor extends down as a pouch behind the prostate. This pouch is ultimately shut off from the peritoneal cavity and exists as two layers of fascia with a potential space between them. These two layers are attached to peritoneum (floor of Douglas' pouch) above, and to the urogenital diaphragm and perineal body below. This is the fascia of Denonvilliers (prostatoperitoneal fascia) (*Fig.* 251). The anterior of these two fascial layers is firmly attached to the prostate. The posterior layer is not quite so firmly blended with the sheath of the rectum (derived from visceral layer of pelvic fascia). The potential space between the two layers of fascia is the space of Denonvilliers.

In the performance of perineal prostatectomy, the surgeon must find his way between these two fascial layers by opening the space of Denonvilliers. This is an essential step of the operation, and failure may mean damage to the rectum.

RECTO-URETHRALIS MUSCLE (OF ROUX): The recto-urethralis muscle of Roux is shown in *Fig.* 255. This consists of two bundles of muscles (recto-urethralis superior and inferior), both derived from the longitudinal

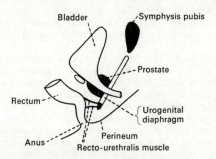

Fig. 255. Diagram of the recto-urethralis muscle.

muscle coat of the gut. They hold the anorectal junction forward, angulating it to form the rectal angle. They are both attached to the upper part of the perineal body. They must be divided in perineal prostatectomy, as only then will the rectum fall back, the muscles constituting the stay which hold it forward. A perineal prostatectomy is now infrequently performed.

Retropubic prostatectomy

A transverse incision is used as described above.

The prostate is exposed in the retropubic space. The dorsal vein of the penis and its branches are ligated as they run on the anterior surface of the prostate. A transverse incision is made through the prostatic capsule and the 'adenoma' is enucleated. In the retropubic operation, visualization of the prostatic cavity is better than in any other exposure.

MALE URETHRA

See Fig. 256.

PROSTATIC URETHRA: This part extends from the bladder to the external sphincter which lies between the two layers of the urogenital diaphragm. It has a small projection on its posterior wall called the 'verumontanum'. The prostatic glands drain into the prostatic sinus, situated alongside the verumontanum. The ejaculatory ducts empty into the posterior urethra at the prostatic utricle situated at the apex of the verumontanum. When 'adenomata' of the prostate enlarge, the verumontanum is pushed downwards towards the external sphincter (see transurethral prostatectomy).

MEMBRANOUS URETHRA: This is the shortest part and is surrounded by the external sphincter consisting of striated muscle innervated by the pudendal nerve. The external sphincter is under voluntary control.

PENILE URETHRA: The penile urethra is enclosed by the corpus spongiosum which itself forms the glans penis. The corpus spongiosum is firmly joined to two other erectile structures, the corpora cavernosa which make up the penis. The bulb is situated at the proximal end of the penile urethra. Because of the change of direction of the urethra at the level of the bulb, urethral instrumentation must be directed posteriorly so that the tip of the instrument can negotiate the membranous and prostatic urethra. At the distal end of the urethra there is slight enlargement of the urethra called the 'fossa navicularis' which contains bacteria, while the more proximal urethra normally does not. The narrowest part of the urethra is just within the external meatus.

The prostatic portion is lined by transitional cell epithelium which changes to stratified columnar epithelium at the membranous part. Near the fossa navicularis, this columnar lining changes to a stratified squamous epithelium. The ducts of the bulbo-urethral glands (Cowper's glands) open into the proximal part of the penile urethra.

Transurethral prostatectomy

Most adenomatous enlargements of the prostate are now resected trans-urethrally using a resectoscope.

The verumontanum is a very important landmark because resection of prostatic tissue distal to this point may cause damage to the external

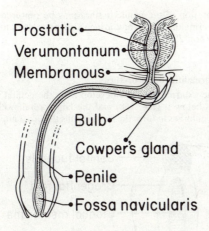

Prostatic

Verumontanum

Membranous

Bulb

Cowper's gland

Penile

Fossa navicularis

Fig. 256. The male urethra.

sphincter. After prostatectomy the external sphincter is the only sphincter left to the urethra because the internal sphincter is destroyed by the operation.

Rupture of the urethra

A fractured pelvis is the usual cause of a ruptured membranous and prostatic urethra. On rectal examination the prostate may be felt higher than its normal position.

Traumatic rupture of the urethra above the urogenital diaphragm results in an extraperitoneal pelvic extravasation of urine (*Fig*. 257A).

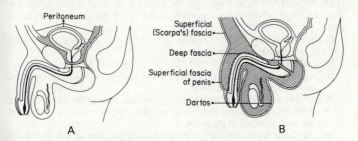

Peritoneum

Superficial (Scarpa's) fascia

Deep fascia

Superficial fascia of penis

Dartos

A   B

Fig. 257. A, Rupture of the urethra above the urogenital diaphragm; B, rupture of the bulbous urethra. The cross-hatching represents extravasation of urine.

The bulbar portion of the penile urethra may be ruptured due to blunt trauma in the perineum. Blood and urine extravasate deep to Scarpa's and Colles' fasciae (*Fig.* 257B).

Congenital abnormalities of the urethra

In the male, the external genitalia develop from the genital tubercle, two urogenital folds below it (*Fig.* 258) and the labioscrotal swellings. As the genital tubercle enlarges to form the penis it pulls the urogenital folds with it.

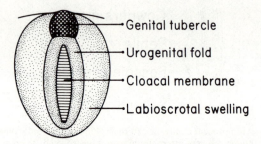

Fig. 258. Early development of the external genitalia in the male.

These folds form the lateral walls of the urethral groove which is on the ventral surface of the penis. The urogenital folds fuse with each other along the ventral surface of the penis to form the spongy urethra. As a result the external urethral orifice moves progressively towards the glans penis. The labioscrotal swellings grow together and fuse to form the scrotum.

HYPOSPADIAS: In hypospadias the external urethral orifice is on the ventral surface of the penis instead of at the tip of the glans. The penis is curved ventrally which is a condition known as 'chordee'.

In all types of hypospadias the prepuce is deformed, forming a triangular hood on the dorsum of the penis.

Hypospadias may be balanic, penile or perineoscrotal.

Balanic: The urethra ends at the base of the glans penis. The glans is often grooved on its undersurface.

Penile: The urethra ends anywhere between the base of the glans and the front of the scrotum. Extending forward from its orifice is a gutter on the undersurface of the penis.

In both these types, the fault is partial failure of fusion of the lips of the groove on the undersurface of the genital tubercle.

Perineoscrotal: The lips of the groove on the undersurface of the genital tubercle entirely fail to fuse and the urogenital folds remain separate. The individual has remained in the indifferent sexual stage. The labioscrotal folds also fail to fuse and the external urethral orifice is located between the unfused halves of the scrotum.

EPISPADIAS: The urethra opens on the dorsal surface of the penis. It is often associated with exstrophy of the bladder. In this condition the anterior wall of the bladder is missing and the pubes remain separate so that no symphysis exists (ectopia vesicae or exstrophy).

CONGENITAL CAUSES OF OBSTRUCTION OF THE OUTFLOW OF URINE: Narrowing of the channel or congenital valves causing obstruction may occur at the following sites (*Fig.* 259):
From one kidney:

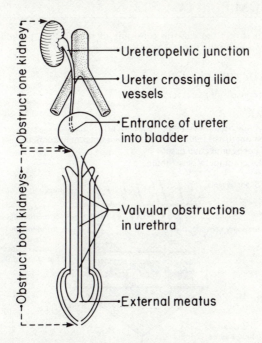

Fig. 259. Diagram to show possible sites of congenital obstruction to flow of urine from one kidney or both.

    1. At the junction of the renal pelvis with ureter.
    2. Where the ureter crosses the brim of the pelvis.
    3. Where the ureter opens into the bladder.
From both kidneys:
    1. At the internal urethral meatus.
    2. Congenital valves occur in the male urethra below the verumonta-
       num (the site of opening of the ejaculatory ducts). The valves are
       semilunar in shape and present no obstruction to an instrument
       passed up the urethra. Other forms of narrowing in the male
       urethra are rarely congenital, but most often traumatic in origin.
    3. Pinpoint meatus—the opening of the glans is excessively small.

Chapter 25

THE SCALP

The scalp covers the calvaria consisting of the superior portions of the frontal bones and the parietal and occipital bones.

LAYERS OF THE SCALP

The scalp consists of five layers (*Fig.* 260):

    S   Skin
    C   Connective tissue (superficial fascia)
    A   Aponeurosis (galea aponeurotica or epicranial aponeurosis)
    L   Loose connective tissue
    P   Pericranium or periosteum.

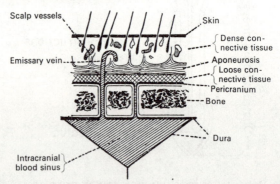

Fig. 260. Diagrammatic representation of the anatomy of the scalp. Note particularly the emissary vein.

SKIN: Epidermis and dermis contain more hair follicles and sebaceous glands than elsewhere in the body. The skin of the scalp is therefore a very common site of epidermoid cysts.

CONNECTIVE TISSUE: This is the layer of superficial fascia consisting of dense fatty connective tissue attaching the skin and the underlying galea aponeurotica by dense fibrous trabeculae.

GALEA APONEUROTICA: This is the flat tendon between the frontalis and occipitalis muscles. The fibres of the galea course from front to back in a sagittal direction, therefore sagittally placed wounds tend to remain closed whereas transversely placed wounds tend to gape. Because of its attachment to the occipitalis and frontalis muscles, the galea extends from the superior nuchal lines posteriorly to the eyebrows. Contraction of the occipital and frontal muscles moves the scalp.

From the surgical standpoint, the skin, connective tissue and aponeurosis are intimately united and should be regarded as a single layer attached to bone posteriorly and the skin anteriorly; this has surgical significance. The layer of loose connective tissue deep to the epicranial aponeurosis allows the first three layers to separate easily from the pericranium. In surgical procedures the first three layers are turned down as a flap.

In a compound fracture of the skull the wound in the scalp may not overlie the fracture site because of the mobility of the epicranial aponeurosis. Blood or pus may accumulate in the subaponeurotic space; these subaponeurotic collections of fluid may extend posteriorly to the superior nuchal lines, laterally to the zygomatic arch and anteriorly it may track into the root of the nose and eyelids.

A 'black eye' can be caused in different ways:

1. It is most commonly due to local violence causing subcutaneous extravasation of blood into the lids; haemorrhage occurs soon after receipt of the injury into upper and lower eyelids. This must be differentiated from a subconjunctival haemorrhage following localized injury to the eyeball.
2. Another cause of 'black eye' is bleeding into the layer of loose connective tissue after a blow on the skull; the blood gravitates slowly under the frontalis muscle and appears first in the upper eyelid and then the lower eyelid over the course of a couple of days.
3. Fracture of the orbital plate of the frontal bone also results in haemorrhage into the orbit; the blood tracks under the conjunctiva appearing as a triangular, flame-shaped haemorrhage, the apex of which is at the margin of the cornea and the posterior limit cannot be seen, which distinguishes it from the subconjunctival haemorrhage.

BLOOD VESSELS OF THE SCALP

Arteries

Five arteries exist (*Fig.* 261) on each side which are derived from the internal and external carotid arteries. They run mainly in the layer of connective tissue between the galea and the skin. Two anterior arteries,

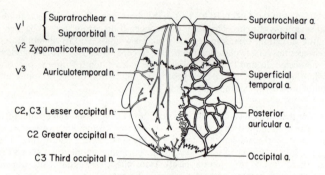

Fig. 261. The arteries and nerves of the scalp.

supra-orbital and supratrochlear, are branches of the ophthalmic artery (from the internal carotid artery). The external carotid artery gives rise to the superficial temporal artery laterally and the posterior auricular and occipital arteries posteriorly. The blood vessels anastomose freely with each other so there is little danger of reducing markedly the blood supply to an area of scalp, unless a skin flap with a narrow inferior pedicle is produced. In performing a craniotomy, the surgeon raises an osteoplastic flap which contains the appropriate portion of skull with the overlying scalp attached. To ensure a good blood supply of the flap, the skin incision is so placed that the base of the flap incorporates one of the arteries supplying the scalp.

Wounds of the scalp bleed profusely. The blood vessels tend to retract into the fibrous trabeculae of the superficial fascia. Bleeding is relatively easily stopped by compressing the scalp upon the underlying skull. When making a surgical incision in the scalp, bleeding is controlled by artery forceps applied to the galea. The vessels are thereby compressed between the skin and galea.

Because of the profuse blood supply, wounds of the scalp heal well and infection is uncommon. Minimal or no débridement is required in scalp wounds.

The direction of blood flow in the supra-orbital and supratrochlear arteries is normally from within the skull in an outward direction. In patients with stenosis or occlusion of the internal carotid artery, the direction of flow is reversed. The external carotid artery and its branches thus form an important collateral arterial supply to the brain. The changed direction of flow can be detected by applying a Doppler flow probe to the supra-orbital margin where the supra-orbital and supratrochlear arteries pass over the bone.

Veins

To some extent, veins (*Fig.* 262) follow the course of the arteries and therefore are divisible into similar groups. Their ultimate outflow is, however, variable. In infants the veins of the scalp are easily seen deep to the skin and are the favoured site of intravenous infusion.

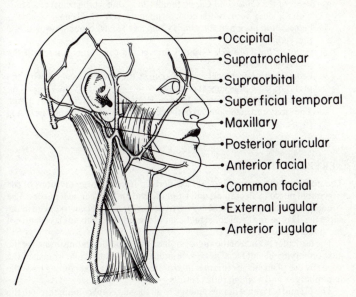

- Occipital
- Supratrochlear
- Supraorbital
- Superficial temporal
- Maxillary
- Posterior auricular
- Anterior facial
- Common facial
- External jugular
- Anterior jugular

Fig. 262. The veins of the scalp.

EMISSARY VEINS: These are veins which link the intracranial venous sinuses with veins outside the cranial cavity. Of necessity, they pass through the potential space between the galea aponeurotica and the pericranium. They are of importance in that they are channels along which infected thrombosis may reach the interior of the cranial cavity from infections outside it.

The following are recognized emissary veins:

1. *Vein of the Foramen Caecum:* Connects the commencement of the superior sagittal or longitudinal sinus with the veins of the frontal sinus and root of the nose.
2. *Ophthalmic Veins:* May be looked upon as large emissary veins connecting the supra-orbital and frontal veins of the forehead with the cavernous sinus of the skull.
3. *Parietal Emissary Vein:* Connects the veins of the scalp with the superior sagittal sinus.
4. *Mastoid Vein:* Connects the posterior auricular vein with the transverse sinus. It is a constant and very important emissary vein.
5. *Veins of the Hypoglossal Canal:* Small veins connect the transverse sinus with the deep veins of the neck through the hypoglossal canal.
6. *Veins of the Condyloid Canal:* Small veins connect the transverse sinus with the deep veins of the neck through the condyloid canal.
7. *Veins of the Foramen Lacerum:* Connect the cavernous sinus with the pterygoid plexus.
8. *Veins of the Foramen Ovale:* Connect the cavernous sinus with the pterygoid plexus.
9. *Veins of the Foramen Vesalii:* Connect the cavernous sinus with the pterygoid and pharyngeal plexuses.
10. *Middle Meningeal Veins or Sinuses:* Run with the artery of that name. They may end in the sinuses of the skull or in the pterygoid plexus, being then emissary veins.

NERVES OF THE SCALP

The nerves of the scalp (*Fig.* 261) are derived from all three divisions of the trigeminal nerve (Vth cranial) and from the 2nd and 3rd cervical nerves. The cutaneous distribution of these nerves is seen in *Fig.* 261. The nerves run in the superficial fascia and local anaesthetic should be injected into this layer and not the subaponeurotic layer.

The auricular branch of the vagus is joined by a communicating branch of the glossopharyngeal and facial nerves. Stimulation of the auricular branch of the vagus by use of an ear speculum is interpreted by the brain as coming from the hypopharynx and a cough reflex results.

The C2 and C3 spinal nerves emerge from the vertebral column through the intervertebral foramina which are often affected with osteo-arthritis of the adjacent joints. Compression or irritation of these nerves may result in pain felt in their distribution and be the cause of occipital headaches. It should be noted that the dura mater of the posterior fossa of the skull is also supplied by the segments C2 and C3 and that infections of the posterior dura, such as meningitis, may result not only in occipital headache but also in the characteristic 'neck rigidity', by reflex activity of the posterior neck muscles.

LYMPH DRAINAGE OF THE SCALP

The lymphatic watershed may be regarded as a line passing over the vertex of the head from ear to ear. The part anterior to the line drains into the parotid lymph nodes and the part posterior to the line drains into the mastoid and occipital lymph nodes. These drain into the upper deep cervical nodes.

Chapter 26

THE ANATOMY OF THE NORMAL AND THE ENLARGED PITUITARY BODY

ERRORS IN THE DEVELOPMENT OF THE HYPOPHYSIS (PITUITARY BODY)

This is developed from two separate parts: (*a*) a downgrowth from the floor of the third ventricle forms the infundibulum and the posterior lobe; (*b*) an upgrowth (Rathke's pouch) from the roof of the primitive pharynx forms the anterior lobe. The site where this upgrowth took place is represented in the adult on the posterior border of the nasal septum, and may be marked by a recess—a remnant of the pouch of Rathke (*Fig.* 263). In the region of the tuberculum sellae in the anterior fossa of the skull there is sometimes a foramen (craniopharyngeal canal) which marks the upper part of the canal made by the upgrowth that goes to form the anterior lobe of the hypophysis.

At the site of the pouch of Rathke or along the craniopharyngeal canal, cysts may grow from portions of the upgrowth which have become sequestrated. These are lined with squamous epithelium and are histologically adamantinomata. When they occur in the skull:

1. They are likely to damage the hypophysis and cause interference with its function, resulting sometimes in a very fat, backward individual without secondary sexual characters—dystrophia adiposogenitalis (Fröhlich's syndrome).
2. They become calcified and may be detected radiologically in 80 per cent of cases in which such a cyst exists.
3. They may press on the optic chiasma and cause bitemporal hemianopia.

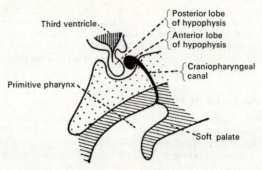

Fig. 263, Schematic representation of development of the hypophysis. The surrounding parts have been shown at a more advanced developmental stage to make the picture clearer.

NORMAL PITUITARY BODY

The pituitary body is suspended from the base of the brain in the region of the floor of the third ventricle by a projecting stalk—the infundibulum. The organ lies in the pituitary fossa of the sella turcica of the sphenoid bone in the middle fossa of the skull. It is completely covered by a fold of dura mater, the diaphragma sellae, which is perforated by a tiny orifice for the passage of the infundibulum.

    Dimensions: $13 \times 8 \times 6$ mm

    Structure: The organ consists of two lobes, anterior and posterior
            (*Fig.* 264).

The anterior lobe

This lobe consists of a pars anterior and a pars intermedia, which are separated from each other by a narrow cleft which is the remnant of the diverticulum from which the lobe develops. The pars intermedia is unimportant in man. The pars anterior is kidney shaped with the concavity posterior, embracing the posterior lobe.

    It is very vascular, the blood vessels reaching the gland along the infundibulum from the circulus arteriosus. Arterial branches from the circle of Willis supply the hypothalamus. From here a network of capillaries extends along the infundibulum and then subdivides to end in another network of capillaries around the cells of the anterior pituitary. The blood supply to the anterior pituitary therefore starts and ends in capillaries without an intermediate heart and is therefore regarded as a portal system. Hormones

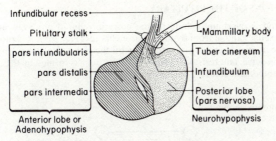

Fig. 264. The gross structure of the pituitary body.

released from the hypothalamus are conveyed to the anterior pituitary by this portal system.

The posterior lobe
The posterior lobe is developed as a downgrowth from the floor of the 3rd ventricle.

HISTOLOGY

Anterior lobe
Depending on their staining characteristics, the cells of the anterior lobe are classified as chromophils or chromophobes. The chromophils contain many granules and are stained either basophilic or eosinophilic, while chromophobes contain no granules and do not stain. It is now thought that the latter cells do not stain because they are actively secreting. When the chromophobes enter a resting phase they become again chromophilic. There is, therefore, only one cell type in varying phases of secretion. Immunologically and on electron microscopy, the chromophils can be subdivided according to the hormones they produce.

Posterior pituitary
Nerve fibres extend from the hypothalamus to the posterior pituitary which is composed mainly of glial-like cells. These cells act as supporting structure for the nerve endings from the hypothalamus which secrete antidiuretic hormone and oxytocin.

RELATIONS OF THE PITUITARY

The gland is overhung behind by the posterior clinoid processes and the dorsum sellae, and in front by the anterior clinoids (*Fig.* 265). It is roofed by a curtain of dura stretching over the fossa for the gland (*Fig.* 266). This dural curtain is dense and resistant. The floor of the fossa is formed by the roof of the sphenoidal air sinus.

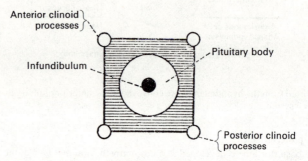

Anterior clinoid processes

Pituitary body

Infundibulum

Posterior clinoid processes

Fig. 265. The 'four-poster bedstead' in which the pituitary body reposes. The cross-hatching represents blood sinuses.

The infundibulum passes up posterior to the chiasma and is in contact with its posterior edge and undersurface. The chiasma is not in contact with the bone.

The immediate superior relation of the chiasma is the anterior communicating artery which connects the two anterior cerebral arteries (*Fig.* 267). Pituitary tumours which grow upwards, particularly the congenital cysts of Rathke's pouch (craniopharyngiomas), push the chiasma up.

Four blood sinuses form a square which encloses the gland (*Fig.* 265): the cavernous sinus on each side and the anterior and posterior intercavernous sinuses in front and behind. In the outer wall of the cavernous sinus lie the IIIrd, IVth, ophthalmic branch of the Vth, and the VIth cranial nerves, and also the internal carotid artery, which is rather beneath the sinus (*Fig.* 268).

ENLARGEMENTS OF THE PITUITARY

Symptoms of pituitary tumours are divisible into two classes: (*a*) endocrine, (*b*) 'neighbourhood symptoms', which are produced by the pressure of the enlarged gland on adjacent parts, especially the optic chiasma.

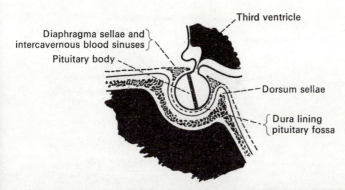

Fig. 266. Sagittal section of the pituitary gland showing the dural relations. Notice the dura between the gland and its fossa.

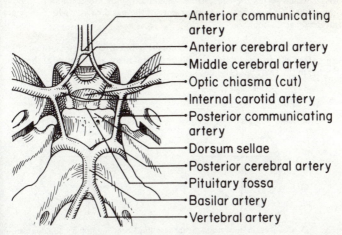

Fig. 267. A figure to show the vascular relations (circle of Willis) of the pituitary fossa. The hypophysis has been removed. (After Cope.)

Neighbourhood symptoms

Only 50 per cent of pituitary tumours give rise to visual signs. These signs are affections of the visual fields and disc changes. A pituitary tumour produces visual symptoms if it can expand upwards through the foramen in the

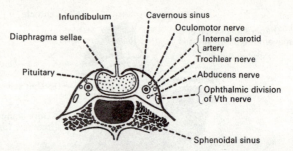

Fig. 268. Coronal section through the pituitary body.

diaphragma sellae and press on the optic chiasma. If it is contained beneath the diaphragma sellae, it tends to bulge through the floor of the pituitary fossa, which forms the roof of the sphenoidal sinus. Such tumours may lie immediately posterior to the upper part of the nasal cavity, where they are surgically accessible.

1. VISUAL CHANGES: The commonest is bitemporal hemianopia which consists of a flattening of the superior temporal fields and is rarely of the same degree in the two eyes (*Fig.* 269).

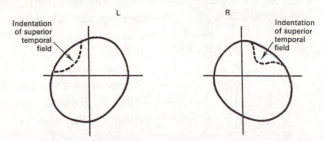

Fig. 269. Changes in the visual fields resulting from a pituitary tumour causing bitemporal hemianopia. The solid line represents the normal field.

2. OTHER EYE SIGNS PRODUCED BY PITUITARY TUMOURS:
    i. The IIIrd nerve, being near the pituitary, may be pressed on, diplopia and IIIrd nerve palsy resulting.
    ii. Palsies of the IVth or VIth nerves are very rare.
    iii. Pressure on the cavernous sinus may cause proptosis with engorgement of the lids.

3. PRESSURE ON OTHER PARTS OF THE BRAIN: With a large growth, pressure may be exerted on the anterior part of the temporal lobe, causing uncinate fits, which produce sensations of smell. Pressure upwards may close the foramen of Monro and produce symptoms of hydrocephalus. Pressure up and backwards by a large tumour may cause interference with the pyramidal tract in the crus, resulting in symptoms referred to the opposite half of the body, e.g. paresis or paralysis. Pressure upwards on the floor of the third ventricle may cause persistent drowsiness. Pressure on the frontal lobes may cause mental dullness.

4. CHANGES IN THE SELLA TURCICA: The pituitary fossa is deepened by an intrasellar growth, and in X-ray photographs characteristic ballooning of the sella is seen. The floor bulges down into the sphenoidal sinus. The clinoid processes may be eroded, though this occurs more usually with tumours arising above the sella from other parts of the brain.

Endocrine changes

Micro-adenomata, usually under 1 cm in size, do not give rise to neighbour-hood symptoms, but only to hormonal changes. This may present as an isolated hormone deficiency or as an excess of one of the anterior pituitary hormones.

HYPOPHYSECTOMY

Pituitary tumours may be removed by the transfrontal operation or by the trans-sphenoidal route. As the tumour does not admit of complete removal, the part left goes on growing and soon causes symptoms again unless this can be prevented. This is best achieved by removing the floor of the sella turcica so that the remains of the tumour tend to be extruded by intracranial pressure into the sphenoidal sinus. The floor of the pituitary fossa can only be removed by the trans-sphenoidal route. This is also the route favoured for the insertion of pellets of radioactive substances into the pituitary.

Trans-sphenoidal operation

A small incision is made in the mucous membrane between the upper lip and gum. The anterior edge of the nasal septum is exposed. The mucoperiosteum is separated from each side of the septum nasi and the whole of the latter removed. The anterior wall of the sphenoidal sinus is cut away, exposing the bulging floor of the sella turcica which is removed. This exposes the dura beneath the pituitary, excision of which exposes the tumour. The cavity of the nose is not entered, so that the approach is not through a septic cavity. (*See Fig.* 270.)

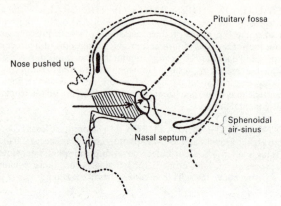

Fig. 270. Nasal route to the pituitary gland is indicated by arrows. (Hugh Cairns, after Cushing.)

Chapter 27

THE MENINGES, CEREBROSPINAL FLUID AND SPINAL CORD

THE MENINGES

These consist, from outside in, of dura mater, arachnoid mater, and pia mater.

Dura mater

Consists over the brain of two layers, named 'periosteal' and 'investing', which are firmly adherent excepting where they split to enclose venous sinuses (*Fig.* 271). These latter are formed in two ways: (*a*) by a separation of the two layers; (*b*) by a reduplication of the inner layer.

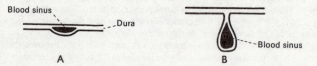

Fig. 271. Showing the methods of formation of the intracranial blood sinuses: A, a split between the two layers of the dura; B, a reduplication of the inner layer.

THE OUTER PERIOSTEAL LAYER: The outer periosteal layer is the periosteum of the inner surface of the skull bones. It ends at the foramen magnum. It is firmly adherent over the base, less so over the vault, except at the sutures, where it is attached to the pericranium by the sutural membrane. It is continuous with the pericranium at the foramina. Owing to the firm fixation of this layer of dura to the base, it is usually torn in fractures of the base of the skull, and as it forms part of the walls of the basal venous sinuses, such as the petrosals, a fractured base is frequently associated with severe bleeding from ear or nose, or into the pharynx.

INVESTING OR INNER LAYER:
1. Gives sheaths to the nerves which leave the skull. The dural sheaths fuse with the epineurium of the cranial nerves outside the skull. This is especially important in the optic nerve where the central artery and veins of the retina cross the subarachnoid space to become enclosed in a space around the posterior part of the optic nerve.
2. Becomes continuous with the dura mater spinalis at the foramen magnum.
3. Sends four processes inwards:
   i. *Falx Cerebri:* A sickle-shaped reduplication which intervenes between medial surface of the two hemispheres. It contains three venous sinuses: (*a*) the superior sagittal along its upper border; (*b*) the inferior sagittal along its lower (free) border; (*c*) the straight sinus along its line of attachment to the tentorium cerebelli.
   ii. *Tentorium:* This is a semilunar reduplication of the dura which intervenes between the cerebellum and the occipital lobes of the brain. It therefore roofs in the posterior fossa of the skull. Its outer convex border is attached to the lips of the transverse sinus on the occipital bone, the mastoid angle of the parietal bone, and the superior border of the petrous temporal; it ends by being attached to the posterior clinoid process. Its inner concave free border extends forward over the attached border to become attached to the anterior clinoid process. This border bounds an oval space ('the door of the tent') which is occupied by the midbrain. Through this opening, cerebrospinal fluid finds it way from the spinal region and base of the brain to the outer surface of the brain, where it is absorbed. The transverse or lateral sinus lies between the two layers of the tentorium along the posterior half of its attached border. The superior petrosal sinus lies along the anterior half of this border.
   iii. *Falx Cerebelli:* A small sickle-shaped fold intervening posteriorly between the two halves of the cerebellum. It contains the occipital sinus.
   iv. *Diaphragma Sellae:* A fold of dura roofing over the pituitary fossa. It has a central aperture for emergence of the infundibulum (stalk) of the pituitary. It encloses the intercavernous sinuses.

BLOOD SINUSES OF CRANIUM: They receive the venous blood from the brain and drain ultimately into the two internal jugular veins. There are some important matters of applied anatomy in relation to these venous channels:

1. Sinus bleeding is usually consequent on fracture of the skull. This occurrence is infrequent as the channels do not lie in bony grooves with the exception of the lower part of the lateral sinus (sigmoid sinus).
2. Pressure in the sinus is low but is readily raised by coughing, struggling etc. As the walls of the sinuses are too rigid to collapse, copious bleeding follows wounds of these channels. Traumatic transection of large sinuses may well be fatal.

The Superior Sagittal Sinus: It begins at the crista galli in the midline in the anterior fossa of the skull by the union of small meningeal veins. Here it communicates with the veins of the nose or frontal sinus by emissary veins traversing the foramen caecum. It passes back over the convexity of the brain lying along the attached border of the falx major and, at the level of the inion (external occipital protuberance), it turns to one or other side (usually the right) to form the lateral sinus.

It receives veins from the medial surface of the hemispheres and from the upper halves of their convex lateral surfaces. These veins enter the sinus in the opposite direction to that of the blood flow in the sinus. The veins from the lower part of the outer surface of the hemispheres drain into the Sylvian system. There is an adequate anastomosis between these two areas of venous drainage.

The veins entering the sinus must pass through the subdural space. Here they are least protected and may be torn as the result of trauma often of a relatively minor nature. This results in the formation of a subdural haematoma.

SPINAL DURA: A single layer continuous with the inner layer of the dura mater of the brain. It is a long tube enclosing the spinal cord but extending five vertebrae lower. Its existence as a tube ends at the 2nd sacral vertebra, but a prolongation of the membrane invests the filum terminale, ending on the back of the coccyx.

Epidural Space: Between the dura and the walls of the vertebral canal lies the epidural (extradural) space, which contains the dural sac, spinal nerve roots, a plexus of veins, the spinal arteries, lymphatics and fat. Local anaesthetic solution which exerts its effects on the spinal nerve roots may be injected into this space.

Subdural Space: This is a capillary space between the dura and arachnoid over both brain and cord. It contains no cerebrospinal fluid.

Arachnoid mater

A delicate avascular membrane which dips into the longitudinal and lateral fissures of the brain. It ends at the 2nd sacral vertebra.

ARACHNOIDAL PROCESSES:

1. *The Arachnoidal Villi:* These are fine tortuous processes which arise from the surface of the arachnoid, push the dura before them, eventually perforating it and projecting into the venous sinuses and large veins. They are covered by specialized mesothelial cells which convey the cerebrospinal fluid to the bloodstream.

2. *The Arachnoidal Granulations (Pacchionian Bodies):* These are merely aggregations of arachnoidal villi clumped together. They have the same functions and relations as the villi, but are found only in adults, not in children.

Pia mater

Very thin and delicate. All the blood vessels to the brain and cord run on it before entering the brain or cord, yet the pia itself is avascular.

PROCESSES GIVEN OFF BY THE PIA:

1. The perivascular space: the blood vessels going to the brain lie in the subarachnoid space before piercing the pia.

2. Septa dip into all the sulci and fissures of the brain.

3. Sheaths to all cranial and spinal nerves.

4. Tela choroidea of the 4th ventricle is the name given to the pia over the lower part of the roof of the 4th ventricle. The choroid plexuses of the 4th ventricle lie in it.

5. Tela choroidea of the 3rd ventricle is the pia which lies above the roof of the 3rd ventricle. The choroid plexus of the 3rd ventricle and the choroid plexus of each lateral ventricle are invested by this pial process.

6. A septum into the anterior median fissure of the spinal cord is given off by the pia. Where this process is given off the pia presents a thickening—linea splendens.

7. Ligamenta denticulata: twenty-one toothed processes, on each side, extend from the pia to the dura, pushing the arachnoid before them. They leave the pia midway between the anterior and posterior nerve roots and serve to suspend the cord in the midline. The lowest ligamentum denticulatum is forked, and the posterior root of the first lumbar nerve lies on the outer prong of the fork (*Fig.* 272). In the lower region of the cord it is the surgeon's guide to the 1st lumbar nerve and gives him a nerve root of known number from which he may determine the position of whatever nerve roots he is in search of.

SUBARACHNOID SPACE: This contains the cerebrospinal fluid. It is traversed by septa lined with flat arachnoidal cells. It is also traversed by the vessels going to the brain and cord. It presents certain dilatations (cisterns) which act as a waterbed to the brain:

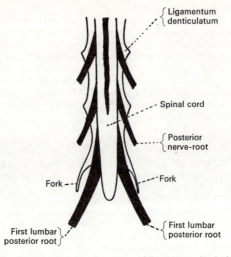

Fig. 272. 'Fork' made by lowest process of ligamentum denticulatum.

1. Cisterna magna: situated posteriorly between the cerebellum and medulla.
2. Cisterna pontis: in front of the pons.
3. Cisterna interpeduncularis at the base of the brain. It contains the circulus arteriosus (circle of Willis).
4. Smaller less important cisterns.

Communications between the Cavities of the Brain and the Subarachnoid Space:

1. Median aperture of 4th ventricle (foramen of Magendie): the median aperture in the roof of the 4th ventricle.
2. Lateral apertures of 4th ventricle (foramina of Luschka): two lateral apertures, one in each lateral recess of the 4th ventricle.

CEREBROSPINAL FLUID

In an adult, the total volume of cerebrospinal fluid (CSF) is about 150 ml while the rate of production is 500 ml per day.

The choroid plexus of the ventricles, especially the lateral ventricles, is a major source of CSF and the cerebral interstitial fluid is an important additional source. As the brain has no lymphatic system, the CSF drains into the ventricular system or subarachnoid space.

The fluid is passed into the venous sinuses through the arachnoidal villi and granulations. This absorption takes place on the outer surface of the hemispheres, the fluid passing through the opening in the tentorium cerebelli to attain this situation.

Cisternal puncture

The patient is sitting or lying on one side with the head flexed forwards. The needle is entered in the midline just above the first palpable cervical spinous

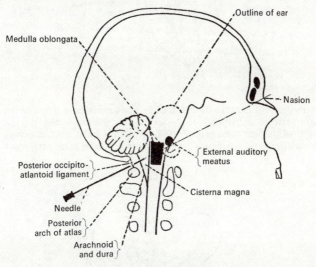

Fig. 273.   Cisternal puncture.

process—that of the axis or 2nd vertebrae (*Fig*. 273). It is directed forwards and upwards, parallel to an imaginary line joining the external auditory meatus with the nasion. The point of the needle strikes the atlanto-occipital ligament in the adult at a depth of 4–5 cm from the surface and is felt to pierce the ligament and enter the cistern. The posterior surface of the medulla is fully 2·5 cm anterior to the posterior atlanto-occipital ligament.

Lumbar puncture

In this procedure, the spinal subarachnoid space is tapped below the 2nd lumbar vertebra at which level the spinal cord ends (*Fig*. 274). The needle is

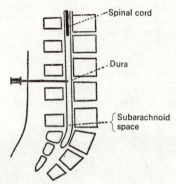

Fig. 274. Route of needle in performing lumbar puncture. The cord is out of danger. The cauda equina is not shown.

inserted usually between the 3rd and 4th lumbar vertebrae. The spine of the latter vertebra corresponds to the level of the line connecting the highest points of the iliac crest (*Fig.* 275). The patient's spine must be maximally flexed to open the space between the spinous processes of the vertebrae.

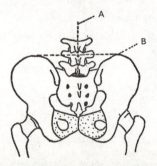

Fig. 275. Determining the usual site for lumbar puncture in the region of intersection of mid-vertical line (A) with line joining points of iliac crests (B).

Loculation syndrome (Froin's)

If a block occurs anywhere in the vertebral canal preventing fluid passing the obstruction, the fluid below has special properties: (*a*) it may coagulate spontaneously as the percentage of protein in it is greatly increased; (*b*) it may be yellow (xanthochromia) like plasma.

Sudden increase of the intracranial venous pressure is not transmitted to the fluid below the block. In Queckenstedt's test both internal jugular veins are compressed in the neck. Blood dams back in the skull and raises the intracranial pressure with the patient in the lateral position. Should the circulation of cerebrospinal fluid in the subarachnoid space be cut off by a tumour, the change in pressure will not be transmitted to the subarachnoid space below the tumour.

SPINAL CORD

Blood supply

The spinal cord derives its blood supply from longitudinally directed anterior and posterior spinal arteries supplemented by radicular arteries.

1. THE ANTERIOR SPINAL ARTERY: This vessel (*Fig.* 276) is formed by the union of two small branches of the right and left vertebral arteries in the

Posterior spinal artery

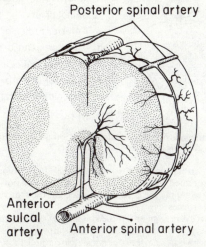

Anterior
sulcal
artery   Anterior spinal artery

Fig. 276. The anterior and posterior spinal arteries.

upper cervical canal. It runs caudally in the ventral median sulcus and terminates along the filum terminale. The anterior spinal artery supplies the anterior two-thirds of the cord.

2. POSTERIOR SPINAL ARTERIES: There are two posterior spinal arteries (*Fig.* 276), each arising from a small branch of either the vertebral or posterior inferior cerebellar arteries. Each posterior spinal artery runs on the posterolateral aspect of the cord and together they supply the posterior third of the cord. The anterior and posterior spinal arteries anastomose with each other in the pia around the cord.

3. RADICULAR ARTERIES: Radicular arteries (*Fig.* 277) are derived from spinal branches of the vertebral, deep cervical and ascending cervical arteries which stem from the proximal aorta. The intermediate area of the aorta provides radicular arteries through the spinal branches of the intercostal arteries and the terminal portion of the aorta performs this function through spinal branches of the lumbar and lateral sacral arteries.

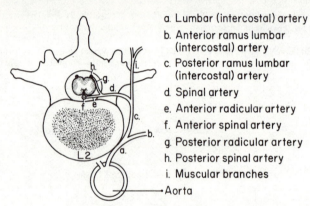

a. Lumbar (intercostal) artery

b. Anterior ramus lumbar (intercostal) artery

c. Posterior ramus lumbar (intercostal) artery

d. Spinal artery

e. Anterior radicular artery

f. Anterior spinal artery

g. Posterior radicular artery

h. Posterior spinal artery

i. Muscular branches

Aorta

Fig. 277. The distribution of a lumbar or intercostal artery. The anterior and posterior radicular arteries are branches of the intercostal artery.

Each spinal artery enters the spinal canal by passing through an intervertebral foramen and then dividing into an anterior and posterior radicular artery to supply the cord and supplement the tenuous anterior and posterior spinal arteries.

In the embryo every segment of the spinal cord receives paired radicular arteries, but many of these segmental branches atrophy or disappear so that the adult is left with only one or two cervical, two or three thoracic, and one or two lumbar radicular arteries (*Fig.* 278). The best developed of these radicular arteries is the great radicular artery, or the artery of Adamkiewicz. In 75 per cent of cases, this artery arises from an intercostal artery between T9 and T12 usually on the left side. This artery is the main supply to the lower thoracic segment and the cord distal to it.

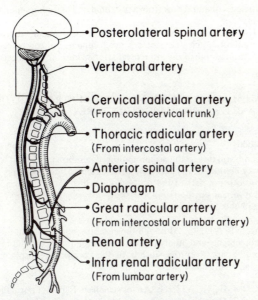

Fig. 278. The blood supply of the spinal cord. The main radicular arteries are shown.

The anterior and posterior spinal arteries are small arteries which are dependent on their anastomoses with the radicular arteries to sustain the flow of blood along the cord. The wide spacing of the radicular arteries, especially from intercostal arteries (intermediate area), renders the spinal cord vulnerable to ischaemic damage if the flow of blood through one of the radicular arteries is interrupted.

Paraplegia following Abdominal Aortic Surgery: The great radicular artery (arteria radicularis magna) (artery of Adamkiewicz) may arise as low as L4 and as high as T8. Depending on its site of origin, the blood flow through this artery may be interfered with during aortic surgery, particularly if the vessel has an abnormally distal origin. The suggestion that the artery of Adamkiewicz should be identified during abdominal aortic aneurysmectomy has been found to be of questionable value.

Occlusion of the artery may produce ischaemia of the cord which results in paraplegia. Fortunately this is a very uncommon (1 in 400) complication following aortic surgery which suggests that, even if an anomalously low Adamkiewicz artery is occluded, there is usually sufficient collateral flow from a proximal or distal companion radicular artery.

The prevalence of paraplegia following aneurysmectomy for abdominothoracic aneurysms is much higher, but can be reduced by implanting some of the intercostal arteries into the prosthesis.

CONGENITAL MALFORMATIONS OF THE CENTRAL NERVOUS SYSTEM AND ITS SUPPORTING STRUCTURES

Hydrocephalus

This is a condition due to the accumulation of cerebrospinal fluid within the skull. It may be due to: (a) excessive production of fluid, which is rare; (b) obstruction in some part of the route along which the fluid circulates; (c) interference with absorption of fluid.

Hydrocephalus can be classified into:

1. COMMUNICATING: Although the cerebrospinal fluid can escape into the cisterna magna and lumbar area, it cannot reach the supratentorial subarachnoid space over the surface of the cerebral hemispheres where absorption normally takes place.

2. NON-COMMUNICATING: An obstruction is present usually in the midline in the 3rd ventricle, aqueduct or 4th ventricle. The obstruction causes distension of one or more ventricles. The site of obstruction may be demonstrated by withdrawing cerebrospinal fluid and injecting air into the ventricles (ventriculography), or by computerized axial tomography.

Shunting Procedures: In both a communicating and non-communicating hydrocephalus, a shunt may be created from the ventricles to the blood stream directly, as in a ventriculo-atrial shunt, or indirectly via the peritoneal cavity, as in a ventriculoperitoneal shunt. In both procedures, a tube is passed from the dilated lateral ventricle subcutaneously into the peritoneal cavity, or via the external jugular vein into the atrium. A third shunt is the ventriculosubarachnoid shunt to bypass an obstruction in the ventricular system. A tube passes from the ventricle into the cervical subarachnoid space.

Spina bifida

This results from incomplete closure of the spinal canal, the commonest site being the lumbosacral region. It is classified as shown in *Fig.* 279 into:

SPINA BIFIDA OCCULTA: Radiologically there is a failure of fusion of the posterior arches of a lumbar vertebra. If it is associated with a cutaneous

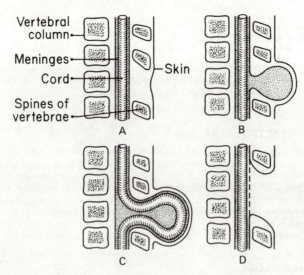

Fig. 279. Spina bifida. A, Spina bifida occulta; B, meningocele; C, meningomyelocele; D, myelocele.

marker in the lumbar region, such as a lumbosacral lipoma, dermal sinus, hairy patch or an angiomatous malformation, then the lower end of the spinal cord is at risk from traction injuries resulting from tethering due to congenital anomalies in the spinal canal. The traction injury to the cord can result in motor, sensory or sphincter disturbances.

SPINA BIFIDA CYSTICA:
  1. *Meningocele:* The pia and arachnoid protrude through the posterior arches. The dura stops at the margin of the bony defect.
  2. *Meningomyelocele:* The cord and the meninges protrude through the defect. There is always a lesion of the cauda equina or the cord.
  3. *Myelocele:* The neural canal remains open so that the cord can be seen as a reddened area through the defect in skin and bone. When this type of defect is present throughout the cord it is called rachischisis.

In spina bifida cystica there may be partial or complete paralysis of the anal and urinary sphincters and the limbs.

Many of the affected children develop hydrocephalus as a result of a concomitant anomaly in the midbrain, known as the Arnold–Chiari malformation. In this condition, there is herniation of the cerebellar tonsils through the foramen magnum with elongation and kinking of the brain stem.

Chapter 28

THE CRANIAL NERVES

A cranial nerve palsy may be the first sign of a space-occupying intracranial lesion. Knowledge of the anatomy of a paralysed cranial nerve is essential in the clinical evaluation of where the lesion is situated.

THE OLFACTORY NERVE (Ist)

The olfactory cells reside in the mucosa of the superior nasal concha and the upper part of the nasal septum. The axons of these cells pass through the sieve-like cribriform plate of the ethmoid bone to reach the overlying olfactory bulb in the anterior cranial fossa which, strictly speaking, is an appendage of the brain. The olfactory tracts pass from the olfactory bulb to the medial surface of the cerebral hemisphere and the temporal lobe.

Lesions of the olfactory nerve result in a loss of the sense of smell (anosmia). Smell is also responsible for the finer appreciation of taste.

Causes of anosmia

1. Head injuries: a sudden shift of the cerebral hemisphere results in avulsion of the olfactory bulb from the brain or from the cribriform plate. The olfactory nerves may also be damaged by a fracture of the cribriform plate which may result in CSF rhinorrhoea.
2. Tumours of the frontal lobe, or those arising near the pituitary gland.
3. Chronic tuberculous meningitis.

OPTIC NERVE (IInd)

Axons of ganglion cells of the retina make up the optic nerve. The optic disc is the central collecting point for these axons. The optic disc is a blind spot because it is made up of nerve fibres only, there being no rods and cones.

The orbital portion of the optic nerve extends from where the optic nerve pierces the sclera to the optic foramen in the skull. The optic nerve is covered by a sheath of dura, arachnoid and pia mater. The retinal artery and vein pierce the dural and arachnoid sheaths about 1 cm behind the eyeball and run a short course in the subarachnoid space before piercing the optic nerve.

The optic nerves leave the orbit through the optic foramen and then unite with each other to form the optic chiasma. Within the chiasma fibres from the nasal half of each retina cross to the opposite side but the temporal fibres remain uncrossed.

The optic chiasma lies superior to the hypophysis cerebri and the 3rd ventricle lies above the chiasma. Laterally the termination of the internal carotid artery is related to the chiasma.

Posterior to the optic chiasma, the optic nerves are continued as the optic tract and most of the nerve fibres form synapses with the neurones in the lateral geniculate body in the thalamus. From the lateral geniculate body some of the nerve fibres go via the optic radiation to the occipital cortex in the region of the calcarine fissure and those concerned with pupillary reflex activity go to the midbrain.

Nerve fibres to the lateral geniculate body therefore conduct fibres for visual appreciation and pupillary light reflexes, while nerve fibres between the lateral geniculate body and the occipital cortex conduct only visual fibres.

Impulses from the right half of the visual field land on the left half of each retina and are conducted by the left optic nerve and vice versa.

Clinical examination of the optic nerve

    a. Inspection of the optic disc (optic nerve head) with an ophthalmoscope. Abnormal pallor or hyperaemia of the disc is noted. The edges of the disc are inspected to see whether they are blurred or well defined. Swelling of the optic nerve head results in loss of cupping of the disc (papilloedema). Papilloedema is a classic sign of raised intracranial pressure which was previously thought to be due to pressure exerted on the central vein of the retina where it crosses the subarachnoid space, but which is now thought to be due to obstruction of axoplasmic flow.

    b. Visual acuity is measured for near and distant vision.

    c. Examination for visual field defects.

It is clinically important to know the anatomy of the visual pathway because it is then possible to determine the location of a lesion producing a visual field defect. Damage to the visual pathway between the eye and the lateral geniculate body causes a visual field defect and loss of pupillary reflexes, whereas more proximal lesions result in a visual defect only.

The following lesions can be identified (*Fig.* 280):

    1. *Damage to the Optic Nerve:* This results in total blindness of the ipsilateral eye. A light shone in the affected eye produces no pupillary reflex in either eye, while a light shone in the normal eye produces a pupillary reflex in both eyes (the consensual light reflex).

    2. *Lesions of the Chiasma:*

        i. Sagittally placed lesions cause bitemporal hemianopia. This may be caused by upward expanding pituitary tumours.

        ii. Laterally placed lesions produce nasal hemianopia.

        The lengths of the optic nerve and optic tract are variable. If the optic nerve is short (prefixed) the chiasma is situated more anteriorly. The chiasma is postfixed when the optic nerve is long and the tract short. This anatomical variation makes it uncertain whether a compressing mass is anterior or posterior to the chiasma.

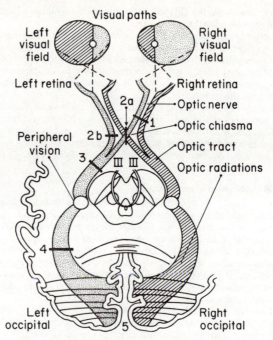

Fig. 280. Situations of injuries to the optic nerve and its central connections. (1) The optic nerve; (2a) sagittally placed lesion of the chiasma; (2b) laterally placed lesion of the chiasma; (3) lesion of the optic tract; (4) lesion of the optic radiation; (5) lesion of the occipital cortex.

3. *Lesions of the Optic Tract:* These lesions result in hemianopia of the ipsilateral nasal and the contralateral temporal visual field (homonymous hemianopia).
4. *Lesions of the Optic Radiation:* A lesion of the lowermost fibres of the optic radiation results in upper quadrantic hemianopia and the uppermost fibres in a lower quadrantic hemianopia.

     Middle cerebral artery occlusion and occlusion of the thalamogeniculate branches of the posterior cerebral artery can destroy the entire optic radiation producing an homonymous hemianopia.
5. *Lesions of the Occipital Cortex:* The upper half of the retina (lower visual field) is connected to the visual cortex above the calcarine fissure and the lower half of the retina (upper visual field) to the visual

cortex below the calcarine fissure. The macula lutea, a small yellowish area lateral to the disc, is the site of most acute vision. This is explained by the fact that nerve fibres coming from the macula lutea occupy 25 per cent of the visual cortex.

Occlusion of the terminal branch of the posterior cerebral artery which supplies the calcarine (visual) cortex also produces homonymous hemianopia but the macula is spared so that reading is possible.

Bilateral ischaemia of the occipital lobes due to spasm in basilar migraine or degenerative arterial disease produces complete loss of vision.

OCULOMOTOR NERVE (IIIrd)

This nerve is the motor nerve to the levator palpebrae superioris muscle of the eyelid and the superior, medial and inferior rectus and inferior oblique muscles of the eyeball. Important parasympathetic pupilloconstrictor fibres run on the upper surface of the oculomotor nerve.

The nucleus of the oculomotor nerve lies in the midbrain. The nerve emerges from the midbrain between the posterior cerebral and superior cerebellar arteries, and passes on the lateral side of the posterior communicating artery. After piercing the dura mater, it lies in the lateral wall of the cavernous sinus before passing through the superior orbital fissure.

Parasympathetic fibres synapse in the ciliary ganglion (of the trigeminal nerve) from where postganglionic fibres supply the ciliary muscle (accommodation) and constrictor muscles of the pupil.

Sympathetic fibres arise in the hypothalamus and run through the brain stem (midbrain pons and medulla) and cervical cord, and emerge through the ventral roots of the 1st, 2nd or 3rd segments of the thoracic spinal cord. These fibres ascend through the sympathetic chain to the superior cervical ganglion from where postganglionic fibres ascend in the carotid plexus and enter the orbit with the ophthalamic artery. These fibres traverse the ciliary ganglion to terminate in the radial (dilator) muscle of the iris. The superior tarsal muscle also receives sympathetic fibres.

Lesions of the oculomotor nerve

These result in:

1. Ptosis (drooping of the upper eyelid). The patient is unable to elevate the lid, unlike ptosis due to lesions of cervical sympathetic trunk where the voluntary motor supply is intact.
2. The patient is unable to look up, down or medially with the affected eye.
3. The pupil is dilated and a light shone in either eye produces no constriction of the dilated pupil.

Causes of IIIrd nerve lesions

1. Raised intracranial pressure, as may occur after intracranial haemorrhage, displaces and distorts the brain. A 'pressure cone' develops at the tentorium cerebelli resulting in pressure on the IIIrd nerve. With stimulation of the parasympathetic fibres running on the oculomotor nerve there is transient constriction followed by dilatation on the side of the lesion. If distortion continues, the contralateral oculomotor nerve may also be involved which results in the same sequence eventually leading to bilateral fixed dilated pupils.

2. Aneurysms of the posterior communicating artery may press on the oculomotor nerve.

3. Internal carotid artery aneurysm in the cavernous sinus. The IVth and VIth cranial nerves and the first two divisions of the Vth nerve may also be involved.

4. Injury to one cerebral peduncle causes a IIIrd nerve palsy with contralateral hemiparesis (Weber's syndrome).

TROCHLEAR NERVE (IVth)

The trochlear is a motor nerve which supplies the superior oblique muscle. The nucleus is in the midbrain and the nerve fibres cross the midline. It is the only cranial nerve that arises from the dorsal aspect of the brain. It passes forwards in the subarachnoid space and pierces the dura mater to lie in the lateral wall of the cavernous sinus (*Fig.* 281). The nerve enters the orbit through the superior orbital fissure.

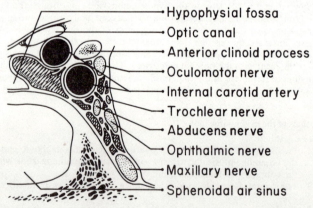

- Hypophysial fossa
- Optic canal
- Anterior clinoid process
- Oculomotor nerve
- Internal carotid artery
- Trochlear nerve
- Abducens nerve
- Ophthalmic nerve
- Maxillary nerve
- Sphenoidal air sinus

Fig. 281. Relation of the oculomotor, trochlear, the ophthalmic and maxillary and the abducens nerves to the cavernous sinus (coronal section).

Paralysis of the superior oblique muscle

The ocular muscles do not act individually but contract in groups and the action of a muscle at any moment will depend on the position of the eye when muscle contraction occurs. When the trochlear nerve is injured there is limitation of movement when the patient is asked to look downward with the eye adducted; in this position the action of the inferior rectus is minimal while that of the superior oblique should be maximal. The patient is unable to look at the tip of his nose.

THE TRIGEMINAL NERVE (Vth)

The trigeminal nerve emerges from the pons by a large sensory and a small motor root. The two roots pass forward in the posterior cranial fossa to the trigeminal ganglion in the middle cranial fossa. Motor fibres leave the pons superior to the site of entry of the sensory fibres but come to lie inferior to the sensory fibres in the trigeminal (Gasserian) ganglion.

As the roots run forward beneath the dural floor of the middle cranial fossa, they carry with them a loose sleeve of dura and arachnoid mater which lines the trigeminal (Meckel's) cave. The dura and arachnoid fuse with the epineurium of the trigeminal ganglion in its anterior half so that only the posterior half, the sensory roots and motor nerve are bathed in cerebrospinal fluid.

The anterior half of the ganglion and its three divisions, ophthalmic, maxillary and mandibular nerves, lie anterior to the trigeminal cave. The upper part of the ganglion with the ophthalmic and maxillary nerves lie in the lateral wall of the cavernous sinus (*Fig.* 281). The lower part of the ganglion and the mandibular nerve lie between two layers of dura mater lateral to the cavernous sinus.

The ophthalmic nerve passes through the superior orbital fissure and is distributed to the cornea, conjunctiva, upper eyelid, forehead, the nose and anterior half of the scalp.

The maxillary nerve leaves the middle cranial fossa through the foramen rotundum, passes through the pterygopalatine fossa and the inferior orbital fissure, crosses the floor of the orbit, and emerges through the infra-orbital foramen. It supplies sensory innervation to the skin of the cheek, lateral aspect of the nose, upper lip, upper teeth, and maxilla. It also supplies the mucosal surfaces of the uvula, hard palate, nasopharynx and inferior part of the nasal cavity.

The mandibular nerve leaves the skull via the foramen ovale. It is a mixed nerve, as the motor nerve has fused with the sensory fibres. Sensory distribution is to the skin over the mandible, the skin of the auricle, the anterior part of the external auditory meatus, the buccal surface of the cheek, the lower lip, the gingivae, the lower teeth, the floor of the mouth and the lateral side of the tongue. The motor component supplies the muscles of mastication, excepting the buccinator muscle.

Trigeminal neuralgia (tic douloureux)

There is lancinating facial pain, usually situated in the lower face.

Surgery is required in cases not responding to medical treatment. A variety of procedures has been proposed:

1. Thermocoagulation of the roots of the trigeminal nerve or of the ganglion. A needle is inserted through the foramen ovale under radiological control. The stilette of the needle is replaced with an electrode and a radiofrequency thermal lesion is produced until analgesia, and not anaesthesia, occurs in the appropriate area of the face.

2. Trigeminal root section: the trigeminal nerve roots are approached either through the middle or posterior cranial fossa. The division of the trigeminal nerve roots is done with microsurgical techniques.

   These procedures have a few serious complications; there is a high incidence of recurrence, corneal anaesthesia with neurotrophic keratitis may occur if the ophthalmic component is damaged and serious paraesthesia may result.

3. Relief of vascular compression: with arterial degeneration and elongation due to atherosclerosis small arteries around the base of the brain may cause compression of cranial nerves in the cerebropontine angle. Some cases of tic douloureux are examples of such cranial nerve vascular compression syndromes. With the use of microsurgical techniques, the small vessel causing the symptoms can be separated from the affected cranial nerve by the interposition of a small sponge.

4. Cryotherapy: under general anaesthesia, the affected branches of the peripheral nerves are exposed and then subjected to cycles of cryotherapy using a modified cryoprobe tip. This has given relief of symptoms for periods of 3–6 months. In some patients the pain cycle may be broken permanently.

Ganglia associated with the trigeminal nerve

The ganglia belong to the cranial part of the parasympathetic nervous system; preganglionic fibres which have a secretory function synapse in the ganglia. Sympathetic and sensory fibres pass through the ganglia without synapse. The sensory root is the peripheral process of a cell body in the trigeminal ganglion.

CILIARY GANGLION: The ciliary ganglion (*Fig.* 282) is the size of a pin-head. It is situated near the apex of the orbit, between the optic nerve medially and the lateral rectus on the outer side. It receives three roots and its terminal branches contain fibres from all three roots.

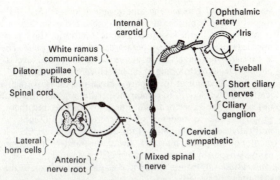

Fig. 282. Ciliary ganglion. Dotted line represents course of sympathetic fibres which supply dilator pupillae muscle.

Roots: Motor (parasympathetic) root from the inferior branch of the oculomotor nerve. Preganglionic fibres are relayed in the ciliary ganglion and supply the sphincter of the pupil and ciliary muscle.

Sensory fibres from the eyeball to the maxillary nerve which is a branch of the ophthalmic nerve.

Sympathetic postganglionic fibres from the superior cervical ganglion to supply the dilator muscle of the pupil and the superior and inferior tarsal muscles.

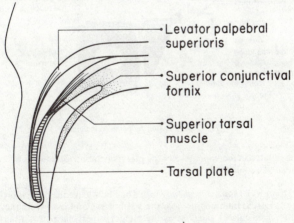

Fig. 283. The superior tarsal muscle.

The Superior Tarsal Muscle: The superior tarsal muscle (*Fig.* 283) is a thin sheet of smooth muscle attached to the inferior surface of a larger voluntary muscle, the levator palpebrae superioris. The superior tarsal muscle is inserted into the upper border of the tarsal plate. The muscle is probably not involved in active elevation of the eyelid, but its paralysis leads to drooping of the lid (Horner's syndrome).

In hyperthyroidism the superior tarsal muscle is overactive which leads to lid retraction. In primary hyperthyroidism (Graves' disease), not only is the superior tarsal muscle overactive, but there may be proptosis due to oedema of the retro-orbital tissues, so called infiltrative ophthalmopathy. Lid retraction is reversible with treatment but proptosis may not always respond to the treatment of primary hyperthyroidism and may in fact get worse.

Branches: Fifteen to twenty ciliary nerves pass to the back of the eyeball with the optic nerve.

PTERYGOPALATINE OR MECKEL'S GANGLION: This ganglion (*Fig.* 284) is connected with the maxillary division of the Vth nerve and is the parasympathetic relay station between the superior salivary nucleus in the pons and the lacrimal gland and mucous and serous glands of the palate, nose and paranasal sinuses.

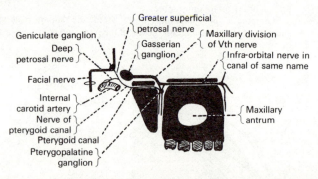

Fig. 284. The pterygopalatine ganglion.

It is situated in the upper part of the pterygopalatine fossa and is the size of the head of a small tack.

Roots:

Motor root (parasympathetic root): The fibres leave the brain stem in the nervus intermedius, join the VIIth nerve and issue from the facial (geniculate) ganglion as the greater superficial petrosal nerve. It enters the pterygopalatine ganglion in common with the sympathetic.

Sympathetic root: The cell bodies are in the superior cervical ganglion, from which nerve fibres pass to the internal carotid plexus, leaving this plexus in the deep petrosal nerve which joins the greater superficial petrosal nerve to form the nerve of the pterygoid canal.

Sensory root: The short thick branches, with their cell bodies in the trigeminal ganglion, come from the maxillary nerve.

Branches:

1. Postganglionic parasympathetic fibres to the lacrimal gland which it reaches through the zygomaticotemporal branch of the maxillary nerve and lacrimal branch of the ophthalmic nerve.
2. Orbital branches to the periosteum and the orbitalis muscle.
3. Palatine nerves to the roof of the mouth, soft palate, tonsil and nasal mucosa. A few taste fibres from the palate are carried by the greater superficial petrosal nerve to the geniculate ganglion of the facial nerve.
4. Nasal branches, one of which, the nasopalatine nerve, reaches the anterior part of the hard palate.
5. Pharyngeal branch to the nasal part of the pharynx behind the auditory tube.

OTIC GANGLION: The otic ganglion (*Fig.* 285) is connected to the mandibular division of the Vth nerve. It is the size of a pin-head.

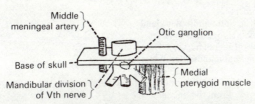

Fig. 285. Schematic representation of mandibular division of Vth nerve showing, as a dotted circle, the otic ganglion medial to the nerve.

It is situated medial to the trunk of the 3rd division of the Vth nerve at the base of the skull just outside the foramen ovale.

Relations:

Lateral: Mandibular nerve.

Medial: Tensor palati muscle.

Posterior: Middle meningeal artery.

Anterior: Internal pterygoid muscle.

Roots:

Motor root: Parasympathetic preganglionic fibres to the parotid salivary gland from the inferior salivary nucleus leave the brain stem in the glossopharyngeal nerve and reach the ganglion in the lesser superficial petrosal nerve.

The nerve to the medial pterygoid is a muscular motor nerve which passes through the ganglion without synapse, to supply the tensor palati and tensor tympani.

Sympathetic root: From the plexus on the middle meningeal artery.

Sensory: Five twigs from the auriculotemporal nerve.

Branches: With the exception of the two motor branches supplying the two tensor muscles, all branches are distributed to the parotid gland, travelling with the auriculotemporal nerve.

SUBMANDIBULAR OR LANGLEY'S GANGLION: This ganglion (*Fig.* 286) is the size of a pin-head. It is situated on the outer surface of the hyoglossus muscle suspended from the lingual nerve.

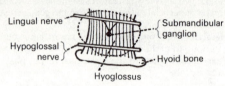

Lingual nerve

Submandibular ganglion

Hypoglossal nerve

Hyoid bone

Hyoglossus

Fig. 286. Submandibular or Langley's ganglion. The dotted line is the submandibular gland.

Relations:

Lateral: Submandibular gland.

Medial: Hyoglossus muscle.

Above: Lingual nerve.

Below: Submandibular duct.

Roots:

Motor (secretory): From the chorda tympani (facial) through the lingual.

Sensory: From the lingual.

Sympathetic: From the plexus round the facial artery.

Branches: It hangs from the lingual nerve by two filaments, the posterior going from the lingual to the ganglion, the anterior going from the ganglion to the lingual, to be distributed through it: (*a*) to the submandibular gland and duct; (*b*) to the sublingual gland; (*c*) to the mucous membrane of the mouth and tongue (through the lingual nerve).

Pathway for Taste:

1. Taste sensation in the anterior two-thirds of the tongue passes via the lingual nerve to the chorda tympani, thence to the facial nerve in the canal for the facial nerve, and so to the geniculate ganglion, whence the impulses go in the nervus intermedius to the pons.

2. From the posterior third of the tongue taste sensation passes via the glossopharyngeal nerve to the brain stem. Temporary loss of taste over the anterior two-thirds of the tongue may follow

removal of the trigeminal ganglion. This is due to swelling of the axons of the lingual nerve consequent on their degeneration.

ABDUCENS NERVE (VIth)

This is the motor nerve to the lateral rectus muscle. It has a long intracranial course and emerges from the brain stem at the junction of the pons and the pyramid of the medulla. It runs upwards, forwards and laterally, in the subarachnoid space and traverses the cavernous sinus, lying at first lateral then inferolateral to the internal carotid artery (*see Fig*. 281). The nerve enters the orbital cavity through the medial part of the superior orbital fissure.

Lesions of the abducens nerve

Abducens nerve paralysis results in the patient being unable to turn the eyeball laterally.

Tentorial herniation may result in abducens nerve paralysis. It is seen more commonly with posterior fossa lesions, such as a slowly accumulating posterior fossa haematoma which results in reversed tentorial coning. The patient may remain conscious while the nerve palsy occurs, which makes diplopia an important symptom.

A caroticocavernous fistula may also result in abducens nerve paralysis.

THE FACIAL NERVE (VIIth)

Two roots, a large voluntary motor root, situated anterior and cranial to a small mixed sensory and parasympathetic root (nervus intermedius), arise from the lateral surface of the brain stem close to the lower border of the pons. These roots are situated anterior and ventral to the vestibulocochlear nerve (VIIIth) to which they are closely related (*Fig*. 287).

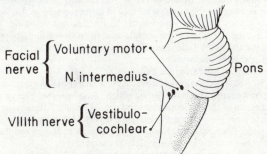

Fig. 287. The facial and vestibulocochlear nerves in the brain stem.

The VIIth and VIIIth cranial nerves pass through the subarachnoid space to enter the internal acoustic meatus. The anterior inferior cerebellar artery may lie anterior or posterior to the nerves and may loop round or pass between the nerves. In operations in the region of the cerebellopontine angle this artery must be preserved. The artery supplies the labyrinthine artery which runs with the nerves in the internal acoustic meatus.

At the outer end of the internal acoustic meatus the two components of the facial nerve form one nerve which now follows a devious course in the facial canal through the temporal bone. This part of the facial nerve is of great importance to the aural surgeon (*Fig.* 288).

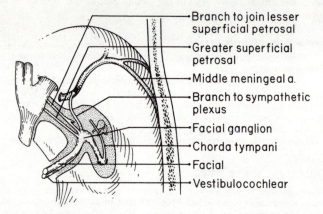

Fig. 288. The course and connections of the facial nerve in the temporal bone.

The initial direction of the nerve in the canal is laterally and slightly forwards, covered by the superior surface of the petrous bone. In this part of its course it runs over the junction of the cochlea and vestibule. When it reaches the medial wall of the middle ear an oval swelling on the nerve indicates the site of the facial ganglion. At this point, the genu (L. knee), the nerve turns sharply backwards.

Three branches arise from the ganglion:

1. The greater superficial petrosal nerve which contains parasympathetic secretomotor efferent fibres which relay in the pterygopalatine ganglion to the lacrimal, nasal and palatal glands. Afferent impulses of taste from the palate are routed in a reverse direction.
2. A small filament joins the tympanic branch of the glossopharyngeal nerve to form the lesser superficial petrosal nerve.
3. A branch to the sympathetic plexus on the middle meningeal artery.

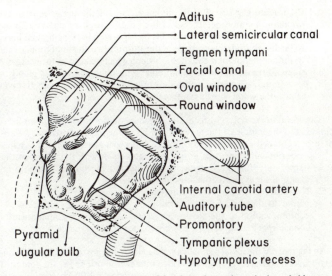

Aditus
Lateral semicircular canal
Tegmen tympani
Facial canal
Oval window
Round window

Internal carotid artery
Auditory tube
Promontory
Tympanic plexus
Hypotympanic recess

Pyramid
Jugular bulb

Fig. 289. The tympanic cavity and facial canal seen from the lateral side.

The second part of its course (*Fig.* 289) starts at the genu. It runs backwards as a prominence on the medial wall of the middle ear. The bony covering of the facial canal is thin and may be defective in places or the nerve may be uncovered by erosion of bone due to disease. In this part of its course the nerve lies above the promontory (basal turn of the cochlea) and the fenestra vestibuli (oval window). Above the nerve lies the ampullary end of the lateral semicircular canal.

The third part of its course commences when it reaches the posterior end of the fenestra vestibuli. Here the nerve runs into the bony posterior wall of the middle ear in a downward and slightly lateral direction. It is closely related to the mastoid antrum and air cells which lie posterior to it and is vulnerable during surgical procedures on this area. The lateral inclination of the nerve brings it to a level of the tympanic membrane at which point it enters the stylomastoid canal. It emerges immediately behind the root of the styloid process.

In the descending part of its course the nerve gives off three branches:

1. The nerve to the stapedius muscle.
2. The chorda tympani branch arises about 5 mm above the stylomastoid foramen.

    It runs upwards and forwards in a separate bony canal and crosses the middle ear fused to the inner surface of the upper part of the tympanic membrane. It leaves the anterior wall of the middle ear through another bony canal and is incorporated into the lingual nerve to be distributed to taste buds of the anterior two-thirds of tongue, and to the submandibular ganglion, through which secretomotor postganglionic fibres reach the submandibular and sublingual salivary glands.

3. A communicating branch with the auricular branch of the vagus is given off just below the chorda tympani nerve.

The facial nerve emerges from the stylomastoid foramen at a point 2·5–4 cm deep to the middle of the anterior border of the mastoid process. Almost at once it enters the parotid gland. Before doing so it gives off three branches:

1. Posterior auricular: this nerve associates itself with the artery of that name, and runs back in the groove behind the pinna to supply the occipitalis muscle and the auricularis posterior.
2. Nerve to stylohyoid: a long thin twig.
3. Nerve to digastric (posterior belly): a short fat twig, which gives a communication to the glossopharyngeal nerve, which communication soon leaves this latter, as the nerve to the stylopharyngeus.

In the parotid the facial nerve lies superficial to the posterior facial vein and external carotid artery. It soon divides into two divisions (*a*) the temporofacial which runs sharply upward; (*b*) the cervicofacial which continues the course of the parent trunk downwards, forwards and outwards (*Fig.* 290).

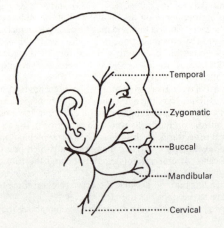

Fig. 290. The facial nerve after its emergence from the stylomastoid foramen.

These divisions in turn divide to form the goose's foot (pes anserinus), the branches of which leave the anterior border of the parotid and pass as five twigs to the (i) temporal, (ii) zygomatic, (iii) buccal, (iv) mandibular, and (v) cervical regions, to supply the muscles of expression, which include the buccinator, the frontalis, and the platysma. All these nerves communicate on the face with branches of the Vth cranial.

The mandibular branch of the facial

This has important relations. It passes down, continuing the course of the main trunk, just behind the angle of the mandible. It then lies deep to the platysma, between it and the deep cervical fascia, crossing the inferolateral surface of the submandibular gland. It turns up and crosses the lower border of the mandible to supply the quadratus labii inferioris muscle. Incisions made behind the angle of the jaw, e.g. mastoid process to hyoid bone, will cut this branch of the facial unless the cut is made at least 2·5 cm behind the angle. The result of division of the nerve is paralysis of the muscle, so that the mouth will be asymmetrical.

Facial nerve in relation to the parotid gland

The gland is divided by the nerve into suprafacial and subfacial parts and parotid tumours should be removed by an anatomical dissection of the gland leaving the nerve intact. The nerve is followed forwards or its terminal branches are traced back. The former procedure entails exposing the trunk of the facial nerve at its emergence from the stylomastoid foramen; there is about 1 cm of nerve trunk before it enters the parotid and another centimetre before it divides into its temporofacial and cervicofacial divisions. It and its branches are followed into the parotid gland and the plane of the cleavage developed between the superficial and deep portions of the gland. Thus the suprafacial portion alone, or together with part of the subfacial parotid, is removed, according to the needs of the case. The nerve is under observation throughout.

Lesions of the facial nerve

It is important to pinpoint the anatomical site of the lesion that has produced the loss of functions.

UPPER MOTOR NEURONE LESIONS: Upper motor neurone lesions (above the facial nerve nucleus in the pons) produce paralysis of the muscles of the lower half of the face only because the upper facial muscles (forehead and eyebrow) are innervated from both cerebral hemispheres. The patient is able to wrinkle the skin of his forehead while the lower facial muscles are paralysed.

LOWER MOTOR NEURONE LESIONS: These include lesions of the facial nerve nucleus or distal to it, and the site can be determined by testing the function of the branches of the nerve. These branches are concerned with homolateral lacrimation, the stapedius reflex, homolateral submandibular salivary gland secretion, and taste function from the homolateral anterior two-thirds of the tongue.

1. A lesion at or proximal to the geniculate ganglion (trans-labyrinthine) (*Fig.* 291A) produces diminished lacrimation on the homolateral side as well as disturbance in function of the other branches.

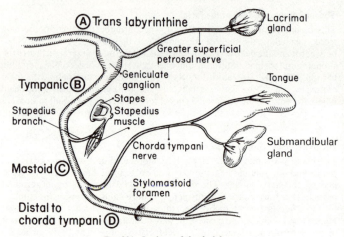

Fig. 291. Lesions of the facial nerve.

2. A lesion in the middle ear segment of the nerve (tympanic) (*Fig.* 291B) does not affect lacrimation but interferes with the homolateral stapedial reflex, submandibular salivary gland secretion on that side, and taste function from the homolateral anterior third of the tongue.

3. If the lesion is in the vertical course of the facial nerve within the mastoid bone (*Fig.* 291C), there will be a reduction in taste function on the anterior two-thirds of the tongue on that side as well as diminished homolateral submandibular salivary gland secretion; however, lacrimation and the stapedius reflex would be normal.

4. If the involvement of the facial nerve is at the stylomastoid foramen or distal to it (*Fig.* 291D), all the branches just mentioned will reflect normal function on testing.

5. If the lesion is distal to the stylomastoid foramen, the extent of involvement of the facial nerve branches is determined by asking the patient to raise his eyebrows (temporal branch), close the eye (temporal and zygomatic), flare the nostrils (buccal), smile (mandibular).

THE VESTIBULOCOCHLEAR NERVE (VIIIth)

The intracranial course of this nerve has been discussed with the facial nerve above. It is a sensory nerve consisting of two components.

1. The cochlear nerve is the sensory nerve for hearing and consists of the central processes of bipolar neurones which have their cell bodies in the petrous temporal bone. The peripheral processes end in relation to the hair cells of the spiral organ of Corti.

2. The vestibular nerve is the nerve of balance which detects movements of the head. The peripheral processes of the vestibular nerve are distributed to the semicircular canals, the utricle and the saccule.

The vestibular and cochlear components enter the internal auditory meatus with the facial nerve and run in the petrous temporal bone to the inner ear.

Fractures of the middle cranial fossa which involve the internal acoustic meatus may cause permanent deafness.

THE GLOSSOPHARYNGEAL NERVE (IXth)

This nerve arises from the lateral aspect of the medulla just caudal to the pons in the groove between the olive and inferior cerebellar peduncle. The rootlets forming the nerve are in the same line as those of the vagus and accessory nerves. From its origin the nerve runs laterally and separates from the vagus nerve as it pierces the dura to enter the anterior compartment of the jugular foramen. Outside the foramen, it passes forwards between the internal jugular vein and internal carotid artery. There is a superior and inferior ganglion where it lies in the jugular foramen.

It is a predominantly sensory nerve but also contains voluntary motor fibres to the stylopharyngeus muscle and preganglionic parasympathetic fibres, which run in the tympanic branch and contribute to the formation of the tympanic plexus in the middle ear. A branch from the tympanic plexus is joined by a branch from the facial (geniculate) ganglion to form the lesser superficial petrosal nerve, which relays in the otic ganglion and reaches the parotid salivary gland in the auriculotemporal branch of the mandibular nerve.

The sensory fibres are distributed to the tympanic cavity and the auditory (Eustachian) tube, the tonsillar region, posterior third of the tongue and to a limited portion of the skin of the external auditory meatus and the pinna.

The distribution of the glossopharyngeal nerve is shown in *Fig*. 292.

Lesions of the glossopharyngeal nerve

These are rare in isolation. Interruption of all the fibres results in:

1. Loss of sensation including taste, in the posterior third of the tongue.
2. Unilateral loss of the gag reflex (produced by stimulating the posterior pharyngeal wall).
3. Difficulty with swallowing.

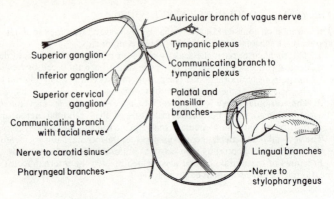

Fig. 292. The glossopharyngeal nerve showing its distribution and connections.

Glossopharyngeal neuralgia

This is much rarer than trigeminal neuralgia and the diagnosis is often overlooked. Paroxysms of pain are felt in the sensory distribution of the glossopharyngeal nerve. In cases not responding to medical treatment intracranial section of the nerve root is performed.

THE VAGUS NERVE (Xth)

This is a mixed nerve containing both motor and sensory fibres. Its fibres arise from the medulla by about ten rootlets, below the glossopharyngeal nerve in the groove between the olive and the inferior cerebellar peduncle.

The vagus nerves pursues a perfectly straight course from the jugular foramen to where it enters the thorax by crossing anterior to the subclavian artery. At the base of the skull it is posterior to the internal carotid, in front of the internal jugular, and associated with the IXth, XIth, and XIIth cranial nerves; it soon comes to lies in the groove between the jugular and carotid in the carotid sheath, and keeps this position in relation first to the internal and then to the common carotid (*Fig.* 293). It presents, therefore, very much the same relationship as the common and internal carotids lying in front of the cervical sympathetic trunk. It has two important ganglia on it: (1) the superior ganglion, and (2) the inferior ganglion.

1. The superior ganglion

This is in the jugular foramen and contains cell bodies of neurones

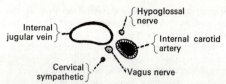

Fig. 293. Showing immediate relations of right internal carotid a little below base of skull.

concerned with general visceral sensation. It gives off the following branches:

i. The auricular (alderman's nerve or Arnold's nerve) passes outwards across the bulb of the internal jugular vein and enters a canal in the outer wall of the jugular foramen. It emerges between the anterior border of the mastoid process and the external acoustic meatus. It communicates three times with the facial nerve, twice in the bone, and once behind the ear. It supplies the posterior half of the skin lining the acoustic meatus and tympanic membrane.

The auricular branch of the vagus was once known as the alderman's nerve. Aldermen, those lovers of good cheer, were said, when replete at banquets, to stimulate their jaded appetites by dropping cold water behind the ear. Apparently this acted by reflexly encouraging gastric peristalsis because of the vagal supply to the stomach.

ii. The meningeal branch goes in a recurrent direction to the dura of the posterior cranial fossa through the jugular foramen.

iii. The superior ganglion is a kind of nerve exchange, as communications reach it from the VIIth, IXth, and XIth cranial nerves and superior sympathetic ganglion.

2. The inferior ganglion

This is the second largest ganglion in the neck, being second only to the superior cervical sympathetic ganglion. It is 1·8 cm long and lies just below the base of the skull. It is formed where the accessory portion of the spinal accessory joins the vagus, and is connected by big communications with the first loop of the cervical plexus, the superior cervical sympathetic ganglion, and the hypoglossal nerve.

It gives off two important nerves:

i. The pharyngeal branch of the vagus passes between the internal and external carotids to the pharyngeal plexus on the middle constrictor. These motor fibres to the constrictor muscles of the pharynx come from the accessory nerve.

ii. The superior laryngeal nerve passes deep to both the internal and external carotids. It divides deep to the internal carotid into the internal and external laryngeal nerves.

The internal nerve pierces the thyrohyoid membrane together with the superior laryngeal vessels, and supplies the mucous membrane of the larynx (superior laryngeal—sensory to the larynx).

The external laryngeal nerve passes downwards on the inferior constrictor deep to and parallel to the superior thyroid artery and supplies the cricothyroid muscle and the inferior constrictor. The cricothyroid muscle is the tensor of the vocal cords. The external laryngeal nerve may be damaged during thyroidectomy if it is included in the ligature of the superior thyroid artery. There may be no noticeable change in speech but singing is affected.

Vagal trunk branches

1. The superior cervical cardiac branches, usually two on each side, run downwards and medially often joining sympathetic cardiac branches to the cardiac plexus.

2. The recurrent nerve: on the right side this nerve arises as the vagus crosses the subclavian artery. It hooks round that vessel, and, passing up behind the common carotid, reaches the groove between the oesophagus and trachea, and running along the medial surface of the lobe of the thyroid gland, where it may be damaged during thyroidectomy. It disappears under the lower border of the inferior constrictor, behind the cricothyroid joint, into the larynx, being called the 'inferior laryngeal nerve'. It is accompanied under the constrictor by the inferior laryngeal branch of the inferior thyroid artery, and is motor to all the muscles of the larynx except the cricothyroid. On the left side, when it enters the neck, the recurrent nerve already lies in the groove between the trachea and oesophagus.

The recurrent nerves supply the inferior cervical cardiac branches of the vagus to the deep cardiac plexus, and in addition to supplying the muscles of the larynx, they give branches to the inferior constrictor, trachea and oesophagus.

Lesions of the vagus nerve

The external and the recurrent laryngeal nerves may be damaged during thyroidectomy or sometimes during other operations in the region.

The effect of damage to the external laryngeal is inability to tense the cord which will be particularly noticeable in singing. Breathing is not affected.

Damage to the recurrent laryngeal nerve, however, will result in the cord being pulled by the cricothyroid muscle into the paramedian position. This decreases the airway and, if both recurrent laryngeal nerves are damaged, the airway becomes inadequate necessitating a tracheostomy.

If both the external and the recurrent laryngeal nerves are injured, the vocal cord is fixed in the intermediate or cadaveric position. The airway is good but the patient is unable to approximate the vocal cords, resulting in a poor voice.

ACCESSORY NERVE (XIth)

This nerve consists of a spinal nerve and a cranial nerve. The spinal part of the nerve emerges from the lateral surface of the upper five segments of the cervical cord behind the ligamentum denticulatum. It enters the posterior fossa lateral to the vertebral artery and unites with the cranial root medial to the jugular foramen.

The cranial root consists of axons which leave the lateral surface of the medulla caudal to the rootlets of the vagus nerve. The cranial root is an accessory part of the vagus nerve which it joins just below the base of the skull to be distributed to the striped muscles of the pharynx, palate and larynx.

The spinal part of the accessory nerve descends between the internal jugular and internal carotid, then turns and passes over or under the internal jugular, to cross the transverse process of the atlas. It passes under the posterior belly of the digastric and the occipital artery, and enters the anterior

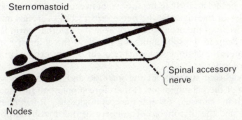

Fig. 294. Transverse section through right sternomastoid. Relation of the lymph nodes to the spinal accessory nerve.

border of the sternomastoid muscle (*Fig*. 294). It emerges from the posterior border of this muscle and, in this situation, is related to lymph nodes of the upper deep cervical chain. The nerve then crosses the posterior triangle, enters the trapezius, and ends in the substance of this muscle at the lowest point of origin of the trapezius (i.e. the 12th thoracic vertebral spine).

The spinal part of the accessory nerve supplies, therefore, only the sternomastoid and the trapezius. Whilst in the sternomastoid it communicates with C2, and in the trapezius with C3 and 4. Where it is crossed by the occipital artery, the artery gives off a sternomastoid branch which accompanies the nerve into the sternomastoid muscle. This blood vessel may be used as a guide to the nerve in operations in this region.

Lesions of the accessory nerves

Paralysis of the sternomastoid muscle causes weakness on turning the head away from the paralysed muscle. The patient is unable to shrug his shoulders against resistance when the trapezius muscle is paralysed.

Isolated lower motor neurone lesions of the accessory nerve may occur after lymph node dissection in the neck. Lesion due to trauma to the base of the skull are usually associated with other cranial nerves lesions of the IXth, Xth and XIIth cranial nerves.

HYPOGLOSSAL NERVE (XIIth)

The hypoglossal nerve arises from the medulla between the olive and the pyramid as 10–15 rootlets. The fibres pass anterolaterally and leave the posterior cranial fossa via the hypoglossal canal just in front of the foramen magnum. The rootlets unite to form a single nerve after traversing the canal and it passes medial to the internal jugular and the internal carotid. It then curves laterally, working round the inferior ganglion of the vagus, and comes to lie in front in the groove between the internal carotid and internal jugular. (The vagus lies posteriorly in the groove between these two vessels.) At the lower border of the digastric the nerve crosses both carotids and, hooking round the origin of the occipital artery from the external carotid, lies on the hyoglossus deep to the submandibular gland; at the anterior border of this muscle it enters the genioglossus and breaks up into its terminal branches. It is a purely motor nerve.

The hypoglossal supplies all the intrinsic and extrinsic muscles of the tongue except the palatoglossus. It therefore supplies all the muscles whose names end in -glossus, except the palatoglossus. It supplies also the geniohyoid and the thyrohyoid. The nerve to the thyrohyoid is a separate branch.

The hypoglossal receives a communication from the 1st cervical nerve. At the point where it hooks round the occipital artery it gives off a nerve which is called the descendens hypoglossi. This nerve takes part in the formation of the ansa hypoglossi, and it, together with the nerves to the thyrohyoid and geniohyoid, is derived from the fibres which the hypoglossal receives from C1.

Lesions of the hypoglossal nerve

Unilateral weakness of the tongue results in deviation on protrusion to the paralysed side. Isolated lower motor neurone lesions of the hypoglossal nerve are uncommon.

Chapter 29

PERIPHERAL NERVES

ANATOMY OF A PERIPHERAL NERVE

Separate nerve fibres are loosely bound together by the endoneurium, a fine collagen network. Bundles of nerve fibres (fasciculi) are enclosed by a connective tissue sheath known as the perineurium and the entire nerve is surrounded by a sheath of connective tissue called the epineurium, in which run the blood vessels supplying the nerve. (*See Fig.* 295.)

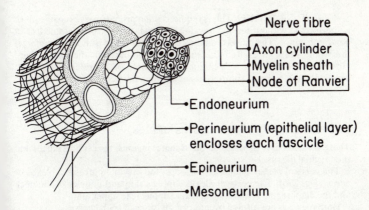

Fig. 295. The anatomy of a peripheral nerve.

INTERRUPTION OF A NERVE

Division of a peripheral nerve may be complete (neurotmesis) or incomplete with damage to nerve fibres, but some of the supporting structures are preserved (axonotmesis). Where the interruption of the nerve is purely a physiological phenomenon, a minimal lesion is produced with paralysis which is usually incomplete or transient (neuropraxia).

Nerve repair

Where repair is indicated, for instance in fresh complete division of the nerve, three techniques of restoring nerve continuity are available:

1. EPINEURIAL REPAIR: Alignment of the proximal and distal ends of the nerve is ensured by inspection of the pattern of longitudinally running blood vessels in the epineurium and the fascicular pattern of each cut surface. The epineurium is coapted with fine non-absorbable sutures, maintaining the appropriate alignment.

2. INTERFASCICULAR REPAIR: Using the operating microscope, the epineurium is trimmed away from the cut surfaces, exposing the fasciculi. The fascicular pattern of the proximal and distal ends are matched and orientated in terms of rotation (this can be achieved correctly in over 90 per cent of cases) and appropriate fasciculi coapted by sutures passing through the peri-neurium. Microsurgeons consider this to be the treatment of choice for cleanly incised fresh nerve injuries with no loss of nerve substance.

3. NERVE GRAFTING: This is required when primary nerve repair cannot be performed without tension because there has been a considerable loss of nerve substance. The most commonly used donor nerve is the sural nerve. If the whole nerve is grafted the sutures will go through the epineurium. However, if microsurgical technique is available, it is preferable to graft individual fasciculi with sutures passing through the perineurium.

THE PLEXUSES ON THE SCALENUS MEDIUS

There are two nerve plexuses on the scalenus medius: the cervical plexus and the brachial plexus.

The cervical plexus is a plexus of loops, the brachial plexus is a plexus of cords (*Fig.* 296). The cervical plexus supplies skin and muscles of the neck and the diaphragm. The brachial plexus supplies the upper limb.

Both plexuses are formed by anterior divisions of spinal nerves.

Cervical plexus

Lies on the scalenus medius and levator scapulae under cover of the sternomastoid. It is formed by the upper four cervical nerves, each of which divides into two, except the 1st. The 1st nerve joins the upper branch of C2, the adjoining upper and lower branches fuse, and the lower branch of C4 joins C5 in the formation of the brachial plexus. In this way, three loops are formed, the first of which is directed forwards in front of the transverse process of the atlas, the other two are directed backwards (*Fig.* 297).

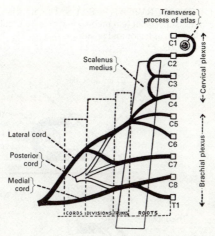

Fig. 296. To show continuity of cervical and brachial plexuses and their relationship to the middle scalene.

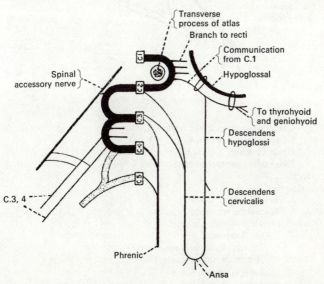

Fig. 297. Cervical plexus and ansa hypoglossi. Observe that the first loop of plexus is directed forwards.

BRANCHES OF THE CERVICAL PLEXUS: The branches of the plexus consist of two groups, superficial (cutaneous) and deep (muscular). The deep branches are divided into anterior and posterior.
Superficial: see Fig. 298.

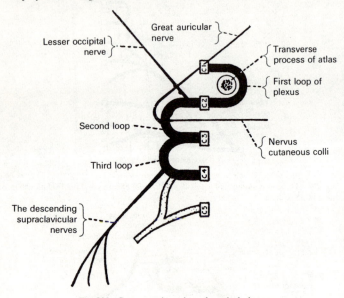

Fig. 298. Cutaneous branches of cervical plexus.

      Cutaneous nerves of the neck: C2, 3
      Lesser occipital nerve: C2
      Great auricular nerves: C2, 3
      Descending supraclavicular nerves: C3, 4
Deep:
  Anterior:
      Phrenic nerves: C3–5
      Muscular branches to:
          Thyrohyoid: C1
          Geniohyoid: C1
          Rectus capitis lateralis: C1
          Rectus capitis superior: C1
          Longus capitis: C1–4
          Longus colli: C3–8

Scalenus anterior: C4–6
Intertransversales: C1–8
Posterior:
Sternomastoid: C2
Levator scapulae: C3, 4
Trapezius: C3, 4
Scalenus medius: C3–7
Communications:
1. With sympathetic: each of the four nerves taking part in the formation of the plexus receives a grey ramus communicans from the superior cervical sympathetic ganglion.
2. With hypoglossal from C1. This nerve may be called the communicans hypoglossi. It joins the hypoglossal and, after a short course with this nerve, leaves it as the nerve to the geniohyoid, thyrohyoid, and the descendens hypoglossi nerve. The latter nerve runs down on the front of the carotid sheath and, having supplied the anterior belly of the omohyoid, it joins the descendens cervicalis nerve (formed by the junction of the communicantes cervicalis nerves from C2, 3) to form a loop, lying in front of the carotid sheath, known as the ansa hypoglossi (*Fig.* 299). This loop supplies the sternohyoid, sternothyroid, and the posterior belly of the omohyoid. The ansa hypoglossi is derived therefore from C1, 2, 3.

Brachial plexus

It is made up of the anterior rami of C5, 6, 7 and 8, and T1, with communications from C4 and T2. It consists of roots, trunks, divisions, cords and branches. The roots and trunks lie in the neck, the divisions behind the clavicle, and the cords and branches in the axilla. Therefore the subclavian artery is related to roots and trunks, and the axillary artery to cords and branches. The cords end by giving off their terminal branches at the lower border of the pectoralis minor, therefore the first and second parts of the axillary artery are related to cords, and the third part to branches; for the same reason all the terminal branches of the cords (i.e. all the long nerves to the arm and forearm) commence at the lower border of the pectoralis minor.

PLAN OF THE PLEXUS: *See Fig.* 300.
1. C5 and 6 roots join to form the upper trunk.
   C7 alone forms the middle trunk.
   C8 and T1 join to form the lower trunk.
2. Each trunk divides into an anterior and posterior division.
3. All the posterior divisions join to form the posterior cord.
   The upper two anterior divisions join to form the outer or lateral cord.
   The lowest anterior division alone forms the inner or medial cord.

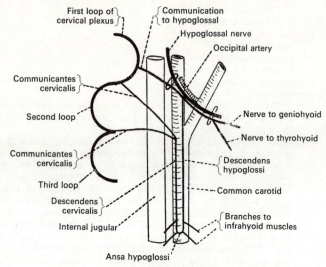

Fig. 299. The ansa hypoglossi.

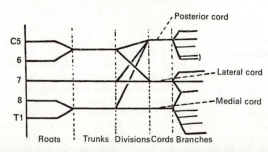

Fig. 300. Diagram showing method of construction of brachial plexus. The constituent parts—roots, trunks, divisions, cords and branches—are indicated.

BRANCHES OF THE BRACHIAL PLEXUS: The plexus gives off three sets of branches: from the roots, from the trunks, and from the cords.

1. *Branches from the Roots:*
    i. Nerve to serratus anterior (long thoracic nerve of Bell).
    ii. Dorsal scapular nerve.
    iii. Muscular branches to the three scaleni and longus colli.

2. *Branches from the Trunks:* Only two, both from the upper trunk, both begin with 'S':
    i. Suprascapular nerve: C5, 6
    ii. Subclavius nerve: C5, 6
3. *Branches from the Cords:*
    i. *Medial cord:*
        Medial head of median: C8, T1
        Medial pectoral: C8, T1
        Ulnar nerve: C8, T1
        Medial cutaneous of forearm: C8, T1
        Medial cutaneous of arm: T1
    ii. *Lateral cord:*
        Lateral pectoral: C5, 6, 7
        Lateral head of median: C5, 6, 7
        Musculocutaneous: C5, 6, 7
    iii. *Posterior cord:*
        Radial: C5, 6, 7, 8, T1
        Axillary: C5, 6
        Nerve to latissimus dorsi: C6, 7, 8
        Subscapular: upper and lower: C5, 6

Most of the branches of the plexus are grouped round the third part of the axillary artery (*Fig*. 301). The artery and plexus are covered proximally by the skin, fascia, and pectoralis major; distally by skin and fascia only. The medial head of the median nerve crosses the artery from within out to join the outer head, so that the formed median nerve is lateral to the artery.

In the groove between the artery and the vein, there is, in front, the medial cutaneous nerve of the forearm and, behind, the ulnar nerve. Along the inner border of the vein is the medial cutaneous nerve of the arm.

The radial and axillary nerves both separate the axillary artery from the subscapularis. The radial alone separates it from the latissimus dorsi and the teres major.

ERB'S POINT: The spot where six nerves meet (*Fig*. 302): the 5th and 6th cervical roots join to form the upper trunk, which is very short, gives off the suprascapular nerve and the nerve to subclavius, and then divides into anterior and posterior divisions. It is here that the upper trunk usually stretches or tears in the upper-arm type (Erb's) of birth paralysis.

ABNORMAL COMMUNICATIONS TO THE BRACHIAL PLEXUS: Occasionally the communications to the plexus from T2 may be abnormally large, so that the plexus may be said to be pushed one spinal segment lower down (a postfixed plexus). The plexus is said to be prefixed when it is one nerve (cord segment) higher than usual and the C4 contribution is abnormally

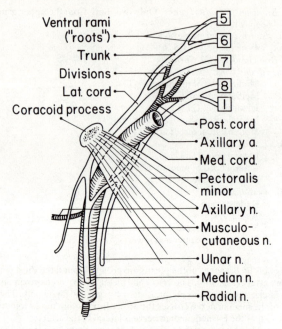

Ventral rami ("roots")
Trunk
Divisions
Lat. cord
Coracoid process

5
6
7
8
1

Post. cord
Axillary a.
Med. cord
Pectoralis minor
Axillary n.
Musculo-cutaneous n.
Ulnar n.
Median n.
Radial n.

Fig. 301. Relation of the brachial plexus to the axillary artery.

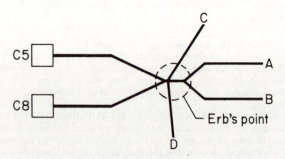

C5

C8

C

A

B

D

Erb's point

Fig. 302. Erb's point.

large. Note that the contribution which is given by T2 to the plexus is made up largely of sympathetic (autonomic) nerve fibres.

CERVICAL RIB: At their exit from the neck, the brachial plexus and the subclavian artery pass through a narrow triangle, bounded by the two scalene muscles and the 1st rib. Thus these two structures are bound to be angulated, if not compressed, when the base of this triangle is raised by the presence of a cervical rib, forcing its way between the nerve and the 1st rib.

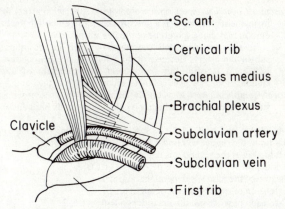

Fig. 303. A cervical rib.

A cervical rib (*Fig.* 303) is an additional rib which arises from the 7th cervical vertebra and which is usually attached to the 1st rib, close to the insertion of scalenus anterior. The anomaly, which is present in less than 0·5 per cent of the population, may consist of a complete rib, but more often the bone is present for a variable distance only, the anterior part being made up of a fibrous band (*Fig.* 304).

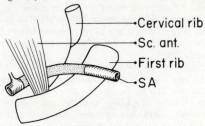

Fig. 304. A short cervical rib with a fibrous attachment to the first rib.

Cervical rib is more often unilateral and somewhat more frequent on the right. In 90 per cent of cases, cervical rib probably causes no trouble. In the remainder, complications may be neurological, vascular or local.

Neurological Complications: Tingling along the distribution of the lowest part of the brachial plexus, along the ulnar border of the forearm and the hand. Many people, especially in middle age, complain of severe symptoms, but it is now thought that this is often due to cervical osteo-arthritis causing pressure on nerve roots, rather than the cervical rib.

Vascular Complications: Compression of the subclavian artery may result in an aneurysm, which is a potential source of emboli to the hand. The emboli may cause gangrene of the finger tips.

In addition, repeated trauma may result in thrombosis of the subclavian artery. Because of the good collateral circulation, critical ischaemia is rare, but the patient will complain of upper limb claudication, as well as coldness and numbness in the hand.

Local Complications: Occasionally the patient will present with a tender supraclavicular lump which, on palpation, is bony hard and fixed.

BRACHIAL PLEXUS LESIONS: Before considering nerve lesions of the upper limb, the reader will find it helpful to observe that:

Abduction at the shoulder is dependent on C5.

Adduction at the shoulder is dependent on C6, 7.

Flexion of the elbow is dependent on C5, 6.

Extension of the elbow is dependent on C7, 8.

Extension of wrist and fingers is dependent on C6, 7.

Flexion of wrist and fingers is dependent on C8, T1.

Stretched between two mobile structures (the cervical spine and the shoulder), the brachial plexus can be damaged or even torn apart by violent injury to these structures. It is convenient to consider brachial plexus injuries as follows:

1. *Upper Plexus Injury (Erb's Paralysis):* Caused by forcible widening of the angle between the head and the shoulder. This can be caused by traction on arm at birth, or by severe injuries, commonly motorcycle accidents. C5, C6 and sometimes C7 are involved. This leads to a typical ('porter's tip') deformity with: adduction and medial rotation of humerus (deltoid and lateral rotators paralysed C5, C6), extension of elbow (flexors paralysed C5, C6), pronation of forearm (supinator paralysed C5, C6).

This injury can be the result of avulsion of the roots from the cord, which carries a poorer prognosis for recovery than truncal lesions. Such avulsion can be recognized clinically by paralysis of serratus anterior, levator scapulae, and the rhomboid muscles, and by myelography, which demonstrates extravasation of contrast medium at the exit of the nerve roots (traumatic meningocele).

2. *Lower Plexus Injuries (Klumpke's Paralysis):* Caused by hyperabduction of the arm such as may occur during delivery (extended arm in a breech delivery), a fall on an outstretched arm, or an arm pulled into machinery. C8, T1 and sometimes C7 are involved.

   The result is clawing of the hand due to paralysis of the flexors of the wrist and fingers (C6, C7, C8) and all the intrinsic muscles of the hand (C8, T1).

3. *Injury at the Level of the Roots:* Injury at the level of the roots is associated with cervical sympathetic paralysis (Horner's syndrome) and has a poorer prognosis for recovery. This condition presents clinically with miosis (contraction of the pupil), ptosis (drooping of the upper eyelid due to paralysis of the superior tarsal muscle), apparent enophthalmos (due to ptosis and miosis, the eyeball appears to be sunken but true enophthalmos does not occur), and lack of sweating (anhidrosis) on the affected side of the face, neck and arm.

4. *Cord Injury:* These are usually caused by traction (e.g. road traffic accidents) or penetrating wounds (e.g. knife and gunshot wounds).

   Lateral cord injury:

   Motor loss:

   Biceps and brachialis (musculocutaneous nerve).

   Flexor carpi radialis and pronator teres (lateral head of median nerve).

   Sensory loss:

   Of lateral side of forearm.

   Posterior cord injury:

   Motor loss:

   Internal rotation and abduction of humerus (axillary and subscapular nerves).

   Extension of elbow, wrist and metacarpophalangeal joints (radial nerve).

   Sensory loss:

   Over shoulder, posterior part of arm and dorsum of 1st and 2nd metacarpals and first web space.

   Medial cord injury:

   Motor loss:

   Flexors of the wrist (except flexor carpi radialis).

   Long flexors of fingers.

   All intrinsic muscles of hand; essentially a combined median and ulnar nerve paralysis.

   Sensory loss over:

   Front and medial side of arm.

   Medial side of forearm.

   Anterior surface of palm and fingers.

   Posterior surface of palm and fingers, except over 1st and 2nd metacarpals and first web space.

PERIPHERAL NERVE LESIONS

Radial nerve

This nerve is often injured in the radial groove of the humerus, when the bone is fractured or by pressure of a crutch in the axilla. Complete division of the nerve before branching causes:

Motor Paralysis of:
1. Extensors of elbow, wrist, knuckles, and all joints of thumb.
2. Supinator and brachioradialis (chiefly a flexor of the elbow).
   The motor loss causes a typical drop-wrist (*Fig.* 305).

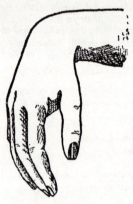

Fig. 305. Drop-wrist resulting from radial nerve palsy.

Sensory Loss: Anaesthesia over the dorsum of the 1st, 2nd and 3rd metacarpals. There may be considerable variation in the amount of sensory disturbance (*Fig.* 306) and the area involved may be so small as to affect the index knuckle only. This is because of the overlapping of adjacent sensory areas, but will only occur if the injury is below the axilla and leaves the dorsal cutaneous nerve of the forearm and the superficial branch of the radial intact. The muscles affected show loss of pain and muscle sense. Joint sense is usually unaffected.

Median nerve

INJURY: This nerve may be injured by penetrating wounds of the forearm. Complete severance causes:

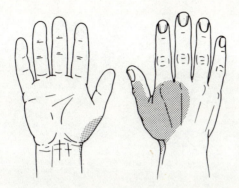

Fig. 306. Area of sensory loss following division of the radial nerve above the elbow.

Motor Paralysis of:
   1. The pronators.
   2. The radial flexor of the wrist.
   3. Flexors of all the proximal interphalangeal joints.
   4. Flexors of the terminal joints of the thumb and index and middle fingers.
   5. Flexors of the 1st and 2nd metacarpophalangeal joints (including flexor pollicis brevis).
   6. Abductor and opponens pollicis—loss of the power to rotate thumb opposite index finger for the 'pincer action' in picking up objects.

The median is the nerve which is responsible for powerful coarse hand movements, which are executed by the long muscles coming from the forearm.

In injury at the level of the wrist, the muscular paralysis may go unnoticed, but the sensory loss will reveal the serious nature of the lesion.

Sensory Loss: C6 and C7 are the vital sensory posterior nerve roots of the median nerve distribution.

   Deep pressure pain is lost in the above muscles.

   Joint sense is lost in interphalangeal joints of index, and last joints of thumb and middle finger.

   Cutaneous loss, as shown in *Fig.* 307. The loss of sensation over the thumb and index finger renders the hand virtually useless in fine movement, e.g. buttoning a coat. (Hence the term 'the eye of the hand' has been applied to the median.)

   Trophic changes are prominent because the median carries most of the sympathetic nerve supply of the hand.

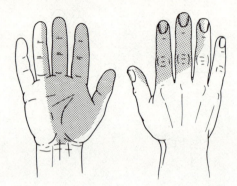

Fig. 307. Area of sensory loss following division of the median nerve.

CARPAL TUNNEL SYNDROME: The median nerve may be compressed at the wrist by the inelastic transverse carpal ligament. Although a significant portion of the carpal tunnel syndromes is due to the size and shape of the carpal tunnel itself, other factors are oedema (especially in pregnancy), synovial swelling (associated with rheumatoid arthritis), bony encroachment (osteo-arthritis or injury) and myxoedema.

Presenting symptoms are painful paraesthesia and numbness affecting the radial three and a half digits of the hand, which characteristically wakes the patient up at night, presumably because of tissue fluid accumulation in the absence of the forearm muscle pump action with the arm at rest. Motor symptoms, including inability to perform fine movement and clumsiness, follow later.

Examination reveals wasting of the thenar eminence, hypo-aesthesia to light touch and pinprick over the palmar aspect of radial three and a half digits. Note, however, that the skin over the thenar eminence is not affected, as it is supplied by the palmar cutaneous branch of the median which arises proximal to the carpal tunnel.

The most reliable clinical diagnostic test of carpal tunnel compression involves inflation of a sphygmomanometer cuff around the arm to a point above systolic pressure. This reproduces the patient's symptoms within one minute, presumably as a result of ischaemia superimposed on an irritable nerve.

Electrical conductivity tests confirm the diagnosis and should be performed prior to surgery to demonstrate a reduced conduction velocity in the nerve as it crosses the wrist. The normal conduction velocity of motor nerve fibres is of the order of 50 m/s, thus values below 40 m/s are suspicious, and below 30 m/s are diagnostic of carpal tunnel syndrome.

Ulnar nerve

INJURY: This nerve is most commonly injured in penetrating wounds of the forearm and fractures involving the medial epicondyle of the humerus.

Complete division causes:

Motor Paralysis of:
1. Ulnar flexor of wrist (flexor carpi ulnaris).
2. Flexors of terminal phalanges of the ring and little fingers, i.e. profundus digitorum.
3. Muscles of the hypothenar eminence, i.e. abductor, flexor, and opponens digiti minimi.
4. Adductor pollicis.
5. Palmaris brevis.
6. All the interossei and inner two lumbricals. This loss results in a mild degree of clawing of the hand in which the 1st phalanges of the fingers are extended and the 2nd and 3rd flexed. It is not a true claw-hand (*Fig.* 308).

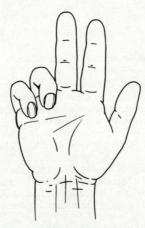

Fig. 308. Position of fingers in an ulnar 'claw-hand'.

There is a characteristic flattening of the hypothenar eminence and depression of the interosseous spaces due to atrophy of hypothenar and interosseous muscles.

Sensory Loss:
Deep:
1. Muscle pain—lost in all above muscles.

2. Joint sense—lost in all joints of little finger and interphalangeal joints of ring finger.
3. Pressure sense—lost on ulnar border of hand and whole of little finger.

Cutaneous: Loss of light touch, pinprick and temperature sensation over area shown in *Fig.* 309.

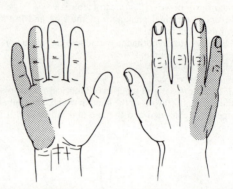

Fig. 309. Area of sensory loss following division of the ulnar nerve.

The functional disability following ulnar nerve transection is slight, the motor disability being mostly loss of fine movements of the fingers (which can be improved by tendon transfers around the wrist and hand) with the sensory loss being restricted to the two ulnar digits only.

COMPRESSION OF THE ULNAR NERVE (TRAUMATIC ULNAR NEURITIS):

1. *At the Wrist:* Compression may occur where the nerve passes deeply into the muscle of the hypothenar eminence through the trough formed by the pisiform medially and the hook of the hamate laterally. Ganglion formation and a tight pisohamate ligament may aggravate the condition.

   The symptoms are then of pain and paraesthesia over the 4th and 5th digits and weakness of the medial interosseous muscles. Nerve conduction studies will confirm the diagnosis by showing slowing of nerve conduction over the zone of nerve compression.

2. *At the Elbow:* Compression may occur behind the medial epicondyle at the elbow after an old treated fracture or, immediately distal to this point, as the nerve passes between the two heads of the flexor carpi ulnaris.

   In the case of compression behind the medial epicondyle transposition of the ulnar nerve to a position in front of the epicondyle may be effective (*Fig.* 310). This manoeuvre may also be utilized to gain length for nerve suture in the arm or forearm.

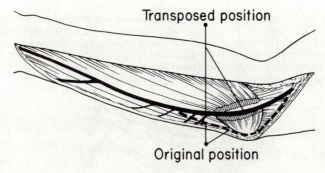

Transposed position

Original position

Fig. 310. Transposition of the ulnar nerve.

COMBINED LESIONS OF MEDIAN AND ULNAR NERVES:

Motor Paralysis of:

1. Intrinsic muscles of the hand.
2. Flexor carpi ulnaris.
3. All the flexors of the digits.
4. The pronators.
5. All the flexors of the wrist.

A scheme represents this as follows:

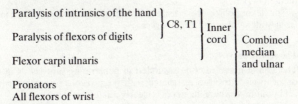

Sensory Loss:

1. Total anaesthesia over all the ulnar area and in the two terminal phalanges of the middle and index fingers.
2. The thumb, outer half of the palm of the hand, and sometimes the palmar aspect of the proximal phalanges of the 2nd and 3rd fingers remain sensitive to a very deep pinprick. This sensibility is

accounted for by the probable assistance given by the fibres of the superficial branch of the radial and lateral cutaneous nerves of the forearm.

3. All the median area may be completely anaesthetic.

CLAW-HAND: A combined median and ulnar lesion at the elbow causes a true claw-hand (*Fig.* 311) of severe type. This results in hyperextended wrist and metacarpophalangeal joints and flexion of interphalangeal joints. The same type of clawing is produced by a lesion of the medial cord of the brachial plexus and by Klumpke's paralysis. The position taken up by the hand is the result of paralysis of the interosseous and lumbrical muscles.

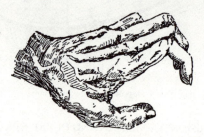

Fig. 311. Claw-hand.

Anomalous nerve supply to the muscles of the hand

These may be variations in the nerve supply to intrinsic muscles of the hand with all gradations from complete ulnar to complete median innervation, e.g. the 1st (or 1st and 2nd) dorsal interosseous muscle may be supplied by the median nerve.

The flexor pollicis brevis usually has a dual nerve supply with a contribution from both median and ulnar nerves.

The sciatic nerve

The sciatic nerve may be wounded in penetrating injuries or in posterior dislocation of the hip associated with fracture of the posterior lip of the acetabulum to which the nerve is clearly related.

Severance of the nerve at its origin causes:

Motor Paralysis of:

1. All the hamstrings, i.e. all flexors of the knee, except sartorius.
2. All leg muscles.
3. All foot muscles.

A condition known as foot-drop results, and ultimately the toes become clawed.

Sensory:
   Deep:
       Loss of joint sense in ankle and all foot and toe joints.
       Loss to pressure beyond the metatarsal heads.
       Loss of deep pressure pain in all the paralysed muscles.
   Cutaneous: As in diagram (*Fig.* 312). Trophic ulcers occur especially on
   points subjected to pressure, i.e. heel and balls of toes.

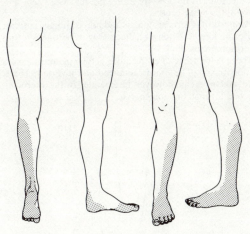

Fig. 312. Areas of sensory loss following division of sciatic nerve near its origin.

Tibial (medial popliteal) nerve

INJURY: Division of this nerve results in:
   Motor Paralysis of:
       Leg: Popliteus, soleus, gastrocnemius, tibialis posterior, flexor digi-
           torum longus, flexor hallucis longus.
       Foot: All the muscles of the foot excepting only the extensor digitorum
           brevis.
   If this nerve is divided, the foot is held dorsiflexed at the ankle and everted,
and the tendo Achillis prominence is lost. No movement for lowering the foot
can be made. Severe disability results; the intrinsic muscles of the foot are
paralysed and the patient cannot stand on his toes. He walks with a splay foot
without elasticity or spring.
   Sensory: Sensibility is lost on the sole of the foot and on the dorsal aspect of
       their last phalanges. Trophic ulcers are common.

TARSAL TUNNEL SYNDROME: Compression of the tibial nerve within the fibro-osseous tunnel under the flexor retinaculum of the ankle joint. This causes pain and paraesthesia in the sole of the foot, often worse at night.

Common peroneal (lateral popliteal nerve)

The most commonly injured nerve in the lower limb, because it winds superficially around the neck of the fibula where it is vulnerable to injury, by fracture of the fibula or by pressure from a plaster cast.

Severance of the nerve causes:

Motor Paralysis of: Peroneus longus and brevis, tibialis anterior, extensor digitorum longus, extensor hallucis longus, peroneus tertius, extensor digitorum brevis.

There is foot-drop, i.e. the ankle is fully plantar-flexed and cannot be dorsiflexed. The foot is adducted and inverted. The second and third phalanges can, however, be extended by the interossei, which are supplied through the tibial nerve.

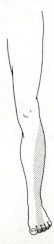

Fig. 313. Area of sensory loss following division of the common peroneal nerve.

Sensory: There is sensory loss on the dorsum of the foot and on the outer surface of the leg (*Fig.* 313).

Anterior tibial syndrome

This arises usually in young men, as a result of unaccustomed exertion or trauma, followed by increased pressure within the anterior tibial compartment, impaired muscle blood supply and ischaemic necrosis. The deep peroneal (anterior tibial) nerve is involved initially by compression (in which case recovery is rapid after decompression) but later by ischaemia (in which case permanent loss of function results).

Chapter 30

PROLAPSE OF THE UTERUS, VAGINAL EXAMINATION AND HYSTERECTOMY

PROLAPSE

The term is used to signify the protrusion of a viscus through an anatomical aperture normally present, and also to imply the protrusion of a structure through an aperture not normally existent, e.g. through a wound. Examples of the latter are prolapse of the iris through a corneal wound and prolapse of the testis through a skin wound. We are here concerned solely with prolapse through a pre-existent aperture.

Prolapse of the uterus and vagina

LIGAMENTS OF THE UTERUS: These (*see Fig.* 314) are:

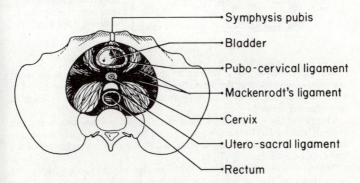

- Symphysis pubis
- Bladder
- Pubo-cervical ligament
- Mackenrodt's ligament
- Cervix
- Utero-sacral ligament
- Rectum

Fig. 314. Ligaments of the uterus.

1. The transverse ligament of the cervix or Mackenrodt's ligaments.
2. The round ligament.

3. The uterosacral ligament.
4. The pubocervical ligament.

They are strong fibromuscular ligaments, formed from condensation of connective tissue surrounding the uterine and vaginal arteries.

The ligaments radiate fanwise from the cervix at the level of the internal os and cervicovaginal junction, to the side walls of the pelvis. Mackenrodt's ligaments are by far the strongest and most important of these ligaments.

SUPPORTS OF THE UTERUS: Notice particularly that the term 'supports of the uterus' (*Fig.* 315) is not synonymous with the 'ligaments of the uterus', which play a minor part in supporting the organ in its correct position. The main support to the uterus is, in fact, the pelvic diaphragm, which forms a fibromuscular floor to the pelvis.

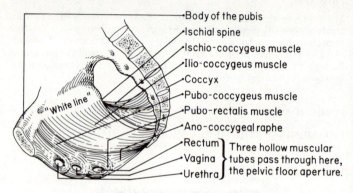

Fig. 315. The pelvic diaphragm.

The pelvic diaphragm is formed by the levator ani, which is the most important constituent of the pelvic floor. It is constantly being subjected to strains due to increase of intra-abdominal pressure by such acts as laughing and straining at stool.

The pelvic floor, formed by the levator muscle system, presents a gap behind, traversed by the rectum, and another in front, traversed by the vagina and urethra. The anterior gap is protected by the muscles and fascia of the urogenital diaphragm.

Typical Position of the Uterus: With the bladder and rectum empty, the body of the uterus, in the standing individual, should lie almost horizontally forward in the anteverted position. The body and the cervix form an angle of 90–100 degrees with each other and it may be said that, normally, the long axis of the uterus forms a right-angle with the long axis of the vagina (*Fig.* 316A).

Version implies an alteration in the direction of the uterus as a whole, the organ rotating round a coronal axis passing through the external os. It is often associated with inflammatory change.

Flexion implies an increase or a decrease in the angle between body and cervix.

The direction of the cervix in the pelvis may be normal or altered in these conditions. If the position of the body is altered, the cervix naturally lies in front of or behind its typical situation.

Retroversion is apt to bring the uterine axis into line with the vaginal axis and this factor facilitates prolapse.

VARIETIES OF PROLAPSE:

1. *Prolapse of the Posterior Vaginal Wall:* If this is associated with prolapse of the rectum, the condition is termed a 'rectocele' and, if there is an associated prolapse of the peritoneum of the pouch of Douglas, it is then known as an 'enterocele'.

2. *Prolapse of the Anterior Wall of the Vagina:* This usually involves the bladder and is then termed a 'cystocele'—a condition commonly associated with 'stress' incontinence of urine.

3. *Prolapse of the Uterus:* If this prolapse is complete, i.e. the uterus presents outside the introitus, it is termed 'a procidentia'.

CAUSATION OF PROLAPSE: Obstetric injury is the main factor in causation. If this results in injury to the pelvic floor from laceration of the perineum and damage to and separation of the levator muscles, the vagina, being relatively unsupported below, tends to sag downwards and the rectum tends to bulge forwards into the vagina. A rectocele is not necessarily present owing to the loose attachment between rectum and posterior vaginal wall.

Damage and separation of the levator and fasciae in front of the uterus and around the base of the bladder will remove the normal support in that region, and this lack of support is more pronounced if perineal damage also exists. This is the genesis of prolapse of the anterior vaginal wall.

For the uterus to descend it first becomes retroverted so far as to bring the axis of uterus and vagina into line (*Fig.* 316B). The uterus will then be able to descend along the vaginal canal, gradually inverting the vagina from above downwards, as its weight, constantly thrown on the ligaments, weakens them till they are no longer able to support it alone. Further, the damaged pelvic floor, perineum, levator ani, and fasciae no longer close the pelvic outlet in the normal manner. Should vaginal prolapse precede uterine prolapse, as is often the case, the drag of the vagina on the uterus will also tend to bring down this organ. The extruded body of the uterus is covered by the vagina.

All the uterovaginal supports share a tissue sensitivity to oestrogen which maintains their tone and elasticity. Thus, while childbirth is responsible for the initial tearing and stretching of these supports, it is usually only in the postmenopausal period, when oestrogen is deficient, that symptomatic prolapse presents.

PROLAPSE OF THE FEMALE URETHRA: This condition is due to loss of tone in the sphincteric musculature permitting the mucosa to glide on the underlying tissues and ultimately prolapse or herniate through the meatus. It is found in emaciated children and as a result of parturition in adults. Tumours growing from the mucous membrane may project to the exterior and pull the mucosa after them.

VAGINAL EXAMINATION

Inspection of the vulva
1. Look for signs of infection.
2. Ulceration due to a carcinoma.
3. Bartholin's abscess: a painful swelling appears at the posterior part of the vulva.
4. Evidence of uterine prolapse.

Inspection of the cervix
A vaginal speculum is inserted. If a vaginal or cervical smear is to be made to look for exfoliated cells, no lubricant apart from water should be used on the speculum.

Digital examination
1. The vagina—abnormalities of its entrance or walls.
2. The urethra—is felt as a cord in the anterior wall.
3. The rectum—if it contains faeces or a foreign body, or is the site of a tumour. Faeces may be indented by the vaginal finger.
4. The cervix uteri and external os. The cervix slopes downwards and backwards.
5. The vault of the vagina, divided by the cervix into anterior, posterior, right and left lateral fornices.
6. The recto-uterine pouch—the finger in the posterior fornix is separated from this pouch by the thickness of the vaginal wall, pelvic fascia and peritoneum. The pouch is normally empty except for coils of gut. It may contain the uterus, prolapsed ovaries and tubes, inflammatory collections of fluid, tumours, and almost any abdominal viscus. The floor of the recto-uterine pouch varies in distance from the skin of the perineum being 5–7·5 cm above it. In complete prolapse of the rectum, the pouch lies in the rectum or prolapses through the anus.

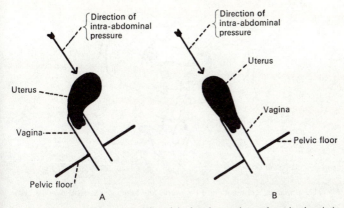

Fig. 316. Diagrammatic representation of the fact that uterine prolapse is a herniation of the viscus through the pelvic floor via the vagina. In (A), the normal relationship is shown, the uterus being anteverted, lying parallel with the pelvic floor and at right-angles to the vagina; intra-abdominal pressure is indicated by the arrow. In (B), the uterus has straightened out and is now lying in the axis of the vagina and at right-angles to the pelvic floor; the direction of intra-abdominal pressure is such that it tends to push the uterus into the vagina.

7. In late pregnancy vaginal examination can be used to assess the size and shape of the pelvis.

Bimanual examination

This examination (*Fig.* 317) is conducted with one or two fingers of the right hand in the vagina and the left hand on the lower abdomen, and palpating the structures between the two hands. By this means the pelvic organs may be examined.

Rectovaginal examination

The index finger is in the vagina and the middle finger is in the rectum. This examination may help to distinguish between a lesion in the rectum and one between the rectum and vagina.

TOTAL ABDOMINAL HYSTERECTOMY

The bladder is catheterized before the operation. The uterus is mobilized by dividing the ovarian ligaments, the Fallopian tubes and the round ligaments.

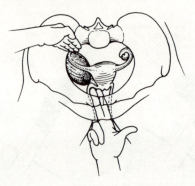

Fig. 317. Bimanual examination of the uterus and adnexa. The right ovary is cystic.

The uterus is now separated from its extraperitoneal attachments. The peritoneum of the uterovesical pouch is incised, from the round ligament of one side to the round ligament of the opposite side. The bladder is now pushed down off the front and sides of the cervix. The vesicocervical ligament, which is a fascial condensation in the midline, is divided and the ureters are moved away from the side of the cervix where they may be damaged when the uterine arteries are ligated. Mackenrodt's ligament and the uterosacral ligament are divided and the uterine artery ligated close to the cervix. The uterus can now be removed by transecting the vagina.

The vagina is closed with sutures. At the lateral angles of the vagina, there is a plexus of veins which requires a separate suture.

The pelvic floor is reconstituted by suturing the uterosacral, Mackenrodt's and the round ligaments to the lateral angles of the vaginal vault, which prevents subsequent vaginal prolapse. The raw surface is covered with peritoneum.

VAGINAL HYSTERECTOMY

This is an alternative approach, which is much favoured by many gynaecologists although the procedure has some very definite contraindications. The anatomical structures encountered are obviously the same as for abdominal hysterectomy, but are dealt with in a different sequence.

Chapter 31

THE ANATOMY OF THE CHILD

HEAD

At birth the circumference of the infant's head averages 33–35 cm. It gains 7–6 cm in the first six months. At the end of the first year it is 45 cm; at five years it is 50 cm; at ten years it is 53 cm.

Fontanelles

The skull at birth is only partly ossified; gaps or fontanelles exist between the bones which are filled in by a membranous structure which consists of three layers. The inner is the outer layer of the dura, the middle is the future periosteum of the skull bones, the superficial layer is the aponeurosis joining the occipitalis and frontalis muscles. The fontanelles serve two very important purposes: (*a*) they permit some overlapping of the skull bones during the moulding and pressure which the skull undergoes during birth; and (*b*) they permit growth of the brain.

It is of the utmost importance to note that the normal skull only develops round a normal brain (the term 'normal' is here used as implying absence of gross anatomical defect). There are six fontanelles at birth. One is situated at each angle of a parietal bone. Two are therefore median and four are lateral. The four lateral fontanelles close within a few weeks of birth. The median fontanelles are posterior and anterior.

THE POSTERIOR FONTANELLE: This is situated where the two parietal bones meet the occipital bone. It closes soon after birth.

THE ANTERIOR FONTANELLE: This is the most important. It is situated at the place where the two parietal bones and the two halves of the frontal bone come close together (*Fig.* 318).

Fig. 318. Shape of the anterior fontanelle.

Shape: It is rhomboid in shape. Each of its four angles marks the end of a suture.

Size: It measures about 3–8 cm in length by 2–5 cm in breadth.

Significance:

Developmental significance: For two years after birth there is a non-rigid area which permits increase in size of the brain.

Clinical significance: Valuable information is obtained from the fontanelle. The degree of tenseness of the membrane gives an index of the intracranial pressure. On the other hand, abnormal depression of the membrane indicates an insufficiency of body fluids. The fontanelle is of service for further purposes; through its lateral angle a needle may be passed into the lateral ventricle of the brain and the superior sagittal sinus may be approached through the membrane in the midline.

Tympanic antrum and mastoid process

The tympanic antrum is a well-developed cavity at birth. The mastoid process does not begin to develop until the end of the second year, the same age at which the mastoid air cells begin to develop (*Fig.* 319).

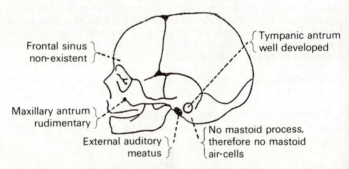

Fig. 319. Condition of the air sinuses at birth.

Before the mastoid process develops, the facial nerve is a subcutaneous structure and is in danger of being cut by an incision behind the ear which extends too far down (*Fig.* 320). In the adult the nerve is 2·5–3·8 cm from the surface, being pushed to the base of the skull by the development of the mastoid process.

There is, in the infant, a strip of cartilage uniting the squamous and petrous parts of the temporal bone. This cartilaginous strip is very thin and lies under the dura and temporal lobe of the brain. Infection of the middle ear spreads

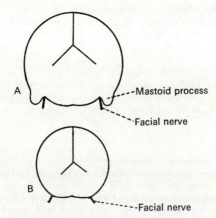

Fig. 320. Adult skull. A, Demonstrating the protection afforded to the facial nerve in the adult by the mastoid process. B, Infant's skull; the nerve is superficial, as the mastoid process is undeveloped in the infant.

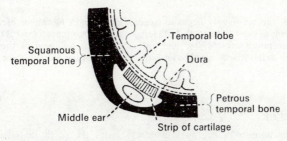

Fig. 321. Scheme to show the readiness with which disease of the middle ear in the infant may cause intracranial complications.

through this cartilage to cause an extradural or temporal lobe abscess (*Fig.* 321).

Frontal sinus

This does not exist at birth. It begins to develop as an outgrowth from the nose during the first year. It is rarely evident before the seventh or eighth year. It reaches full development between the fifteenth and twentieth years.

Maxillary antrum (sinus)

At birth the maxillary antrum is rudimentary. It reaches full development between the fifteenth and twentieth years.

The mandible

All traces of the cartilage uniting the two halves of the mandible at the symphysis menti have disappeared at birth. At this time they are united by fibrous tissue. Ossification is complete within the first year.

Suctorial pad

The roundness and fullness of the infant's cheeks are due to the presence in the cheek of a large pad of fat known as the suctorial pad. This lies anterior to the masseter, on the buccinator. It is pierced by the parotid duct and is represented in adults by the buccal pad of fat which is relatively much smaller. It is of assistance in the act of sucking. The newborn child, though edentulous, does not present the unsightly appearance of the toothless adult because the suctorial pad prevents infalling of the cheeks.

Teeth

Though the teeth only begin to appear at the sixth month of life, the rudiments of most of the teeth, both temporary and permanent, exist at birth. The exceptions are the 2nd and 3rd molars. The rudiment of the 2nd appears at the fourth month after birth, and that of the 3rd about the fifth year.

THE NECK

The newborn baby has no visible neck, with the result that the left brachiocephalic (innominate) vein crosses the trachea so high in the superior mediastinum that it encroaches on the tissues of the neck above the suprasternal notch, especially when the neck is extended, as it would be during tracheostomy. The vein is, therefore, at risk during this procedure in an infant.

Larynx and trachea

The larynx and trachea are of small bore at birth. The vocal cords are about 5 mm long by the end of the first year. Because of the narrow lumen, stridor is a common symptom of laryngitis and tracheitis in infants.

THORAX

The thorax at birth and for two years after is circular on section; the adult thorax is oval. The diameter of the adult thorax may therefore be increased by thoracic breathing. This is impossible in the child, as the surface area of a circle cannot be increased within a circumference the length of which remains constant. For this reason respiration in the first two years of life is almost entirely abdominal (diaphragmatic), and only in later years does intercostal (thoracic) respiration take much part in breathing.

HIBERNATING GLAND

There lies in the posterior triangle of the neck of the infant a mass of fat which extends down behind the trapezius towards the scapula. This is said to be the remains of a collection of fat which exists here in hibernating animals. This fat is histologically different from ordinary fat and may give rise to a special form of tumour. In humans this structure is important in non-shivering thermo-genesis.

SUBCUTANEOUS FAT

This has a very firm feel in the healthy child. In the newborn baby an episode of severe hypothermia could cause this layer to gel. When present this is detected as an abnormal hardening of the tissues and is known as sclerema neonatorum.

THE SPINAL COLUMN

The spine of the neonate is disposed in the shape of a long kyphotic or C-shaped curve, concave forwards. When the head is held up after the age of three months, its weight causes the neck to be curved with a convexity forwards. On sitting up at the age of six months, a similar curve with convexity forwards develops in the lumbar region. These two latter curves are called 'secondary curves'.

SPINAL CORD

The cord ends at a level one vertebra lower in the newborn child than in the adult. It therefore ends at the 3rd lumbar vertebra.

THYMUS GLAND

At birth the organ extends from the cricoid to the 4th costal cartilage, lying anterior to the trachea, great vessels of the thorax, and the pericardium. It is of pyramidal shape, greyish-white in colour, and has anterior, posterior, and right and left lateral surfaces. It has a definite connective-tissue sheath.

ABDOMINAL CAVITY

Liver

The liver is relatively large at birth and can be felt beneath the right costal margin. This is a normal finding until the child is between 2 to 3 years old.

Perirenal fat

There is a very little perirenal fat in infants and young children. This means that the kidney is much more intimately related to the peritoneum in young children than it is in adults.

Kidneys

The kidneys are lobulated at birth. The external evidence of lobes of the kidneys disappears during infancy as cortical growth of nephrons occurs.

Adrenal gland

At birth adrenal glands are nearly as large as the kidneys themselves. During the first two weeks after birth the adrenals reduce to about half their former size.

The bladder

In infants and children the normal bladder, even when empty, is in the abdomen. It begins to enter the pelvis at about 6 years of age. Needle puncture of the bladder is a convenient way to obtain an uncontaminated specimen of urine for culture in an infant.

The omentum

The omentum is short in length and relatively underdeveloped in infancy. The omentum, once called the 'policeman of the abdomen', is a factor concerned in localizing inflammatory processes in the abdominal cavity, i.e. acute appendicitis. The underdevelopment of the omentum in the child is one of the factors which make inflammatory disease so serious in the abdomen of the child.

PREPUCE

The prepuce is fused to the glans and is usually not retractable at birth. Breakdown of the fused surfaces normally occurs during infancy.

Chapter 32

BONES AND AMPUTATIONS

DEVELOPMENT OF BONES

In the fetus, bones develop from condensations of mesenchyme (embryonic connective tissue). This mesenchyme may undergo ossification directly, intramembranous ossification (membrane bone formation), or the mesenchyme is initially replaced by dense cellular cartilage which subsequently becomes ossified by intracartilaginous ossification. The final histological structure of bone formed in membrane or in cartilage is identical.

Membrane bones

Intramembranous ossification occurs rapidly and is found in bones which are required for protection such as the flat bones of the skull and face. The clavicle and mandible are also membrane bones.

Cartilage bones

These are of different shapes and lengths, e.g. long, short, flat and irregular bones. All, except some of the irregular bones, have a primary and secondary ossification centre. Most primary centres appear when the fetus is 7–12 weeks old and virtually all are present by birth. A secondary ossification centre appears at about the time of birth at the cartilaginous end of the bone. The epiphysis is that part of bone ossified from a secondary centre.

The constituent parts of a long bone before the completion of growth

The bone (*Fig.* 322) consists of:

1. DIAPHYSIS: The diaphysis or shaft is ossified from the primary centre.

2. EPIPHYSIS: Each long bone has at least one epiphysis at either end, and

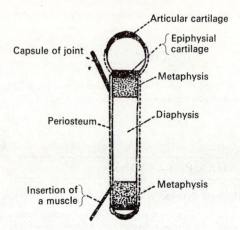

Fig. 322. Some features of the anatomy of bone. Observe: (1) dipping in of periosteum at epiphysial line; (2) fusion of capsule with periosteum; (3) attachment of the tendon of a muscle to the bone in the metaphysial region.

often several. One of the epiphyses at each end is covered with articular cartilage, and all or part of this epiphysis is inside the capsule of the joint.

3. EPIPHYSIAL CARTILAGE: The epiphysial cartilage is a plate of cartilage intervening between the epiphysis and the end of the diaphysis. From this cartilage the growth in length of the bone occurs by additions of osseous tissue to the related parts of the epiphysis and diaphysis.

4. METAPHYSIS: The metaphysis is that part of the diaphysis which abuts on the epiphysial plate. It is highly vascular and it is not as strong as the rest of the diaphysis.

The metaphysis has important characteristics when considered from a surgical point of view:

 i. It is the area of greatest growth activity in the bone.
 ii. It has an extremely profuse blood supply, as the different sets of blood vessels supplying the bone anastomose in this region. It has been aptly called 'a lake of blood'.
 iii. The muscles, tendons, and joint capsules and ligaments are attached to, or near it, so that it is an area which is very likely to suffer damage in strains, whether these come directly through the bone or through the ligaments attached to the metaphysis.
 iv. Because of its great vascularity, and the delicate nature of the lamellae

of which it is composed, 'separation of epiphysis' takes place through the part of the metaphysis which abuts immediately on the epiphysial cartilage, namely the zone of calcification. As this cartilage is separated from the shaft with the epiphysis, angular or longitudinal growth disturbance may occur.

v. A part of the metaphysis is often inside the capsule of a joint, so that disease of the metaphysis is very likely to invade the joint in such circumstances, or vice versa.

5. PERIOSTEUM: The periosteum consists of two layers, the inner of which is tacked down to the epiphysial line, continuing on over the epiphysis to blend with the articular cartilage. The outer layer is continuous with the joint capsule. Pus deep to both layers is prevented, therefore, by the above-mentioned 'tacking down' from extending onto the epiphysis (*Fig*. 323). The periosteum is a vascular membrane assisting in the blood supply of the bone, and is an osteogenic structure, depositing bone on the surface of the shaft and thus adding to its girth.

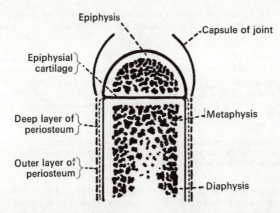

Fig. 323. Figure showing relation of periosteum to epiphysial cartilage and capsule of the joint. Observe that pus between periosteum and bone cannot spread beyond the epiphysial cartilage because the deep layer of the periosteum blends with this structure; notice also that the outer layer of the periosteum is continuous with the capsule of the joint.

Long bones after growth is complete

The bone consists now of a solid osseous structure without epiphyses, metaphyses, or epiphysial cartilages.

Ossification

Certain features of the development of bone have clinical and surgical applications.

SKULL: Centres of ossification, additional to the usual ones, may appear in the membrane from which the vault of the skull develops, and give rise to small bones situated between the named ones. These are the so-called 'Wormian bones' or 'sutural bones'. They are most common where the occipital bone joins the parietals (lambdoid suture).

Ossification may fail to extend across the membrane which at an early stage unites the two halves of the frontal bone. This results in a vertical suture called the 'metopic suture', which occurs in 8 per cent of skulls and which may be mistaken for a skull fracture on X-ray.

MANDIBLE: A bone developed in membrane. It is the second bone in the body to begin the ossify. A single centre appears in each half at the sixth week. All traces of symphysial cartilage are gone at birth.

CLAVICLE: The ossification of the clavicle (*Fig.* 324) is more complicated than was at one time thought. During the seventh week, two centres of

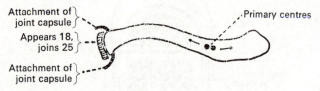

Fig. 324. Ossification of clavicle (Fawcett). Observe the two primary centres at the junction of the middle and outer thirds of the bone. They soon fuse. The arrows show how ossification extends from the centre.

chondrification appear quite close to each other at the junction of the outer third with the inner two-thirds. Centres of ossification soon appear in these foci and the two ossific centres soon unite. From this double centre, ossification spreads towards the acromion and towards the sternum, being preceded by a formation of cartilage. At the eighteenth year, a secondary centre appears in cartilage at the sternal end of the bone. This epiphysis unites at the age of 25. It is intracapsular.

The clavicle is the first bone to ossify and its epiphysis is the last to appear.

The elucidation of the development of the clavicle has enabled the many variations to which the bone is subject to be better understood:

1. The clavicle may be absent.
2. The outer one-third may be absent.

3. The inner two-thirds may be absent—half as often as (2).
4. A fissure may divide the outer one-third from the inner two-thirds.
5. The rhomboid fossa of the collar bone has an unusual X-ray appearance in the clavicle(s) of adult males which resembles an erosion of part of the bone. It is situated on the inferior surface of one or both clavicles in the area of attachment of the costoclavicular (rhomboid) ligament. It is a broad rough surface about 2·5 cm long, commencing about a centimetre from the sternoclavicular joint (*Fig*. 325).

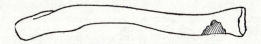

Fig. 325. The rhomboid fossa of the clavicle.

SCAPULA: It has a complicated development. The only fact of practical importance in this development is concerned with the acromion. Two or more centres appear for the acromion at puberty. They may fail to unite with the rest of the bone. This failure of union may be interpreted in an X-ray picture as a fracture. In such cases, a radiograph of the acromion of the opposite side will in all likelihood show the same failure of union.

LONG BONES OF THE LIMBS: According to the law of ossification where a bone has an epiphysis at either end, the epiphysis which is the first to appear is the last to join, and the epiphysis which is the last to appear is the first to join. The fibula is the only exception to this rule.

Growth continues longest at the shoulder and wrist in the upper limb, and longest at the knee in the lower limb. That means that the epiphyses of:

The upper end of the humerus ⎫
The lower end of the radius   ⎪ Unite later than the
The lower end of the ulna   ⎬ epiphyses at the other
The upper end of the tibia   ⎪ ends of these bones.
The lower end of the femur   ⎭

The nutrient foramina of the limb bones are directed according to the rhyme 'to the elbow I go, from the knee I flee'. The nutrient foramina are originally directed in the opposite direction to that which they take in the adult, but, growth being more active at the shoulder, wrist, and knee, the arteries are pushed farther and farther away from the ends of the bones, and ultimately the foramina are deflected towards the other (and slower growing) ones.

HIP BONE: By fusion of its three constituent elements at the acetabulum, this becomes one bone at the age of 12–16 years (*Fig.* 326). The skeletal maturity of the vertebral column may be assessed by the progress of ossification in the secondary centre of the crest of the ilium—the iliac apophysis. Ossification begins at the anterior superior iliac spine and extends backwards. When it reaches the posterior superior iliac spine, ossification of the vertebral column is complete. Radiographs supply the information which is a guide in the handling of cases of structural scoliosis, as lateral curvature of the spinal column usually ceases to progress when the column is skeletally mature.

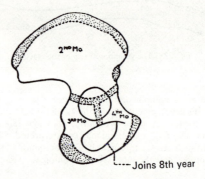

Fig. 326. Ossification of the hip joint. Dates of appearance of primary centres for the three constituent parts of the bone are shown in the figure. Portions developed from secondary centres, five in number, are stippled. These centres appear at puberty and fuse between the ages of 18 and 25, except a triradiate strip of cartilage in the acetabulum, which is completely ossified by 16, through the intervention of a secondary centre known as the os acetabuli.

The secondary centre for the lower end of the femur occurs in the ninth month just before birth. It indicates that the infant has developed to a viable size and is therefore of important medicolegal significance.

THE BLOOD SUPPLY OF BONES

There is a regular standardized plan of blood supply for each type of bone. In general each bone has a nutrient artery, which supplies mainly the bone marrow, and branches from the periosteum, which arise from muscular, ligamentous and capsular attachments, which supply mainly the compact and cancellous bone.

Before union of an epiphysis, it is supplied from the circulus vasculosus, a vascular plexus which surrounds the epiphysis and supplies the joint structures. After fusion of the epiphysis, an anastomosis is established between these latter vessels and those of the bone.

The blood supply of a long bone

The blood supply of a long bone is derived from the following four sources (*Fig.* 327):

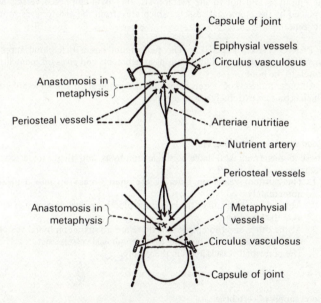

Fig. 327. Schematic representation of the blood supply of a long bone.

1. NUTRIENT ARTERY: Before entering the bone, this vessel is very tortuous, which allows movement without damage to the nutrient vessel. On entering the bone the vessel divides into two branches, one running towards each end of the bone. Each soon divides into a leash of parallel vessels which

run to the metaphysis where they terminate as end arteries. When the epiphysial plate ossifies, these vessels establish communications with the epiphysial vessels and then are no longer end arteries. At this stage, infarction from embolism will no longer occur and the predilection of the metaphysis to osteomyelitis ceases.

2. METAPHYSIAL VESSELS: These are numerous small vessels derived from the anastomosis round the joint. They pierce the metaphysis along the line of the attachment of the joint capsule.

3. EPIPHYSIAL VESSELS: In those cases where the capsule is attached to the epiphysis and not to the metaphysis, the juxta-epiphysial vessels are replaced by the epiphysial vessels, which arise from the anastomosis round the joint.

4. PERIOSTEAL VESSELS: The periosteum has a rich blood supply, provided by muscular and ligamentous attachments and gives off many little vessels to the bone.

All these four sets of vessels come into communication at the metaphysis, which is thus an extremely vascular zone.

Blood supply of short long bones

These bones (*Fig.* 328) have a single epiphysis and therefore a single metaphysis.
1. The nutrient vessel on entering the shaft breaks up into a plexus immediately.
2. At the epiphysial end of the bone, the blood supply is arranged exactly as in the long bones.
3. At the other end (no epiphysis), there are no juxta-epiphysial vessels, and only vessels corresponding to the epiphysial vessels exist.
4. The periosteal vessels assist in the supply.

Blood supply of vertebrae

See Fig. 329.

BODY:
1. Two large vessels enter the body from behind.
2. Smaller vessels enter the body from in front.

ARCH: A vessel enters at the root of the transverse process and sends branches to lamina, pedicle, spine, and transverse process.

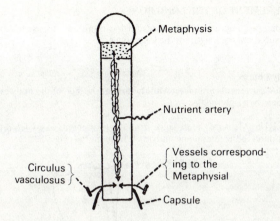

Fig. 328. Blood supply of a short long bone. The periosteal vessels are omitted for simplicity. Only the blood supply of the end devoid of epiphysis is shown. At the epiphysial end, the blood supply corresponds to that at the end of a long bone.

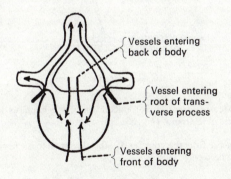

Fig. 329. Blood supply of a vertebra.

Blood supply of flat bones, e.g. scapula, ileum, mandible and ribs

These have nutrient vessels, but the periosteal blood supply from the surrounding muscles assumes particular importance and ensures a rich blood supply.

MEASUREMENT OF THE LONG BONES

It is sometimes important in fractures, dislocations, and disease to compare by measurement the lengths of the long bones.

The upper limbs

These measurements are taken with the arm at the side of the body and the elbow bent to a right-angle.

HUMERUS: Measure the distance from the prominent, easily felt angle of the acromion to the lateral epicondyle of the humerus (*Fig*. 330).

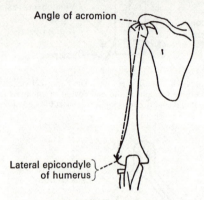

Angle of acromion

Lateral epicondyle of humerus

Fig. 330. Measuring the humerus.

RADIUS: Measure from lateral epicondyle of the humerus to the tip of styloid process of the radius (*Fig*. 331).

ULNA: Measure from the upper end of the olecranon to the head of the ulna or tip of its styloid (*Fig*. 332).

The relative levels of the radial and ulnar styloids may be of value in the diagnosis of fractures of the radius. The radial styloid should project 0·6 cm distal to the ulnar styloid. The best method of determining the levels of the styloids of the radius and ulna is as follows (*Fig*. 333): facing the patient, whose hand is palm downwards, the nail of one of the examiner's index fingers is pushed against the tip of the ulnar styloid and the nail of the other index finger is pushed against the tip of the radial styloid, the examiner's index fingers being flexed at the proximal interphalangeal joints.

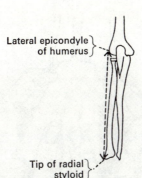

Lateral epicondyle of humerus

Tip of radial styloid

Fig. 331. Method of determining relative lengths of the radii.

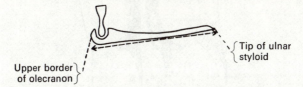

Tip of ulnar styloid

Upper border of olecranon

Fig. 332. Method of measuring the ulna.

Lower limbs

The relative lengths of the lower limbs are equal in only 10 per cent of cases. The femur is more liable to inequality than the tibia. A variation of a centimetre in the comparative length of the lower limbs may, therefore, be looked upon as within the limits of normal. The conclusion that the inequality is not due to injury or disease will only be arrived at after a careful process of exclusion.

The relative lengths of the entire lower limbs are measured from the anterior superior iliac spines because the upper end of the femur is inaccessible. This is also used in measuring the length of the femur.

The anterior superior iliac spines must be exactly on the same horizontal level and the lower limbs extended and symmetrically positioned. The measurement is made from the anterior superior iliac spine to the tip of the medial malleolus.

FEMUR: Measurement is made from the anterior superior iliac spine to one of the following bony points: (*a*) adductor tubercle, (*b*) the lower limit of the medial condyle (joint line) or (*c*) the upper border of the patella (a movable and therefore not very accurate point) (*Fig.* 334).

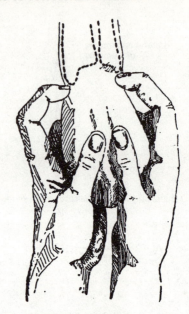

Fig. 333. Method of palpating styloid processes of radius and ulna.

Relative Heights of the Upper Borders of the Greater Trochanters:

Bryant's triangle: With the patient on his back, the lower limbs parallel, and spines of the ilia on the same horizontal level, mark out the anterior superior iliac spine, and mark out the posterior superior angle of the greater trochanter. Drop a vertical line from the anterior superior iliac spine. Measure the shortest distance between this line to the posterior superior angle of the greater trochanter. This length should be the same on both sides. If it is not, it denotes one of four things: (i) dislocation of the upper end of the femur; (ii) fracture of the femoral neck; (iii) alteration of neck-shaft angle of the femur, e.g. coxa vara or valga; (iv) destruction of the head of the femur, e.g. avascular necrosis. (*See Fig.* 335.)

Nélaton's line: The same information may be gained by drawing a line joining the anterior superior iliac spine to the tuberosity of the ischium (*Fig.* 336). This line should touch the upper border of the greater trochanter. If the trochanter is above this line, it means that one of the above four conditions exists.

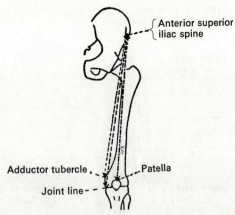

Anterior superior
iliac spine

Adductor tubercle   Patella

Joint line

Fig. 334. Determining relative lengths of the femora. Measurements may be made from the anterior superior iliac spine to one of the following bony landmarks: adductor tubercle, joint line or upper border of patella. Measurement obtained is compared with length between corresponding points on the other side.

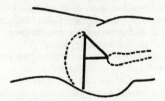

Fig. 335. Bryant's triangle.

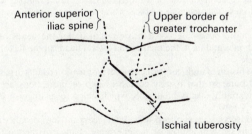

Anterior superior
iliac spine

Upper border of
greater trochanter

Ischial tuberosity

Fig. 336. Nélaton's line.

TIBIA AND FIBULA: They are readily measured as they are subcutaneous and their extremities can be felt (*Fig.* 337).

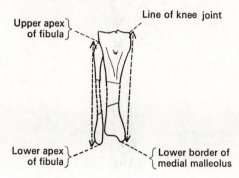

Fig. 337. Determining the actual lengths of the tibia and fibula.

SESAMOID BONES

These small structures, which consist of fibrous tissue, cartilage or bone, derive their name from their alleged resemblance to sesame seeds. They are persistent structures in mammals and do not represent residual primitive bones. They are formed in separate cartilaginous centres in certain tendons. Ossification occurs in the second decade of life except in the case of the patella which ossifies between the third and sixth year of life.

Sesamoid bones are found where a change in direction of pull of a tendon occurs. They give a mechanical advantage to the tendon and protect it from excessive wear.

The patella, which forms in the quadriceps tendon, and the pisiform, which forms in the tendon of the flexor carpi ulnaris, are examples of larger sesamoid bones. The articular surface of the sesamoid bone is covered with cartilage.

Two sesamoid bones are constantly present under the heads of the 1st metatarsal bones and lie in the medial and lateral heads of the flexor hallucis brevis muscle.

Failure of fusion of multicentric centres of ossification results in partition of a sesamoid bone so that it may consist of two or more bony areas. This anomaly invariably occurs bilaterally which helps to distinguish it from a fracture on X-ray.

Repeated stress, such as occurs in ballet dancers and long distance runners, may result in stress fractures or degenerative change of the cartilaginous surface of the sesamoid bone (chondromalacia). The latter condition usually involves the medial sesamoid bone of the flexor hallucis brevis muscle when it is bipartite.

ACCESSORY (SUPERNUMERARY) BONES

These result from an additional ossification centre which develops in a bone or when one of the usual ossification centres fails to fuse with the main bone. The separated bone gives the appearance of an additional bone. These abnormal ossicles are especially common in the foot and, if not recognized, may be mistaken as evidence of a fracture on X-ray.

Os tibiale externum or accessory navicular

Note that, despite the name, the bone (*Fig.* 338) occurs on the internal border of the foot. It occurs in 10–12 per cent of persons, on the inner aspect of the navicular, as a separate navicular tuberosity. It is usually bilateral, but may be unilateral.

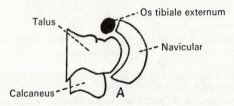

Fig. 338. The os tibiale externum. (Redrawn from Holland.)

This accessory ossicle may be associated with pain and redness on the inner side of the navicular which has been precipitated or aggravated by footwear.

Os trigonum or accessory talus (astragalus)

This bone (*Fig.* 339) exists usually as the lateral tubercle of the posterior border of the talus. In 7 per cent of cases, the lateral tubercle is a separate bone which is known as the os trigonum. In a radiograph it is seen as a separate ossicle in the angle between the posterior border of the talus and the upper surface of the calcaneus. Very exceptionally the ossicle may be fused with the upper surface of the calcaneus.

PATHOLOGY OF BONE

Diseases of bone show a decided predilection for certain anatomical sites, and the same may be said of tumours affecting bone. Similarly, some diseases

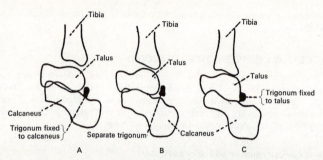

Fig. 339. The os trigonum; A, Os trigonum fused to calcaneus; B, Separate os trigonum; C, Trigonum fused to talus. (Redrawn from Holland.)

attack membrane bones out of choice, others select cartilage bones.

Membrane bones

1. Although frequently complicated in shape, their ossification is for the most part simple, e.g. one or two ossific centres only, as they are protective and not weight bearing.
2. They have very poor regenerative powers; thus the bone of the skull vault shows no regenerative power, so that the defects occasioned by trauma or disease are permanent unless filled in by bone grafting. The mandible, however, shows, strong regenerative powers.
3. Association with special pathological conditions:
   i. They escape pathological change in the disease of achondroplasia.
   ii. They are the only bones affected in the disease of craniocleido-dysostosis.
   iii. They may be affected by acute pyogenic osteomyelitis though this is uncommon.
   iv. They are the only bones affected by creeping periostitis (leontiasis).
   v. They are common sites of ivory osteoma.

Cartilage bones

1. CONGENITAL BONE DISEASE:
   i. Cartilage-capped exostosis grows from the region of the metaphysis of a long bone. It is usually single.
   ii. Multiple exostoses, or diaphysial aclasia, also grow from the ends of the shaft of a long bone, but affect only those parts of the skeleton where a

core of bone formed in cartilage becomes ensheathed in a layer of bone formed by the periosteum.

iii. Achondroplasia affects the bones formed in cartilage.

2. TRAUMA: Separation of the epiphysis is never a pure separation but rather a fracture separation.

3. INFECTION:

i. Acute osteomyelitis is a disease of childhood. It has a marked predilection for the long bones. The part of the bone affected is the metaphysis, because of the rich blood supply and the fact that the arteries are end arteries in this region. These considerations, in the presence of mild injury to the bone and a symptomless bacteraemia, may precipitate the formation of acute infection in the bone.

ii. Chronic osteomyelitis, due to causes like tuberculosis, typhoid etc.; often chooses the metaphysis of a long bone, but has a tendency also to affect bones like vertebrae, ribs, hip bone and sternum.

iii. Tuberculosis of the short long bones (metacarpals and phalanges) is located in the middle of the diaphysis instead of at the metaphysis because of the peculiarities of the blood supply of these bones.

iv. Tuberculosis of a vertebra begins in one of three sites:

   a. In the upper or lower metaphysis of the body of the bone, i.e. just beneath the plate of cartilage in relation to the epiphysis of the upper or lower surface of the body.

   b. Just beneath the anterior longitudinal ligament where the vessels supplying the front of the body of the bone enter it.

   c. In one of the vertebral processes. This is rare.

v. The epiphysis is relatively immune to bone disease except by extension from the shaft or neighbouring joint, but osteomyelitis, especially syphilitic, sometimes attacks this part of the bone.

vi. The metaphysis is frequently partly or wholly intracapsular. It follows that bone diseases may readily erupt into a joint and vice versa.

vii. Inflammation often destroys large parts of a bone. The dead bone is cast off in the form of sequestra. The restoration of the bone depends on the bone-forming functions of the periosteum. This structure is therefore treated with the greatest care by the surgeon.

viii. Bone differs from other tissues in the body in that it cannot contract because of its rigidity. It follows that cavities in bone often go on discharging unless some surgical method of obliterating the cavity is resorted to.

4. TUMOURS: Tumours often show a remarkable constancy in the bony sites which they choose (*Fig.* 340).

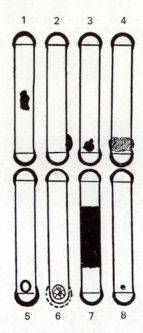

Fig. 340. Pathology of bone in terms of anatomy. The characteristic situations of the various types of tumours of bone. The cross-line is the epiphysial cartilage. (1) Metastatic carcinoma; (2) periosteal fibrosarcoma; (3) solitary chondroma; (4) osteogenic sarcoma; (5) solitary cyst of osteitis fibrosa; (6) benign giant-cell tumour; (7) Ewing's tumour; (8) acute osteomyelitis.

SURGICAL APPROACH TO THE LONG BONES

Humerus

The shaft of this bone is much more difficult to expose than that of the femur. The reasons are:

1. The axillary and brachial neurovascular bundle is related to the inner part of the shaft above, and the front of the shaft below.
2. The musculocutaneous nerve crosses the front of the shaft very obliquely from medial to lateral.
3. The radial nerve crosses the back of the shaft from medial to lateral.

UPPER THIRD: The incision is the same as that for the anterior exposure of the shoulder joint, i.e. between contiguous borders of deltoid and pectoralis major, along the upper part of the cephalic vein.

LOWER TWO-THIRDS: An incision is made in the line of the medial or lateral intermuscular septum. If the incision is a lateral one, the radial nerve is in the same line as the cut. If it is medial, the incision is between the median and ulnar nerves.

WHOLE SHAFT: To expose the whole shaft, the skin incision follows the cephalic vein from the tip of the coracoid process to the level of the bend of the elbow, and continues in the midline of the flexor aspect of the forearm in its upper third (*Fig.* 341). (The incision will of course be shorter if it is required to expose less of the shaft.)

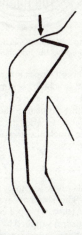

Fig. 341. Henry's incision for exposure of whole length of the humeral shaft. The black line represents the cut through the skin and deep fascia. The arrow marks the acromioclavicular joint. If it is desired to expose the shoulder joint an incision is carried outwards (from the upper end of the main incision) along the anterior border of the clavicle, and the deltoid is detached from this bone and thrown laterally as a muscle flap.

The incision is deepened between the deltoid and pectoralis major above, and then along the outer edge of the biceps. The outer one-quarter of the brachialis muscle projects lateral to the biceps. This part of the brachialis is separated from the rest of this muscle by deepening the incision to the bone

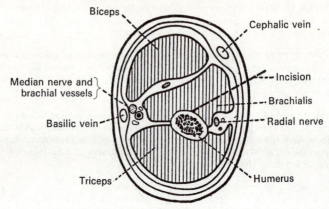

Fig. 342. To show the manner in which Henry's incision for exposure of the humeral shaft avoids the radial nerve by splitting the brachialis.

(*Fig.* 342). This part of the incision slopes inwards, reaching the bone in the midline. The outer part of the brachialis is in reality a migrated part of the triceps and is supplied by the radial nerve. Thus the nerve supply of the brachialis is not impaired by this exposure. The outer part of the brachialis forms a protection for the radial nerve when the muscles are stripped from the shaft. The incision through the brachialis stops 4 cm above the epicondyle so as not to enter the elbow joint.

Radius

This bone may be exposed in its whole length by an incision along the anterior border of the brachioradialis. This landmark is the frontier line between the structures on the medial side (flexors) supplied by the median nerve, and those on the lateral side (extensors) supplied by the radial. The incision in its lower two-thirds is also that for exposure of the radial artery. This artery, and the superficial branch of the radial nerve, lie in the line of the cut and are actually exposed by it. In the lower half of the forearm the radial nerve is retracted laterally and the artery medially, as here the nerve is passing posteriorly and laterally. The supinator is exposed proximally and its fibres are detached and retracted laterally, care being taken of the dorsal interosseous nerve which is in the muscle at the level of the neck of the radius. The pronator quadratus distally is detached and retracted medially.

Ulna

The dorsal border is subcutaneous throughout its length. The bone may be exposed by an incision in this line, the extensor carpi ulnaris being lateral and the flexor carpi ulnaris medial.

Femur
See Fig. 343.

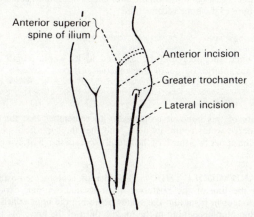

Fig. 343. Showing the anterior and lateral incisions of the femoral shaft.

LATERAL APPROACH: The shaft may safely be exposed by an incision from the greater trochanter to the outer condyle. This incision divides the iliotibial band and is deepened to the bone along the posterior border of the vastus lateralis, i.e. in the line of the lateral intermuscular septum. The vastus lateralis is detached from the linea aspera and any perforating vessels that may be encountered are ligated. The incision cuts the transverse branch of the lateral femoral circumflex artery above and the superior lateral geniculate artery below.

ANTERIOR APPROACH: The femoral shaft is exposed along its anterior surface below the level of the lesser trochanter. Excellent exposure is obtained and no important structures are damaged. The incision extends from the anterior superior iliac spine to the outer border of the patella. The deep fascia being divided, the vastus lateralis is separated from the rectus femoris. Under these muscles lies the vastus intermedius. The nerve to the vastus lateralis and the descending branch of the lateral circumflex artery form a neurovascular bundle crossing the upper part of the vastus intermedius. They are retracted up and the muscle is divided down to the bone. The suprapatellar pouch extends three finger-breadths above the upper patellar border. The cut is not extended so far down. If necessary the pouch may be separated from the femur without injury and this part of the shaft exposed, though efforts to free the pouch from the overlying quadriceps tendon will result in injury to the bursa and an opening into the knee joint. Because of the existence of this extension from the knee joint there can be no question that in cases of infection the lateral incision is safer, at least as far as the lower third of the bone is concerned.

Tibia

Like the ulna, the tibia may be exposed in its whole length along its subcutaneous anterior border or anteromedial surface.

Fibula

In exposure of this bone, it is necessary to remember that the common peroneal nerve winds round its neck, and that the superficial peroneal is related to the upper two-thirds of the lateral aspect of the shaft, lying between the peronei.

UPPER AND MIDDLE THIRDS: The incision is along the posterolateral border in the line of the posterior intermuscular septum, exposing the peroneus longus in front and the soleus behind in the upper third, and the flexor hallucis longus behind in the middle third of the bone. At the upper part of the incision care is taken of the common peroneal nerve.

LOWER THIRD: The incision extends along the anterolateral border between the peroneus tertius in front and peroneus brevis behind.

WHOLE SHAFT: This may be exposed by an incision behind the peroneal muscles (Kocher).

AMPUTATIONS

The indications for amputation of a limb are that the limb is dead, dangerous or useless. The following general principles should be kept in mind:

1. LEVEL OF AMPUTATION: The level of amputation is influenced by the following factors:
   i. *Healing of the Stump:* This is especially important in vascular disease where healing of the stump is dependent on the collateral circulation. If the collateral circulation is inadequate for the length of the stump, healing will not occur. The collateral circulation can be judged

clinically by the appearance of the skin and underlying tissues, hair growth and skin temperature. Intra-operatively, bleeding from vessels in the skin and muscle suggest that healing will occur. Laboratory methods such as measuring the skin oxygen tension have also been used.

ii. *Age of the Patient:* In an elderly patient with central nervous disease where there is no hope of a prosthesis ever being worn, a more proximal level of amputation is chosen to ensure primary healing.

In children the main problems that arise from amputation are those that are associated with subsequent growth. A midthigh or forearm amputation in a child does not grow in proportion to the rest of the body because growth would have continued longer at the knee and wrist. The opposite applies to below-knee and above-elbow stumps which become progressively longer. A revision of the amputation may be necessary before cessation of growth.

iii. *Joint Contractures:* These are particularly common in the knee and hip joints. A fixed flexion contracture will make the wearing of a prosthesis impossible so that the level of amputation is influenced by other factors.

iv. *Cosmesis:* Disarticulation of the knee provides a strong end-bearing stump, but the jointed side steels of the prosthesis are unattractive. This type of amputation is more suitable for the elderly patient.

v. *Lower Limb:* In the lower limb return of function is much better after a below-knee than after an above-knee amputation.

2. TISSUES:
  i. *Skin Flaps:* The skin flaps are comprised of skin and fascia and are usually of equal length with their bases at the level of bone section. The combined length of the skin flaps is slightly more than the diameter of the limb. An exception is a below-knee amputation which has a long posterior flap because the main blood supply is found posteriorly.

  ii. *The Muscle:* The muscles are cut back obliquely from the skin incision to the site of bone section.

In lower limb amputations the muscles are sutured over the bone ends (myoplasty) or the muscles are sutured to a hole drilled in the bone (myodesis). A myoplasty or myodesis keeps the muscles at approximately their resting length and preserves muscle balance around the proximal joint. The stump is therefore better able to move the artificial limb.

  iii. *Bone:* The periosteum is cut circumferentially at the level of bone section. The bone must not be devascularized by being stripped of its periosteum.

  iv. *Vessels:* The major arteries and veins are doubly ligated.

  v. *Nerves:* The nerves are gently stretched and then divided to allow them to retract into the muscles. The sciatic, tibial and median nerves each have a companion artery of supply which may require ligation after dissecting it away from the nerve.

Lower limb amputations

TOES:
1. Amputations through the first interphalangeal joint of the outer four toes or through the 1st phalanx are not advised, as the remaining stump is of little use and may form a troublesome projection.
2. Even if single toes are amputated there is a tendency for secondary deformities to develop. Amputation of the 2nd toe leads to a hallux valgus deformity of the big toe. Amputation of the 5th toe leads to trauma of the head of the 5th metatarsal which predisposes to the formation of a tender bursa.

RAY EXCISION OF A TOE: This is a very useful amputation in diabetics with infection of a toe. A circular incision is made round the dorsal aspect of the toe, then through the webspace on either side of the affected toe to meet halfway along the length of the plantar aspect of the foot. The ligaments on either side of the metatarsal head are divided and the shaft of the metatarsal bone is sectioned as far proximally as necessary. In diabetics the wound is not sutured.

TRANSMETATARSAL AMPUTATION: This amputation (*Fig.* 344) is recommended in diabetics with gangrene of two or more toes, but in whom the peripheral pulses are palpable.

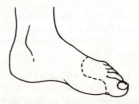

Fig. 344. Transmetatarsal amputation.

The incision passes across the dorsum of the foot, just distal to the anticipated level of the bone section. The plantar incision extends to a level 1 cm proximal and parallel to the flexion creases of the toes. The plantar flap is longer, on the medial side, to cover the greater thickness of the foot on this side.

The dorsal incision is carried down to bone and the plantar incision down to the joint capsule. The soft tissues on the plantar aspect are separated from the metatarsals with a periosteal elevator up to the level of bone section. The metatarsals are divided individually with a Gigli saw. The flexor and extensor tendons are pulled down and divided.

The fascia and skin of the plantar flap are sutured to the fascia and skin of the dorsal flap; alternatively the flap may be left open for secondary suture.

SYME'S AMPUTATION: This is a classic example of an end-bearing stump. The amputation is so designed that the heel pad covers the lower end of the tibia after section of the malleoli and the distal articular surface of the tibia. The operation cannot be performed in diabetics because a neuropathy will result in ulceration of the heel pad.

BELOW-KNEE AMPUTATION: The anterior skin flap is formed by a transverse skin incision which extends two-thirds of the circumference of the leg at a level 14 cm from the joint line of the knee (*see Fig.* 345). The bone is also sectioned at this level which is the optimal length, but even a stump 5 cm in length can be fitted with a prosthesis. The posterior skin flap extends distally to a point where the gastrocnemius and soleus muscles become tendinous. The posterior skin flap should be rectangular and not tapered.

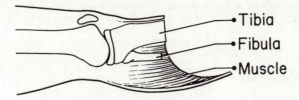

Fig. 345. Below-knee amputation.

The anterior tibial and peroneal muscles are divided in the line of the anterior skin flap. The periosteum of the tibia is raised proximally for a short distance and the tibia is divided with a Gigli saw; the anterior subcutaneous border of the tibia is bevelled to avoid pressure on the skin.

The fibula is divided 1·5 cm proximal to the tibia. The deep muscles of the calf are divided at the level of bone section, but the soleus and gastrocnemius muscles are left attached to the fascia down to the level of the posterior skin incision. The fascia of the gastrocnemius is sutured to the periosteum of the tibia and the fascia of the anterior compartment.

THROUGH-KNEE AMPUTATION: *See* Chapter 38.

TRANSFEMORAL AMPUTATION: Equal anterior and posterior skin flaps are used. The bone is sectioned 25 cm distal to the greater trochanter. The muscles are cut obliquely back to the level of bone section.

The extensor muscles are sutured to the hamstring muscles, and the lateral and medial muscle bellies are sutured to these muscles (myoplastic amputation). The fascia and then the skin flaps are sutured.

The shorter the thigh stump the more inefficient does it become as a lever to activate an artificial limb. The irreducible limit for a useful stump is a bone section 6·5 cm below the perineum or 11·5–12·5 cm distal to the tip of the greater trochanter.

SUBTROCHANTERIC AMPUTATION: The bone is sectioned just below the level of the lesser trochanter. Such amputees are fitted with a limb on the top of which is a platform called a 'tilting table'. If the hip joint is disarticulated (as may be necessary, e.g. in sarcoma of the femur), then the outer surface of the hip bone is so smooth that the patient has a constant sensation of slipping in his splint. If the upper end of the femur is left, then the stump has a square end on which the patient sits much more securely. In these amputations, most of the muscles are cut away from the hip bone, and the flap is a single posterior one with the scar lying below and parallel to the inguinal ligament.

HINDQUARTER AMPUTATION: This amputation is performed almost exclusively for malignant disease of the bone or soft tissues of the pelvis and thigh. The lower limb together with the hip bone are removed from the patient.

The upper limbs

AMPUTATION OF THE FINGERS: *See* Chapter 36.

FOREARM AMPUTATION: Equal anterior and posterior flaps are marked out with the forearm in supination. If the arm is in pronation, the elasticity of the skin draws the flaps into an oblique position.

The optimum length of radius and ulna should be 17 cm measured from the olecranon prominence. Short forearm stumps may also be of value, but the shortest length compatible with the efficient activation of a prosthesis is a stump with 8 cm of ulna. Pronation and supination should be retained in forearm amputations whenever possible. Ability to rotate adds considerably to the value of a forearm stump. Rotation is lost if the bone ends become joined by fibrous or bony ankylosis.

THROUGH-ARM AMPUTATION: The optimum length of an arm stump measured from the tip of the acromion is 20 cm. The shortest length of humerus which can be fitted with a useful prosthesis is a 13-cm stump, measured from the tip of the acromion.

FOREQUARTER AMPUTATION: In this amputation the upper limb, scapula and lateral two-thirds of the clavicle are removed from the patient. It is performed for malignant disease.

ARTIFICIAL LIMBS

Site of weight bearing

1. END-BEARING PROSTHESIS: In a through-knee disarticulation the patient 'stands' in the socket of the artificial limb, the weight being distributed over the lower surfaces of the femoral condyles.

2. PROXIMAL-BEARING PROSTHESIS: In a transfemoral amputation, the weight is borne by the ischial tuberosity and in a below-knee amputation by the middle of the patellar ligament, the lower border of the patella, the anteromedial flared end of the proximal tibia, and the fibula below the head.

Sockets

1. SUCTION-SOCKETED LIMB: The above-knee prosthesis contains a total contact-bearing socket which fits so perfectly that it is held in place partly by a vacuum created between the stump and the socket. It is most suitable for the young or middle-aged amputee.

2. NON-SUCTION LIMB: There is a less intimate fit of the stump in the socket and the limb is suspended by a waist band.

Chapter 33

SHOULDER JOINT

The shoulder joint should not be considered as a single entity but as a component of the whole shoulder girdle, comprising the scapula, clavicle and humerus with five linkages (*Fig.* 346).
  1. Glenohumeral joint.
  2. A functional linkage between the scapula and the thorax (scapulothoracic linkage).
  3. A functional linkage between the head of the humerus and the coraco-acromial arch (the suprahumeral articulation).

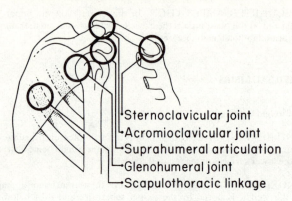

- Sternoclavicular joint
- Acromioclavicular joint
- Suprahumeral articulation
- Glenohumeral joint
- Scapulothoracic linkage

Fig. 346. The shoulder joint.

    4. Acromioclavicular joint.
    5. Sternoclavicular joint.

Normal function of the shoulder girdle requires the smooth coordination of all these joints and linkages. Impairment in any one joint leads to functional impairment of the whole complex.

The main function of the shoulder in man is to enable him to place his hand where he wishes to use it, in a coordinated and controlled manner.

From a weight-bearing front leg of a quadruped to the highly mobile and adaptive shoulder girdle of man, substantial phylogenetic changes have had to occur. The shoulder girdle in man has sacrificed stability for mobility, which gives rise to much of the pathology in the shoulder joint.

GLENOHUMERAL JOINT

The glenohumeral joint is a ball-and-socket joint, but with a very shallow socket allowing considerable mobility.

Movement in a 'congruous' ball-and-socket joint, such as the hip, takes place about a more or less fixed central axis. This affords stability to a joint. In an 'incongruous' ball-and-socket joint there is no fixed axis of rotation but rather an ever-changing axis of rotation. This fact has two important implications:

    1. The capsule in an 'incongruous' joint must be sufficiently flexible to allow this changing axis of movement to occur.
    2. The muscles that move the joint must also provide stability to the joint.

Bone

The glenoid fossa faces upwards laterally and forwards. The area of the glenoid is increased by the glenoid labrum which is a fibrous structure (not fibrocartilage as previously thought).

Capsule

The glenohumeral capsule is a thin-walled capacious structure with several outpouchings, which are seen on arthrography. It attaches around the perimeter of the glenoid rim and around the anatomical neck of the humerus. A portion of the epiphysial line of the proximal humerus is intracapsular, thus explaining the occasional appearance of septic arthritis following metaphysial osteomyelitis.

Ligaments

The anterior glenohumeral ligaments are condensations in the anterior capsule. These may be divided into three bands: the superior, middle and lower glenohumeral ligaments. A defect exists between the superior and middle band. This defect acquires importance in anterior dislocation of the shoulder.

Muscles of the glenohumeral joint

There are five prime movers of the glenohumeral joint. These are the deltoid muscle and four other muscles which are known collectively as the rotator cuff. They are: subscapularis, supraspinatus, infraspinatus and teres minor (*Fig.* 347).

These muscles constitute rotators of the humerus but are also of great importance in abduction.

THE SUPRASPINATUS: The supraspinatus originates from the supraspina-tus fossa of the scapula and passes under the coraco-acromial arch and inserts on the greater tubercle of the humeral head just lateral to the bicipital groove. It is innervated by the suprascapular nerve, C4, C5 and C6.

THE INFRASPINATUS: The infraspinatus originates from the infraspinatus fossa of the scapula and inserts into the greater tubercle of the humerus adjacent to the supraspinatus.

TERES MINOR: The teres minor originates from the superior half of the axillary border of the scapula and inserts into the greater tubercle just behind and below the infraspinatus. It is innervated by the axillary nerve, C5 and C6.

THE SUBSCAPULARIS: The subscapularis originates from the entire anterior surface of the scapula and inserts into the lesser tubercle of the

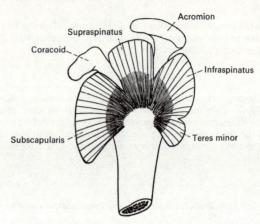

Fig. 347. The black shading shows the musculotendinous cuff.

humerus anterior and medial to the bicipital groove. The subscapularis is separated from the neck of the scapula by a bursa. It is innervated by the upper and lower subscapular nerves.

THE DELTOID MUSCLE: The deltoid muscle is a multipennate muscle with three main portions. Each portion can act independently or it can act in harmony with the other portions. To achieve smooth action of the shoulder, it has to work in close coordination with the rotator cuff.

The anterior portion originates from the anterior border of the clavicle and acts as a flexor and abductor of the arm. The middle portion originates from the lateral border of the acromion process and acts as an abductor. The posterior portion originates from the lower border of the spine of the scapula and acts as an extensor and abductor of the arm. The whole muscle inserts into deltoid tubercle on the anterolateral surface of the humerus. The nerve supply is the axillary nerve, C5 and C6.

Nerve supply

Attention should be drawn to Hilton's law, which states that a joint is supplied by branches from the nerves which supply the muscles moving the joint and the skin over the joint. In joint disease, therefore, the irritation of the nerves causes a reflex spasm of the muscles which fixes the joint in the position of greatest comfort and may cause pain referred to the overlying skin.

The sensory branches of the suprascapular nerve constitute the main sensory nerve supply to the acromioclavicular and glenohumeral joints. In conditions of severe shoulder pain, this nerve can be easily blocked by injecting local anaesthetic solution 0·5 cm above a point on the scapular spine. This point is defined by bisecting the scapular spine and again bisecting the lateral half.

Glenohumeral movement

Movements that can occur at the glenohumeral joint are flexion (forward), extension (backward), abduction, internal rotation and external rotation. The deltoid is the main mover of the shoulder. In patients with axillary nerve paralysis, and thus no deltoid action, all movements are exceedingly weak.

With the arm by the side, the deltoid acting in isolation elevates the humeral head in the glenoid socket against the acromion. It cannot initiate abduction (*Fig.* 348).

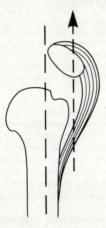

Fig. 348. With the arm, dependent contraction of the deltoid elevates the humeral head in the glenoid socket against the humerus.

Abduction at the shoulder

This is a complex movement (*Fig.* 349) which can for convenience be separated into two coordinated events.

Firstly: at the glenohumeral joint which allows for only about 120 degrees abduction, being limited by impingement of the greater tubercle of the humerus on the acromion process.

Secondly: at the scapulothoracic linkage which allows further abduction.

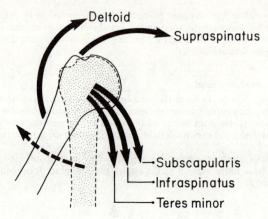

Fig. 349. Combined rotator cuff and deltoid action upon the glenohumeral articulation. Abduction of the humerus is the result of combined action of the supraspinatus adducting the head into the fossa, the teres minor, infraspinatus and subscapularis adducting and depressing the head, and the deltoid acting as an abductor when working with these cuff muscles. There is a downward gliding movement of the head of the humerus.

1. Abduction at the glenohumeral joint is a coordinated movement involving the deltoid muscle and the rotator cuff. The latter holds the head in the glenoid socket while the deltoid, assisted by the supraspinatus, produces abduction. This movement will only allow 90 degrees of abduction, when the greater tubercle of the humerus impinges on the acromion. For a further 30 degrees of abduction to occur the humerus must be externally rotated allowing the greater tubercle to pass posterior to the acromion. This external rotation is produced by the short external rotators.

   Glenohumeral movement must be associated with a downward slide of the head of the humerus at the socket, because the head is larger than the socket. This downward slide is produced by the infraspinatus, teres minor and subscapular muscles. The infraspinatus and teres minor also act as short external rotators while the subscapularis acts as an internal rotator.

   It is to be noted that in internal rotation of the humerus, only 60 degrees of abduction can occur at the glenohumeral joint. This is one of the reasons why abduction is limited by operations for recurrent dislocation of the shoulder that deliberately shorten the subscapularis muscle preventing external rotation.

   Total abduction at the glenohumeral joint is 120 degrees. The shoulder girdle, however, can be abducted 180 degrees. The additional 60 degrees of abduction takes place at the scapulothoracic linkage.

2. Abduction at the scapulothoracic linkage is an important component. While the scapulothoracic movement is being described here as if it occurs only after full glenohumeral abduction has occurred, it should be stressed that the glenohumeral and the scapulothoracic movements in fact occur concurrently and not sequentially.

The scapula glides on the posterior thoracic wall. Upward rotation is accomplished by the synchronous action of two muscles, trapezius and serratus anterior.

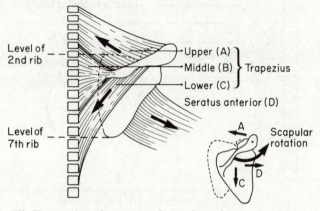

Fig. 350. The trapezius and serratus anterior muscles produce rotation of the scapula.

The trapezius is a fan-shaped muscle and consists of an upper, middle and lower part (*Fig.* 350). The upper part originates from the ligamentum nuchae of the lower cervical spine, the posterior spinous processes of the cervical spine and upper thoracic spine. It inserts into the upper border of the spine of the scapula. Their action is to elevate the scapula and rotate it upwards about the axis of the acromioclavicular joint.

The middle fibres originate from the spinous processes of the upper thoracic vertebrae and insert into the medial border of the scapular spine. Their action is to stabilize the scapula during abduction.

The lower fibres originate from the spinous processes of the lower thoracic spine and insert into the lower border of the medial half of the scapular spine. Their action is to depress the scapula and rotate the glenoid fossa upwards.

The combined action of the trapezius is to rotate the scapula resulting in the glenoid fossa pointing upward.

The serratus anterior originates from the upper eight ribs on the anterolateral chest wall and inserts into the lower medial border of the scapula. It also produces upward rotation of the glenoid.

The other muscles acting on the scapula are of less importance. They are levator scapulae, rhomboid major and minor. Their combined action is to rotate the glenoid fossa downwards (*Fig.* 351). This downward movement of the glenoid is supplemented by latissimus dorsi and pectoralis major acting indirectly via their humeral attachments.

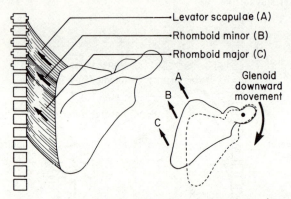

Levator scapulae (A)

Rhomboid minor (B)

Rhomboid major (C)

Glenoid downward movement

Fig. 351. The levator scapulae, rhomboid major and minor elevate the vertebral border of the scapula and produce downward rotation of the glenoid fossa.

The total range of rotation of the scapula is 60 degrees. This rotation takes place about the acromioclavicular joint.

THE SUPRAHUMERAL ARTICULATION

This consists of the coraco-acromial arch above (*Fig.* 352), protecting the head of the humerus below, with the subdeltoid/subacromial bursa (*Fig.* 353) interposed to provide smooth movement between these bony components. The coraco-acromial arch consists of the coracoid process, the acromion and the coraco-acromial ligament joining the two. The arch would prevent upward dislocation if abnormal upward force is exerted on the humerus, but under normal circumstances there is a space of about 1·5 cm between the bony components of the articulation. However, in the process of abduction the upper end of the humerus would tend to impinge on the arch at about 90 degrees of abduction.

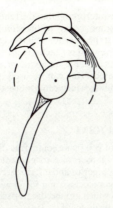

Fig. 352. The coraco-acromial arch.

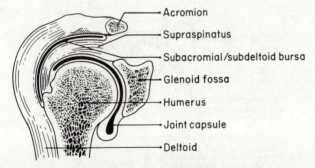

Acromion

Supraspinatus

Subacromial/subdeltoid bursa

Glenoid fossa

Humerus

Joint capsule

Deltoid

Fig. 353. The subacromial/subdeltoid bursa.

Between the humeral head and the coraco-acromial arch there is the rotator cuff formed by fusion of the tendons of the subscapularis anteriorly, supraspinatus superiorly and infraspinatus and teres minor posteriorly. In the event of impingement, this rotator cuff would be jammed between the bones to cause a potential irritation of the supraspinatus tendon at that site.

The subacromial/subdeltoid bursa is situated superior to the rotator cuff and communicates with the shoulder joint in 10 per cent of people; this must not be misinterpreted in arthrography.

The long head of biceps muscle arises from the supraglenoid tubercle of the scapula. Its tendon crosses the humeral head within the capsule of the shoulder joint, but is extrasynovial, and descends in the intertubercular sulcus of the humerus. It could be interpreted that the tendon slides up and down in the bicipital groove during movement of the shoulder, but a more correct interpretation would be that the intertubercular sulcus is sliding up and down on a fixed tendon. This movement is a factor in attrition of the tendon.

The long head of biceps can act as an abductor of the shoulder when the humerus is externally rotated. This can be used as a 'trick movement' in patients with abductor paralysis which can confuse the clinician.

ACROMIOCLAVICULAR JOINT

The acromioclavicular joint is a plane joint. It is divided into two by a disc analogous to a meniscus. It is prone to early degeneration. Stability is accomplished by the strong superior and inferior acromioclavicular ligaments and also by the important coracoclavicular ligaments. These latter ligaments consist of two components which are the flat trapezoid ligament lying lateral to the cone-shaped conoid ligament (*Fig.* 354).

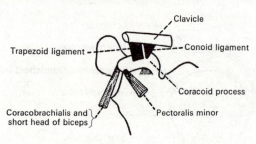

Fig. 354. The coracoclavicular ligaments.

For acromioclavicular dislocation to occur, all these ligaments must be ruptured. The function of these ligaments is to hold the scapula to the clavicle.

THE STERNOCLAVICULAR JOINT

The sternoclavicular joint is a plane joint that acts like a ball-and-socket joint. Degeneration in this joint is uncommon.

Movement at the acromioclavicular and sternoclavicular joints

The scapula is able to rotate 60 degrees of which 30 degrees can be accommodated by simple clavicular evelation at the sternoclavicular joint

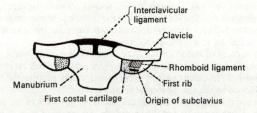

Fig. 355. The sternoclavicular joint and its ligaments.

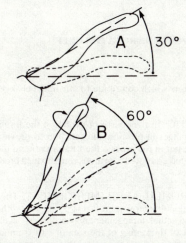

Fig. 356. A, The first 30 degrees of scapular rotation is associated with 30 degrees of clavicular elevation. B, The next 30 degrees of scapular rotation is associated with rotation of the 'crank-shaped' clavicle about its long axis.

(*Fig.* 355). The remaining 30 degrees of scapular rotation occurs by rotation of the 'crank-shaped' clavicle about its long axis (*Fig.* 356).

COMPOSITE SHOULDER GIRDLE MOVEMENT

The movement of each of the components of the shoulder girdle has been considered individually. In fact, movement of the shoulder is a smooth integrated movement which has been called 'scapulohumeral rhythm'.

Of every 3 degrees of abduction of the arm, 2 degrees take place at the glenohumeral joint and 1 degree at the scapulothoracic linkage. This 2:1 relationship remains constant throughout the full range of movement. Thus at 180 degrees, or full elevation, 60 degrees has occurred at the scapulothoracic linkage and 120 degress at the glenohumeral joint.

Only 60 degrees of abduction can take place at the glenohumeral joint with the humerus in internal rotation. At this point, the arm will be elevated 90 degrees; further elevation can only occur by externally rotating the humerus. This is achieved by the short external rotators.

Rotation of the scapula is accompanied first by elevation of the clavicle to 30 degrees. Further rotation of the scapula is accompanied by rotation of the clavicle in its long axis.

LESIONS INVOLVING THE ROTATOR CUFF

Aetiology

There are four factors which contribute to attritional changes in the rotator cuff.

1. PHYLOGENETIC: In the course of evolution the forelimb has undergone significant changes in position and function to provide a remarkable degree of mobility, but in the process the rotator cuff and the tendon of the long head of biceps have adopted a tortuous course which predisposes them to attritional influences.

2. CORACO-ACROMIAL ARCH IMPINGEMENT: The space between the arch and the glenohumeral joint is 1–1·5 cm, but with abduction this space is reduced and actual impingement may occur, especially if this space is reduced as a result of thickening of the rotator cuff from acute or chronic inflammation or bony spurs secondary to chronic arthritis of the shoulder joint.

3. BLOOD SUPPLY TO THE ROTATOR CUFF: A 'critical zone' of relatively decreased blood supply has been identified in the supraspinatus tendon about 1 cm proximal to its insertion into the greater tubercle of the humerus (*Fig.* 357). Traction on the supraspinatus tendon by contraction of its muscle or by the dependent position of the humerus attenuates the vessels in the critical zone which becomes relatively ischaemic. This is the most common site of attritional change.

4. STRUCTURAL CHANGES WITH AGEING: With advancing age there is a decrease in the number and size of the tenoblasts and tenocytes, as well as a decrease in water and mucopolysaccharide content.

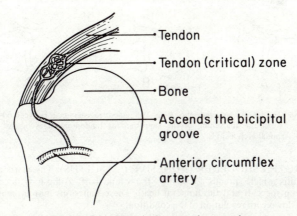

Fig. 357. Critical zone in the supraspinatus tendon.

Pathology

This follows a sequence of 'wear and tear and repair'. Degeneration takes place in the 'critical zone' with resultant inflammatory swelling of the cuff which may, in turn, cause impingement in abduction. Progressive degeneration may lead to small or large tears in the supraspinatus tendon. Small tears may heal, but major tears are irreversible, with persistent symptoms.

Clinical syndromes

1. ACUTE CALCIFIC TENDINITIS: The patient presents with acute severe pain in his shoulder. Calcium hydroxyapatite crystals deposit in the 'critical zone'. An intense vascular reaction occurs causing the calcium to become resorbed and within a few weeks the patient is back to normal.

2. CHRONIC TENDINITIS (PAINFUL ARC SYNDROME): This syndrome (*Fig.* 358) is characterized by a chronic thickening of the tendon of the supraspinatus resulting in a typical impingement syndrome with pain experienced between 60 and 120 degrees abduction.

The inflamed area can be identified by locating a tender spot to palpation in the shoulder, but in full abduction the tender spot will be under the coraco-acromial arch and will then not be found on examination.

This condition usually subsides with conservative (anti-inflammatory) treatment, but may require decompression of the subacromial space by acromionectomy, acromioclavicular ligament resection or acromioplasty which prevent repeated impingement with abduction.

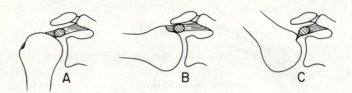

Fig. 358. The painful arc syndrome, A–C, The patient registers pain between 60–120 degrees, when the thickening of the supraspinatus tendon impinges against the coraco-acromial arch as in B.

3. FROZEN SHOULDER (ADHESIVE CAPSULITIS): This starts as a tendinitis which spreads to involve the whole cuff. Adhesions develop between the cuff and the humeral head. These adhesions may ultimately break down with resolution of the condition.

4. ROTATOR CUFF TEARS: These usually occur in association with the unresolving chronic tendinitis. The tear may be partial, disrupting only the deep surface of the tendon, or complete, so that the joint communicates with the subacromial bursa. Partial tears can heal, but with complete tears healing does not occur.

In a younger patient with a normal rotator cuff, tearing can occur from an inappropriate load being placed on an unprepared joint such as when falling onto the shoulder. Pain is felt immediately, radiating from the deltoid insertion. In a partial tear there is greater limitation of active (to 60 degrees) than of passive abduction in the presence of a normally contracting deltoid. If the arm is passively abducted to above 90 degrees, the patient will be able to hold it in this position and even abduct it further, because the tear will have moved beyond the site of impingement and pain will no longer limit movement.

Active and passive abduction are painful in both partial and complete tears. The pain is abolished by injecting local anaesthetic. If relief of pain makes active abduction possible the tear is only partial.

Complete tears in young patients should be sutured. In elderly patients surgery is not usually indicated.

LESIONS OF THE BICEPS TENDON

Tendinitis

Because the long head of biceps tendon is intimately involved with the capsule of the shoulder joint, it is frequently involved by inflammatory processes affecting this joint. The patient experiences pain in the shoulder and the tendon is tender to palpation in the intertubercular sulcus.

Rupture

A patient over the age of 50 feels something snap while lifting a heavy weight. The belly of the muscle is situated more distally than normal. Disability is surprisingly small and treatment is usually conservative.

CONGENITAL ANOMALIES OF THE SCAPULA

Sprengel's deformity

The scapulohumeral complex normally migrates from a cervical to a thoracic position from about the fifth week. Failure of descent results in congenital elevation of the scapula (Sprengel's deformity).

Two-thirds of children with Sprengel's deformity have associated skeletal anomalies such as abnormal vertebrae, renal anomalies or hypoplasia of the muscles of the pectoral girdle.

In more than a quarter of the patients there is a fibrous band, cartilaginous bar, or omovertebral bone, extending from the superior scapular angle to a posterior element of the 4th to 7th cervical vertebrae. Scapulocostal movement is limited but passive glenohumeral movement is almost normal in most cases.

Klippel–Feil syndrome

There is bilateral failure of scapular descent associated with marked anomalies of the cervical spine and failure of fusion of the occipital bones.

Clinically there is a low hairline in the neck and it looks as if the patient has no neck. The neck is webbed bilaterally and there is gross limitation of neck movement.

SUBLUXATION AND DISLOCATION

Dislocation of the glenohumeral joint takes place largely as a result of its inherent instability. Dislocation may be either anterior or posterior.

Anterior dislocation

Anterior dislocation accounts for about 97 per cent of dislocations because of the flimsy anterior capsule. It may occur at any age but, in the younger individual, the rate of recurrence is very high.

There are four types of anterior dislocation:
1. Subcoracoid.
2. Subglenoid.
3. Luxatio-erecta—an anterior dislocation in which the arm is abducted above the head.
4. Subclavicular.

Luxatio-erecta and subclavicular dislocations are very rare.

The mechanism of injury is either a direct injury to the shoulder or an indirect force usually from falling onto the outstretched hand.

The structures damaged in anterior dislocation of the shoulder include:
1. The glenoid labrum which is often torn off the glenoid. This usually starts antero-inferiorly and is called the 'Bankart lesion' after the man who described it.
2. The anterior capsular structures, including the subscapularis muscle.
3. A depressed fracture or dent in the posterolateral part of the head.
4. Fractures of the anterior rim of the glenoid.

Clinically the dislocation is usually obvious. The patient's arm is held in a position of external rotation. The shoulder appears flattened which in turn makes the acromion appear more prominent than usual.

Reduction of anterior dislocation of the shoulder joint

The basic principle of reduction is longitudinal traction to overcome muscle spasm and gentle manipulation of the head of the humerus into the glenoid cavity. Forced rotational movements of the humerus should be avoided because of the risk of fracture of the shaft of the humerus, especially in the older patient; therefore Kocher's manipulation is not favoured.

In recurrent dislocation the patient is often able to reduce his own dislocation. Treatment of this condition is surgical.

Posterior dislocation

Posterior dislocation of the shoulder is a rare condition accounting for less than 3 per cent of all shoulder dislocations. It occurs specifically in patients having epileptic fits and electric shocks such as lightning injuries.

Reduction of a posterior dislocation of the shoulder is performed according to the same principles as for anterior dislocation. The dislocation is reduced by applying traction to the limb.

Nerve damage associated with dislocations of the shoulder

The axillary nerve lies immediately below the humeral head. This nerve may occasionally be damaged by the dislocating shoulder. Its motor supply is to the deltoid muscle which often is difficult to test due to pain-restricting movement.

The axillary nerve, however, terminates by supplying sensation to a small area of skin 2·5 cm in diameter anterior to the deltoid tuberosity of the humerus. Sensation in this area should always be tested in patients with a dislocated shoulder.

The force producing the dislocation may continue after the dislocation has occurred. In such an event severe injuries of the brachial plexus may occur.

ASPIRATION OF THE SHOULDER JOINT

The shoulder joint can be aspirated anteriorly, posteriorly or laterally. The anterior approach is most convenient because, when the joint is distended with fluid, a fluctuant area is palpable anteriorly. The needle is inserted 1 cm inferior and 1 cm lateral to the coracoid process.

SURGICAL APPROACHES TO SHOULDER

In approaching the shoulder there are several important principles:
1. The surgeon must be clear what he wishes to expose.
2. The patient should be operated on in a 'sitting' position with a sandbag behind the scapula.
3. The arm should be draped separately to facilitate free movement of the limb.
4. An extra assistant is often required.
5. Blood should be readily available.

The shoulder can be approached from the front or the back. The following approaches will be considered.
1. Anterior exposure.
2. Axillary exposure.
3. Transacromial exposure.

Anterior exposure

INDICATIONS:
1. Irreducible anterior dislocation of the shoulder.
2. Recurrent anterior dislocation of the shoulder.
3. Fractures of the proximal humerus.
4. Arthroplasty.
5. Septic arthritis or tuberculosis of the shoulder.

POSITION OF THE PATIENT: The patient is placed in a semisitting position with a sandbag under the lowest part of the scapula of the affected shoulder.

INCISION: A 'shoulder-strap' incision is made from the deltoid tubercle anteriorly extending over the superior aspect of the shoulder to the spine of the scapula posteriorly (*Fig.* 359).

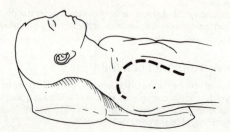

Fig. 359. The shoulder-strap incision.

DISSECTION: The deltopectoral groove, cephalic vein, and the deltoid branches of the thoraco-acromial vessels are identified. The deltopectoral groove is opened on the lateral side of the cephalic vein. It is usually unnecessary to divide this vein. The origin of the deltoid muscle on the clavicle is defined and this portion of the muscle, together with the adjacent periosteum or with part of the clavicle, is detached as a myoperiosteal or a myo-osteal flap, which can subsequently be repaired.

Structures encountered in the depths of the wound from above down are:

a. Tip of the coracoid giving origin to the coracobrachialis.
b. Tubercles of the humerus on rotating the limb in and out.
c. Surgical neck of humerus, mostly covered by (*d*).
d. Tendon of the pectoralis major.
e. Bicipital (intertubercular) sulcus containing the long tendon of the biceps which is covered by the pectoral tendon.

The muscles attached to the tubercles (subscapularis to lesser, and supraspinatus, infraspinatus, and teres minor to the greater) conceal the joint capsule. The latter is exposed by detaching the muscles from the tubercles or by detaching the tubercles themselves. The joint can then be opened.

If access to the anterior part of the rotator cuff is particularly required, exposure can be improved considerably by performing an osteotomy of the coracoid process and reflecting medially the tip of the coracoid process with the attached origins of the pectoralis minor, coracobrachialis and the short head of biceps. At the end of the operation, the tip of the coracoid process is screwed back into position, or the tip is excised subperiosteally and the muscles are sutured to the coracoid process.

The incision can be extended into the neck by dividing the clavicle three finger-breadths from its sternal end. It can also be extended distally by continuing the incision along the groove between the lateral edge of the biceps muscle and the brachialis muscle.

Axillary approach

This exposure is a cosmetically excellent, bloodless exposure of the anterior part of the glenohumeral joint and no important structures are damaged or traversed.

INDICATIONS: Recurrent antero-inferior dislocation of the shoulder particularly in young females (for whom an inconspicuous scar is important).

PROCEDURE: An 8-cm incision is made across the edge of the anterior fold of the axilla extending across the axilla (*Fig.* 360).

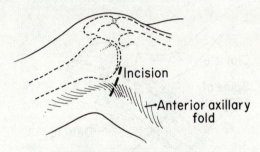

Fig. 360. The axillary incision.

The arm, which is free-draped, is held in a position of abduction and external rotation. The pectoralis major is retracted superiorly. The short head of biceps and coracobrachialis muscle will be noted laterally in the wound. The neurovascular bundle will be identified by palpation. Dissection follows the short head of biceps to beneath the coracoid process. The subscapularis will be noted posteriorly with the axillary nerve at its lower border. Extreme care must be taken to avoid the neurovascular bundle and the axillary nerve.

If further exposure is required, the coracoid process and the subscapularis tendon can be detached with ease.

Transacromial approach

INDICATIONS:
1. Rupture of the rotator cuff requiring repair or reconstruction.

2. Displaced fractures of the greater tubercle of the humerus.
3. Persistent painful arc syndrome requiring major decompression.

ADVANTAGES: The major complication of other exposures of the rotator cuff is dehiscence of the origin of the deltoid muscle. As this exposure is transacromial, this complication does not occur.

PROCEDURE:
1. The patient is placed in a semisitting position with a sandbag under the scapula.
2. The skin incision bisects the angle between the spine of the scapula and the back of the clavicle. It extends 4 cm proximal and 5 cm distal to tip of acromion (*Fig*. 361).

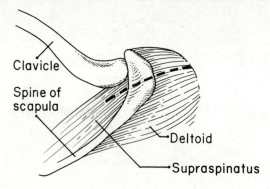

Clavicle

Spine of scapula

Deltoid

Supraspinatus

Fig. 361. The transacromial approach.

3. The trapezius and the deltoid muscles are split in the line of their fibres. Injury to the axillary nerve can be avoided by limiting the lateral extent of the incision; the nerve lies about 3 cm distal to the insertion of the rotator cuff.
4. Beneath the trapezius is the supraspinatus separated from the trapezius by a fat pad.
5. An oscillating saw is used to divide the acromion in the line of incision.
Exposure is obtained by using a self-retaining retractor. In this way the entire rotator cuff is easily seen.

CLOSURE: This may be achieved in three ways:
1. The detached portion of the acromion may be reattached by using Kirschner wire or a small screw.

2. The distal half of the acromion may be excised.
3. The divided acromion may simply be left apart. This affords effective decompression of the rotator cuff.

ARTHRODESIS OF THE SHOULDER

The optimum position is 45 degrees to 90 degrees abduction and 20 degrees flexion in front of the coronal plane (*Fig.* 362). The younger the patient, the greater the abduction angle made at the shoulder joint. In the position of

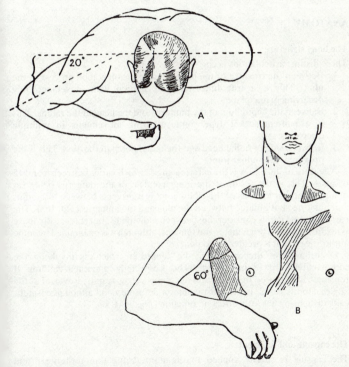

Fig. 362. Optimum position for ankylosis of shoulder joint. A, Seen from above; B, seen from the front.

partial abduction, the arm may be brought to the side by movements of the scapula on the chest wall; the younger the patient, the freer this movement.

Chapter 34

THE ELBOW

The elbow is a complex joint allowing flexion and extension of the arm and also rotating movements of the forearm.

ANATOMY

The bony structure

Three distinct articulations occur:

1. Between the trochlea of the humerus and the olecranon process of the ulna. This is a true hinge-type articulation with movement only occurring in one plane.
2. Between the capitellum of the humerus and the head of the radius. This is a ball-and-socket type joint, allowing movements in multiple directions.
3. Between side of radial head and the radial notch of the ulna. This is the proximal radio-ulnar joint.

A feature of the elbow is the carrying angle, which varies between 5 and 15 degrees. This is the result of the inner condyle of the humerus being set obliquely so that the axis of the elbow joint is transverse between the radius and humerus, but oblique between the ulna and the humerus (*Fig.* 363). The carrying angle varies considerably between individuals, but statistically there is no difference between males and females, although it is maintained by some authorities that it is greater in women.

Disturbance of the angle may be caused by fractures involving the supracondylar area of the humerus. This is especially common in children. If the angle is increased the condition of cubitus valgus results. Reversal of the angle, cubitus varus, is the most common deformity and although cosmetically disfiguring has little effect on function (*Fig.* 364).

The capsule and ligaments

The capsule is closely applied to the joint, being thin posteriorly and anteriorly so as not to obstruct flexion and extension, but thickened medially and laterally to give stability to the joint in the form of collateral ligaments.

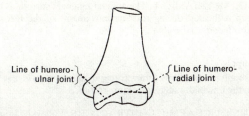

Fig. 363. Demonstrating the obliquity of humero-ulnar joint in comparison with transverse humeroradial joint. It is this obliquity which pushes the ulna laterally, producing the carrying angle.

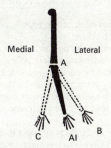

Fig. 364. AA1, the normal carrying angle; **AB**, increase of carrying angle—cubitus valgus; AC, the opposite condition—cubitus varus.

ULNAR COLLATERAL LIGAMENT:

Superior Attachments: To the distal part of the medial epicondyle of the humerus.

Inferior Attachments: To the medial margins of the olecranon and coronoid processes and to a band which stretches across between these bony processes.

It gives origin to some fibres of the flexor digitorum sublimis. This ligament plays an important part in preventing lateral movement at the elbow joint. If it is broken, there is lateral movement at the joint towards the opposite side.

RADIAL COLLATERAL LIGAMENT:

Superior Attachments: To the distal part of the lateral epicondyle of the humerus.

Inferior Attachments: To the annular ligament of the head of the radius.

THE ANNULAR LIGAMENT: The annular ligament surrounds the radial head to keep it located during rotating movements of the forearm. It is attached at both ends to the ulna.

The blood supply

The blood supply to the elbow comes from the numerous articular branches arising from the brachial, radial and ulnar arteries.

VOLKMANN'S ISCHAEMIC CONTRACTURE: Following injury of the arm, particularly of the elbow, injury to the brachial artery with associated spasm of the main artery and the collateral circulation results in ischaemia of the muscles of the forearm. Usually the flexor digitorum profundus and flexor pollicis longus are most severely affected, but the other flexors may also be affected.

In the acute stage degeneration of the muscle belly occurs and later this undergoes fibrosis with contracture.

In the early stage there is pain, aggravated by passive extension of the fingers, and in the stage of contracture there is flexion of the interphalangeal joints of the fingers which can be partially extended when the wrist is flexed. This demonstrates that the contracture is in the flexor group of muscles and enables this condiition to be differentiated from Dupuytren's contracture which affects the palmar fascia, and the contracture is thus not influenced by flexion of the wrist.

Pressure by haemorrhage and tight plasters or bandages may interfere with the blood supply of muscles to produce ischaemia and later contractures and these must be avoided, recognized, and treated promptly before irreversible damage has been done.

Bursae related to the joint

These consist of:
1. Two in relation to the triceps insertion.
2. Two in relation to the biceps insertion.

BURSAE IN RELATION TO THE TRICEPS INSERTION: *See Fig.* 365. An upper one between the triceps tendon and the upper surface of the olecranon is small and of little importance. A lower one between the triceps expansion and subcutaneous triangular area on the dorsal surface of the olecranon is large and may become inflamed.

BURSAE IN RELATION TO THE BICEPS INSERTION: These are both small. One separates the biceps tendon from the smooth anterior part of the bicipital tuberosity of the radius; the other separates the tendon from the oblique cord.

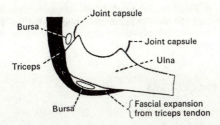

Fig. 365. Bursae in relation to the triceps tendon.

The nerve supply

The nerve supply to the joint is derived from all the major nerves which cross the joint: the radial, ulnar, median and the musculocutaneous nerves.

NERVE ENTRAPMENT SYNDROMES: Nerve entrapment syndromes are fairly common about the elbow. This causes pain, muscle atrophy and weakness in the area supplied by the entrapped nerve.

Entrapments which occur about the elbow are:

1. *Median Nerve:* The median nerve may be compressed by the hypertrophied pronator muscle where it passes through the pronator teres muscle or by an abnormally dense aponeurotic edge of the sublimus ridge where it dips under the sublimus.

2. *Ulnar Nerve:* The ulnar nerve may be compressed in the cubital tunnel against the posterior aspect of the medial epicondyle of the humerus in cases of cubitus valgus or by external compression when a patient is on the operating table, in bed, or in an armchair.

3. *Posterior Interosseous Nerve:* The posterior interosseous nerve may be compressed just distal to the elbow where it goes beneath the aponeurotic bridge of the extensor carpi radialis brevis or as it penetrates the supinator muscle. This is a motor nerve and compression results in deep, poorly localized pain in the lateral part of the elbow aggravated by rotation and extension of the wrist.

DISLOCATIONS OF THE ELBOW

Dislocations of the elbow occur in adults (children being more prone to fractures) and are caused invariably by falling on an outstretched arm. The joint dislocates posteriorly, usually fracturing the coronoid process as it does so. Reduction, if done early, is achieved fairly easily by traction to overcome the spasm, and flexion to lever the joint back into place.

In the child, dislocation of the radial head occurs as a result of the head subluxating through the annular ligament by pulling on the forearm (pulled elbow). Reduction is accomplished by firmly supinating the elbow, which spontaneously reduces the subluxation.

OPERATIVE PROCEDURES

1. Aspiration

The part of the joint which is nearest the surface lies posteriorly, between the head of the radius and the capitellum (lateral condyle) of the humerus. The head of the radius can always be distinguished and the needle is entered just proximal to the head, in a direction directly forwards (anteriorly), the joint being flexed to a right-angle and the forearm semipronated (*Fig.* 366). When the elbow joint is distended with pus the capsule bulges to either side of the triceps and may be easily and efficiently drained in this situation.

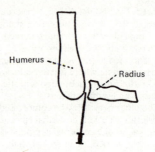

Humerus

Radius

Fig. 366. Aspiration of the elbow joint.

2. Approaches to the joint

Two methods are in general use: Kocher's method—used for wide exposure of the joint, e.g. to excise the whole articulation; Langenbeck's method—used for a lesser degree of exposure, e.g. to remove a piece of loose bone from the joint.

KOCHER'S METHOD: Incision commences 5 cm above the joint line over the lateral epicondylar ridge and extends vertically down to the head of the radius between the brachioradialis and radial extensors laterally and the triceps medially (*Fig.* 367). It then trends inwards, passing along the outer border of the anconeus between that muscle and the extensor carpi ulnaris, tailing off on to the inner aspect of the forearm.

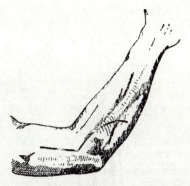

Fig. 367. Posterolateral aspect of right arm and forearm showing Kocher's method of approach to elbow joint.

The muscles around the back and sides of the joint are separated from the bones, exposing the whole posterior aspect of the capsule and the bone ends. No structures are exposed other than those mentioned; the supinator and the interosseous recurrent artery may lie between the anconeus and the extensor carpi ulnaris, though they are usually under the anconeus.

The planning of the incision was a surgical inspiration. It passes between those muscles supplied by the radial nerve before it pierces the lateral intermuscular septum, which is medial to it, while the muscles lateral to the incision are supplied by the nerve after it has pierced the septum.

LANGENBECK'S METHOD (POSTERIOR APPROACH): A vertical centrally placed incision is made at the back of the elbow (*Fig.* 368). Its centre is at the tip of the olecranon. It divides the triceps in the direction of its fibres above and the anconeus below. The joint is exposed by separating the muscles from the bones. The incision may injure the nerve to the anconeus, which runs in the line of the incision in the substance of the triceps.

This exposure is also used for internal fixation of fractures involving the distal humerus and proximal ulna.

3. Fusion

Loss of movement at the elbow is a great disability. Fusion should only be done when all else fails. The optimal position is about 100 degrees of flexion, with the forearm in neutral rotation.

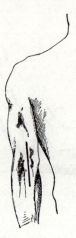

Fig. 368. Langenbeck's approach to elbow joint.

Chapter 35

THE WRIST COMPLEX

The wrist complex consists of two joints, namely, the radiocarpal joint and the midcarpal joint (*Fig*. 369).

The radiocarpal joint

This lies between the concave lower articular surface of the radius and the triangular fibrocartilage of the lower radio-ulnar joint proximally, and the convex articular surface of the scaphoid, lunate and triquetral bones distally. Note that the head of the ulna does not form part of the joint and it can be excised without interfering with wrist function. The pisiform bone, which is one of the proximal carpal bones, also does not form part of the joint surface; it functions entirely as a sesamoid bone in the insertion of the tendon of flexor carpi ulnaris.

The midcarpal joint

This lies between the scaphoid, lunate and triquetral bones proximally, and the trapezius, trapezoid, capitate and hamate distally.

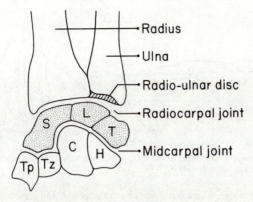

Fig. 369. The radiocarpal and midcarpal joints. *See text*.

Stability of the wrist complex

1. CAPSULES: The radiocarpal joint is enclosed by a strong but somewhat loose capsule. The capsule of the midcarpal joint is anatomically separate from the radiocarpal joint. The fibres of the joint capsule merge with the ligaments.

2. LIGAMENTS: The carpal bones are firmly bound together by interosseous, palmar and dorsal radiocarpal ligaments and ulnar and radial collateral ligaments. The palmar radiocarpal ligament is the strongest and most important in stabilizing the wrist complex. If this ligament is torn, the patient has carpal instability.

3. TENDONS: The tendons passing to the hand add some stability to the joint.

4. BONE SHAPE: With the exception of the lunate bone, the carpal bones are broad on their dorsal aspect, and narrower on their palmar aspect, which possibly accounts for the joint being more stable when the palm is flexed.

Movements of the wrist complex

These (*Fig.* 370) are dorsiflexion, palmar flexion, radial and ulnar deviation. When palmar flexion, ulnar deviation, dorsiflexion and radial deviation occur, in sequence, circumduction occurs.

It should be noted that there are no active muscular forces applied to the proximal row of carpal bones, which serve as a mechanical link between the radius and the distal carpals to which muscular forces are applied. Movement of the distal row of carpal bones must be transmitted to the proximal row by an

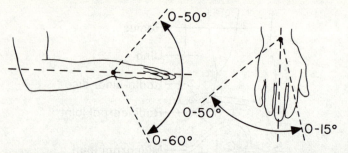

Fig. 370. Range of movement at the wrist joint. Most hand functions are performed with the wrist in ulnar deviation.

intracarpal bridge, which is provided by the scaphoid, and supported by the wrist ligaments. Reference to *Fig.* 369 shows that on the radial side the midcarpal joint is braced by the scaphoid which passes across this joint line.

Although the articular surfaces are comparatively small, movement at two levels imparts a wide range of mobility to the wrist complex.

The extensor and flexor retinaculum

These are discussed in the chapter on the Hand (Chapter 36).

Nerve supply of the wrist complex

Many muscles act on the wrist complex. The nerves supplying these muscles are the anterior interosseous branch of the median, the posterior interosseous branch of the radial and the dorsal and deep branches of the ulnar. Articular branches are supplied by each of these nerves (Hilton's law).

FRACTURE OF THE SCAPHOID BONE

A fall on the dorsiflexed wrist may fracture the scaphoid (*Fig.* 371). The

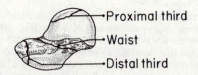

Fig. 371. Fracture of the scaphoid.

fracture usually occurs through the waist of the scaphoid (70 per cent), because the scaphoid lies partly in each row of carpal bones. In other cases the fracture occurs through the distal third, or the proximal third of the bone.

Nutrient vessels enter the bone through multiple foramina in the ridge between the two main articular surfaces. In two-thirds of the bones, the vessels are distributed throughout the length of the ridge and in the other third there are no vessels entering the proximal half which is supplied by branches of the distal nutrient vessels running backwards in the bone. Under these circumstances, a fracture of the waist, sometimes, and a fracture of the proximal third always results in avascular necrosis of the proximal fragment.

ASPIRATION OF THE RADIOCARPAL JOINT

The needle is introduced posteriorly, immediately below the lower end of the radius, between the tendons of extensor indicis and extensor pollicis longus.

SURGICAL APPROACH TO THE WRIST JOINT

Dorsal approach
See Fig. 372.

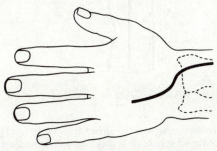

Fig. 372. Incision for dorsal approach to the wrist joint.

INCISION: A longitudinal curvilinear incision is centred over the dorsal tubercle of the radius.

STRUCTURES ENCOUNTERED: The extensor retinaculum which is divided between the tendon of extensor pollicis longus and the tendons of the extensor digitorum muscle. The latter is retracted to the ulnar side of the wrist and a transverse incision is made in the capsule of the radiocarpal joint.

Medial approach
See Fig. 373.

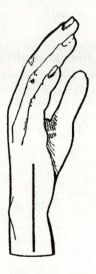

Fig. 373.   Incision for medial approach to the wrist joint.

INCISION: A vertical incision on the ulnar border of the hand and forearm with its centre at the wrist joint. It begins 5 cm above the ulnar styloid and extends to the middle of the 5th metacarpal bone.

STRUCTURES ENCOUNTERED: The dorsal branch of the ulnar nerve winds around the dorsum of the wrist immediately distal to the head of the ulna. It supplies the little finger and the ulnar half of the ring finger with sensory fibres and must be preserved.

The incision passes between the extensor and flexor carpi ulnaris. The capsule is opened longitudinally; injury to the triangular fibrocartilage attached to the ulna must be avoided.

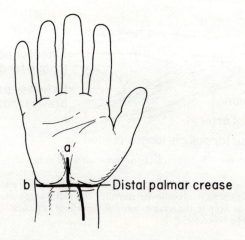

Fig. 374. Incision for volar approach to the wrist joint.

Volar approach
See Fig. 374.

INCISION: Curved longitudinal (a), or a transverse incision (b) in the distal palmar crease.

STRUCTURES ENCOUNTERED: Palmaris longus tendon, median nerve and flexor pollicis longus tendon are gently retracted to the radial side and the flexores sublimis and profundus tendons to the ulnar side. The joint capsule is incised, revealing the distal end of the radius and lunate.

Lateral approach
See Fig. 375.

INCISION: Curvilinear, extending from the base of the 2nd metacarpal distally, crossing the radial styloid process, to the prominent ridge on the anterior surface of the lower end of the radius proximally.

STRUCTURES ENCOUNTERED: The extensor pollicis brevis and abductor pollicis longus tendons, which form the anterior boundary of the anatomical snuff box, the radial artery and the lateral terminal branch of the superficial branch of the radial nerve, are retracted anteriorly; the extensor pollicis longus tendon which forms the posterior boundary of the snuff box is

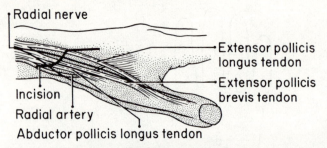

Fig. 375. Incision for lateral approach to the wrist joint.

retracted posteriorly. The tubercle of the scaphoid is exposed and the radial collateral ligament is incised longitudinally. The radial artery which crosses the snuff box deep to the tendons and the superficial branches of the radial nerve must be protected.

Chapter 36

THE HAND

THE SKIN

The overlying skin of the palm of the hand is firmly fixed to the underlying palmar aponeurosis by fibrous bands which extend through the subcutaneous fat. This tethering of the palmar skin prevents bunching of the palmar skin when the hand is clenched.

The overlying skin on the dorsum of the hand is lax, lying on loose areolar tissue, which forms the dorsal subcutaneous space, through which pass veins, lymphatics and sensory nerves. The dorsal surface receives most of the lymphatic drainage of the hand, including that from the palmar surface. It is for this reason that the oedema from a palmar infection occurs on the dorsum of the hand.

LIGAMENTS AND APONEUROSES

The superficial transverse metacarpal ligament

The superficial transverse metacarpal ligament of the palm (interdigital ligament) lies deep to palmar skin, in the superficial fascia, across the free margins of the web spaces. Its fibres lie transversely and extend as far proximally as the metacarpophalangeal joints. The two ends, and parts that lie across the fibrous flexor sheaths continue along the fingers, resulting in a tethering of the overlying skin to the phalanges.

The palmar aponeurosis (fascia)

The palmar aponeurosis (*Fig.* 376) represents the deep fascia of other parts of the body, and is superficial to the vessels, nerves, muscles and tendons. It

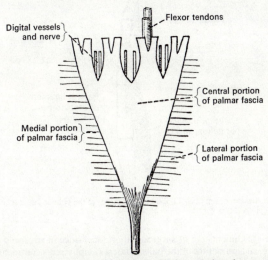

Digital vessels and nerve

Flexor tendons

Central portion of palmar fascia

Medial portion of palmar fascia

Lateral portion of palmar fascia

Fig. 376. General arrangement of palmar fascia. The central triangular process is seen dividing into four digital processes, each of which splits into two. The superficial components of the digital processes are not shown.

consists of a central triangular-shaped portion of considerable strength with thinner and weaker medial and lateral extensions over the hypothenar and thenar eminences.

ATTACHMENTS OF THE PALMAR APONEUROSIS:

Apex: Attached to the transverse carpal ligament (flexor retinaculum) and the palmaris longus tendon from which it is derived.

Base: It divides opposite the heads of the metacarpals into four slips, one going to each one of the four fingers. Each one of the four slips divides into superficial and deep components. The superficial part is attached to the skin of the palm and fingers and the deep component divides into two processes which are continuous with the fibrous flexor sheaths and has expansions to:

1. The deep transverse metacarpal ligament.
2. The whole length of the inner and outer borders of the proximal phalanx.
3. The proximal part of the inner and outer borders of the middle phalanx (*Fig.* 377).

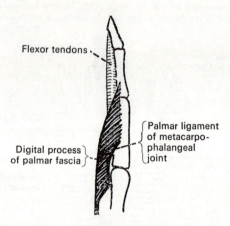

Fig. 377. Attachment of one of the digital processes of the palmar fascia seen from the side.

These attachments are of surgical importance, since in advanced cases of pathological contracture of the palmar fascia (Dupuytren's contracture), the proximal and intermediate phalanges of the fingers are acutely flexed because the palmar fascia is attached to them. The distal phalanx is extended, as the fascia has no attachment to it.

Each pair of processes, passing deeply to the fibrous flexor sheaths, forms a canal allowing the passage of the tendons for that finger. Between these run the lumbrical muscles, digital vessels, and nerves.

When carrying out a dissection for removal of the aponeurosis in Dupuytren's contracture, it is essential first to isolate these important structures in the intertendinous compartments before resecting the fascia.

The deep transverse metacarpal ligament

The deep transverse metacarpal ligament binds the four fingers together. It is attached to the palmar (volar accessory) ligaments of the metacarpophalangeal joints and prevents separation of the four inner metacarpal bones from each other. The transverse metatarsal ligament has a precisely similar arrangement except that it binds together all five metatarsals. The interossei are dorsal to this ligament; the lumbricals, flexor tendons, and palmar or plantar vessels and nerves are volar to the ligament.

THE LONG FLEXOR TENDONS IN THE HAND

The grasping action of the hand is dependent on the combined action of the flexor digitorum superficialis (sublimis) and flexor digitorum profundus muscles in the forearm. The tendons begin in the distal third of the forearm and pass through the carpal canal to the respective fingers. The superficialis tendon inserts on the middle phalanx and the profundus at the base of the distal phalanx.

The profundus muscle has only one muscle belly, but the superficialis tendon has individual bellies for each of the four fingers. This fact is used in the test for integrity of these tendons.

The patient's hand is laid on the table, palm upwards and the surgeon holds the fingers flat on the table with the exception of the one to be tested. Flexion of the proximal interphalangeal joint of the finger being tested is indicative of an intact superficialis tendon because the profundus has been rendered inactive by holding the other fingers in extension.

The integrity of the profundus tendon can be demonstrated by the ability to flex the distal interphalangeal joint while the middle phalanx is immobilized with the proximal interphalangeal joint in extension (*Fig.* 378).

INTRINSIC MUSCLES OF THE HAND

Small muscles of the thumb

ABDUCTOR POLLICIS BREVIS: An important muscle.
  Action: It pulls the thumb directly forwards away from the palm in a plane at right-angles to the palm (*Fig.* 379).

OPPONENS:
  Action: It enables the pad of the last phalanx of the thumb to be approximated to that of any other finger.

The abductor pollicis brevis and opponens are together responsible for the action of rotating the thumb opposite the index finger for the pincer action in picking up objects.

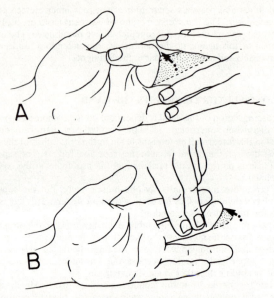

Fig. 378. A, The correct method of testing for flexor digitorum superficialis: the intact superficialis tendon actively flexes the PIP joint, while the profundus unit is inactivated by passive extension of the other fingers. B, The correct method of testing the flexor digitorum profundus. The intact profundus tendon actively flexes the DIP joint.

ADDUCTOR POLLICIS:

Action: It pulls the thumb across the palm in a plane parallel to the palm.

Test (Froment's Sign): Give the patient a thin book and tell him to grasp it firmly between the last phalanges of the thumb and forefinger. If the muscle is acting, the thumb will be straight. If the muscle is not acting, the last phalanx of the thumb will be fully flexed (*Fig.* 380). The reason is that with weakness of the adductor, the flexor pollicis longus substitutes for it.

The muscle is supplied by the deep branch of the ulnar nerve.

Lumbricals and interossei

LUMBRICALS: Four muscles arise from the tendons of the flexor profundus. They wind around the radial (lateral) sides of the fingers (*Fig.* 381).

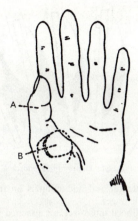

Fig. 379. Action of abductor pollicis brevis. A, Thumb in line with fingers; B, thumb pulled directly forwards by the short abductor at right-angles to plane of palm.

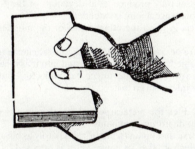

Fig. 380. Testing the adductor pollicis. Interphalangeal joint of upper thumb is flexed, showing paralysis of the adductor. In the lower thumb it is acting normally and thumb is straight.

INTEROSSEI:
1. There are seven interossei in each hand.
2. Four are dorsal, of which each arises from two adjacent metacarpal bones. Three are palmar, of which each arises from one metacarpal bone only.
3. The dorsal interossei are abductors from the central axis ('DAB').
4. The palmar interossei are adductors towards the axis ('PAD').

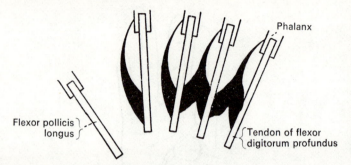

Fig. 381. The lumbrical muscles.

5. The axis of abduction and adduction is an imaginary line passing through the middle finger.
6. The palmar and dorsal interossei are attached to the dorsal extensor expansion and the bases of the 1st phalanges.
7. The interossei are the extensors of the 2nd and 3rd phalanges of the fingers.
8. The interossei only produce axial deviation of the fingers when the metacarpophalangeal joint is extended.

With these facts in mind the attachments of the muscles can be readily identified.

The muscles are best represented by a simple scheme (*Figs* 382 and 383). Note that the thumb has no interossei inserted into it as it has abductors and adductors of its own. The little finger has abductors but no adductors, therefore palmar interossei go to it.

Actions:

Lumbricals: Flex the metacarpophalangeal joint. Its opponent is the extensor digitorum communis.

Observe that though a lumbrical is hardly as big as an earthworm, from which it takes its name, yet it is opposed by a muscle which extends from the humerus. Also flexion is a stronger action than extension.

The extensor digitorum communis has, as its prime function, extension of the metacarpophalangeal joint (*Fig.* 384). When, however, the knuckles are bent, extension of the interphalangeal joint is a combined function of the long extensors and intrinsic muscles of the hand, which insert into the extensor expansion.

Interossei: Besides being abductors, the interossei are extensors of the middle and terminal phalanges.

The interossei are inserted into the extensor tendon expansion at the back of the first phalanx. The firm attachment of the extensor

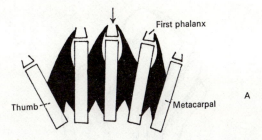

Fig. 382. The dorsal interossei.

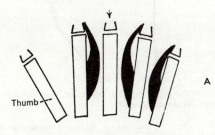

Fig. 383. The palmar interossei.

tendon to the back of the 1st phalanx is the insertion of the extensor tendon proper, and the extensor, therefore, extends this phalanx and does nothing more. The distal expansion of the tendon divides into three slips, one short central and two long laterals (*Fig.* 385). These slips are really extensions of the interossei tendons, and are inserted into the second and third phalanges, which are therefore extended by the interossei.

The opponents of the interossei acting as extensors are the flexores digitorum sublimis (which flexes the 2nd phalanx) and profundus (which flexes the 3rd phalanx).

Nerve Supply:

   Lumbricals: 1st and 2nd supplied by the median; 3rd and 4th supplied by the ulnar.

   Interossei: All are supplied by the deep branch of the ulnar nerve. Occasionally the 1st, or 1st and 2nd dorsal interossei in the hand may be supplied by the median nerve.

      The median is the nerve mainly responsible for coarse movements of the hand, as it supplies most of the long muscles on the front of the forearm. It is the 'labourer's' nerve.

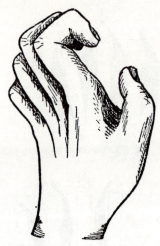

Fig. 384. Shows that the prime function of the extensor digitorum communis is extension of the metacarpophalangeal joint.

The ulnar is the nerve mainly responsible for the fine movements of the hand, as it supplies most of the small muscles of the hand. It is the 'musician's' nerve (hence the old name for the lumbricals was musculi fidicinales). If the ulnar nerve which supplies the interossei is paralysed, then the two distal phalanges cannot be extended.

The interosseous muscles can be tested by letting the patient grasp a piece of paper between the sides of two adjacent fingers. If the muscles are acting, this paper will be firmly held and some resistance will be offered to its withdrawal (*Fig.* 386). Extension of the 2nd and 3rd phalanges is also a test for the muscles.

Summary:

Metatacarpophalangeal joint:
    Flexed by   :   Lumbrical.
    Extended by   :   Extensor digitorum.
Proximal interphalangeal joint:
    Flexed by   :   Sublimis
    Extended by   :   Interossei.
Distal interphalangeal joint:
    Flexed by   :   Profundus
    Extended by   :   Interossei.

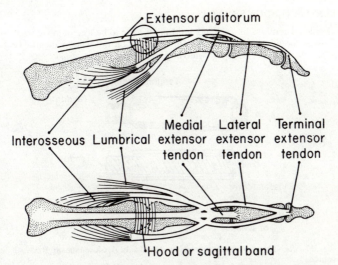

Fig. 385. The extensor expansion at the back of the first phalanx breaks up into one short central and two long lateral processes. Note the attachment (ringed) of the extensor tendon to the base of the proximal phalanx in the lateral view.

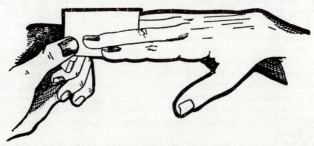

Fig. 386. Test for interossei. The wrist should be dorsiflexed to cut out the action of the long flexors of the fingers.

The small muscles of the thumb are abductor, adductor, flexor brevis and opponens.

The small muscles of the 5th finger are abductor (no adductor), flexor brevis and opponens.

FLEXOR TENDON SHEATHS

The flexor tendons in the hand and fingers have to be free to move so as to provide mobility of the fingers. This depends on the tendon sheaths (*Fig.* 387), which are of two types: synovial and fibrous.

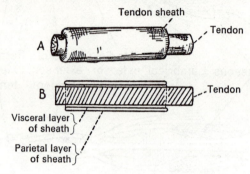

Fig. 387. The arrangement of a synovial tendon sheath. A, Closed sheath; B, sheath on section.

Synovial sheaths

The tendon is invested by a glistening endothelial-lined membrane, which plays inside a second endothelial-lined membrane, the two layers being joined at their extremities. The sheath thus forms a sac, closed at both ends.

The sublimis and profundus slips to each of the 2nd, 3rd, 4th and 5th digits have a common sheath which extends from the neck of the metacarpal bone to the base of the distal phalanx, where the profundus ends. Over the middle third of the metacarpals these tendons, with the exception of those to the 5th digit, have no sheaths. Proximal to this the tendons are invested by another sheath which extends upwards as far as 2·5 cm above the wrist joint (*Fig.* 388). The sheath investing the tendons to the 5th digit continues proximally without interruption to join the common flexor sheath at the wrist. The common flexor sheath with its extension along the little finger tendons is the ulnar bursa.

Not infrequently, there may be an interruption in the ulnar bursa, the arrangement of the sheath of the 5th digit then being identical to that of the other fingers. A tenosynovitis of the little finger would, in such cases, be held up by such an interruption. When operating on any case of tenosynovitis the arrangement of the sheath should be carefully examined under a bloodless field, so that operation can be planned accordingly.

The flexor pollicis longus has a sheath which extends from the base of the distal phalanx to a point 2·5 cm above the upper border of the wrist joint.

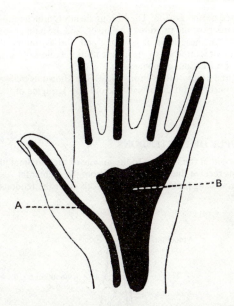

Fig. 388. Synovial sheaths of flexor tendons of wrist and fingers. A, Radial bursa or synovial sheath of flexor longus pollicis; B, ulnar bursa or synovial sheath of flexores sublimis and profundus at wrist, and its extension to little finger.

This is called the 'radial bursa'. The radial and ulnar bursae pass under the flexor retinaculum (transverse carpal ligament).

It should be noted that the synovial sheaths are found where the tendon has to glide round a bend. In areas where there are no synovial sheaths the tendon is able to move by virtue of loose connective tissue called the 'paratenon'. This is seen particularly where the tendon has to move in a straight line.

The flexor sheath, therefore, is a double-walled hollow synovial-lined connective tissue tube, which encloses the flexor tendons. This complicates surgical repair of a ruptured tendon which requires special care for a successful result. In contrast the extensor tendons are devoid of sheaths and surgical repair is easy to achieve.

Fibrous sheaths

In the fingers the flexor tendons also have fibrous sheaths which form an osteofascial tunnel with the underlying bone. Its main function is to hold the tendon in place during flexion. The fibrous sheath is attached to the medial and lateral borders of the proximal phalanges, and the palmar surface of the distal phalanx. In these areas it is strong and fibrous, unlike the areas in between, where it is attached to the ligaments of the joints of the fingers, and is weak, to allow freedom of movement.

The thickened areas of the fibrous sheath are known as pulleys and must always be reconstituted if disturbed to avoid bow stringing of the tendon in flexion.

BLOOD SUPPLY OF THE TENDONS

From their origin in the forearm to the middle of the proximal phalanx, the flexor tendons receive their blood supply from the segmental vessels arising from the surrounding paratenon. These vessels enter the tendons and travel longitudinally.

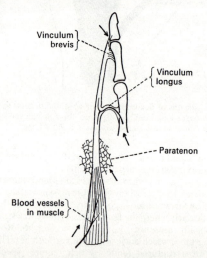

Fig. 389. The nature of the blood supply to tendons. The four arrows indicate the vascular mechanisms.

From the middle of the proximal phalanx distally, the blood supply is related to the vincula of the phalanx (*Fig.* 389). These are folds of mesotenon which carry the blood supply to both flexor superficialis and flexor profundus. Although there are common variations, there is a short and a long vinculum for each tendon. This system exists on the dorsal surface of each tendon, and is supplied by the transverse communicating branches of the common digital artery.

When exploring an intact pulley/tendon system, it is therefore preferable to enter the tendon sheath away from the thickened areas, and it must be borne in mind that the blood supply to the vincula also enters at these areas.

DIGITAL JOINTS

At the metacarpophalangeal joint the head of the metacarpal articulates with the 1st phalanx, forming a condyloid joint, allowing flexion, extension and slight side-to-side movement. The interphalangeal joints are plane or hinge joints permitting only flexion and extension.

The metacarpal head is narrow on its dorsal surface, and has a widened volar plate giving progressive contact with the base of the proximal phalanx in flexion.

All these joints have weak capsular ligaments, defective posteriorly, where the extensor expansion, assisted by the lumbrical and interosseous component, fill the gap.

The front of the joint is formed by the volar plate. This is a strong fibrocartilaginous plate with which the head of the metacarpal articulates. It is continuous, laterally, with the deep transverse metacarpal ligament. The volar plate has a thick fibrocartilaginous distal portion, and a thin, membranous, proximal portion. The plate is firmly attached to the base of the proximal phalanx, and thins out proximally to gain a much weaker attachment to the metacarpal, just proximal to the head.

This arrangement allows flexion at the joint as the thin part of the volar plate can buckle (*Fig.* 390). If these joints are dislocated and the volar plate is avulsed the tear is much more likely to occur at the weak proximal attachment. It may be displaced between the bone ends and interfere with reduction (*Fig.* 391). Dislocation of any finger joint implies, therefore, the rupture of ligaments.

The volar plate checks the extension of the joint. If the volar plate is torn, it remains firmly attached to the distal bone.

Collateral ligaments of metacarpophalangeal and interphalangeal joints

These ligaments are attached to the side of the head of the proximal bone and to the side of the base of the distal bone. These ligaments prevent lateral mobility.

The ligaments of the metacarpophalangeal joint are only at full stretch when the joint is fully flexed to 90 degrees.

The ligaments of the interphalangeal joints are stretched when the joint is fully extended.

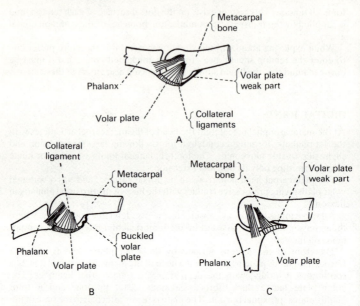

Fig. 390. These diagrams show the anatomy of the accessory ligaments of the metacarpophalangeal joints in different positions. **A**, The joint is extended, the volar plate is tense, the collateral ligament is lax. Note the attachment of the latter structure to the former. **B**, The joint is semiflexed; the thin part of the volar plate is buckled; the collateral ligament is lax. **C**, The joint is fully flexed; the volar plate and collateral ligament are tense. (Modified from Moberg.)

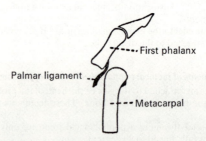

Fig. 391. Illustrating the usual type of metacarpophalangeal dislocation: 1st phalanx passing back, and the palmar ligament remaining attached to phalanx and frequently offering a bar to reduction.

This is vital when immobilizing a hand, as contracture of the joints occurs within 14 days, and if the joints are immobilized in a position allowing the ligaments laxity, then the resultant shortening will lead to irreversible joint contractures.

1. POSITION OF IMMOBILIZATION: As indicated above, the metacarpophalangeal joints are immobilized fully flexed (*Fig.* 392), while the interphalangeal joints are fully extended.

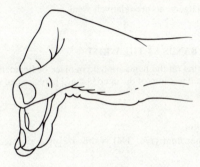

Fig. 392. Position of immobilization.

2. POSITION OF ARTHRODESIS: The wrist joint is moderately dorsiflexed. The metacarpophalangeal and interphalangeal joints are set in neutral position. (*See Fig.* 393.)

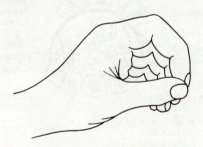

Fig. 393. Position of arthrodesis.

COLLATERAL LIGAMENTS OF THE WRIST JOINT

The ligaments of the wrist joint provide the structural integrity to the complex movements of this joint.

The major ligaments are intracapsular, and are thus very difficult to visualize at operation.

The volar ligaments are much more substantial, their general configuration being a double V-shaped structure with an area of potential weakness between them (the space of Poirier). This weak area lies directly over the capitolunate articulation.

The collateral ligaments are relatively weak.

THE BINDING BANDS AT THE WRIST

The tendons acting on the hand are held in place by ligaments which are all merely specialized portions of the deep fascia. There are two such specialized bands:

Flexor retinaculum

The flexor retinaculum (*Fig.* 394) is the size of a 'postage stamp' (to be

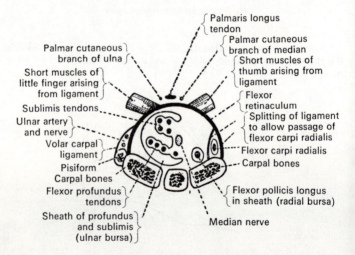

Fig. 394. The flexor retinaculum.

remembered in the surface marking of the ligament). Like a postage stamp, it has two surfaces and four borders.

BORDERS:
Superior: The deep fascia of the forearm is attached to it.
Inferior: The central portion of the palmar fascia is attached here.
Medial: Is attached to the pisiform and hook of the hamate.
Lateral: Is attached to the tubercle of the scaphoid and the ridge on the trapezium. This attachment is by two processes so arranged as to leave a gap for the passage of the tendon of the flexor carpi radialis.

SURFACES:
Palmar: This surface is crossed by those structures entering the palm superficial to the ligament; centrally is the palmaris longus tendon with a nerve on each side: the palmar cutaneous branch of the median on the radial side, the palmar cutaneous branch of the ulnar on the ulnar side. The ulnar vessels and nerve cross the ligament under cover of the pisiform bone. They are held in place by a fascial process named the 'volar carpal ligament', which is attached to the pisiform medially and the flexor retinaculum laterally. In addition, this surface gives partial insertion to the flexor carpi ulnaris and palmaris longus, and partial origin to all the small muscles of the thenar and hypothenar eminences except the abductor digiti minimi, i.e. the abductor pollicis brevis, the flexor pollicis brevis, opponens pollicis, opponens minimi digiti, and the palmaris brevis.

The muscular attachments entirely hide the volar surface of the ligament, which is much farther from the skin surface than the surgeon is apt to think.

Dorsal: This surface forms a tunnel with the carpal bones. This tunnel is traversed by the flexors of the fingers, sublimis and profundus, the long flexor of the thumb, and the median nerve. The flexors of the fingers are invaginated into a synovial bag (named the 'ulnar bursa') from its outer side, which bag is therefore open laterally. In this gap lies the median nerve. The arrangement of the tendons under the ligament is as follows:

The sublimis tendons are all separate, being arranged in two pairs: the upper pair consists of one to each of the middle and ring fingers; the lower pair consists of one to each of the index and little fingers.

The profundus tendons: only the slip to the index finger is separate; the other three are still fused and lie medial to the index slip.

The flexor pollicis longus tendon is on the radial side in a separate synovial sheath called the 'radial bursa'. In 50 per cent of cases there is a communication between the radial and ulnar bursae in this situation.

The flexor carpi radialis tendon passes through a separate canal deep to the lateral part of the flexor retinaculum and runs on a groove in the trapezium. The tendon attaches to the base of the 2nd metacarpal.

Extensor retinaculum

The extensor retinaculum (*Fig.* 395) is oblique in direction at the back of the wrist. It has four borders and two surfaces.

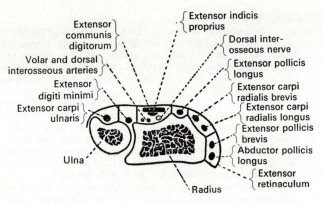

Fig. 395. The extensor retinaculum and the structures passing beneath it.

BORDERS:
Superior and Inferior: Are continuous with the deep fascia.
Medial: Is attached to the triquetrum and pisiform.
Lateral: Is attached to the lower 2–5 cm of the volar (anterior) border of the radius.
It is not attached to the lower end of the ulna by its medial border. If it were, it would interfere with the movements of the radius round the ulna (pronation and supination).

SURFACES:
Dorsal: The dorsal surface is crossed by veins draining the dorsal carpal arch (i.e. the commencement of cephalic and basilic veins) and by four cutaneous nerves, viz. the dorsal branch of the ulnar nerve, the superficial branch of the radial, and the terminations of the posterior branches of the medial and lateral cutaneous nerves of the forearm.

Deep or Anterior: This surface is related to the extensor tendons. Fascial processes pass from it to the radius and ulna, which divide the space between the ligament and the bones into six compartments for the tendons. These six compartments house from lateral to medial:

1. Abductor pollicis longus and extensor pollicis brevis.
2. Extensor carpi radialis longus and extensor carpi radialis brevis.
3. Extensor pollicis longus.
4. Extensor communis digitorum and extensor indicis proprius. The terminations of the volar and dorsal interosseous arteries and the dorsal interosseous nerve go through this compartment lying between it and the bone.
5. Extensor digiti minimi.
6. Extensor carpi ulnaris.

FASCIAL SPACES OF THE HAND

These are: (i) midpalmar; (ii) thenar; (iii) forearm space; (iv) dorsal subcutaneous space; (v) dorsal subaponeurotic space. The midpalmar, thenar, and forearm spaces all lie deep to the flexor tendons and their synovial sheaths, which therefore form the anterior boundaries of these spaces.

Midpalmar space

This space lies under the inner half of the hollow of the hand (between the thenar and the hypothenar eminences). Its shape is triangular.

BOUNDARIES: *See Figs 396–398.*

Anterior:
1. Flexor tendons (with their synovial sheaths) of the little, ring, and middle fingers. The tendons of the middle finger are anterior relations of the thenar space also, but are more intimately related to the midpalmar space.
2. The lumbrical muscles related to the tendons of the ring and little fingers, i.e. 3rd and 4th lumbricals.

Posterior: The dense fascia covering the interossei and metacarpal bones.

Radial: The fibrous partition between the thenar and the midpalmar spaces. This partition extends between the fascia on the undersurface of the flexor tendons and the fascia covering the interossei and adductor of the thumb.

Ulnar: The hypothenar muscles.

Proximal: It reaches the level of the distal margin of the transverse carpal ligament. Sometimes this space is continuous with the forearm space by a small tunnel behind the flexor sheaths at the wrist.

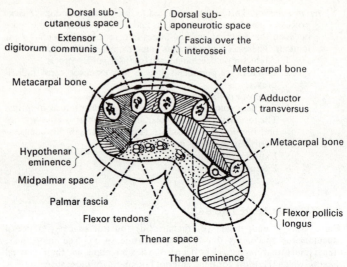

Fig. 396. Section through the palm to show thenar and midpalmar spaces. The dorsal subcutaneous and subaponeurotic spaces are also shown.

Distal: It reaches almost to the level of the distal palmar crease.

The lumbrical muscles have delicate fascial sheaths which are so intimately related to the palmar spaces that infection of the space causes infection of the related lumbrical sheaths. Each lumbrical sheath may therefore be looked on almost as a diverticulum of the space to which it is related. The 3rd and 4th lumbrical sheaths would therefore be diverticula of the midpalmar space. The 1st lumbrical sheath would be a diverticulum of the thenar space. The 2nd lumbrical sheath may be a diverticulum of either the thenar or midpalmar space. Pus in the midpalmar space can be drained by slitting the web between the 3rd and 4th or 4th and 5th digits and opening the sheath of the lumbrical in the space.

Thenar space

The thenar space (*Figs* 396–398) lies under the outer half of the hollow of the palm. It is triangular in shape.

BOUNDARIES:
Anterior:
    1. Short muscles of the thumb.

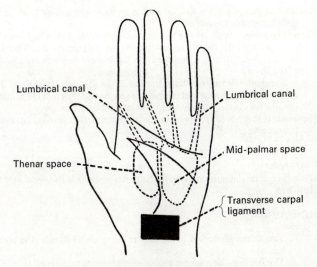

Fig. 397. The dotted lines indicate the fascial spaces of the palm. The prolongations of the spaces along the lumbrical canals are shown.

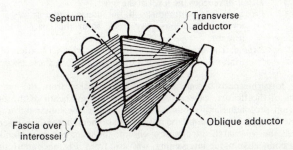

Fig. 398. The soft tissues of the palm have been removed to show the posterior boundary of the thenar and midpalmar spaces. On the left is the fascia overlying the interossei which bounds the midpalmar space. On the right is the transverse part of the adductor pollicis which bounds the thenar space. The black line is the septum between the spaces.

    2. Flexor tendons of index finger.
    3. 1st and 2nd lumbricals.
Posterior: The adductor pollicis, mainly its transverse head.

Radial: The flexor pollicis longus tendon in its synovial sheath which is called the 'radial bursa'.

Ulnar: The septum between the two spaces, midpalmar and thenar.

Distal: It reaches to the proximal transverse palmar crease. The 1st lumbrical sheath and sometimes the 2nd extend as distal diverticula of the space.

   The digital flexor sheaths of the 2nd, 3rd and 4th digits begin at the level where the thenar and midpalmar spaces end. Pus in these tendon sheaths may therefore burst into and infect the palmar spaces.

Proximal: It reaches to the distal border of the anterior annular ligament (transverse carpal).

Forearm space

This is merely a fascial interval deep to the flexor tendons in the distal part of the forearm.

BOUNDARIES:
   Anterior:
      1. The flexor digitorum profundus in its synovial sheath (the ulnar bursa).
      2. The flexor pollicis longus in its synovial sheath (the radial bursa).
         Posterior: The pronator quadratus and the interosseous membrane.
         Distal: It reaches the level of the wrist.
         Proximal: It is continuous with the intermuscular spaces of the forearm, and pus may track from the space into the forearm.
         Lateral: The space extends to the outer and inner borders of the forearm, and is drained by incisions along these borders.

The forearm space becomes infected by extension from the synovial sheaths of the flexors, especially from the common sheath of the flexor digitorum profundus and sublimis, which is called the 'ulnar bursa'. Pus presents behind these tendons and not in front of them, because, as is seen in *Fig.* 399, the synovial sheath almost opens into the space behind the tendons, a little connective tissue intervening, whilst in front it is much more firmly attached to the tendons.

Dorsal spaces

On the dorsum of the hand the areolar tissue is much looser than in the palm. The extensors of the fingers are connected to each other by fibrous tissue, which forms, with the extensor tendons, an aponeurotic barrier between two spaces—the dorsal subcutaneous and the dorsal subaponeurotic spaces (*Fig.* 396). These spaces are both triangular, with the apex of the triangle at the wrist and the base at the knuckles.

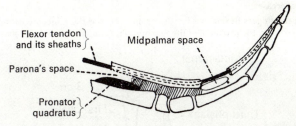

Fig. 399. Section in the long axis of the hand to show the forearm space—Parona's.

BOUNDARIES:
  Proximal: They are continuous with the subcutaneous tissue of the forearm.
  Distal: They are continuous with the subcutaneous tissue of the webs of the fingers.
  Medial and lateral: They are continuous with the subcutaneous tissue around the ulnar border of the hand and 2nd metacarpal, respectively.
      These two spaces are therefore much more extensive and less well circumscribed than the palmar spaces.

CREASES OF THE HAND AND FINGERS

Palmar creases

WRIST CREASES: These are two creases just proximal to the thenar and hypothenar eminences:
  1. The proximal marks the level of the wrist joint.
  2. The distal marks the level of the proximal border of the transverse carpal ligament. The superficial palmar arch is three finger-breadths distal to this crease. The deep palmar arch is two finger-breadths distal to this crease.

METACARPOPHALANGEAL CREASES: The creases between the palm and fingers are not at the level of the metacarpophalangeal joints. These joints are 2 cm proximal to the creases.

INTERPHALANGEAL CREASES: Of the two creases between the 1st and 2nd phalanges, the proximal marks the joint. The crease between the 2nd and 3rd phalanges marks the joint.

Dorsal creases

With the fingers flexed to a fist the prominences at the joints are formed in every case by the proximal of the two bones forming that joint (*Fig*. 400).

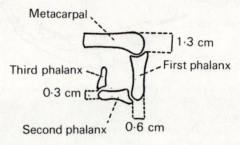

Fig. 400. To show that when the fingers are clenched the prominence of the knuckle is always formed by the proximal bone. The distance of the joint from the knuckle is shown.

1. The metacarpophalangeal joint is 1·3 cm distal to the prominences of the knuckle.
2. The proximal interphalangeal joint is 0·6 cm distal to the prominence at the joint.
3. The distal interphalangeal joint is 0·3 cm distal to the prominence at the joint.

INFECTIONS OF THE HAND

Skin

See Fig. 401.

INTRACUTICULAR: An abscess in the epidermis is usually referred to as an intracuticular abscess. An infected traumatic blister is an example of such an infection.

SUBCUTICULAR INFECTION: A furuncle (boil) due to a staphylococcal infection of a hair follicle is an example of a subcuticular infection. These infections usually occur on the dorsum of the hand.

SUBCUTANEOUS ABSCESS: This may arise as a result of a penetrating injury of the hand or an extension from a superficial infection.

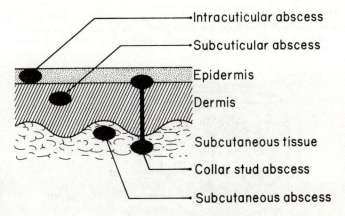

Fig. 401. Skin infection of the hand.

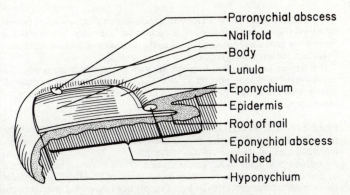

Fig. 402. Nail sectioned in sagittal plane.

COLLAR STUD ABSCESS: An infected blister may penetrate through the dermis to the subcutaneous space or deeper; alternatively a deep-seated infection may extend superficially. In either case a collar stud abscess is formed which should always be suspected when the apparently trivial superficial component of the abscess is associated with a severe tissue reaction.

Terminal phalanges

More than half of all hand infections involve the terminal phalanges of the fingers. These may occur around the nail fold (*Fig.* 402) or the pulp space (*Fig.* 403).

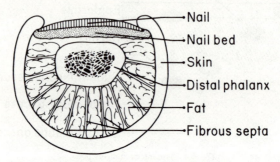

Nail
Nail bed
Skin
Distal phalanx
Fat
Fibrous septa

Fig. 403. Transverse section through the pulp space of distal phalanx.

NAIL FOLD INFECTION: Paronychial and eponychial infections are caused by trivial trauma and initially are intracuticular infections. When pus has formed it is quite simply drained by lifting the nail fold with a sterile needle: no anaesthetic of any kind is required.

If infection has extended beneath the nail, the eponychium (cuticle) is pushed back and that portion of the nail overlying the pus is excised. Anaesthesia either by regional block or inhalation is obviously necessary in these cases.

PULP SPACE INFECTION: Pulp spaces occur on the volar aspect of all the phalanges but the pulp space over the terminal phalanx is most commonly infected usually as the result of minor trauma.

Over the front of the distal phalanx the skin is bound down to the periosteum by dense fibrous processes with fatty tissue between. The distal four-fifths of the terminal phalanx receives its blood supply from the digital arteries at the sides of the finger. These vessels to the bone reach it by penetrating the dense fibrous processes mentioned (*Fig.* 404). Should infection of this tissue occur, there is no provision for expansion because of its fibrous nature. The arteries to the bone are compressed by the inflammatory pressure, which may result in necrosis of the part of the bone they supply, i.e. the distal four-fifths.

The pus is drained through an incision over the point of maximal tenderness or through a subcuticular blister if present. The abscess must be explored to determine whether the terminal phalanx feels roughened which is suggestive of an osteitis. No drains are used.

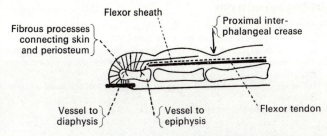

Fig. 404. A figure to show: (1) The fibrous bands binding skin to periosteum over the last phalanx, and the blood supply to the shaft of the phalanx traversing these bands. The vessels to the epiphysis do not go through this area. (2) The fact that the flexor sheath is immediately subjacent to the proximal interphalangeal crease, so that a pin-prick in the direction of the arrow may cause tenosynovitis.

> *Digital Nerve Block:* Provided the infection is confined to the distal phalanx, satisfactory anaesthesia is achieved with a digital nerve block. The needle is inserted into the loose tissue of the web at the base of the finger and then directed forwards. About 2–3 ml of local anaesthetic without adrenaline is injected around each digital nerve.

Tendon sheath infections (tenosynovitis)

The skin of the creases of the proximal interphalangeal joints of the fingers is closely bound down to the underlying fibrous flexor sheaths. Pricks in these creases may, therefore, cause tenosynovitis, as the sheath is so intimately related to the skin (*Fig.* 404).

Tenosynovitis is usually due to a haemolytic streptococcus. The finger is swollen and passive extension of the finger is very painful. If seen early most cases respond to antibiotics. Tendon sheaths may be drained by transverse incisions into both ends of the sheath.

Fascial space infections

Infections in these spaces, midpalmar and thenar, are now uncommon. If there is a collar stud abscess this is explored, but if no superficial abscess is present an incision is made over the point of maximal tenderness parallel to a palmar crease if possible. Once the thick palmar skin has been incised, a closed sinus forceps is pushed through the subcutaneous tissue until the abscess cavity is entered. The forceps displace important structures without damaging them. If the infection points in one of the web spaces the incision is made in the web space and forceps used to locate the pus.

INCISIONS IN THE HAND

Certain principles are applicable to all incisions of the hand:
1. An incision in the palm of the hand should be longer than an incision on the dorsum of the hand, because the palmar skin lacks mobility.
2. The incision should be of adequate length to avoid unnecessary retraction.
3. Incisions should be parallel to major skin creases of the hand as far as possible.
4. An incision should not cross a skin crease at a right-angle.

Finger incisions

1. MIDLATERAL INCISIONS: This incision (*Fig*. 405) is placed on the side of the finger dorsal to the posterior limits of the flexor creases. The incision continues through the subcutaneous fat and is then directed between the bone dorsally and the neurovascular bundle ventrally. The flexor tendon sheath is then exposed.

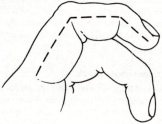

Fig. 405. Midlateral incision just dorsal to flexor creases.

This incision heals well but the dorsal branches of the digital nerves are severed and the incision may injure the collateral and retinacular ligaments. An extension of the incision into the palm may damage the neurovascular bundle. Exposure of the flexor tendon is also somewhat restricted.

2. VOLAR ZIG-ZAG INCISION: The volar skin incisions (*Fig*. 406) form an angle (hinge) of about 135 degrees at the skin creases of the fingers. The incisions should extend only to a point anterior to the neurovascular bundle. Proximally the incision can be extended into the palm.

Volar zig-zag incisions provide adequate exposure and do not interfere with the neurovascular bundle.

In tendon injuries of the flexor tendons (*Fig*. 407), associated with oblique wounds, additional exposure is obtained by extending the wound to a flexor crease to form the hinge of a zig-zag incision.

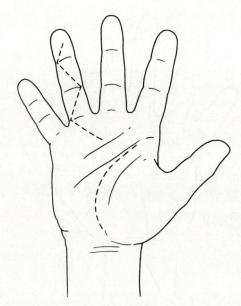

Fig. 406. Volar zig-zag incision and palmar incision parallel to skin crease.

In transverse wounds of the finger, the wound should not be enlarged by zig-zag extensions immediately adjacent to the primary wound, because this would create skin flaps with acute angles and compromise the blood supply. The initial extension of the wound is in the long axis of the finger to the next skin crease.

If one digital artery is severed, the distal extension of the incision must be on the same side as the injury or a skin slough will occur.

3. PALMAR INCISIONS: Zig-zag incisions from the fingers may be made until a palmar crease is reached. In the palm particular care must be taken to avoid damaging the recurrent branch of the median nerve which emerges 3·5 cm distal to a point on the distal wrist crease at the junction of its lateral third with its medial two-thirds.

The palmar incision can be extended onto the wrist by making a longitudinal incision with a small zig-zag at wrist level to reduce the scar (*Fig.* 407).

Scars do not stretch, but hypertrophy as the result of intermittent tension and must not, therefore, cross flexion creases.

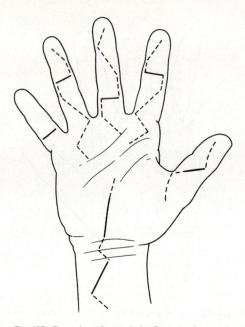

Fig. 407. Extension of wounds for flexor tendon repair.

AMPUTATIONS

In general, in the hand, consideration must be given to saving the maximum amount consistent with function and a pain-free state.

Thumb

The value of this member is almost as great as the rest of the fingers combined. As much as possible must be saved.

Index finger

This is the finger most commonly used to oppose with the thumb. Hence, maximum length must be maintained where possible.

An exception to this might be where cosmetic priorities exist in a young female of sedentary occupation, where a ray amputation, with a deepening of the first web and resultant three-finger hand, gives an excellent cosmetic and functional result.

In a manual labourer where grip is important, only an oblique removal of the head of the metacarpal should be contemplated to preserve the deep transverse metacarpal ligament which provides strength and stability of the grip (*Fig.* 408).

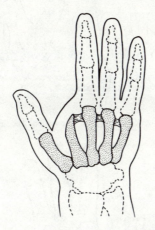

Fig. 408. Amputation through the metacarpal head of index finger.

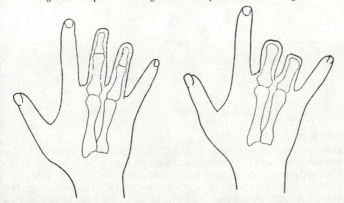

Fig. 409. Commendable amputations of the middle and ring fingers. They would also be sound in principle if amputation was confined to but one of the digits.

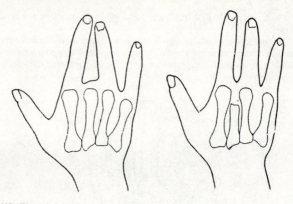

Fig. 410. The left-hand figure shows a poor amputation. The defect is rectified in the right-hand figure.

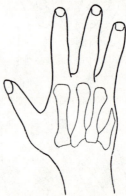

Fig. 411. Sound amputation of the little finger.

Middle and ring fingers

Here conditions are different. Amputations at all levels are acceptable as far proximally as the first interphalangeal joint. The stump lends strength to the hand and prevents the adjacent fingers from falling together (*Fig.* 409).

Amputation through the metacarpophalangeal joint is unsatisfactory. The adjacent fingers fall together and the metacarpal head tends to be displaced dorsally. This is prevented by removing the metacarpal head (*Fig.* 410).

Little finger

Amputation may be carried out at any level where good flaps are available. Metacarpophalangeal amputation leaves an unsightly projection which is readily injured. Removal of the metacarpal head is advisable (*Fig*. 411). This, however, will weaken the grip due to damage to the deep transverse metacarpal ligament and should, therefore, not be done in labourers requiring a firm grip.

Chapter 37

THE HIP

The hip joint is the largest joint in the body and is notable for both its stability and mobility. The bony ball-and-socket configuration supported by the surrounding soft tissues provides most of the stability, but also allows for its mobility.

Dislocations are thus not common but when they do occur are usually associated with violent injuries.

The joint is synovial in nature, consisting of the spherical femoral head articulating in a bony cup, the acetabulum.

The head is attached to the shaft of the femur by a neck which is angled at 135 degrees, anteverted (points anteriorly), and which is of smaller circumference than the head (*Fig*. 412). These factors contribute to the exceptional mobility of the joint.

The acetabulum is deficient of articular cartilage centrally and inferiorly and is deepened by its deformable fibrocartilaginous labrum. The head is joined to the acetabulum by a strong ligament extending from the fovea centralis (a depression on the medial aspect of the head) to the transverse ligament of the acetabulum which spans its deficient inferior border.

The function of the joint is dependent on these skeletal parameters. Abnormalities occur on both acetabular and femoral sides of the joint, and these inevitably lead to pain, deformity and disability.

The acetabulum may be congenitally shallow and not contain the head well—a condition known as 'acetabular dysplasia'.

The femoral neck is biomechanically more susceptible to fractures than the shaft of the femur, especially in any condition resulting in osteoporosis. The neck shaft angle may be reduced (coxa vara) (*Fig*. 413) as a result of slipped upper femoral epiphysis, malunited fracture, and bending of the upper femoral shaft in rickets and fibrous dysplasia.

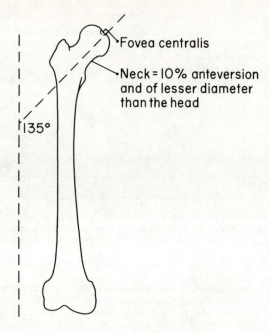

Fig. 412. Angle of the neck of the femur.

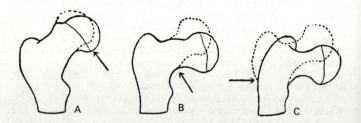

Fig. 413. Coxa vara. The dotted lines represent the normal. The arrows indicate the site of the origin of the deformity. A, Epiphysial type; B, cervical type; C, bending of the shaft of the femur.

The neck shaft angle may be increased—coxa valga. This is either congenital or acquired. The limb is held in a position of abduction and external rotation. Coxa valga is seen in congenital dislocation of the hip.

CONGENITAL DISLOCATION OF THE HEAD OF THE FEMUR

In this condition, the child is born with the head of the femur outside its socket, resting usually on the dorsum ilii behind the acetabulum. This condition is associated with important changes in the upper end of the femur:

1. The neck of the femur is short and in valgus.
2. The forward (anteversion) angle is considerably increased, being anything from 30 degrees to 90 degrees instead of the normal 12 degrees.

The result of this is that in a radiograph of the joint with the toes pointing forward, no neck of the femur can be seen, the epiphysis appearing to sit on the top of the vertical shaft (*Fig.* 414). If, however, the limb is rotated fully inward so that the toes point inwards at a right-angle, and another plate is taken, the neck will be seen.

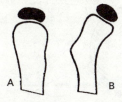

Fig. 414. Radiographs of upper end of femur in congenital dislocation of hip joint. A, Schematic representation of upper end of femur with toes directed forwards; the neck of the bone is not seen. B, With the foot rotated in as far as possible; the neck is seen.

This condition must be diagnosed at birth because at this early stage treatment is simple and the results are excellent. Failure to make an early diagnosis results in delayed treatment, with poor development of the femoral and acetabular components of the joint.

A valuable clinical test is the Ortolani test where the infant lies on its back, with the hips and knees flexed and, with abduction at the hips, a click is felt as the head is reduced. On reversing this manoeuvre the head is once again dislocated (which is the principle of Barlow's test).

TRAUMATIC DISLOCATIONS OF THE HIP

Posterior dislocations are the most common (80 per cent) and are usually due to a direct blow to the knee with the hip in a flexed position, e.g. a passenger in a motor vehicle accident striking his knee against the dashboard at the time of impact. The sciatic nerve may be injured in this type of dislocation.

Anterior dislocations occur infrequently and involve disruption of the capsule and the iliofemoral ligament.

In all dislocations, the blood supply to the head of the femur may be compromised with resulting avascular necrosis of the head of the femur.

THE CAPSULE AND LIGAMENTS OF THE JOINT

The capsule (*Fig*. 415) attaches proximally to the rim of the bony acetabulum except inferiorly where it is attached to the transverse ligament. Distally the capsule attaches to the femoral neck posteriorly and to the intertrochanteric line anteriorly. The fibres from here are reflected along the neck to the femoral head.

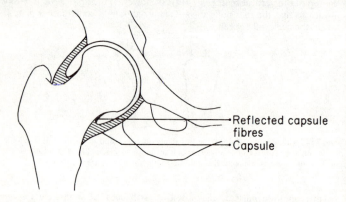

Fig. 415. The capsule of the hip joint.

The anterior aspect of the capsule is reinforced by:

1. The iliofemoral ligament (*Fig*. 416): this is shaped like an inverted Y and is one of the strongest ligaments in the body. Its attachment anteriorly is the anterior inferior iliac spine and distally the intertrochanteric line. Its function is to resist hyperextension of the hip.

2. Pubofemoral ligament: the fibres pass from the superior ramus of the pubis to the lowest part of the capsule. The posterior part of the capsule is reinforced by the ischiofemoral ligament which extends from the ischium just below the acetabulum to the posterior surface of the acetabulum.

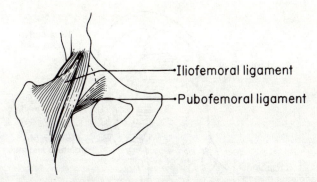

Iliofemoral ligament

Pubofemoral ligament

Fig. 416. Iliofemoral and pubofemoral ligaments of the hip joint.

SESAMOID OF THE RECTUS FEMORIS

This bone is important as it may be mistaken for a fracture. In radiographs of the hip joint a small nodule of bone is frequently seen just below the anterior inferior iliac spine. It is a sesamoid bone in the reflected head of the rectus femoris. It is seen in adult hip joints long after acetabular ossification is complete (*Fig.* 417).

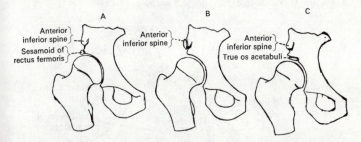

Fig. 417. A, The sesamoid of the rectus femoris; B, avulsed anterior inferior spine; C, os acetabuli.

The anterior inferior iliac spine may be avulsed by the powerful iliofemoral ligament. It is obvious, therefore, that compensation cases may centre round the question of whether a loose portion of bone is a sesamoid or a fracture.

Very rarely the superior portion of the acetabulum may persist as a separate bone, the os acetabuli, which is in the hip joint and not external to it.

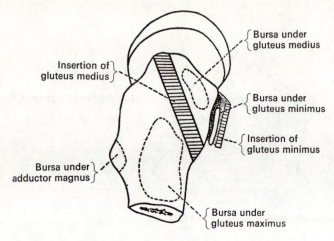

Fig. 418. Bursae on the greater trochanter of the femur.

BURSAE AROUND THE HIP

These are: (1) subgluteal (*Fig.* 418); (2) subpsoas (*Fig.* 419).

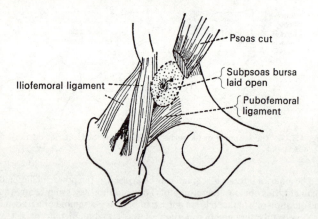

Fig. 419. Showing a communication between the subpsoas bursa and the hip joint.

1. Subgluteal

Four bursae occur under the gluteus maximus:

1. Between the gluteus maximus and the smooth part of the ilium lying between the posterior curved line and the outer lip of the iliac crest.
2. Between the gluteus maximus and the lower part of the outer aspect of the greater trochanter of the femur. It is large.
3. Between the gluteus maximus and the ischial tuberosity. It may enlarge in persons who follow sedentary occupations (weaver's bottom). It is small and often absent.
4. Between the tendon of the gluteus maximus and vastus lateralis.

One under the gluteus medius: between it and the upper part of the lateral aspect of the greater trochanter.

One under the gluteus minimus: in relation to its insertion into the front of the greater trochanter.

2. Subpsoas

This important bursa is found between the iliopectineal eminence and the psoas tendon. In 10 per cent of cases it communicates with the hip joint through the thin part of the capsule between the iliofemoral and pubofemoral ligaments.

BLOOD SUPPLY OF THE HEAD OF THE FEMUR

The femoral head gets its blood supply principally from the circumflex and gluteal arteries which form a vascular ring about the base of the neck (*Fig.*

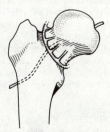

Fig. 420. Blood supply of the head of the femur.

420). From here 'intracapsular' vessels pass up in the reflected retinacular fibres of the capsule and enter the head at its junction with the neck. The most important vessels are found in the superior lateral aspect of the neck fibres.

These vessels are subject to:

a. Occlusion by effusion (blood, pus etc.) which might increase the joint space pressure.

b. Disruption by fractures occurring in the neck of the femur, hence the high association of the avascular necrosis of the femoral head seen in fractures occurring in this area, especially if displacement has occurred.

The head also receives a small blood supply from the endosteal, metaphysial vessels and an insignificant amount via the ligamentum teres.

NERVE SUPPLY

This arises from all three major nerves of the lower limb: the femoral, obturator and sciatic. It is therefore not surprising that pain in the hip joint can present as referred pain in the back, the knee, or rarely in the calf and about the ankle.

ANATOMICAL BASES OF CLINICAL TESTS

Trendelenburg's hip test

Two sets of muscles go from the hip bone to the femur:

1. THE ILIOTROCHANTERIC: These are short powerful muscles which go from the ilium to the region of the greater trochanter, e.g. glutei, obturators, piriformis, quadratus femoris etc. These are the muscles which maintain the pelvis at a horizontal level with the patient standing on one leg, provided the head of the femur is in its socket (and the bone intact).

2. THE ILIOFEMORAL: Long muscles going from the hip bone to the femur, e.g. adductors and hamstrings. (These muscles do not really arise from the ilium but from the pubis and ischium.) They are not concerned with the balancing of the pelvis in standing on one limb apart from their function as stays to the joints.

PERFORMANCE OF THE TEST: The patient stands on one leg. If the hip joint on that side is normal, the pelvis rises slightly on the opposite side as determined by the level of the anterior superior iliac spine. If the patient bears weight on the pathological hip, then the pelvis sinks on the opposite side as shown by the level of the spines (*Fig.* 421). The iliotrochanteric muscles are not powerful enough to maintain the horizontal position of the pelvis, and the opposite side may be seen to drop lower the longer the patient stands on the affected limb. This is a positive Trendelenburg test.

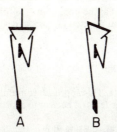

Fig. 421. Trendelenburg's hip test. A, Normal; B, pathological hip.

Thomas' hip flexion test

ANATOMICAL BASIS OF THE TEST: Full flexion of the normal hip joint with the patient recumbent brings the anterior aspect of the thigh into contact with the anterior abdominal wall and flattens out the normal lumbar curve, so that the hand cannot be pushed through between the lumbar region of the spine and the mattress. The opposite thigh meanwhile remains in the same plane as the trunk, i.e. flat on the mattress, if the hip joint on that side is also normal.

When a hip joint is diseased, e.g. by tuberculosis, the thigh takes up a position of flexion. A considerable degree of flexion of the thigh may be disguised by increasing the forward bend or lordosis of the lumbar spine. The patient may then be seen lying in bed with both lower limbs resting on the mattress, thus entirely hiding the flexion deformity of the hip.

PERFORMANCE OF THE TEST: Flexion may be clearly indicated by flexing the sound thigh firmly on the abdomen. This flattens out the forward bend of the lumbar spine and the affected thigh is bent up to whatever degree of true flexion exists.

In performing the test the free hand is between the spine and the mattress. As soon as the back touches the hand the pressure on the sound side is discontinued, thus preventing the misleading result which would ensue should the sacrum be tilted off the bed.

SURGERY OF THE HIP

Aspiration

    a. The needle is inserted at a point 2 cm lateral to the femoral artery just below the inguinal ligament and pushed directly posteriorly, or *b.* The needle is entered at the upper border of the greater trochanter in the midlateral line and directed inwards and slightly upwards, in a line parallel with the femoral neck.

Surgical approaches to the hip

ANTERIOR APPROACH: This approach is useful if it is desired to do an osteotomy or division of the femoral neck or to approximate the fragments in fracture of the neck.

Incision: Almost vertical, passing down the thigh from the anterior superior iliac spine (*Fig.* 422).

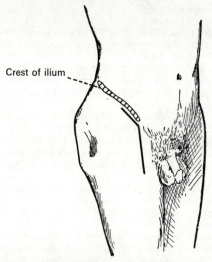

Crest of ilium

Fig. 422. The lower limb of the incision is the anterior approach to the hip joint. The addition of the lateral extension at the upper end of the incision transforms it into the anterolateral approach.

Structures Encountered: The fascia lata is exposed. The lateral cutaneous nerve is to the inner side of the upper end of the incision, but is cut a little below as it passes outwards. The cut extends deep between the sartorius and rectus femoris on the inner side, and the tensor fasciae latae and the gluteus minimus on the outer side. The transverse branch of the lateral femoral circumflex artery is cut. The capsule of the joint is then exposed. The structures in front of the joint (enumerated above) are very tense and poor exposure is obtained, so that no very extensive procedure can be attempted by this route.

ANTEROLATERAL APPROACH: The addition of an external limb to the vertical incision gives vastly better access than the anterior approach. This method (*Fig*. 422) is especially useful for an operation in congenital dislocation of the femoral head, e.g. making a ledge above the acetabulum to prevent the head slipping out.

Incision: Precisely as in the anterior method, with the addition of a 7·5 cm extension backwards from the upper end along the crest of the ilium.

Structures Encountered: The same as in the vertical part of the cut. The external limb of the incision goes through tensor fasciae latae down to the bone, and this muscle and the anterior parts of the two lesser glutei are stripped off the outer aspect of the dorsum ilii, carrying with them the superior gluteal nerve. Thus the superior surface of the joint and femoral neck is exposed in addition to the front of the joint.

LATERAL APPROACH: This is probably the most used approach to the hip today as most total hip arthroplasties are done through this exposure (*Fig*. 423).

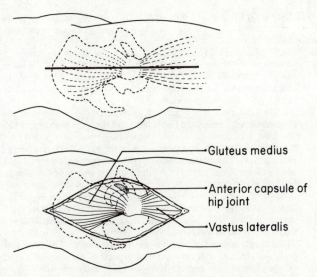

Gluteus medius

Anterior capsule of hip joint

Vastus lateralis

Fig. 423. The lateral approach to the hip joint.

Incision: With the patient in the supine position a horizontal incision is made over the greater trochanter approximately 20 cm in length, equal proportions above and below it.

Structures Encountered: The fascia lata (iliotibial tract) is the first structure encountered; above the trochanter the tract becomes the tensor fasciae latae muscle. The incision is carried through this muscle and fascial tract in the same line as the skin incision, thus entering the large bursa over the greater trochanter and revealing the gluteus medius fibres attaching to the trochanter superiorly and to vastus lateralis inferiorly.

The hip joint itself can now be approached by:

a. A trochanteric osteotomy of the greater trochanter, lifting off the gluteal abductor mechanism and exposing the anterior and superior aspects of the joint.

b. Anterior capsulectomy by retracting the glutei superiorly and all structures anterior to the joint medially.

c. Transgluteally by elevating the anterior half of the gluteal fibres together with the anterior fibres of the vastus lateralis and capsule of the joint from the anterior aspect of the greater trochanter and femoral neck right up to the acetabular margin.

POSTERIOR APPROACH: This approach is much the best and most popular for extensive operative procedures on the joint, e.g. treatment of fracture dislocations.

Incision: This is angled (*Fig.* 424) with the angle at the tip (anterior or posterior) of the greater trochanter. The lower limb of the incision extends vertically down the limb axis for 7·5 cm. The upper limb extends towards the posterior superior iliac spine in the direction of the fibres of the gluteus maximus.

Structures Encountered: The tendinous insertion of the gluteus maximus is divided where it meets the fascia lata, and here are found branches of the lateral circumflex artery. The gluteus itself is divided in the direction of its fibres, many branches of the gluteal arteries being cut in the process. When the gluteus maximus is poorly developed it need not be divided, but its upper border exposed and pulled downwards. Having dealt with the gluteus maximus and with a layer of fat beneath it, there appears the interval between the two minor glutei above and the piriformis below. The two former muscles are detached from their trochanteric attachments, or alternatively the trochanter with its muscles is chiselled off and retracted up and back. The obturators and piriformis are pulled down. Thus the entire posterior, lateral, and even anterior aspects of the capsule and neck of the femur are displayed. No large vessel or nerve is seen throughout.

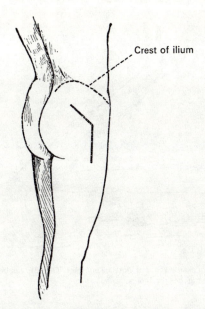

Crest of ilium

Fig. 424. The posterior approach to the hip joint.

Incision through the capsule is vascular as a significant amount of the blood supply to the head arises from vessels situated in the capsule posteriorly.

Osteotomy

This can be done on either side of the joint:

A. PELVIC: Alteration to direction of or the anatomy of the acetabulum.

B. FEMORAL: Alteration of neck direction thereby changing the loading pattern of the femoral head. This is done at an intratrochanteric level because of rich blood supply to this area, thus ensuring subsequent union.

Excision (Girdlestone operation)

The head and neck of the femur are excised. A fibrous joint develops, retaining some movement although lacking stability, but enabling the patient to walk and sit.

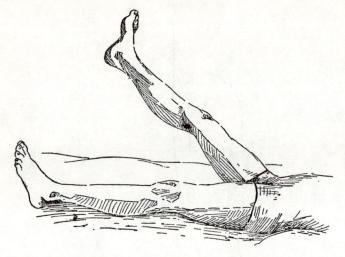

Fig. 425. Optimum position for ankylosis of hip joint. The limb can be brought on the couch if the patient arches the lumbar spine.

Fusion

Fusion (*Fig*. 425) can be achieved either intra- or extracapsularly. The optimal position of fusion is:

Flexion, 15–20 degrees.
Abduction, 5–10 degrees.
Rotation, 0 degrees.

Joint replacement

Probably one of the most successful reconstruction procedures done today. In total joint replacement, both the femoral and acetabular components are replaced. If the femoral head only is replaced, this is known as an endoprosthesis or a hemiarthroplasty.

Amputations about the hip

At the hip joint: this should be modified, if possible, to retain the head, neck and part of the greater trochanter of the femur in the stump (transtrochanteric amputation) as it leaves a stump which is more comfortable to the patient. Such amputees are fitted with a limb on the top of which is a platform called 'a tilting table'.

If the hip joint is disarticulated (as may be necessary, e.g. in sarcoma of the femur), then the outer surface of the hip bone is so smooth that the patient has a constant sensation of slipping in his splint. If the upper end of the femur is left, then the stump has a square end on which the patient sits much more securely.

In these amputations most of the muscles are cut away from the hip bone, and the flap is a single posterior one with the scar lying below and parallel to the inguinal ligament.

Chapter 38

THE KNEE JOINT

The knee joint is a modified hinge joint. The mobility of the joint is provided by its bony structure and the stability by its soft tissues.

MOVEMENTS AT THE KNEE JOINT

The extensibility of the ligaments, muscles and the joint capsule determines the extent of movement that is possible at the knee joint.

Flexion and extension take place around a transverse axis, but because the femoral condyles, on which the tibia is hinged, are not truly spherical, the axis is not constant. The curve of the condyles presents a changing radius that is smallest when the knee is flexed and increases with extension (*Fig.* 426).

Because of this change in radius there is a shifting axis during flexion and extension which results in tightening of the collateral ligaments in full extension.

The shape of the medial condyle of the femur (*Fig.* 427) determines that as the tibia glides on the femur, from the fully flexed to the fully extended position, it follows the curve of the medial femoral condyle and as a result the tibia rotates outwards.

In the fully extended position the tibial tubercles are lodged in the intercondylar notch, the menisci are tightly wedged between the femoral and tibial condyles and this, with tightening of the collateral ligaments, results in 'locking' of the knee in which position no rotation of the tibia on the femur is possible. This provides mechanical stability to the knee joint and enables the person to stand erect without quadriceps muscle contraction, but the inability to rotate renders it vulnerable to injury.

When the tibia is fixed, as in rising from the sitting position, the rotation in the process of extension has to take place by the femur rotating medially on the tibia. This mechanism may result in injury to the hip joint.

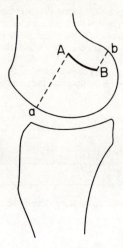

Fig. 426. The changing radius of the femoral condyles. Radius B–b is small in flexion and increases in extension A–a.

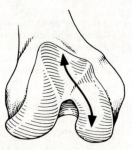

Fig. 427. The articular surface of the medial condyle of the femur.

During the flexion and extension of the knee there is not only the rolling of the femur on the tibia and the rotation produced in full extension, but there is also a sliding effect of the condyles of the femur on the tibia, which prevents the femur rolling off the tibial plateau. This sliding phenomenon occurs in association with movement of the menisci posteriorly in flexion and anteriorly in extension, like a pip squeezed between the fingers. This renders the menisci vulnerable to injury.

The quadriceps muscle is the main extensor of the knee and the vastus medialis is the most important component responsible for the last 10 degrees of extension. The quadriceps also constitutes an important structure, which is responsible for the stability of the knee and weakness results in pain and recurrent effusions which can be prevented by quadriceps exercises.

LIGAMENTS OF THE KNEE JOINT

Fibrous capsule

It is strengthened in parts by strong expansions from the tendons and muscles which surround the knee joint. Anteriorly it blends with extensions from the

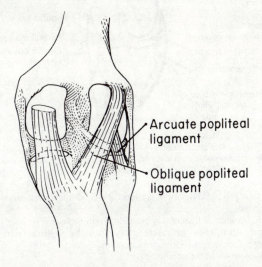

Arcuate popliteal
ligament

Oblique popliteal
ligament

Fig. 428. Posterior reinforcing ligaments of the capsule.

vastus medialis and vastus lateralis. Posteriorly (*Fig.* 428), on the medial side the posterior capsule is reinforced by recurrent fibres of the semimembranosus tendon which form the oblique popliteal ligament.

On the lateral side, the posterior capsule is reinforced by the Y-shaped arcuate popliteal ligament. The stem of the ligament arises from the posterior aspect of the head of the fibula. The medial portion of this ligament is inserted into the intercondylar area of the femur and the lateral portion to the posterior aspect of the lateral epicondyle of the femur.

The collateral ligaments

The collateral ligaments (*Fig.* 429) are very strong structures which prevent lateral movements at the joint. If they are torn or even stretched, the integrity of the joint is lost.

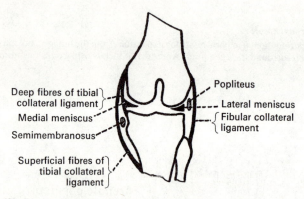

Fig. 429. Diagram showing splitting of tibial collateral ligament into deep and superficial fibres. The former anchor the medial meniscus, and the tendon of the semimembranosus insinuates itself between the two sets of fibres. The lateral meniscus has no attachment to the fibular collateral ligament.

The fibular collateral ligament is round and cord-like and stands well away from the bone.

The tibial collateral ligament is broad and strap-like and is closely applied to the bone. An inferior geniculate artery (from the popliteal) passes under each ligament, running in a forward direction.

The attachments of the two ligaments are:

1. FIBULAR COLLATERAL LIGAMENT:
   Superior: To the lateral epicondyle of the femur just above the groove for the popliteus.
   Inferior: To the head of the fibula anterior to the apex. It divides the biceps femoris tendon into two; the popliteus passes out beneath it.

2. TIBIAL COLLATERAL LIGAMENT: This ligament (*Fig.* 430) consists of superficial, oblique and deep parts:

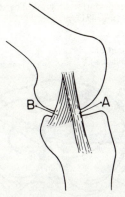

Fig. 430. The medial ligament. A, Superficial part; B, oblique part: The deep part cannot be seen.

Superficial (anterior) part is a vertical band extending from the medial epicondyle to the medial surface of the tibia about 3 cm from the joint line and then extends further down the tibia.

The deep (posterior) part is derived from the joint capsule deep to the superficial part and is attached to the femoral and tibial condyles. It is thick and strong. The peripheral edge of the medial meniscus is firmly attached to it.

The oblique part arises from the medial femoral condyle behind the attachment of the superficial part. It fans out to be attached to the posterior half of the medial condyle. The peripheral edge of the medial meniscus is also attached to this part of the medial ligament. The posterior part of the oblique portion blends with the capsule of the knee joint.

A tear of the tibial collateral ligament is often associated with a medial meniscus tear because of the attachment of the meniscus to the collateral ligament.

The tendons of sartorius, gracilis and semitendinosus cross the tibial collateral ligament. A bursa separates the tendons from the ligament.

Test of Lateral Stability: The collateral ligaments of the knee are tested by the valgus and varus stress tests at 0 and 30 degrees of flexion. At 0 degrees, one tests both the stability of the collateral ligaments and the posterior capsule. At 30 degrees of flexion, the effects of the posterior capsule are eliminated.

The cruciate ligaments

Very powerful cord-like structures. They prevent movement of the two bones on each other in an anteroposterior direction. The attachments of the cruciate ligaments are as follows (*Fig.* 431):

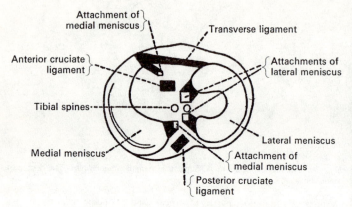

Fig. 431. Attachments to the upper surface of the tibia.

ANTERIOR CRUCIATE:

Below: To the anterior intercondylar fossa of the tibia behind the anterior horn of the medial meniscus.

Above: To the posterior aspect of the medial surface of the lateral condyle of the femur.

It is now thought that part of the anterior cruciate ligament is under tension in any position of the knee.

POSTERIOR CRUCIATE:

Below: To the posterior intercondylar fossa and popliteal surface of the tibia behind the posterior horn of the medial meniscus.

Above: To the anterior aspect of the lateral surface of the medial condyle of the femur. It is joined by a slip from the posterior part of the lateral meniscus.

The posterior cruciate ligament is taut in flexion.

The anterior cruciate passes backwards and outwards. The posterior cruciate passes inwards and forwards; therefore, in opening the knee joint from the inner side the posterior cruciate is seen first.

The anterior cruciate prevents the tibia from being moved forwards on the femur in extension. The posterior cruciate prevents the tibia from being moved backwards on the femur in flexion.

ANTEROPOSTERIOR STABILITY: The anterior cruciate and tibial collateral ligaments are responsible for anterior stability of the knee joint. When the tibial collateral ligament is torn the medial tibial condyle subluxates forwards, while forward subluxation of the lateral femoral condyle occurs with a tear of the anterior cruciate ligament. Forward subluxation of the whole tibia therefore occurs only when both the tibial collateral and anterior cruciate ligaments are torn.

Posterior stability is dependent on the posterior cruciate, the oblique popliteal ligament which is an extension from the semimembranosus tendon and the arcuate popliteal ligament.

The classical test for the integrity of the cruciate ligaments is the 'drawer' test when the examiner can subluxate the tibia on the femur with the knee flexed to 90 degrees.

In tears of the anterior cruciate and tibial collateral ligaments the tibia is drawn forwards from its normal to an abnormal position—the anterior 'drawer' (*Fig.* 432).

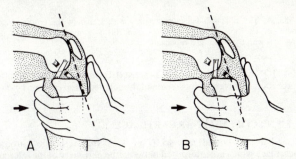

Fig. 432. A, The tibia is drawn forwards from its normal relationship to the femur. B, When the anterior cruciate is torn the tibia moves forwards in relation to the femur.

This test is not sufficiently sensitive and instability is commonly missed. A preferable test is the Lachman test, in which the knee is flexed between 5 and 10 degrees and an attempt is made to pull the tibia forwards on the femur. If the anterior cruciate ligament only is torn the lateral tibial condyle alone subluxates.

An isolated injury of the anterior cruciate ligament, either a partial or complete rupture, is now thought to occur frequently. Such an injury is suspected when an acutely injured knee contains blood and it can be confirmed by doing an arthroscopy.

In a tear of the posterior cruciate, the tibia subluxates posteriorly. The tibia can be drawn forward from this abnormal to a normal position. Unless the initial posterior (abnormal) position of the tibia is recognized, this test may be misinterpreted as a positive anterior drawer sign (*Fig.* 433).

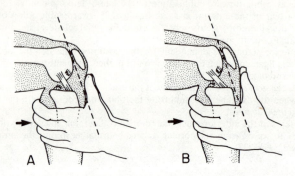

Fig. 433. **A**, The tibia subluxates posteriorly with a tear of the posterior cruciate ligament. **B**, The tibia is drawn forwards from this abnormal position to its normal relationship with the femoral condyles.

ROTATIONAL STABILITY OF THE KNEE: In full extension rotation at the knee joint is prevented by tension of the collateral and cruciate ligaments.

THE MENISCI (SEMILUNAR CARTILAGES)

The medial and lateral menisci (*Fig.* 431) are crescentic portions of fibrocartilage which are interposed between the periphery of the intercondylar surfaces of the tibia and femur. The medial meniscus is C-shaped and the lateral meniscus is more nearly circular. They are firmly attached at the anterior and posterior horns of the intercondylar surface of the tibia. The menisci are attached to the joint capsule by the coronary ligaments and they are joined to each other anteriorly by the transverse ligament.

The posterior half of the medial meniscus is firmly attached to the deep and oblique portions of the tibial collateral ligament. The anterior half is relatively mobile.

The lateral meniscus is not attached to the fibular collateral ligament and is more mobile than the medial meniscus.

Movement of the menisci

The menisci are moved passively by displacement between the tibial and femoral condyles and actively as a result of their attachments to muscles and ligaments. They are pushed anteriorly as the knee extends and posteriorly during flexion. During axial rotation the menisci follow the movement of the femoral condyles. With lateral rotation of the tibia on the femur the medial meniscus moves posteriorly and the lateral meniscus anteriorly.

Functions of the menisci

The following functions have been attributed to the menisci:

1. They increase the stability of the joint by increasing the articular surface of the tibia and by interposing tightly between the joint surfaces when the knee is in extension.
2. They distribute the total load carried by the knee.
3. They spread synovial fluid and provide a slipping surface during knee movement.
4. They prevent the capsule and the synovium being pinched between the articular surfaces during movement of the knee.

Tears of the menisci

A tear is caused by a twisting force with the knee flexed (*Fig*. 434). If the meniscus does not move with the femoral condyles it is crushed or torn by the condyles.

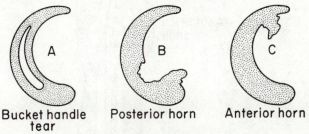

Bucket handle tear   **Posterior horn**   **Anterior horn**

Fig. 434. Tears of the menisci.

The commonest injury is a longitudinal split of the cartilage (bucket-handle tear). The central fragment is displaced to the middle of the joint where it limits full extension (locking) although the joint can still be flexed.

In the elderly, the menisci degenerate and then a transverse tear of the meniscus occurs often with minimal trauma.

The medial meniscus is torn more frequently than the lateral meniscus because the C-shaped meniscus is firmly attached at three widely separated points: the anterior horn, posterior horn and the medial collateral ligament. The lateral meniscus is more circular so that the anterior and posterior horns are closer to each other.

Menisectomy

The periphery of the meniscus receives its blood supply from its attachment to the capsule and ligaments. Repair of a damaged cartilage will occur only in peripheral lesions because the central portion is avascular.

A modern trend in meniscus surgery is an accurate pre-operative diagnosis of the type of injury by arthroscopy or arthrography. A partial menisectomy, in which only the detached portion of the cartilage is removed, is performed. After total menisectomy, local stresses on the articular cartilage are significantly increased with subsequent development of osteo-arthritis.

KNEE ALIGNMENT AND DEFORMITIES

The anatomical axes of a bone is defined as a line that runs along the shaft of the bone. Normally, the femoral and tibial axes meet at the knee to form an

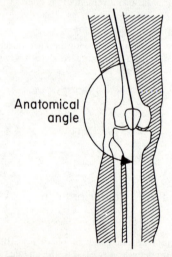

Fig. 435. The physiological valgus angle of the knee joint.

obtuse angle of about 170–175 degrees, which opens laterally (*Fig.* 435). This angle is the physiological valgus angle of the knee joint. If the valgus angle is less than 165 degrees, genu valgum or knock knees exist. If the anatomical angle exceeds 180 degrees, the resulting abnormality is called genu varum or bow legs. These two deformities are important predisposing conditions to joint overload which results in osteo-arthritis.

PATELLOFEMORAL JOINT

The patellofemoral joint is part of the quadriceps mechanism. The patella is anchored distally to the tuberosity of the tibia by the patellar tendon and superiorly to the tendon of the quadriceps muscle, and by medial and lateral retinacula to the knee joint capsule. These structures form a strong bony and fibrous covering for the anterior compartment of the knee. The function of the patella is to increase the leverage of the quadriceps muscle.

The relative medial or lateral insertion of the quadriceps mechanism is determined by the Q angle. This is the angle formed by the line of pull of the quadriceps mechanism and that of the patellar tendon as they intersect at the centre of the patella. Clinically the angle is represented by the intersection of a line drawn from the anterior superior iliac to the centre of the patella with a second line from the centre of the tibial tuberosity to the centre of the patella

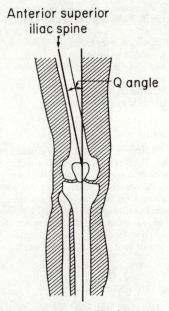

Fig. 436. The Q angle.

(*Fig.* 436). When the angle becomes greater than 15 degrees the contracting quadriceps exerts increasing lateral forces on the patella which predisposes to subluxation of the patella.

Dislocations of the patella

Classified as:
1. Congenital.
2. Traumatic.
3. Recurrent.

1. CONGENITAL: The congenital variety is very rare. It is usually unilateral and is due to an abnormality in the quadriceps. The patella is dislocated laterally and there is an inability to flex the knee.

2. TRAUMATIC: This type is always lateral and is due to either direct trauma or muscular activity, often in those patients who have a predisposition to recurrent dislocation.

3. RECURRENT: Recurrent dislocation is the most common variety. It is always lateral, except in those rare instances where a surgical overcorrection has been performed, when it may be medial. It occurs almost exclusively in females. The predisposing factors are:
   a. Generalized ligamentous laxity.
   b. Localized ligamentous laxity (as following acute trauma).
   c. Increased Q angle.
   d. Patella alta (high-riding patella).
   e. Hypoplastic lateral femoral condyle.

Infrapatellar pad of fat

The infrapatellar fat pad is situated behind and on either side of the ligamentum patellae. The fat is pliable and has a high content of elastic tissue. The fat acts as a cushion during extension of the knee and is protected from injury by alar folds of synovium which cover the joint surface. The fat is connected to the front ends of the semilunar cartilages.

The fat is a mobile structure in the knee joint. Fibrous scars as the result of surgery or adherence to surrounding structures interfere with the mobility of the fat pad which then becomes compressed during straightening of the knee. This results in swelling of the fat and a painful knee.

BURSAE AROUND THE KNEE JOINT

There are twelve bursae (*Fig.* 437): two are posterior; three are medial; three are lateral; four are anterior.

Two posterior bursae

One between each head of origin of the gastrocnemius and the capsule of the

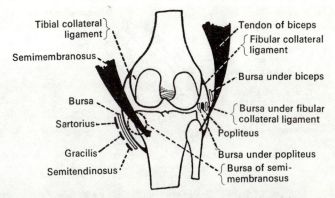

Fig. 437. Bursae on the inner and outer aspects of the knee joint.

joint. They often communicate with the joint. The bursa between the medial head of the gastrocnemius and the capsule sends a prolongation between the gastrocnemius and semimembranosus. This bursa is often enlarged, forming a swelling at the medial side of the popliteal space, which is spoken of as enlargement of the semimembranosus bursa.

Three medial bursae

The first separates the sartorius, gracilis, and semitendinosus from the tibial collateral ligament as they cross it.

The second and third separate the tendon of the semimembranosus from the tibial collateral ligament medially and the condyle of the tibia laterally. The semimembranosus tendon is sandwiched between the ligament medially and the condyle of the tibia laterally.

Three lateral bursae

1. Between the biceps tendon and the fibular collateral ligament.
2. Between the fibular collateral ligament and the popliteus tendon.
3. Between the popliteus tendon and the lateral condyle of the femur. This bursa is really a tube of synovial membrane around the popliteus tendon like that around the long head of the biceps at the shoulder joint. The bursa therefore communicates with the joint.

Four anterior bursae

See Fig. 438.

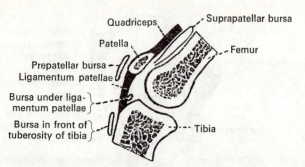

Fig. 438. Bursae on the front of the knee joint.

1. The suprapatellar bursa lies between the anterior surface of the lower part of the femur and the deep surface of the quadriceps muscle. It extends exactly three finger-breadths above the upper border of the patella when the limb is at rest in extension. It always communicates with the knee joint.
2. Prepatellar bursa: the bursa of housemaid's knee. It lies in front of the lower half of the patella and the upper half of the patellar ligament, in the same area where the patellar nerve plexus is situated between the bursa and the skin. Enlargement of this bursa is called housemaid's knee because in scrubbing the floor the bursa is in contact with the ground. This often causes inflammation (bursitis). Such a bursa may get very large and drop by its weight much below its original situation.
3. Between the patellar ligament and the tibia.
4. Between the skin and the smooth lower part of the tuberosity of the tibia. This bursa enlarges in priests and board surfers.

DISLOCATION OF THE KNEE

Dislocation is possible only if all or some of the ligaments are ruptured. Complete dislocation can cause injury to the popliteal vessels, tibial and peroneal nerves.

ASPIRATION OF THE KNEE

1. When the knee joint contains fluid the needle is inserted into the suprapatellar bursa through the quadriceps expansion of the vastus lateralis (*Fig.* 439).

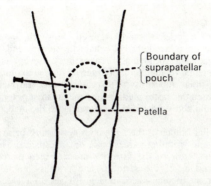

Fig. 439. Puncture of suprapatellar pouch. The needle is entered through the vastus lateralis, in an inward and backward direction.

2. The needle is introduced at any point along the lateral or medial border of the patella. The needle passes obliquely between the patella and the femur (*Fig.* 440).

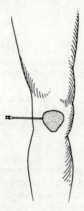

Fig. 440. Aspiration of the knee deep to the patella.

SURGICAL APPROACHES TO THE KNEE JOINT

This may be anteromedial, anterolateral, anterior, posteromedial, posterolateral or posterior, and may be by opening the joint or through an arthroscope.

Anteromedial

OPEN: The entire incision is seldom used. More commonly, only the parapatellar portion is needed. The whole incision extends from 10 cm proximal to the patella at the medial border of the quadriceps tendon, curving medially 2 cm medial to the medial border of the patella and ending just medial to the tibial tuberosity. Dissection passes through the fascia proximally between the vastus medialis and the quadriceps tendon, through the medial capsule and synovium 1–2 cm medial to the medial edge of the patella.

The infrapatellar branch of the saphenous nerve must be avoided; injury can cause pain and irritating paraesthesia or anaesthesia. The saphenous nerve courses posterior to the sartorius muscle, then pierces the fascia between the tendons of the sartorius and gracilis muscles to become subcutaneous on the medial side of the leg. It gives off a large infrapatellar branch on the medial side of the knee. Because the position of this branch is inconstant, blunt dissection between the skin and joint capsule should be used to locate the nerve and to retract it out of harm's way.

ARTHROSCOPIC: The portal of entry is usually medial to the tip of the patella missing the patellar tendon and aiming for the intercondylar notch.

Anterolateral

OPEN: Inspection of the joint is more difficult from this side, because the patella dislocates medially with difficulty. Once again it is unusual to require the whole length of the incision, and commonly only the parapatellar portion is used.

The incision begins proximal to the patella at the insertion of the vastus lateralis. It should pass 2·5 cm lateral to the outer border of the patella and ends 2·5 cm below the tibial tuberosity. Fascia, capsule and synovium are opened in the line of the incision.

ARTHROSCOPIC: This is the most commonly used portal. With the knee flexed a palpable depression is felt in the angle between the patellar tendon and the lateral tibial plateau. The arthroscope is introduced into the centre of the small depression in a posteromedial direction, to enter the intercondylar notch.

Anterior

OPEN: Midline longitudinal incisions have increased in popularity, particularly for joint replacement. The incision heals better and stretches less than parapatellar incisions. The skin incision is centred over the middle of the patella, the length depending on the degree of exposure required. The joint may be entered either by a medial parapatellar incision or by a midline incision, shelling out the medial half of the patella from the retinaculum.

The incision extends proximally through the quadriceps tendon and distally it is usually medial to the patellar tendon.

ARTHROSCOPIC: The transpatellar tendon approach of Gilquist is 1 cm below the tip of the patella in the middle of the knee joint and also through the patellar tendon (but not through the centre of the tendon, which is usually more lateral).

Posteromedial

OPEN: This is done with the knee at 90 degrees. The incision is from the adductor tubercle, parallel and just posterior to the posterior border of the medial collateral ligament and anterior to the medial hamstrings. The capsule is incised posterior to the ligament. This incision is commonly used in combination with a medial parapatellar incision; a curved artery forceps passed from the medial parapatellar incision, deep to the medial collateral ligament, quickly determines the extent of the ligament and a safe point for entry.

ARTHROSCOPIC: The point of entry is below the medial femoral condyle and above the tibial plateau. One can palpate this gap with the knee distended with saline and in 90 degrees of flexion with a varus stress. Enter first with a fine needle; if saline is obtained, introduce the trocar and sheath in the same direction which is slightly anterior and inferior. The popliteal vessels must be avoided.

Posterolateral

OPEN: The skin incision is made with the knee flexed 90 degrees. It runs anterior to the tendon of biceps femoris and the head of the fibula. Proximally, one dissects anterior to the lateral intermuscular septum and exposes the lateral femoral condyle together with the fibular collateral ligament. Identify the tendon of popliteus deep to the biceps tendon; retract it posteriorly and enter the joint capsule posterolaterally.

ARTHROSCOPIC: An unusual portal of entry. The point of entry is at the bisection of two lines; the one in line with the lateral intermuscular septum and the other projected in the line of the fibula and its styloid process.

Posterior

OPEN: The posterior approach requires a knowledge of the anatomy of the popliteal space. The incision is 10–15 cm in length and centred in the fossa. Proximally, the incision is close to the semimembranosus muscle and curves laterally at the level of the joint for about 5 cm, and then runs distally along the lateral head of the gastrocnemius.

One must locate the posterior cutaneous nerve of the calf and the short saphenous vein between the heads of the gastrocnemii. Trace the nerve to its parent trunk, the tibial nerve. Dissecting the tibial nerve distally, one defines branches to the gastrocnemii, soleus and plantaris. Proximally the nerve joins the common peroneal nerve. The space between the tibial nerve and the semimembranosus muscle is avascular and no nerves cross it. This is a good plane to follow to enter the joint. Do so with the leg extended. Once inside, flex the knee slightly to allow a finger to enter the joint.

THROUGH KNEE (DISARTICULATION) AMPUTATION

This is a quick amputation in which no bone is cut. Provided equal lateral flaps are fashioned healing is satisfactory. There is improved proprioception in an end-bearing stump. It is the amputation of choice in a child because the epiphysis at the lower end of the femur is not removed.

Chapter 39

THE ANKLE–FOOT COMPLEX

THE ANKLE JOINT

The ankle joint is a hinge joint between the lower end of the tibia and fibula which accommodates the body of the talus in the mortise formed by the medial and lateral malleoli and the lower articular surface of the tibia. The integrity of the ankle joint is dependent on the inferior tibiofibular ligament supplemented by collateral ligaments. This structure provides stability together with the necessary mobility in one plane only.

Ligaments of the ankle joint

THE INFERIOR TIBULOFIBULAR LIGAMENT: The inferior tibulofibular ligament (*Fig.* 441) which maintains contact between the fibula and tibia is so strong that stresses that tend to separate the bones will fracture the fibula proximal to the ligament before the ligament will tear.

THE MEDIAL COLLATERAL (DELTOID) LIGAMENT: The medial collateral (deltoid) ligament is fan-shaped (*Fig.* 442) and consists of

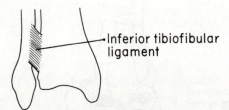

Fig. 441. The inferior tibiofibular joint.

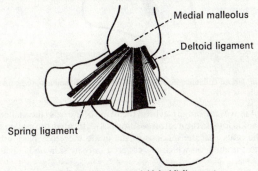

Fig. 442. Medial collateral (deltoid) ligament.

superficial and deep fibres and is extremely strong. Its fibres extend from the borders of the tibial malleolus to the navicular, talus and calcaneus. Stresses opening the medial side of the ankle may avulse the medial malleolus before the ligament tears.

THE LATERAL COLLATERAL LIGAMENT: The lateral collateral ligament (*Fig.* 443) is composed of three separate bands, the anterior and posterior talofibular and calcaneofibular ligaments, which are weaker than the medial collateral ligament.

A partial tear of the lateral ligament occurs when a patient 'twists' (inversion injury) his ankle. A complete tear of the lateral ligament is diagnosed by the X-ray appearance of the ankle with the foot inverted. Because the recent injury is painful this is done under anaesthesia. If the talus tilts out of the mortise 10 degrees more than on the normal side, a complete tear of the lateral ligament is diagnosed.

The ankle joint axis

Because the ankle is a hinge joint which can only move about its axis, no

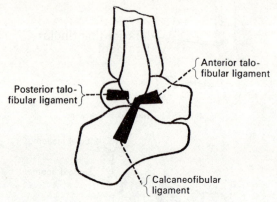

Fig. 443. The lateral collateral ligament. The talofibular ligaments are horizontal, the calcaneofibular is vertical.

tendon that moves the hinge can lie in the plane of the axis (the malleoli). The axis of the ankle joint in the neutral position passes through the malleoli and the body of the talus. All the tendons of the ankle therefore pass anterior or posterior to the malleoli which are covered only by skin and subcutaneous tissue.

Four tendons, the anterior tibial and extensor hallicis longus separated from the extensor digitorum longus and the peroneus tertius laterally by the dorsalis pedis artery, lie anterior to the axis of the ankle joint.

The lateral malleolus acts as a pulley for the peronei longus and brevis and the medial malleolus acts as a pulley for the posterior tibial and flexor digitorum longus muscles enabling these tendons to pass posterior to the axis of the ankle joint. The tendon of the flexor hallucis longus muscle passes posterior to the distal end of the tibia and occupies a broad groove on the posterior surface of the talus which is continuous with a groove on the plantar surface of the sustentaculum tali. The tendo Achillis inserts about 5 cm posterior to the axis of the ankle joint and therefore is a powerful flexor of the ankle.

Range of motion of the ankle is 20 degrees of dorsiflexion and 30–50 degrees of plantar flexion from neutral (the foot at a right-angle to the tibia).

Retinacula around the ankle

These structures prevent bowstringing of the tendons during movements of the ankle.

SUPERIOR EXTENSOR RETINACULUM: This is a thickening of the deep fascia, with which its borders are continuous. Its attachments are the anterior borders of the lower 2·5 cm of the shafts of the tibia and the fibula. Under it pass the structures going from the front of the leg to the dorsum of the foot. These lie in one common compartment except for the tibialis anterior, which lies in a separate compartment. The relation of these structures from medial to lateral is: the tibialis anterior, extensor hallucis longus, the anterior tibial artery with a vein each side, the deep peroneal nerve, the extensor digitorum longus and the peroneus tertius.

The superficial surface is crossed by the commencement of the long saphenous vein, the saphenous nerve, and the superficial peroneal nerve.

INFERIOR EXTENSOR RETINACULUM: This is a Y-shaped structure stretching across the foot in the region of the ankle joint. It is a thickening of the deep fascia.

The stem of the Y is attached to the upper surface of the anterior part of the calcaneus (the extensor digitorum brevis also arises from here and therefore takes origin from the ligament as well).

The upper limb of the Y is attached to the medial malleolus. The lower limb of the Y blends with the deep fascia on the medial border of the foot (plantar aponeurosis).

The structures passing under this ligament are identical with those passing under the superior extensor retinaculum. They are now, however, grouped into two compartments—a medial for the extensor hallucis longus, and a lateral for the extensor digitorum longus and peroneus tertius. The vessels and nerves pass deep to the ligament. The tibialis anterior passes superficial or deep to the inner part of the ligament, not lying in a specialized compartment.

The ligament acts like a sling preventing the tendons from prolapsing to the inner side of the foot (*Fig.* 444).

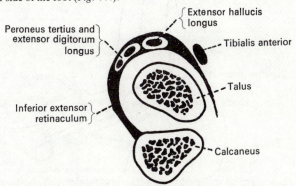

Fig. 444. Arrangement of inferior extensor retinaculum. Note its relation to the tendon of tibialis anterior. (Redrawn from Frazer.)

Flexor retinaculum: Has four borders and two surfaces.
> *Borders:*
>> *Upper:* Is continuous with two layers of fascia: the deep fascia of the leg, and the strong fascia which extends between the superficial and deep muscles of the calf.
>> *Lower:* Is continuous with the medial part of the plantar aponeurosis. The abductor hallucis takes origin from it.
>> *Lateral:* Is attached to the tuberosity of the calcaneus.
>> *Medial:* Is attached to the medial malleolus.
> *Surfaces:*
>> *Superficial or medial:* Is related to the medial calcaneal vessels and nerves, which first pierce it and then cross it.
>> *Deep or lateral:* Is related to the tendons, vessels, and nerves passing from the back of the leg to the sole of the foot. They lie in a common compartment in the following order from the front to the back: tibialis posterior, flexor digitorum longus, posterior tibial artery with a vein each side, posterior tibial nerve, and flexor hallucis longus. Each tendon has a separate synovial sheath.
>> Under the lower part of the ligament the artery and nerve both divide into medial and lateral plantar branches.

PERONEAL RETINACULA: These are thickenings of the deep fascia (*Fig.* 445).

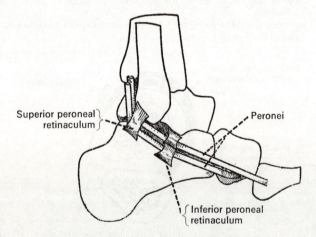

Fig. 445. The peroneal retinacula.

Superior: The superior runs from calcaneus to lateral malleolus and binds the two peronei, longus and brevis, to the back of the lateral malleolus in a common compartment. The brevis is next to the bone.

Inferior: The inferior is attached to the outer surface of the calcaneus. It is divided into two compartments by a septum which is attached to the peroneal tubercle. The brevis is highest.

In the condition of recurrent dislocation of the peroneal tendons, the tendons dislocate forwards over the fibula during dorsiflexion and eversion. In treatment of this condition, the superficial cortex of the lower 5 cm of the fibula is turned backwards and sutured over the peroneal tendons to hold them in their correct position.

Tendon sheaths around the ankle joint
ANTERIOR: Three separate sheaths are found (*Fig*. 446).

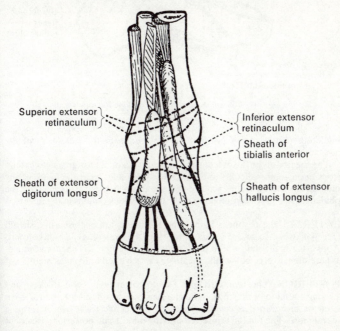

Superior extensor retinaculum

Inferior extensor retinaculum

Sheath of tibialis anterior

Sheath of extensor digitorum longus

Sheath of extensor hallucis longus

Fig. 446. Tendon sheaths anterior to ankle.

The sheath of the tibialis anterior extends from the upper border of the transverse ligament of the leg to just below the ankle joint.

The sheaths of the extensor hallucis longus, extensor digitorum longus, and peroneus tertius extend from the level of the malleoli to the base of the metatarsal bones.

MEDIAL: Three sheaths are found (*Fig.* 447).

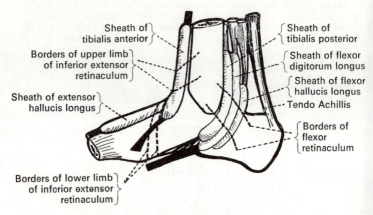

Fig. 447. Tendon sheaths anterior and medial to ankle.

The sheath of tibialis posterior extends from 5 cm above the medial malleolus to the site of insertion of the tendon at the tuberosity of the navicular.

The sheaths of the flexor hallucis longus and flexor digitorum longus extend from the medial malleolus to the middle of the sole. Near the heads of the metatarsals these tendons acquire new sheaths which are arranged over the phalanges in a precisely similar manner to that which obtains in the fingers.

LATERAL: The peroneus longus and the brevis are enclosed in a sheath (*Fig.* 448) which extends 5 cm above the tip of the malleolus and 5 cm below it. Above the malleolus, where the tendons lie together, the sheath is single. Where they diverge below, the sheath gives each a separate investment.

POSTERIOR: The tendo Achillis (tendo calcaneus) is the thickest and strongest tendon of the body. It has no synovial sheath but for about 7·5 cm from its insertion it is covered by loose connective tissue which forms a 'paratenon'. The tendon is inserted into the middle and posterior surfaces of the calcaneus with a bursa intervening (*Fig.* 449). An adventitious bursa

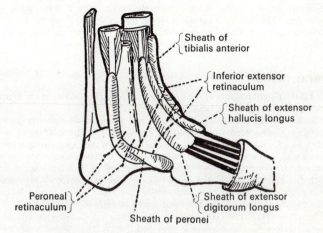

Fig. 448. Tendon sheaths anterior and lateral to ankle.

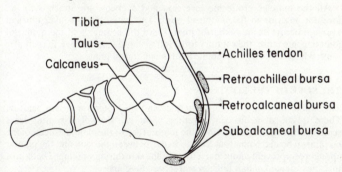

Fig. 449. Bursae around the tendo Achillis.

between the skin and the tendo Achillis (retro-achilleal bursa) may be found and there is also one beneath the calcaneus.

Long distance runners may develop pain, swelling and tenderness around the heel which may be due to:

1. Retrocalcaneal bursitis.
2. Retro-achilleal bursitis.
3. Subcalcaneal bursitis.
4. Irritation of the tendo Achillis paratenon.
5. Small tears in the tendo Achillis.

Rupture of the tendo Achillis probably occurs only if the tendon is degenerate. The patient is unable to stand on tiptoe and a gap can be felt above the insertion of the tendon. With the patient prone the calf is squeezed: the foot plantar flexes if the tendon is intact but not when it has ruptured.

SUBTALAR JOINT

The subtalar joint consists of the anterior and posterior talocalcaneal joints which are separated by the tarsal tunnel.

The movements of inversion and eversion occur in the subtalar joint. Inversion is associated with adduction (movement to the midline of the body), foot supination (in which the lateral border of the foot is brought into contact with the ground) and foot plantar flexion. Eversion is associated with foot abduction (movement away from the midline of the body), pronation (in which the big toe and medial border of the foot are rotated down) and dorsiflexion. The individual components of inversion and eversion always occur together at the subtalar joint and cannot be combined differently.

The transverse tarsal (midtarsal) joint is made up of two anatomically separate joints, the talonavicular joint and the calcaneocuboid joint, but functionally they act together.

All the muscles producing inversion and eversion are attached to the forefoot anterior to the midtarsal joint. The initial part of inversion and eversion occurs at the midtarsal joint. Once the ligaments of the midtarsal joint become tense, the rotatory force is transmitted passively to the subtalar joint, which is much more mobile than the midtarsal joint.

THE SOLE OF THE FOOT

The skin of the sole is about 4 mm thick and is adapted for weight bearing. There are subcutaneous concentrations of fat over the weight-bearing areas such as the heel, lateral margin of the sole and across the plantar aspects of the metatarsal heads. Numerous fibrous bands between the skin and the plantar aponeurosis prevent undue movement of the skin during walking. The skin of the sole is devoid of hair follicles and sebaceous glands.

Incisions on the sole heal well. If there is loss of skin and subcutaneous tissue in weight-bearing areas of the sole as a result of trauma, the defect is best covered by a local flap. If a distant flap containing fat is used from other areas of the body the lack of fibrous septa binding the skin to the underlying tissues result in excessive movement of the skin on walking.

ARCHES OF THE FOOT

The entire body weight is supported by the foot. In weight bearing or jumping from a height the extra strain is taken by the foot. To meet these requirements an elastic structure is supplied which is made up of a number of little bones held together by ligaments, tendons and muscles, which together form longitudinal and transverse arches.

Longitudinal arch

This consists of medial and lateral portions resting on a common pillar posteriorly—the tuberosity of the calcaneus. The medial longitudinal arch is formed by the talus, the navicular, the three cuneiform bones, and the inner three metatarsal and corresponding phalanges. The lateral longitudinal arch is formed by the calcaneus, the cuboid, and outer two metatarsals and corresponding phalanges.

The talus is the keystone of the arch. It receives the body weight and transmits it to the arches below.

The lateral longitudinal arch is very low and rests lightly on the ground. The medial is high and only touches the ground behind (tuberosity of calcaneus) and in front (head of first metatarsal bone, i.e. ball of the great toe).

The parts of the foot which normally bear the body weight and transmit it to the ground are, therefore, the tuberosity of calcaneus, the head of the 1st metatarsal, and the head of the 5th metatarsal.

The inner border of the foot is normally straight or concave inwards when weight is being borne. When the arch collapses, as it does in flat-foot, this concavity becomes a convexity because the head of the talus projects down into it.

The transverse arch

This arch (*Fig.* 450) is a continuous structure formed by the cuboid, three cuneiforms and the bases of the metatarsal bones. The middle cuneiform forms the keystone of the arch. The arch continues distally and can be visualized as a series of arches with a lessening curvature to the level of the metatarsal heads, where the arch is no longer apparent because the metatarsal heads are parallel to the weight-bearing surface. The second metatarsal is recessed into the mortise formed by the lateral, middle and medial cuneiforms, at the apex of the arch.

Maintenance of the arches

The integrity of the bony arches is maintained by:
1. Ligaments and the plantar aponeurosis.
2. The action of extrinsic and intrinsic muscles.
3. The structure of the bones.

1. LIGAMENTS: These are amongst the most important structures which maintain the arches when standing. Electromyographic studies have shown

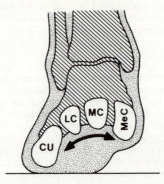

Fig. 450. The transverse arch at the level of the anterior tarsals. Cu, cuboid; LC, lateral cuneiform; MC, middle cuneiform; MeC, medial cuneiform.

that muscles are relatively inactive until walking begins.

Plantar Calcaneonavicular or Spring Ligament: This ligament (*Fig.* 451) is a broad, thick powerful structure, which is the most important ligament in the foot.

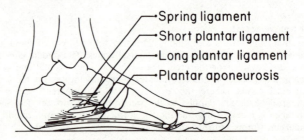

Fig. 451. Ligaments of the longitudinal arch.

Attachments and relations of the spring ligament:

Posteriorly: It is attached to the anterior border of the sustentaculum tali.

Anteriorly: It is attached to the plantar surface of the navicular.

Inner border: The deltoid ligament of the ankle joint is attached to its inner border.

Upper surface: The head of the talus rests on it and the bone has a flat facet on it made by contact with the ligament.

Lower surface: Is crossed by the tendon of the tibialis posterior, which supports the ligament.

The ligament is accessory to the joints between the talus, calcaneus, and navicular, and the capsules of the joints round the head of the talus are blended with the ligament. There is, therefore, a mass of ligamentous tissue around the inner side of the talocalcaneonavicular joint. This ligament supports the keystone of the arch of the foot, the talus.

Long Plantar Ligament: This ligament (*Fig.* 451) is a powerful quadrilateral band which assists in maintaining the longitudinal arch of the foot. Its attachments and relations are:

Posteriorly: It is attached to the undersurface of the calcaneus in front of the tuberosity.

Anteriorly: It is attached to the ridge on the undersurface of the cuboid and to the bases of the 2nd, 3rd, and 4th metatarsal bones.

Undersurface: Is covered by and gives origin to the quadratus plantae, the short flexor of the 5th toe, and the adductor of the great toe.

Upper surface: Crosses the calcaneocuboid joint and supports it. The short plantar ligament is between it and the joint. The peroneus longus is between it and the cuboid. With the cuboid the ligament forms a tunnel for the tendon.

Short Plantar Ligament: This ligament (*Fig.* 451) binds the undersurfaces of calcaneus and cuboid, lying between these bones and the long plantar ligament.

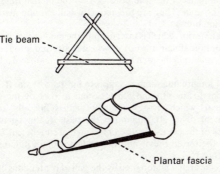

Tie beam

Plantar fascia

Fig. 452. Showing that the plantar fascia acts as the 'tie-beam' of a gable.

Plantar Aponeurosis: The intermediate part of the plantar fascia is very strong and acts as the 'tie-beam' of a gable holding the extremities of the medial and lateral longitudinal arches together (*Fig.* 452). The medial part of the plantar aponeurosis extends from the medial tubercle of the calcaneus to its attachment to the sesamoid bones of the flexor hallucis brevis and strengthens the medial longitudinal arch. The lateral part of the plantar aponeurosis extends from the lateral tubercle of the calcaneus to the tuberosity of the 5th metatarsal bone and helps to maintain the lateral longitudinal arch. Five slips of the aponeurosis are inserted into the base of each proximal phalanx through a plantar pad, which is a conjoint structure consisting of plantar aponeurosis and joint capsule. As the toes undergo dorsiflexion the plantar aponeurosis is stretched around the metatarsal heads. This stabilizes and elevates the longitudinal arch.

Transverse Metatarsal Ligament: Binds the five metatarsals together anteriorly on the plantar aspect and prevents 'spreading' of the heads of the metatarsals.

Interosseous Ligaments: These bind together the non-articular surfaces of adjacent bones. They take a small part in maintaining the arches.

2. EXTRINSIC AND INTRINSIC MUSCLES: Although the ligaments of the foot and the plantar aponeurosis are important in maintenance of the arches, the foot will become flat unless supported by healthy muscles.

The medial longitudinal arch is supported by the flexor hallucis longus and the flexor digitorum longus tendons to the 2nd and 3rd toes. Both these muscles run longitudinally beneath the arch. During walking, strain on the arch is taken up by the tendons of these muscles.

The short muscles of the sole inserted into the medial three toes assist in maintaining the arch. They are the abductor hallucis and medial half of the flexor digitorum brevis.

The tibialis anterior, which is inserted into the medial cuneiform and the 1st metatarsal, and the tibialis posterior, which is inserted into the tuberosity of the navicular, maintain the arch by preventing inversion and adduction of the foot.

The lateral longitudinal arch is supported in part by the flexor digitorum longus tendons to the 4th and 5th toes and in part by the tendon of the peroneus longus which crosses obliquely across the sole under the long plantar ligament to its attachment to the base of the 1st metatarsal and adjoining area of the lateral surface of the medial cuneiform. The lateral half of the flexor digitorum brevis and the abductor digiti minimi also assist in maintaining the arch.

The transverse arch is maintained by the pull of the tendons of the peroneus longus which tends to approximate the medial and lateral borders of the sole of the foot. In walking, the interossei draw the metatarsals together and prevent spread of the foot.

3. BONY STRUCTURE: Interlocking of the articulating bones plays an unimportant role in maintenance of the arches.

CONGENITAL DEFORMITIES OF THE FOOT

Congenital talipes equinovarus (clubfoot)

In the normal infant, the foot can be dorsiflexed and everted until the dorsum of the foot touches the front of the leg.

Congenital clubfoot consists of three elements:

1. Equinus or plantar flexion of the foot at the ankle joint.
2. Varus or inversion deformity of the heel.
3. The forefoot in the varus position.

There is associated wasting of the calf muscle and the heel appears small.

Treatment should start within 3 days of birth and aims to correct each component of the deformity in turn by manipulation and holding the foot in normal position by adhesive strapping.

Congenital metatarsus adductus and varus

This is a common deformity which may be mistaken for a clubfoot, but the heel is normal or sometimes valgus.

In the majority of cases the forefoot can be passively corrected with the heel held in the neutral position. If the dorsiflexors and evertors are functioning normally, the deformity will be corrected by repeated passive stretching.

Deformity of the 1st metatarsal

The 1st metatarsal is the strongest of the metatarsal bones and its head normally lies in a more anterior plane than the others. Weight is borne by the head of the 1st metatarsal as the body is swung forwards on walking.

Developmental anomalies of the 1st metatarsal include:

1. Metatarsus primus varus in which the metatarsal is moved away from the 2nd metatarsal towards the midline of the body. This anomaly is one of the factors responsible for hallux valgus which is discussed below.
2. Short metatarsal in which the head of the 1st metatarsal is situated proximal to the head of the 2nd metatarsal.
3. Excessive mobility of the metatarsal.

These anomalies result in the 2nd and 3rd metatarsals assuming the function of the 1st metatarsal. This may give rise to a stress (march) fracture of the neck of the 2nd metatarsal.

FRACTURES OF THE CALCANEUS

When the patient falls from a height onto his heels, the calcaneus is driven up against the talus and is split or crushed. Normally this bone is set at an angle so that only its tuberosity comes into contact with the ground. In fractures, the bone may be crumpled so that its long axis is horizontal instead of being oblique.

The degree of deformity can be estimated by measuring the calcaneal angle (*Fig.* 453) in a lateral X-ray of the foot.

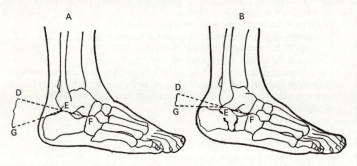

Fig. 453. To show the calcaneal angle. A, The line DEF touches the highest point of the bone and its anterior extremity; GE touches the posterior extremity and the highest point; the resultant angle is the calcaneal angle DEG which is 25–40°. B, The calcaneus has been crushed; the bone lies more horizontally; the calcaneal angle is reduced.

ACQUIRED DEFORMITIES OF THE FOOT

Flat foot

If the medial longitudinal arch touches the ground the foot is described as flat.

It should be differentiated from pseudo-flat foot which is encountered during the process of normal development.

At birth, the smooth convex contours of the sole are due to subcutaneous fat which fills the hollow beneath the medial longitudinal arch. Between 1 and 2 years, when walking becomes established, the child walks on a wide base with the feet turned out and the feet appear to be flat.

Variations in normal development of the lower limb as a whole, such as genu valgum, also cause an apparent flat foot.

AETIOLOGY OF FLAT FOOT:
1. Poor muscle tone in the foot muscles which is seen in children with bad posture, in patients after prolonged bed rest, and in elderly persons whose muscles become flabby and who at the same time gain weight.
2. A short tendo Achillis resists dorsiflexion of the foot on walking and pulls the foot outwards which causes flattening of the medial arch. If the patient stands on tiptoe the arch is restored.

3. Genu valgum and external rotation of the limb cause the body weight to be taken too far medially.

ANATOMICAL FEATURES OF FLAT FOOT: The spring ligament supports the keystone of the arch of the foot, the talus. When the arch drops in flat foot, the head of the talus descends, pushing the spring ligament before it; this stretches the ligament and may produce pain over the ligament immediately posterior to the tubercle of the navicular.

In the early stages of flat foot, there are no recognizable bony changes but, as the spring ligament yields, the body of the talus moves forwards on the upper surface of the calcaneus and the head of the talus is pressed medially and downwards. The head of the talus, sustentaculum tali and navicular are prominent on the medial border of the foot. When the heel is viewed from behind, the tendo Achillis appears to be deviated laterally. The medial part of the sole of the shoe wears more quickly than the lateral.

Pes cavus (claw toes)

The intrinsic muscles of the toes (lumbricals and interossei) produce flexion at the metatarsophalangeal joints and extension at the interphalangeal joints and they are normally in balance with the long tendons of the toes (flexor and extensor digitorum and flexor hallucis longus) which produce extension at the metatarsophalangeal joints and flexion at the interphalangeal joints (clawing).

Weakness of the intrinsic muscles results in unopposed function of the long toe muscles which produces clawing of the toes and an abnormally high longitudinal arch. Callosities will develop due to abnormal pressure under the metatarsal heads.

Hallux valgus

Many aetiological factors have been suggested for this condition, but a striking factor is that 80 per cent of patients with hallux valgus have flat foot. A likely explanation is, therefore, that the flat foot causes splaying of the forefoot, with varus of the 1st metatarsal, and that the shoe pushes the big toe into valgus.

Once established, the intrinsic muscles of the hallux (the adductor hallucis, the flexor hallucis and even the abductor hallucis), which are all inserted into the base of the proximal phalanx, as well as the extensor and flexor hallucis longus, all increase the valgus deformity (*Fig.* 454).

An alternative explanation is that muscle imbalance is the primary factor.

The clinical picture consists of:

1. Varus of the 1st metatarsal.
2. Flat foot (in 80 per cent of cases).
3. Valgus of the big toe.

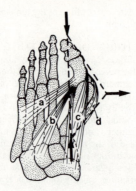

Fig. 454. The imbalance of the muscles inserted into the hallux: (a) transverse belly of adductor hallucis; (b) oblique belly of adductor hallucis; (c) flexor hallucis; (d) abductor hallucis. The arrows indicate the direction of the forces involved.

4. An exostosis on the medial side of the head of the 1st metatarsal.
5. A bursa (bunion) over this prominence.
6. Osteo-arthritis of the metatarsophalangeal joint (in the later stages).

Calcaneal spurs

The attachment of the plantar fascia to the calcaneus may become ossified giving the radiological appearance of a calcaneal spur (*Fig.* 455). A similar spur may occur related to the insertion of the tendo Achillis. Spurs are usually seen in middle age or later and are frequently asymptomatic.

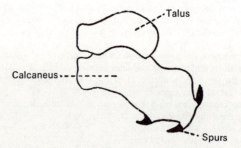

Fig. 455. Varieties of calcaneal spurs. (Redrawn from Holland.)

Morton's metatarsalgia

In this condition there is intermittent sharp pain in the forefoot usually between the 3rd and 4th metatarsals. It is thought to be due to pressure on the digital nerve between the 3rd and 4th metatarsals. The condition responds to the use of a transverse metatarsal bar just proximal to the heads of the metatarsals.

Chapter 40

THE SPINAL COLUMN

The spinal column consists of 24 vertebrae (7 cervical, 12 thoracic, 5 lumbar), together with the intervening discs which in the adult account for 20 per cent of the total length of the spine. The sacrum consists of 5 fused vertebrae and the coccyx is made up of 4 vestigial fused elements.

CURVES OF THE COLUMN

When viewed from its posterior aspect the vertebral column presents a single straight line which bisects the trunk.

When viewed from the side there are a number of curves that vary with age. At birth one long curve, convex posteriorly, is seen. In the adult four distinct anteroposterior curves are seen (*Fig.* 456).

a. Primary curves retain their original posterior convexity (kyphotic) and are found in the thoracic and sacral regions.

b. Secondary curves which are convex anteriorly (lordotic) are found in the cervical and lumbar regions. The cervical curve appears when the infant holds its head up after the third month; the lumbar curve develops when the child begins to walk and hold his trunk upright. These curves continue to develop until growth stops at about the age of 17 years. Wedging of the intervertebral discs contributes to the spinal curves and the sharp angle between the lowest lumbar vertebra and the sacrum.

STRUCTURE OF A TYPICAL VERTEBRA

A cylindrical vertebral body is linked posteriorly to the laminal arch by a pedicle on each side. The laminal arch and the body enclose the spinal canal which transmits the spinal cord, the roots and their coverings. The single spinous process projects backwards from the laminal arch and on each side there is a transverse process with superior and inferior articulating facets

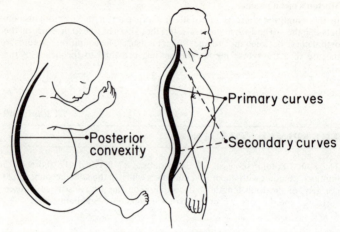

Fig. 456. The vertebral column of an infant exhibits one long curve which is convex posteriorly. In the adult the thoracic, sacral and coccygeal curves are convex posteriorly and are called 'primary curves'. The curves in the cervical and lumbar regions have an anterior convexity and are called 'secondary curves'.

which articulate with the vertebra above and below. The spaces between adjacent vertebrae form the intervertebral foramina through which segmental nerves pass. Each foramen is bounded by a facet joint behind and an intervertebral disc in front and the pedicles constitute the superior and inferior boundaries of the foramen (*Fig*. 457).

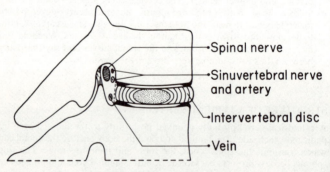

Fig. 457. The intervertebral foramen.

Regional characteristics

CERVICAL VERTEBRAE: There is a foramen (the foramen transversarium) in the transverse processes of all the cervical vertebrae and the vertebral artery ascends through the foramina of C6 to C1, but not that of C7.

C1 vertebra (the atlas) is unique in that it has no body, which forms the odontoid process of C2 vertebra (axis). C7 vertebra is called the vertebra prominens because of its long spinal process.

Surface Landmarks of the Cervical Vertebrae: The transverse process of the atlas is the most prominent transverse process and it can be palpated through the sternomastoid muscle just below and anterior to the mastoid process.

C3 is at the level of the hyoid bone. C4 is opposite the upper border of the thyroid cartilage. C6 is opposite the cricoid cartilage. C7 spinous process is the most prominent and is easily palpable in the midline posteriorly, at the root of the neck.

THORACIC VERTEBRAE: There is one or more articular facets on each side of the body for articulation with the head of the rib. The transverse processes of the upper 10 thoracic vertebrae also have articular facets for the tubercles of the ribs.

LUMBAR VERTEBRAE: The vertebral bodies are larger than those in the cervical and thoracic regions, and have no articular facets for the ribs.

Ossification of a typical vertebra

THREE PRIMARY CENTRES: One in each half of the vertebral arch at the roots of the transverse processes and one in the body (centrum) (*Fig.* 458).

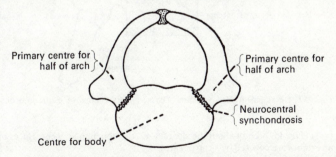

Fig. 458. The development of a vertebra. The primary centres of ossification.

The body (centrum) is occasionally ossified from bilateral centres which may fail to unite. If one of the centres fails to develop, a hemivertebra results which is a cause of lateral curvature of the spine (scoliosis).

At birth the vertebra consists of three bony parts, united by hyaline cartilage at the neurocentral joints and at the junction of the two halves of the vertebral arch in the midline posteriorly.

FIVE SECONDARY OR EPIPHYSIAL CENTRES: These appear about puberty and the epiphyses join the rest of the bone about the age of 25 years. There is one centre for the tip of the spine, one at the tip of each transverse process, and one each in the cartilage on the upper and lower surfaces of the

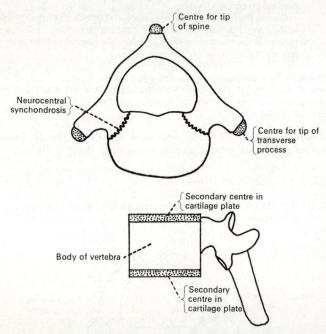

Fig. 459. Development of a vertebra. The secondary centres of ossification of a vertebra.

body (*Fig.* 459). Until about the age of 8–12, the upper and lower surfaces of a vertebra are covered by a cap of cartilage.

Ossification begins in the periphery of these plates and extends so as to form a ring round a central island of cartilage. By the age of 25 this ring has fused with the vertebra, but the central cartilaginous plate remains throughout life as part of the apparatus of the intervertebral disc (*Fig.* 460).

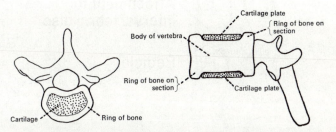

Fig. 460. Development of a vertebra. The vertebra is completely developed and shows diagrammatically the cartilaginous plates on the upper and lower surfaces of the body.

JOINTS AND LIGAMENTS UNITING THE VERTEBRAL BODIES

The anterior and posterior longitudinal ligaments and the intervertebral discs unite the vertebral bodies.

The anterior longitudinal ligament

The anterior longitudinal ligament stretches from the basi-occiput to the sacrum on the anterior aspect of the vertebrae. It is a strong ligament consisting of long (superficial) and short fibres. The superficial fibres bridge several vertebrae and the deep fibres run between single pairs of vertebrae. The deep fibres blend with the intervertebral disc.

The posterior longitudinal ligament

The posterior longitudinal ligament is situated within the vertebral canal and stretches from the basi-occiput to the sacrum. It is wider over the discs than over the bodies (*Fig.* 461). There is a space between the ligaments and the bodies for the paravertebral venous plexus. Superiorly that portion of the ligament which runs from the body of C2, behind the odontoid peg and its transverse ligament, to the occiput is known as the 'tectorial membrane'.

The uncovertebral (Luschka's) joints

Luschka's joints (*Fig.* 462) are probably not true synovial joints, but more likely are false joints which develop as a result of degenerative changes in the edges of the discs in early adult life.

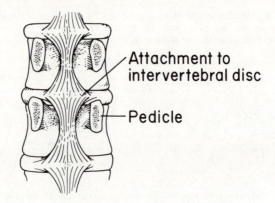

Fig. 461. The posterior longitudinal ligament.

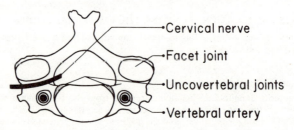

Fig. 462. The uncovertebral joints: osteophytes from these joints may encroach on the nerve and vertebral artery.

These structures lie on the posterolateral aspect of C3 to C7 vertebrae, and form 'articulations' between the vertebral body above and the uncinate process of the superior edge of the vertebra below. They lie just anterior to the cervical intervertebral foramina on the posterolateral aspect of the cervical discs.

Luschka's joints are important because:
1. They are the commonest site of osteophyte formation.
2. The cervical roots lie posterolateral to the joints, so that the osteophytes may produce cervical nerve involvement.
3. The vertebral artery in its course through the foramina transversaria lies lateral to these joints. Osteophytes intruding on the canal can cause distortion of the artery which may lead to vertebrobasilar insufficiency in atherosclerotic vessels.

The occipito-atlanto-axial articulation

This articulation differs considerably from the rest of the spinal column. It controls the movement of the head on the spinal column and has two components.

ATLANTO-OCCIPITAL JOINT: Flexion and extension occur at this joint. The occipital condyles of the skull are convex and fit into reciprocating concave lateral masses of the atlas. The joint is supported by the posterior longitudinal ligament, which here is called the 'membrana tectoria', and the anterior atlanto-occipital membrane, which connects the anterior rim of the foramen magnum with the anterior aspects of the atlas.

The posterior atlanto-occipital membrane is equivalent to the ligamentum flavum elsewhere, and is perforated by the vertebral artery in its inferolateral aspect.

ATLANTO-AXIAL JOINT: Rotation occurs at this joint. Only 50 per cent of rotation occurs at this level, the remainder takes place in the spine. The axis has a stout pillar projecting from its body vertically in the midline. This is called the 'dens' or the 'odontoid process' which articulates with the posterior aspect of the anterior rim of the atlas. There is a synovial joint between it and the anterior arch of the atlas. Posteriorly and at its base, it is embraced by the transverse ligament which attaches to the medial aspects of the lateral masses of the atlas articulation.

The apical ligament attaches the apex of the dens to the foramen magnum. Laterally, there are two alar ligaments which attach the dens to the rim of the foramen magnum. The entire joint is covered by the membrana tectoria.

A fracture of the dens will thus permit forward displacement of the arch of the atlas together with the skull and the ruptured fragment of dens. Similarly, a rupture of the transverse ligament will allow forward displacement of the arch of the atlas to occur in relation to the anterior aspect of the dens. Normally in the adult, this gap is 3 mm (4 mm in children), but with a rupture of the transverse ligament it will be increased.

Only about 15 per cent of injuries at this level produce neurological lesions because the spinal canal is unusually wide in comparison with the lower levels of the spine.

The intervertebral discs

The intervertebral disc (*Fig.* 463) is a fibrocartilaginous complex which forms the strongest bond between the bodies of the vertebrae. The intervertebral discs comprise 20 per cent of the height of the vertebral column. The anterior parts of the discs are wide in the cervical and lumbar region where the shape of the disc contributes to the cervical and lumbar lordosis. Each disc is biconvex and consists of a fibrous outer ring (the annulus fibrosis) and a cartilaginous end plate above and below the disc, with a central nucleus pulposus.

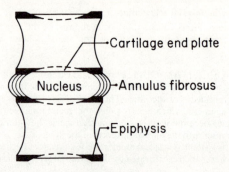

Fig. 463. The intervertebral disc.

THE END PLATE: The end plate is a thin layer of hyaline cartilage adherent to the trabeculae of the cancellous bone of the bodies of the vertebrae from which the disc receives its nutrition. On the vertebral side of the end plate, the cortical bone is very thin and deficient in places. The end plate is surrounded by a circular rim of bone 2 mm thick which is often incomplete posteriorly so that the end plate extends to the back of the vertebral body.

THE ANNULUS FIBROSIS: From the outside in, the annulus consists of concentric rings of collagen, elastic tissue and an inner layer of fibrocartilage where it merges with the nucleus pulposus. The major function of the annulus is to withstand tension which is horizontally directed by the compressed nucleus, to resist twisting strain of the column and to prevent separation of the vertebral bodies on the convex side of a spinal flexure.

The annulus is firmly attached to the outer rings of bone of the vertebrae above and below a disc and to the anterior and posterior longitudinal ligaments. Within the bony ring, fibres from the nucleus and annulus penetrate the end plate (*Fig.* 460).

It has been suggested that in the fetus there are nutritive channels in the annulus which disappear after birth. Degeneration of these channels leaves areas of potential weakness in the posterior annulus through which the nucleus can prolapse.

Sensory nerve fibres are found in the posterior longitudinal ligament and in the adjacent superficial fibres of the annulus. These fibres pass into the sinuvertebral nerve which is the sensory nerve to the structures on the ventral surface of the spinal canal. The sinuvertebral nerve leaves the spinal canal through the vertebral foramen to join the spinal nerve (*Fig.* 457).

THE NUCLEUS PULPOSUS: The nucleus is a sphere of hydrophilic gelatinous tissue, which is derived from mucoid degeneration of the notochord augmented by fibrocartilage. The nucleus occupies an eccentric position closer to the posterior margin of the disc. The nucleus has no blood supply. The cartilage end plates permit the passage of fluid and nutritive substances from within the vertebral bodies to the substance of the disc itself.

The nucleus functions as a 'shock absorber', but some fluid is lost from the nucleus in the upright position. When pressure is reduced in the recumbent position the nucleus re-expands. This explains the diurnal variation in height of up to 1·5 cm. (Astronauts are taller when they return to earth after a period of weightlessness in space.)

JOINTS AND LIGAMENTS UNITING THE LAMINAL ARCHES

Facet joints
The articular facets of adjacent vertebrae form synovial joints which join contiguous borders of adjacent neural arches. The direction of the joint surfaces determines the direction of movements possible between the adjacent vertebrae. Motion at the intervertebral and facet joints is interdependent and the spine as a whole has a considerable range of movement. The changing shape of the intervertebral disc when subjected to pressure contributes to the range of movement.

The greatest range of movement occurs where one type of vertebra changes to another (cervicodorsal and dorsolumbar junctions). The vertebrae at these levels are most liable to injury.

Ligamenta flava (yellow ligaments)
These ligaments run from the lower anterior surface of each lamina to the upper posterior surface of the lamina below. The ligaments are thickest in the lumbar region. Because of their elasticity they remain taught during flexion and extension of the spine. The ligaments have no sensory nerve supply and can therefore be pierced painlessly when a lumbar puncture is performed.

The supraspinous ligament
This is a strong fibrous cord which connects the tips of the spinous processes from C7 to the sacrum. From C7 upwards, it forms the ligamentum nuchae which attaches to the occipital protuberance and gives rise to muscle attachments on each side.

Interspinous ligaments
These blend with the supraspinous ligaments and the ligamenta flava.

The intertransverse ligaments

These extend between the transverse processes; they are generally weak but well developed in the lumbar region.

LESIONS OF THE INTERVERTEBRAL DISC

With the considerable mobility of the spine, degeneration of the intervertebral discs occurs at a relatively young age and continues with advancing years.

The nucleus loses water and elasticity with the result that it can no longer act as a water cushion. Eventually the nucleus becomes fibrous and the shrinking of the disc accounts for the decrease in height with ageing. Fissures open up in the disc and can be outlined by the injection of radio-opaque material into the disc (discography).

The annulus is thinner posteriorly where it may be weakened by the defects created by degeneration of fetal blood vessels.

The cartilage end plates are structurally the weakest part of the disc as can be shown experimentally, because they have to be sufficiently permeable to allow fluid and nutritive substances to pass from the vertebral bodies to the substance of the disc itself.

Clinical syndromes

1. SCHMORL'S NODES: Small defects in the end plate may allow the extension of nuclear material into the body of the vertebra. This is demonstrable radiologically as an area of radiolucency (*Fig*. 464). This condition is common and there is an association with heavy manual work. The condition is usually asymptomatic but is frequently found at routine postmortem examination.

2. DISC DEGENERATION: With the disturbance of the hydrophilic properties of the nucleus, symptoms are produced by stretching the innervated annulus and posterior longitudinal ligament. Comparatively minor strains may result in the protrusion of the contents of the disc.

Degeneration of the intervertebral discs produces a number of secondary changes in related structures (spondylosis).

Osteophyte Formation: As the annulus bulges outwards it elevates the periosteum which then lays down new bone (osteophytes). The osteophytes may occur anteriorly and laterally on the vertebral body. Osteophytes in the spinal canal may cause compression of the nerve root.

Subluxation: The shrinkage of the disc spaces permits subluxation of one vertebra on the other which puts strain on the facet joints and ligaments. This may result in increased dorsal curvature (kyphosis),

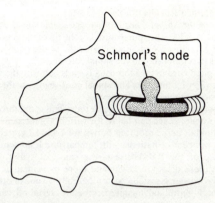

Fig. 464. Schmorl's node.

exaggeration of the lordotic curvature in the cervical or lumbar spine, or a scoliosis if there is asymmetrical degeneration of the disc.

Buckling of the Soft Tissues: As the disc spaces narrow and the vertebrae approximate, infolding of the posterior longitudinal ligament and the ligamentum flavum occurs, which reduces the available space in the spinal canal.

Note: The condition of ballooned discs must not be confused with disc degeneration. The primary defect in ballooned discs is osteoporosis which weakens the vertebral body sufficiently to allow expansion of the intervertebral disc into the upper and lower end plates of the body. It should be emphasized that, for this ballooning to occur, the disc must still have an elastic nucleus (*Fig.* 465).

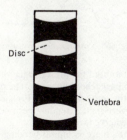

Fig. 465. Ballooning of the disc.

3. LUMBAR DISC PROTRUSION:

Relationship of the Spinal Cord and Nerves to the Spinal Column: At 14 weeks of fetal life, the spinal cord is at the tip of the coccyx. However, skeletal growth exceeds neural growth, so that the cord migrates upwards in relationship to the spinal column.

The spinal cord in an adult usually ends opposite the intervertebral disc between L1 and L2. The spinal cord segments therefore do not correspond with the vertebral levels.

The segmental nerve roots leave the spinal canal through intervertebral foramina, each pair below the vertebra of the same number, e.g. the 1st lumbar nerve root runs between L1 and L2 vertebrae.

In 95 per cent of patients with lumbar disc lesions prolapse of the L4/5 disc or the L5/S1 disc is the cause of symptoms, probably because these discs are larger and more movement occurs at these levels. Protrusion is usually posterolaterally, to one or other side of the posterior longitudinal ligament, into the vertebral canal, where it produces pressure on the nerve root or spinal nerve. A large central rupture may produce pressure on the cauda equina (*Fig.* 466).

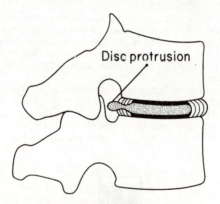

Fig. 466. Posterior disc protrusion.

Clinical Features: Irritation of the posterior longitudinal ligament and the annulus results in backache (lumbago). The pain often radiates to the sacro-iliac joint, the buttock and legs. Pressure on the L5 or S1 nerve root produces severe pain extending peripherally in the dermatome distribution of the nerve (sciatica).

On examination, there is lateral bending of the lumbar spine to relieve the pain. It will be towards or away from the lesion depending on whether the protrusion is medial or lateral to the irritated nerve root (*Fig.* 467).

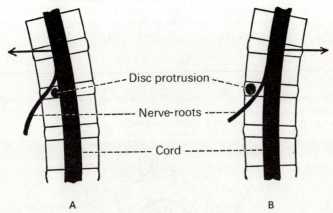

A   B

Fig. 467. The scoliosis will vary, depending on the relationship of the nerve root to the disc protrusion.

The straight-leg raising test (Lasegue's test) is positive if the L4 or L5 nerve roots are affected. The patient's leg is held straight until the patient resists further lifting because of pain. The patient's foot is then sharply dorsiflexed. If this manoeuvre increases the pain then it is produced by increased nerve root tension.

Pain is also produced by coughing. The increased intrathoracic pressure is transmitted to the intracranial venous sinuses which causes a sudden increase in pressure in the subarachnoid space, and to the extradural vertebral venous sinuses through their valveless connections with the trunk veins. The sudden distension of the veins and of the subarachnoid space will jar an irritated nerve root stretched across a disc protrusion.

L5 root compression causes a sensory loss on the outer aspect of the leg, the dorsum of the foot and the cleft between the hallux and the 2nd toe, followed by weakness of the big toe dorsiflexors as the lesion progresses.

S1 root compression results in a reduced or absent ankle reflex, a sensory loss on the outer side of the foot and the lateral two toes and a weakness of eversion of the foot, in this sequence.

4. PROLAPSED CERVICAL DISC: The aetiology and pathology of this condition are similar to those of lumbar disc prolapse. The prolapse usually

involves the disc above or below the 6th cervical vertebra. The nerve roots affected are C6 and C7.

The patient may complain of pain in the neck often radiating to the occiput and scapular region. Pain and paraesthesia may also extend down the outer aspect of the arm and forearm and involve the thumb and fingers. The tendon reflex of biceps (C5–6) and triceps C6–7) may be depressed or absent.

THE VERTEBRAL VENOUS SYSTEM

The vertebral system of veins (*Fig.* 468) is a persistence of the primitive venous plexus of the embryo. There are several plexuses of thin-walled valveless veins in relation to the vertebral bodies.

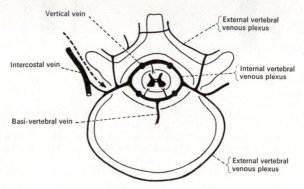

Fig. 468. The vertebral system of veins.

The external vertebral venous plexus consists of anterior vessels in front of the vertebral bodies, and posterior ones on the back of the arches of the vertebrae and in the adjacent muscles.

The internal vertebral plexus consists of a postcentral portion and a prelaminar one, each of these sections being drained by two vertical vessels.

All these plexuses receive the basivertebral veins draining the bodies of the vertebrae and are in free intercommunication with each other. They are drained by the intervertebral veins which drain the spinal cord and pass through the intervertebral foramina with the spinal nerves.

These segmental intervertebral veins pour their blood into vertebral, intercostal, lumbar, and lateral sacral veins and they also communicate with veins of the portal system. Thus all these systems are brought into association by this communicating venous system, making it possible for tumour cells or infected emboli from systemic or portal areas to lodge in vertebrae, spinal cord, skull, or brain.

VERTEBRAL CANAL STENOSIS

This condition is more common in the lumbar spine. One or more roots of the cauda equina are affected due to their constriction in the spinal canal before their exit through the foramina.

Aetiology

1. CONGENITAL NARROWING OF THE CANAL:
    i. The shape of the spinal canal may be oval, triangular or trefoil (*Fig. 469*). A trefoil canal may cause compression of the nerve in the lateral recess of the canal.

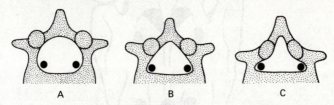

Fig. 469. Shape of the spinal canal: A, oval; B, triangular; C, trefoil.

   ii. Achondroplasia, in which there is early fusion of the centrum and the neural arch, resulting in a narrow spinal canal.

2. ACQUIRED NARROWING OF THE CANAL:
    i. Osteophytes.
    ii. Paget's disease in which there is overgrowth of the vertebral bones.
    iii. Extradural scar tissue which may follow surgical removal of a disc protrusion.
    iv. Spondylolisthesis. This is an important cause in elderly patients.

Clinical features

Patients affected are usually elderly. They complain of backache and sciatica which may be unilateral or bilateral, and is often associated with walking (neurogenic claudication). They may also develop difficulty with micturition.

It is not clear why symptoms are provoked by walking. Relative ischaemia of the nerve roots as a result of compression of the blood vessels in the stenotic canal or increased extension of the lumbar spine which causes compression and rubbing of the nerve roots may play a role.

SACRALIZATION OF THE TRANSVERSE PROCESS OF THE 5TH LUMBAR VERTEBRA

This is a developmental anomaly in which one or both transverse processes of the 5th lumbar vertebra are abnormally large and strong (*Fig*. 470). The transverse process may form a connection with the base of the sacrum or the ilium. A foramen forms between the transverse process and the base of the sacrum.

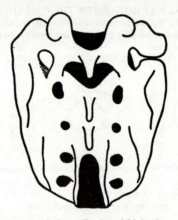

Fig. 470. Asymmetrical sacralization of 5th lumbar vertebra.

This condition only produces low backache when it is unilateral, possibly because it prevents normal lateral flexion. Symptoms commence after the age of 20 when the vertebral column has acquired its final stiffness.

On radiographic examination, an enlarged transverse process is noted and there is a well-marked intervertebral foramen between the body of the vertebra, the sacrum and the transverse process. There is a lumbar scoliosis convex to the affected side.

SPONDYLOLISTHESIS

In the erect posture, because of the normal lumbar lordosis, there is a downward and forward thrust on the lower lumbar vertebrae. This tendency for the lumbar vertebrae to slide forward is counteracted by the articular facets, intact pedicles and the vertebral arch.

Spondylolisthesis designates the slipping forward of a vertebral body. The shift is most commonly between L4 and L5, or between L5 and the sacrum.

Aetiology

1. VERTEBRAL ARCH DEFECT: 'Spondylolysis' is the term used to describe a defect in the vertebral arch in the region of the isthmus. The defect is now thought to be caused by a stress fracture. When associated with disc degeneration at the same vertebral level, the resulting instability gives rise to spondylolisthesis.

2. DEGENERATIVE: Degenerative changes in the facet joints and the discs permit forward movement of the L4/5 level despite intact laminae.

3. CONGENITAL: The lumbosacral pedicles are defective or elongated. Gross vertebral displacement occurs in early childhood or adolescence.

4. MISCELLANEOUS: A single major injury may result in traumatic spondylolisthesis, and bone disease or a tumour may cause pathological spondylolisthesis.

Clinical features of spondylolisthesis

There may be no symptoms but there is usually low backache, with or without sciatica. The trunk is shortened, with a transverse furrow between the ribs and iliac crest, and there is restriction of forward flexion of the spine. The spine of the 5th lumbar vertebra is unduly prominent, with a palpable depression above it (in those cases with a defect in the pars interarticularis) (*Fig.* 471) and the 5th lumbar vertebra may encroach on the brim of the pelvis sufficiently to cause obstructed labour.

On an anteroposterior radiograph the superior surface of the 5th lumbar vertebra is seen (*Fig.* 472), on the lateral view forward slipping is evident and on the oblique view the break in the pars interarticularis may be visible (*Fig.* 471).

TUBERCULOSIS OF THE SPINE

The spine is the commonest site of skeletal tuberculosis. The body of a vertebra is most commonly affected by blood-borne infection. Sometimes two adjacent vertebrae are infected simultaneously. The superimposed

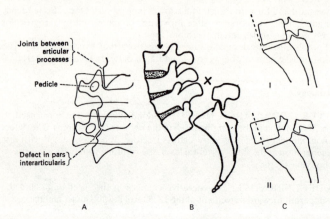

Fig. 471. Spondylolisthesis with a break in the pars interarticularis. A, On the oblique radiograph the defect in the pars interarticularis gives the appearance of a decapitated 'Scots terrier'. B, On the lateral radiograph there is forward slipping of the 5th lumbar vertebra. The prominent 5th lumbar spine and the gap above it (X) can be appreciated. (The arrow indicates the thrust of the body weight.) C, Normally the body of the 5th lumbar vertebra lies behind a perpendicular line drawn from the front of the sacrum, but in spondylolisthesis this line will cut into the body of the 5th lumbar vertebra (*Ullman's sign*). I Normal; II spondylolisthesis.

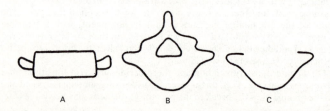

Fig. 472. Diagrammatic representation of X-ray appearances of 5th lumbar vertebra in a case of spondylolisthesis. The bone is seen from the front (anterior-posterior view). A, Appearance of a normal 5th lumbar vertebra. The anterior surface of the body is seen, also transverse processes. B, Upper surface of whole vertebra is seen as the bone has rotated downwards through 90°. This is the appearance in spondylolisthesis. C, Characteristic curve of the body and transverse processes which is the distinguishing feature in (B) as seen in the radiograph.

weight of the vertebral column crushes the body of the infected vertebra which results in an angular deformity (kyphos, gibbus or hunchback). The deformity is most marked in the collapse of a thoracic vertebra because it exaggerates the primary kyphotic curve.

The pus produced by such a disease does not evoke the classic local signs of acute infection (heat and redness) and is therefore called a 'cold abscess'. The pus extends from its site of origin along the paths of least resistance, being guided by fascial attachments, nerves and blood vessels. For instance, a cold abscess in the thoracic area may:

1. Remain prevertebral (in the posterior mediastinum).
2. Track down to the lower end of the posterior mediastinum and escape:
   i. Through the lateral arcuate ligament and down between the anterior layer of the lumbodorsal fascia and the quadratus lumborum. Pus may remain here behind the kidney or extend along the three nerves related to the bed of the kidney—the 12th thoracic, the ilio-inguinal or iliohypogastric—and thus present on the anterior abdominal wall.
   ii. Through the medial arcuate ligament and, having entered the 'stocking' of the psoas sheath, track down to the insertion of the psoas (the lesser trochanter of the femur) and thus present as a swelling in the thigh pushing the femoral artery forwards (*Fig.* 473).

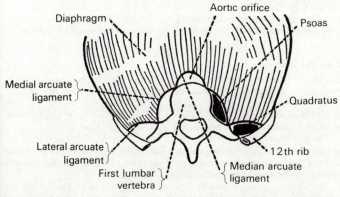

Fig. 473. Diaphragm seen from above showing lumbocostal arches. On the left, the psoas and quadratus are removed. These arches often serve to direct the flow of tuberculous pus.

SCOLIOSIS

This is the name given to a lateral curvature of the spine. There are two clinical types:

1. Non-structural (mobile) scoliosis

This type is non-progressive and the vertebrae are not rotated.

AETIOLOGY:

Postural: This is an important cause in adolescent girls. The curve is usually convex to the left. It disappears when the child bends forwards.

Compensatory: Compensatory to a short leg or a pelvic tilt, due to an abduction or adduction contracture of the hip.

Sciatic: In a lumbar disc lesion there is lateral bending of the spine to relieve the pain.

2. Structural (fixed) scoliosis

There is a major scoliotic curve produced by the lesion and compensatory curves develop to counterbalance the deformity.

Structural scoliosis cannot be voluntarily corrected and is not corrected by bending forward. It is always accompanied by vertebral rotation; the bodies rotate towards the convexity and the spinous processes towards the concavity of the curve.

It is a progressive condition throughout the growth period.

AETIOLOGY:

1. Idiopathic in most instances.
2. Disorders of the bones, muscles and nerves of the vertebral column.

Clinical features

Medical attention is sought because of trunk asymmetry. Common presenting symptoms are a hump on the back, and a prominent shoulder or hip.

RADIOGRAPHIC EXAMINATION: The major curve is the longest curve with the greatest degree of angulation and it is also the least flexible.

The extent of the curve is determined by locating the end vertebrae of the major curve. The end vertebrae are the last vertebrae at the upper and lower ends of the curve which demonstrate a narrower disc space on the concave side of the curve and a wider disc space on the convex side.

The degree of angulation is determined by the angle formed by the intersection of two lines drawn on an X-ray of the back; the first line is perpendicular to the superior surface of the upper end vertebra and the second line is perpendicular to the inferior surface of the lower end vertebra.

Skeletal maturation occurs synchronously with ossification of the iliac crest and the vertebral ring epiphyses. Vertebral growth usually ceases at a bone age of 16 in girls and 18 in boys. No further progression of the scoliosis occurs after skeletal maturation.

SELECTED FURTHER READING

Anderson R. H. and Becker, A. E. (1980) *Cardiac Anatomy*. London: Churchill Livingstone

Duthie R. B. and Bentley G. (1983) *Mercer's Orthopaedic Surgery*, 8th ed. London: Edward Arnold

Goligher J. C. (1980) *Surgery of the Anus, Rectum and Colon*, 4th ed. London: Macmillan

Green D. P. (1982) *Operative Hand Surgery*. New York: Churchill Livingstone

Helfet A. J. and Lee D. M. G. (1982) *Disorders of the Knee*, 2nd ed. Philadelphia: Lippincott

Kapandji I. A. (1970) *The Physiology of Joints*. London: Churchill Livingstone

Klenermann L. K. (ed.) (1982) *The Foot and its Disorders*. Oxford: Blackwell

Nixon H. H. (1976) *The Essentials of Paediatric Surgery*, 3rd ed. London: Heinemann

Nyhus L. M. (ed.) (1977) *Surgery of the Stomach and Duodenum*, 3rd ed. Boston: Little & Brown

Nyhus L. M. (ed.) (1978) *Hernia*, 2nd ed. Philadelphia: Lippincott

Rothman R. H. and Simeone F. A. (1982) *The Spine*, 2nd ed. Philadelphia: W. B. Saunders

Walmsley R. (1978) *Clinical Anatomy of the Heart*. Edinburgh: Churchill

INDEX

Abdominal aneurysm, 266
  resection of, (*Fig.* 186) 243
Abdominal aorta, 226
  exposure of, 243
  surgery, paraplegia following, 349
Abdominal cavity, at birth, 406
Abdominal drainage of pelvic abscess, 49
Abdominal examination, 77
Abdominal hernia, 113
Abdominal hysterectomy, 399–400
Abdominal incisions, (*Figs.* 104–110) 113–118
  for exposure of bladder and prostate, 320
Abdominal inguinal ring, 119, 125
Abdominal musculature deficiency syndromes, errors in gut rotation due to, 28
Abdominal oesophagus, 4–5
Abdominal viscera
  innervation of, 216
  ischaemia of, 226
Abdominal wall
  attachment of gut to, 37
  incision into, 44
  lower, fasciae of, (*Fig.* 113) 123–125
  testis in relation to, 119
Abducens nerve, 268, 338, 363
  relation to cavernous sinus, (*Fig.* 281) 356
Abduction of shoulder, (*Figs.* 349–351) 437–440
Abductor pollicis brevis muscle, (*Fig.* 379) 469
Abscess
  anal, 62
  associated with middle ear infections, 403
  cold, 565
  collar stud, (*Fig.* 401) 491
  eponychial, (*Fig.* 402) 491
  extradural, 403
  extrasphincteric, (*Fig.* 70) 75–76
  horseshoe, 74
  in breast duct, 169–170

Abscess, in cheek, 180
  in ischiorectal fossa, (*Fig.* 68) 75
  in lung, following aspiration, 139
  intersphincteric, 74
  intracuticular, 490
  pelvic, 48–49
  perianal, 74
  subcutaneous, 490
  subphrenic, (*Figs.* 90–91) 99–102
  suprasphincteric, (*Fig.* 69) 75–76
  trans-sphincteric, (*Fig.* 68) 75
Accessory auditory tubercles, 180
Accessory bile duct, 90
Accessory bones, (*Fig.* 338) 421
Accessory breast tissue, 162
Accessory circuit, 224
Accessory hepatic artery, 86
Accessory ligaments of jaw, 188
Accessory lobes of lung, 141–142
Accessory navicular bone, (*Fig.* 338) 421
Accessory nerve, (*Fig.* 294) 373–374
  lesions of, 374
  spinal, 193, 197
Accessory pancreatic duct, 103
Accessory pancreatic tissue, 104
Accessory phrenic nerve, 252
Accessory saphenous vein, 255
Accessory spleens, (*Fig.* 97) 107
Accessory talus, (*Fig.* 339) 421
Accommodation, 355
Acetabulum, 499, 503
  dysplasia of, 499
  fusion at, 411
Acetylcholine, 209
Achalasia, 7
Achilles tendon (*see also* Tendo Achillis), 258, 532
Achondroplasia, 422, 423, 561
Acini, of breast, 161, 163
Aclasia, diaphysial, 422
Acromioclavicular joint, (*Fig.* 341) 425, (*Fig.* 346) 433, 436, 440, (*Fig.* 354) 442
Acromion, 411
  pain referred to skin above, 96

Acromionectomy, 445
Adamkiewicz artery, 348, 349
Adductor pollicis, (*Fig.* 380) 470
Adenohypophysis, (*Fig.* 264) 335
Adenoids, (*Fig.* 157) 189, 192
Adenoma(ta)
    hormonal changes due to, 339
    of parathyroid, 207
    of prostate, 320, 321, 322
Adenosis, sclerosing, of breast, 164
Adherent tonsil, 192
Adhesive capsulitis, 446
Aditus, (*Fig.* 289) 365
Adrenal arteries, 308, 310
Adrenal glands, (*Figs.* 240–242) 311
    at birth, 406
    blood supply to, 308
    embryology of, 307–308
    innervation of, 309
    lymphatic drainage of, 309–310
    relations, (*Fig.* 226) 294, (*Fig.* 241) 308
Adrenal medulla, 208, 308, 311
    nerve endings in, 209
    tumours of, 312
    visceral fibres to, 211
Adrenal tumour, approach to, 310
Adrenal vein, 308, 310
    collateral circulation through, 266
Adrenalectomy, 310
Adrenaline, secreted by phaeochromocy-
    tomata, 312
Adrenergic-blocking agents, 322
Adrenergic receptors, in oesophagus, 7
Adrenocortical carcinoma, 310
Afferent autonomic nerve fibres, 209
Aganglionic megacolon, congenital, 71
Air cells, mastoid, (*Fig.* 319) 402
Air embolism, following hepatic vein
    injuries, 87
Albarran, subcervical glands of, 321
Alcohol, injected to destroy ganglion, 219
Alderman's nerve, 371
Alimentary canal
    before rotation, (*Fig.* 17) 23
    development of, 22
Allantois, in development of bladder, (*Fig.*
    245) 314
Alveolar artery, 181
Alveolar canal, 183

Alveolar nerve, 182, 183, (*Fig.* 154) 184–
    185
    injection for, (*Fig.* 154) 185
Alveolar plate, 186
    innervation of, 185
Alveolar process, 174
Alveolus
    absorption in older people, 197
    blood supply to, 181
Amastia, 162
Ambiguus nucleus, 209
Ampulla of Vater, 89, (*Fig.* 86) 94–95
    carcinoma of, 106
    pancreatic duct joining, 104
    termination of ducts at, 92
Amputation(s), (*Figs.* 322–345) 407–433
    above-knee, 221
    below-knee, (*Fig.* 345) 431
    blood vessels in, 429
    bones in, 429
    hand, (*Figs.* 408–411) 496–498
    hindquarter, 432
    involving hip joint, 512–513
    joint contracture affecting, 429
    level of, 428–429
    lower limb, (*Figs.* 344–345) 430–432
    through knee, 530
    transmetatarsal, (*Fig.* 344) 430
    transtrochanteric, 512
    upper limb, 432–433
Anaemia, haemolytic, 107
Anaesthesia
    corneal, 358
    epidural, 342
    local (*see* Local anaesthetic)
    perineal, 74
Anal..., *see also* Anus
Anal abscesses, development of, 62
Anal canal, 41, (*Figs.* 55–64) 61–71
    anatomy of, (*Figs.* 55–59) 61–66
    development of, (*Fig.* 62) 68–69
    fissure in skin of, 63
    haemorrhoids in, (*Figs.* 60–61) 66–68
    levator ani attached to, 61
    muscles of, 63
    palpation of, 77
    varices of, 84
Anal crypts, 62
Anal cushions, 62

Anal extrasphincteric abscess, (Fig. 70) 75–76

Anal fistula(e), (Figs. 67–70) 74–77
  development of, 62
  intersphincteric, (Fig. 67) 74
  treatment of, 76–77

Anal glands, 62
  infection of, 74

Anal intermuscular groove, palpation of, 77

Anal intersphincteric abscess, 74

Anal intramuscular glands, 65

Anal musculature, 65–66

Anal sinuses, 62

Anal skin, tag of, 68

Anal sphincter, (Fig. 55) 62, (Fig. 56) 63–64
  palpation of, 77
  paralysis associated with spina bifida cystica, 351

Anal suprasphincteric abscess, (Fig. 69) 75–76

Anal trans-sphincteric abscess, (Fig. 68) 75

Anal tubercles, overfusion of, 68

Anal valve, ruptured, 68

Anastomosis, of oesophagus, 10

Aneurysm
  abdominal, (Fig. 186) 243
  false, 289

Aneurysmectomy, 228
  ligation of mesenteric artery in, 52

Angina pectoris, 280

Angioplasty, percutaneous transluminal, 280

Angle of Louis, 137

Angulus venosus, thoracic duct ending in, 271

Anhidrosis, 385

Ankle
  perforating veins of, 262
  pulses of, affected by constriction of popliteal artery, 545
  reflex, affected by S1 root compression, 559
  saphenous vein in, 255
  ulceration of, 259

Ankle joint, (Figs. 442–449) 530–538
  ligaments of, (Figs. 441–442) 530–531, 540

Ankle joint, retinacula around, 532
  tendon sheaths around, (Figs. 446–449) 535–538
  twist injury, 531

Ankylosis, 432
  of hip joint, optimum position for, (Fig. 425) 512

Annular ligament, 456

Annular pancreas, 104

Annulus fibrosis, (Fig. 463) 553–554

Anococcygeal ligament, 50, 61
  attachment of levatores ani to, 65

Anococcygeal raphe, (Fig. 315) 396

Anorectal anomalies, (Figs. 62–64) 68–71

Anorectal canal, 314

Anorectal disease, causing extrasphincteric fistula, 76

Anorectal junction, 63

Anorectal reflex, 65

Anorectal ring, 63
  palpation of, 77

Anorectal varices, 84

Anosmia, 352

Ansa cervicalis, 202

Ansa hypoglossi, 374, (Fig. 297) 377, (Fig. 299) 379

Anterior clinoid process, relation to cavernous sinus, (Fig. 281) 356

Anterior communicating artery, (Fig. 267) 337

Anterior cranial fossa, 352

Anterior facial vein, (Fig. 262) 331

Anterior jugular vein, (Fig. 196) 253, (Fig. 262) 331

Anterior lobe of prostate, 320

Anterior spinal artery, (Fig. 276) 347

Anterior tibial syndrome, 394

Antidiuretic hormone, 335

Antimesocolic taeniae, 53

Anus (see also Anal...)
  absence of ganglia, 71
  anomalies of, (Figs. 62–64) 68–71
  covered, 68
  discharge of mucus through, 49
  ectopic, (Fig. 63) 68
  haematoma of, 67
  imperforate, tracheo-oesophageal fistula associated with, 1
  incomplete migration of, (Fig. 63) 68
  microscopic, 68

Anus, prolapse of rectum through, 50
  varices of, 84
  vestibular, 68
Aorta, 264–267, 286
  abdominal, exposure of, 243
  ascending, 239, 285
  cervical, 287
  coarctation of, (*Fig.* 219) 288
  descending, 239, 289
  dorsal, 286
  occlusion of, 228, 229
  oesophagus in relation to, 3, (*Fig.* 3) 4
  paraplegia following operations on, 289
  partitioning of truncus arteriosus into,
    274
  passage through diaphragm, 156
  position in thorax, 138
  radicular arteries from, 348
  thoracic, rupture of, 289
Aortic aneurysm, 295
  abdominal, 267
Aortic annulus, (*Fig.* 214) 276
Aortic arch, 137, 285–286
  approach to, 239
  double, 287
  malformations of, (*Fig.* 219) 287–288
  right, 287
Aortic atresia, 280
Aortic bodies, (*Fig.* 244) 311
Aortic branches, rupture of, 289
Aortic component of diaphragm, 153
Aortic embolus, 227
Aortic oesophageal arteries, 8
Aortic opening in diaphragm, (*Fig.* 133)
  155
Aortic plexus, 215, 216
Aortic sac, 285
Aortic sinuses of Valsalva, 277
Aortic surgery, abdominal, paraplegia fol-
    lowing, 349
Aortic valve, 276, 279
Aortic valvulitis, 278
Aortic vestibule, 279
Aorticorenal ganglion, 215
Aortobifemoral bypass, 234
Aorto-iliac disease, 229, 234
Aorto-iliac exposure, (*Fig.* 187) 243–244
Apical ligament, 553
Apical vessels of tongue, 196
Aponeurosis, (*Fig.* 260) 328, 329

Appendicectomy, 43–44
Appendicitis
  in infancy, 406
  mimicking cholecystitis, 42
  secondary hypertrophy following, 14
  simulated by diverticulitis, 39
  thrombosis in, 41
Appendicular artery, 41
Appendix, (*Figs.* 34–36) 41–45
  positions of, (*Fig.* 35) 42
Appendix testis, (*Fig.* 112) 123
Arachnoid mater, 342–343
Arachnoid sheath, pierced by retinal ves-
    sels, 352
Arachnoidal granulations, 343
Arachnoidal processes, 343
Arachnoidal villi, 343
Arc syndrome, painful, (*Fig.* 358) 445
Arch of foot, 538–539
Arch of Riolan, (*Fig.* 43) 52, 228
Arch vein, posterior, (*Fig.* 198) 255–256
Arcuate ligament, 214, 226
  median, 6
  popliteal, (*Fig.* 428) 515, 519
Areola, 167
  abscess involving, 170
Arm
  affected by prolapsed cervical disc, 560
  amputation of, 432
  collateral system to, 230
  injury to, 456
  ischaemia of, 231
  raised arterial pressure in, 288
  sensory loss over, 385
  veins of, (*Fig.* 191) 249
Arnold–Chiari malformation, 351
Arnold's nerve, 371
Arrhythmias
  atrial, 281
  following atrial surgery, 278
Arteria auricularis magna, 284
Arterial blood supply to large bowel, (*Figs.*
    43–45) 52–55
Arterial disease, causing loss of vision, 355
Arterial grafting, 256
Arterial pressure, raised in arm, due to
    coarctation of aorta, 288
Arterial pulsation on back, due to coarcta-
    tion of aorta, 288
Arterial supply, to pancreas, (*Fig.* 94) 105

Arteries (*see also specific arteries, and under structures involved*)
  occlusion of, 225–238
Arterioles, vasoconstrictor nerve fibres to, 211
Arteriovenous fistulae, internal, 250
Arthritis, septic, 435
Arthrodesis (*see also* Fusion), (*Fig.* 393) 481
  of shoulder, (*Fig.* 362) 453
Articular disc, of temperomandibular joint, (*Fig.* 156) 187
Artificial limbs, 433
Arytenoid cartilage, 177
Ascending aorta
  approach to, 239
  formation of, 285
Ascending colon
  mesentery to, (*Figs.* 39–40) 46–47
  resection for cancer of, (*Fig.* 47) 56
Aspiration
  lung abscess following, 139
  of chest, 152
  of elbow joint, (*Fig.* 366) 458
  of hip, 507–508
  of radiocarpal joint, 463
  of shoulder joint, 449
Atherosclerosis, 226, 229
  aorto-iliac involvement, 243
Atherosclerotic stenosis, of popliteal artery, 245
Atlanto-axial joint, 553
Atlanto-occipital joint, 553
Atlanto-occipital ligament, (*Fig.* 273) 345
Atlanto-occipital membrane, 553
Atlas, 376, 549, 553
Atresia
  oesophageal, 1, (*Fig.* 1) 2
  of duodenum, 39
  valvular, 280
Atrial appendage, 278
Atrial arrhythmias, 281
Atrial septum, 279
  defect of, 279
Atrioventricular canal, 280
Atrioventricular conduction defect, 277
Atrioventricular nodal artery, 281
Atrioventricular node, 274, (*Fig.* 215) 277
Atrioventricular valves, formation of, 274

Atrium, (*Fig.* 212) 273, (*Fig.* 215) 277, 278
  incorporation of sinus venosus into, 274
Auditory canal, 180
  fistulous track, (*Fig.* 152) 179
Auditory meatus, 179
  lymphatic drainage of, 193
Auditory tube, 369
  lymphatic drainage of, 195
Auditory tubercles, accessory, 180
Auricle, skin, innervation of, 357
Auricular appendages, 180
Auricular artery, posterior, (*Fig.* 261) 330
Auricular branch of vagus nerve, 371
Auricular lymph nodes, (*Fig.* 159) 193–194
Auricular nerves, (*Fig.* 298) 378
Auricular vein, posterior, (*Fig.* 262) 331
Auriculotemporal nerve, 188, (*Fig.* 261) 332, 362
Autonomic nervous system, (*Figs.* 168–176) 207–224
  afferent fibres, 209
  control of rectal muscle by, 63
  efferent fibres, 208–209
  general arrangement, 208–210
  innervating internal sphincter of bladder, 318
  parasympathetic system, (*Fig.* 168) 207–208
  sympathetic system, (*Fig.* 168) 207–208
  transmitter substances in synapses of, 209–210
Autotransplantation, 112
Axillae, excessive sweating of, 219
Axillary approach to shoulder joint, (*Fig.* 360) 451
Axillary artery
  exposure of, 241
  relation of brachial plexus to, (*Fig.* 301) 382
Axillary fascia, 163
Axillary fascial tent, 166–167
Axillary lymph nodes, (*Fig.* 140) 165–166, (*Figs.* 141–142) 167–168, (*Fig.* 211) 272
  of breast, 163
Axillary nerve, 435
  shoulder dislocation causing damage to, 448
Axillary tail of Spence, 163, 165

Axillary vein, (*Fig.* 140) 165, (*Fig.* 192) 250–251
  junction with cephalic vein, 249
  thrombosis of, (*Fig.* 192) 250–251
Axillofemoral bypass, 242
Axonotmesis, 375
Azygos vein, (*Fig.* 124) 83, 138
  caval obstruction involving, (*Fig.* 183) 236–237
  lobes of, (*Fig.* 146) 141–142
  thoracic duct in relation to, 269

B lymphocytes, 106
Back (*see also* Spinal...)
  arterial pulsation on, 288
  hump on, 566
Backache, 558, 561, 562, 563
Balance, nerve of, 369
Balanic hypospadias, 326
Ballooning of intervertebral disc, (*Fig.* 465) 557
Bankart lesion, 448
Barlow's test, 501
Bartholin's abscess, 398
Basal vessels of tongue, 196–197
Basilar artery, (*Fig.* 179) 231, 233, (*Fig.* 267) 337
Basilar migraine, 355
Basilic vein, 242, (*Fig.* 191) 249, 250
Basi-vertebral vein, (*Fig.* 468) 560
Bedsores, covered by myocutaneous flap, 248
Bell, nerve of, 380
Below-knee amputation, (*Fig.* 345) 431
Biceps
  affected by prolapsed cervical disc, 560
  insertion, bursae in relation to, 456
  motor loss to, 385
  relation to brachial artery, 242
  tendon, lesions of, 446–447
Bicipital groove, 435, 436
Bifid nose, 174
Bifid ureter, (*Fig.* 237) 304
Big toe, *see* Hallux valgus
Bile, 79
  in pancreatitis, 90
  obstruction to flow, 89
  reflux of, 90

Bile duct, (*Figs.* 82–86) 88–95
  accessory, 90
  ampulla of Vater, 89
  anomaly of, 39
  blood supply to, 93–94
  cholangiography of, 89
  common, 90
  cystic dilatation of, (*Fig.* 84) 91–92
  development of, 78
  duodenum in relation to, 31
  formation of, 32
  gallstones entering, 91
  Kocher's incision for approach to, 97
  liver arteries in relation to, (*Fig.* 85) 92–93
  liver transplant affecting, 93
  muscles of, 89
  pancreas in relation to, 104
  pancreatic duct joining, 92, 104
  Rutherford Morison incision, 116
  sphincter of Oddi in relation to, 89, (*Fig.* 82) 90
  structure of, 96
  ultrasonography of, 89
  variations in, (*Figs.* 83–84) 90–92
  vascular plexus, 94
  veins of, 94
Biliary colic, 89
Biliary pancreatitis, 90
Biliary system, (*Figs.* 71–91) 78–102
Biliary tree, congenital dilatation of, (*Fig.* 84) 91–92
Biopsy
  needle, of liver, 98
  of prescalene node, 149
Bitemporal hemianopia, 334, (*Fig.* 269) 338, 353
Black eye, causes of, 329
Bladder, (*Figs.* 245–252) 314–320
  abdominal incision for exposure of, 320
  at birth, 406
  blood supply of, 319
  carcinoma of, 319
  exstrophy of, 327
  flow of seminal fluid into, 221
  involved in sliding hernia, 132
  lymphatic drainage of, 319
  muscles of, 318–319
  neck, obstruction of, 321
  nerve supply of, 319–320

Bladder, obstruction to urine flow, 316
  pain in, 320
  peritoneum reflected onto, 48
  plexus supplying, 216
  relations of, (Figs. 250–252) 317–318
  shape of, (Fig. 252) 318
  sphincters of, 318–319, 320
  surgical exposure of, 115, 307
  trigone of (see Trigone of bladder)
  ureter in relation to, (Fig. 235) 302
  uterine ligaments in relation to, (Fig.
    314) 395
Blind spot, 352
Blister, traumatic, 490
Block, sympathetic ganglion, (Figs. 175–
    176) 222–224
Blood
  gases in, chemoreceptors responding to,
    311
  vomiting of, 383
Blood pH, chemoreceptors responding to,
    311
Blood pressure
  affected by coarctation of aorta, 288
  drop due to spinal anaesthetic, 222
  in portal vein, 83
Blood sinuses of cranium, (Fig. 271) 340–
    341, 342
Blood supply
  of bladder, 319
  of bones, (Figs. 327–329) 411–415
  of breast, 164–165
  of common bile duct, 93–94
  of greater omentum, (Figs. 10–11) 15–16
  of ileum, (Fig. 29) 36
  of jejunum, (Fig. 29) 36
  of large bowel, (Figs. 43–45) 52–55
  of liver, (Figs. 74–81) 81–87
  of mandible, 181
  of maxilla, 181–182
  of oesophagus, (Fig. 6) 9
  of palate, 182
  of pancreas, (Fig. 94) 105
  of parathyroid glands, 207
  of rotator cuff, (Fig. 357) 444
  of spinal cord, (Figs. 276–278) 347–350
  of spleen, (Figs. 102–103) 110–112
  of temporomandibular joint, 188
  of thyroid gland, (Figs. 164–165) 202–
    203

Blood supply, of tonsils, (Fig. 158) 191
Blood vessels
  in amputation, 429
  of scalp, (Figs. 261–262) 330–332
  of stomach, (Fig. 9) 14–16
  sensory nerve fibres from, 209
Bochdalek's hernia, 157
Body wall, relation of diaphragm to, 153
Boil, 490
Bone(s), (Figs. 322–345) 407–433
  accessory, (Fig. 338) 421
  blood supply of, (Figs. 327–329) 411–415
  cartilage, 407
  development of, (Figs. 322–326) 407–412
  disease of, 422–423, 563
  in amputation, 429
  membrane, 407
  pathology of, (Figs. 339–340) 421–424
  regenerative powers of, 422
  sesamoid, 420–421
  supernumerary, (Fig. 338) 421
  tumours of, (Fig. 340) 423, 424
Bony ankylosis, 432
Bowel
  fistula from, 68
  large (see Large bowel)
  small (see Small intestine)
  strangulation of, in hernial sac, 132
Bow legs, 522
Bowman's capsule, 297
Brachial artery, 250
  bifurcation of, 242
  exposure of, 242
  injury to, 456
  occlusion of, 231–232
Brachial plexus, 219, 241, (Fig. 193) 251,
    (Figs. 300–303) 379–385
  damage to, 449
  lesions of, 384–385
Brachialis muscle, (Fig. 342) 425
  motor loss to, 385
Brachiocephalic artery, 230
  approach to, 239
  rupture of, 289
Brachiocephalic trunk, formation of, 285
Brachiocephalic vein, 9, 202, 206, 252,
    (Fig. 196) 253
  at birth, 404
  development of, 267
  occlusion of, (Fig. 181) 234

Brachiocephalic vein, relation of great
    lymph trunks to, (*Fig.* 210) 271
  thoracic duct entering, 270
Brachioradialis muscle, 242
Brain
  arachnoid mater, 342–343
  collateral supply to, 232, 331
  dura mater, (*Fig.* 271) 340–342
  pia mater, (*Fig.* 272) 343–344
  venous drainage of, 234
Brain stem, 207, 209, (*Fig.* 173) 218, (*Fig.* 287) 363
Branchial arches, (*Fig.* 150) 174–177, (*Fig.* 218) 285-286
  developmental anomalies of, (*Figs.* 149–152) 175–180
  embryonic rests of, 192
  formation of pinna from, 179
  structures derived from, 176–177
Branchial clefts, 177
Branchial cyst, 177, 179
Branchial fistula, (*Fig.* 151) 177–179
Branchial grooves, 177
  anomalies of, 179
  non-chromaffin paraganglia around, (*Fig.* 244) 311
Branchial pouch, 206
Branchial sinus, 177
Breast (*see also* Mammary...), (*Figs.* 138–144) 161–171
  accessory tissue, 162
  acini of, 161, 163
  amastia, 162
  anatomy of, (*Figs.* 139–143) 163–169
  architecture of, (*Fig.* 139) 163–164
  arterial branch to, 137
  blood supply to, 164–165
  cancer, 164, 171
  congenital abnormalities of, 162–163
  development of, (*Fig.* 138) 161–162
  dimpling of skin, (*Fig.* 144) 170
  ducts of, fibro-adenoma in, 164
  lymphatic drainage of, (*Figs.* 141–143) 167–169
  lymph nodes of, 163
  mastectomy, 171
  Mondor's disease of, 165
  nerve supply to, 165
  nipple, 162
  polymastia of, 162

Breast, polythelia of, 163
  retraction of nipple, (*Fig.* 144) 169–170
  sclerosing adenosis of, 164
  venous drainage of, 165
Breathing, after birth, 405
Bronchial artery, thrombosis associated with, 146
Bronchial tree, (*Fig.* 128) 143–144
Bronchial vessels, 145
Bronchiectasis, causing middle-lobe collapse, 141
Bronchomediastinal trunk, 147
  draining to thoracic duct, 270
  termination of, (*Fig.* 210) 271
Bronchopulmonary circulation, 145–146
Bronchus
  position in thorax, (*Fig.* 124) 138
  supernumerary, 144
Bryant's triangle, (*Fig.* 335) 418
Buccal cortical plate, 186
Buccal mucosa
  innervation of, (*Fig.* 155) 186
  sensory supply to, 183
Buccal nerve, (*Fig.* 153) 182–183
  injection for, 185
Buccal pad of fat, 404
Buccal plate, 184
Buccal salivary glands, innervation of, 182
Buccal soft tissues, blood supply to, 181
Buccal sulcus, 186
Buccinator lymph node group, 194
Buccinator muscle, 181, 182
Bucket-handle incision, (*Fig.* 242) 310–311
Budd–Chiari syndrome, 83
Bulb, urethral, (*Fig.* 256) 325
Bulbo-urethral glands, 324
  inflammation of, 77
Bulbous cordis, 279
Bulbous urethra, rupture of, (*Fig.* 257) 325
Bulboventricular loop, (*Fig.* 212) 273
Bulbus cordis, (*Fig.* 212) 273, 275
Bundle of His, 274
  injury to, 277
Bunion, 546
Bursa(e)
  around hip, (*Figs.* 418–419) 504–505
  around knee joint, (*Figs.* 437–438) 524–526
  around tendo Achillis, (*Fig.* 449) 537
Bursitis, 526

Buttocks
  claudication in, 229
  varices of, 84
Bypass, axillofemoral, 242
Bypass graft, 256
  for arterial occlusion, 234

Caecal artery, 44
Caecal bud, 24
Caecum, 41
  deficient fixation of, 29
  development of, 24
  fossae in relation to, (*Fig.* 36) 44–45
  involved in sliding hernia, (*Fig.* 120) 132
  position of appendix in relation to, (*Fig.* 35) 42
  resection for cancer of, (*Fig.* 47) 56
  volvulus of, 46
Calcaneal angle, (*Fig.* 453) 543
Calcaneal spurs, (*Fig.* 455) 546
Calcaneocuboid joint, 538
Calcaneofibular ligament, (*Fig.* 443) 531
Calcaneus
  fractures of, (*Fig.* 453) 543–544
  making up foot arch, 539
  ossicle fused with, (*Fig.* 339) 421
  retinaculum attached to, (*Fig.* 444) 533
  tendo Achillis in relation to, (*Fig.* 449) 537
Calcarine cortex, 355
Calcarine fissure, 353, 354
Calcific tendinitis, 445
Calcified nodes, in lung, 141
Calcium hydroxyapatite crystals, 445
Calf
  muscles, affected by clubfoot, 543
  pain in, 263
  varicose veins in, 262
  veins, thrombi in, 258
Callosities, associated with pes cavus, 545
Calot's triangle, 97
Camper, fascia of, 123–124
Cancer (*see also* Carcinoma; Fibrosarcoma; Sarcoma; *and under structures involved*)
  causing breast retraction, (*Fig.* 144) 170
  in axillary nodes, 166
  in cervical lymph gland, 149

Cancer, of breast, 164, 167, 171
  of colon, 52
  of gut, resection for, (*Figs.* 47–54) 56–61
  of larynx, 195
  of lip, 196
  of lung, lymphatic spread, 149
  of mouth, 197
  of pancreas, 219
  of skin, removal of plexus on deep fascia, 272
  of thyroid, 205
  of tongue, 194, 197
  requiring removal of submandibular salivary gland, 194
  spread of, 273
Canine teeth
  blood supply to, 181
  innervation of, 183
Cannulation
  in arm, 250
  of internal jugular vein, (*Fig.* 197) 254
  of subclavian vein, (*Fig.* 194) 252–253
Capitate bone, (*Fig.* 369) 460
Capitis muscle, 211
Capsulitis, adhesive, 446
Caput Medusae, (*Fig.* 78) 84
Carcinoma (*see also* Cancer)
  adrenocortical, 310
  bronchogenic, biopsy for, 149
  of bladder, 319
  of bone, (*Fig.* 340) 424
  of cervix, 78
  of oesophagus, 10, 21
  of prostate, 319, 321
  of rectum, 76, 77
  renal, affecting testicular vein, 136
Cardia, (*Fig.* 8) 12, 13
  movement into chest, 160
Cardiac...(*see also* Heart)
Cardiac catheterization, 232
Cardiac chambers, 278
Cardiac injuries, 285
Cardiac lesions, tracheo-oesophageal fistula associated with, 1
Cardiac nerve, (*Fig.* 170) 212, 213
Cardiac notch, (*Fig.* 8) 12
Cardiac plexus, 211, 213
Cardiac tube, looping of, (*Fig.* 212) 273
Cardiac valves, formation of, 274

Cardinal vein
  common, (*Fig.* 212) 273
  development of superior vena cava from, 267
Caroli's disease, 92
Caroticocavernous fistula, resulting in abducens nerve paralysis, 363
Carotid artery, 178, 202, (*Fig.* 165) 203, 211, 230, (*Fig.* 268) 338
  aneurysm of, causing oculomotor nerve lesion, 356
  approach to, 239
  arteries to scalp derived from, (*Fig.* 261) 330
  cavernous sinus in relation to, (*Fig.* 281) 356
  formation of, 285
  in radical neck dissection, 197
  internal (*see* Internal carotid artery)
  occlusion of, 232
  oesophagus in relation to, (*Fig.* 2) 3
  relation to cavernous sinus, (*Fig.* 281) 356
Carotid body, (*Fig.* 244) 311
  tumour of, 313
Carotid nerve, internal, 211
Carotid sheath in relation to nerve trunk, 211
Carotid system in relation to thoracic duct, (*Fig.* 209) 269
Carpal bones, 461
Carpal ligament, 467
Carpal tunnel syndrome, 388
Cartilage
  cricoid, 2, 5
  semilunar, of knee joint, (*Fig.* 434) 520–522, 524
  thyroid, fibres arising from, 5
Cartilage bones, 407
  pathology of, 422–423
Cartilage plate, of spine, (*Fig.* 460) 551
Catecholamines, stored in paraganglia, 311
Catheter, venous, 250
Cauda equina, 561
  pressure on, (*Fig.* 466) 558
Causalgia, 219
Caval opening in diaphragm, (*Fig.* 133) 155

Cavernous sinus, 332, (*Fig.* 268) 338
  cranial nerves in relation to, (*Fig.* 281) 356
  pituitary tumour causing pressure on, 338
Central anastomotic artery, 228
Central fibrous body, (*Fig.* 214) 276
Central nervous system, congenital malformations of, (*Fig.* 279) 350–351
Centrum, (*Fig.* 458) 549, 550
  early fusion of, 561
Cephalic vein, (*Fig.* 191) 249
Cerebellar artery in relation to cranial nerves, 364
Cerebellar tonsils, herniation of, 351
Cerebellum in relation to tentorium, 341
Cerebral artery, 233, (*Fig.* 267) 337
  occlusion of, 354
Cerebral cortex, 207
Cerebral interstitial fluid, 344
Cerebral peduncle, injury to, 356
Cerebrospinal fluid, 343, (*Figs.* 273–275) 344–347, 357
  accumulation of, 350
  in outer surface of brain, 341
Cervical aorta, 287
Cervical arteries, 232
Cervical chain of lymph nodes, 205
Cervical curve, of spinal column, 547
Cervical disc, prolapsed, 559
Cervical ganglion, 211–213, (*Fig.* 173) 218, 361
Cervical lordosis, 553
Cervical lymph nodes, 188, 193, 194–195, 196, 197, (*Fig.* 211) 272, 333
Cervical mediastinoscopy, 149
Cervical nerve, 211, 212
  nerves of scalp derived from, 332
  osteophytes from uncovertebral joints affecting, (*Fig.* 462) 552
Cervical nodes, 10
  in relation to jugular vein, 254
Cervical oesophagus, (*Fig.* 2) 3
Cervical osteo-arthritis, 384
Cervical plexus, (*Figs.* 296–297) 376–377
Cervical radicular artery, (*Fig.* 278) 348–349
Cervical rib, (*Figs.* 303–304) 383–384
Cervical sinus, (*Fig.* 150) 177, 178

Cervical smear, 398
Cervical sympathectomy, 219–220
Cervical sympathetic paralysis, 385
Cervical sympathetic trunk, (*Figs.* 170–171) 211–214
Cervical vertebrae, 549
  Sibson's fascia in relation to, (*Fig.* 134) 156
Cervicodorsal sympathectomy, 219
Cervicomediastinal blood vessels, approach to, (*Fig.* 185) 239–240
Cervicothoracic ganglion, (*Fig.* 171) 213–214, 219
Cervix
  carcinoma of, detected by rectal examination, 78
  inspection of, 398
  palpation of, 77
  ureters in relation to, 305
  uterine ligaments in relation to, (*Fig.* 314) 395
Cheek
  abscess in, 180
  lymphatic drainage of, 194
  sensory innervation of, 357
Chemodectomata, 313
Chemoreceptors, 311
Chest
  accumulation of lymph in, 271
  aspiration of, 152
  reconstruction of wall, 248
  route of lymph from breast into, (*Fig.* 143) 169
  tube drainage of, 271
  wall of, (*Fig.* 124) 137–138
Chevron incision, (*Fig.* 242) 310–311
Child, anatomy of, (*Figs.* 318–321) 401–407
Chin
  numbness of, 184
  skin over, innervation of, 183
Cholangiography, 89, 97
Cholecystectomy, 89, 97–98
  drainage after, 96
  hazard of, 86
Cholecystitis
  causing pain in tip of shoulder, 96–97
  mimicked by appendicitis, 42
Choledochocele, congenital, (*Fig.* 84) 91–92

Cholelithiasis, secondary hypertrophy following, 14
Choleretic effect, 89
Cholinergic receptors, in oesophagus, 7
Chondroma, (*Fig.* 340) 424
Chondromalacia, 420
Chorda tympani, 183, 184, 362, (*Fig.* 288) 364
Chordee, 326
Chromaffin paraganglia, (*Fig.* 243) 311–312
Chylothorax, 271
Chylous ascites, 271
Ciliary ganglion, 217, (*Fig.* 282) 358
  parasympathetic fibres synapsing in, 355
Ciliary muscle, 355
Circle of Willis, 230, (*Fig.* 180) 232–234, 334, (*Fig.* 267) 337, 344
Circulation
  collateral, (*Figs.* 177–184) 224–238
  fetal, 275
Circulus vasculosus, (*Fig.* 327) 413
Circumaortic renal venous cuff, (*Fig.* 205) 265
Circumflex artery
  coronary, 283
  supplying head of femur, 505
Cirrhosis
  causing portal hypertension, 83
  rupture of oesophageal veins in, 156
Cisterna chyli, (*Fig.* 208) 268
Cisterna magna, (*Fig.* 273) 345
Cisternal puncture, (*Fig.* 273) 345
Cisterns, of brain, 343–344
Claudication, intermittent, 225
Clavicle, 407
  ossification of, (*Fig.* 324) 410
  rhomboid fossa of, (*Fig.* 325) 411
  vein crossing, 250
Claw hand, (*Fig.* 311) 392
Claw toe, 545
Cleft palate, (*Fig.* 149) 173–174
Clinoid process, 233, (*Fig.* 265) 336
  anterior, relation to cavernous sinus, (*Fig.* 281) 356
  erosion of, 339
Clitoris, dorsal nerve of, (*Fig.* 66) 73
Cloaca, (*Fig.* 229) 297

Cloaca, development of bladder from, (*Fig.* 245) 314
  ectodermal, development of anal canal from, (*Fig.* 62) 68–69
  entodermal, development of rectum from, (*Fig.* 62) 68-69
  incomplete division of, (*Fig.* 63) 68
Cloacal membrane, (*Fig.* 245) 314, (*Fig.* 258) 326
Clubfoot, 543
Coarctation of aorta, (*Fig.* 219) 288
Coccygeal nerves, 216
Coccygeus muscle, 65
Coccyx, 216, 547
  anal canal in relation to, 61
  insertion of levatores ani into, 65
  palpation of, in rectal examination, 78
  rectum in relation to, 48
Cochlear nerve, 369
Coeliac artery, 22, 226–227
  oesophagus in relation to, (*Fig.* 5) 6
  supplying pancreas, 105
Coeliac ganglion, 215
  excision of, 219
Coeliac nodes, 10
Coeliac plexus, 211, 215
  supplying adrenal glands, 309
Cold abscess, 565
Colic artery, (*Fig.* 37) 45, (*Fig.* 43) 52, (*Fig.* 178) 227
Colic vein, 47
Colitis, ulcerative, palpation for, 77
Collar stud abscess, (*Fig.* 401) 491
Collateral circulation, (*Figs.* 177–184) 224–238
  factors affecting, 225–226
  to brain, 232
Collateral ganglia, 208
Collateral ligament(s)
  lateral, (*Fig.* 443) 531
  medial, (*Fig.* 442) 530
  of finger, 479
  of knee joint, (*Figs.* 429–430) 516–517
  of wrist joint, 482
Colles, fascia of, (*Fig.* 113) 123–125
  extravasation to, 326
Colon (*see also* Large bowel), 41
  ascending, *see* Ascending colon
  dilatation due to aganglionic mega-colon, 71

Colon, infarction of, 47, 228
  mobility of, 29
  movement during development of, 26–28
  resection of, (*Fig.* 51) 59, 228
  transverse, *see* Transverse colon
  tumour, palpation of, 78
  veins of, effect of portal hypertension, 84
  venous drainage of, 47
Colostomy
  barium study after, 71
  rod, 53
  site of, 114
Commando resection of neck, 198
Common bile duct (*see* Bile duct)
Common cardinal vein, (*Fig.* 212) 273
Common carotid artery
  formation of, 285
  occlusion of, 232
  oesophagus in relation to, (*Fig.* 2) 3
Common facial vein, (*Fig.* 262) 331
Common hepatic duct, 90
Common hepatic nodes, 10
Common peroneal nerve, 428
  injuries to, 394
Communicans hypoglossi, 379
Communicating artery, 233, (*Fig.* 267) 337
Communicating veins, 262
  test for competence of, 263
Compartmental syndrome, (*Fig.* 184) 236–238
Concha, nasal, 352
Condylar processes, blood supply to, 181
Condyles, femoral, (*Fig.* 426) 513
Condyloid canal, veins of, 332
Condyloid joint, 479
Congenital abnormalities (*see under structures involved*)
Coning, reversed tentorial, 363
Conjoint tendon, 126, 129, 130
Conjunctiva
  innervation of, 357
  lymphatic drainage of, 194
Conoid ligament, (*Fig.* 354) 442
Consensual light reflex, 353
Constrictors of pharynx, 177
Continence
  faecal, 68
  maintenance of, 66

Continence, mechanism, (*Fig.* 58) 63–64
  muscle control of, 318
Conus ligament, (*Fig.* 214) 276
Cooper, ligament of, 126, 130, (*Fig.* 139) 164
  sutured to inguinal ligament, 134
Coraco-acromial arch, 433, (*Fig.* 352) 440, 444
Coracoclavicular ligaments, (*Fig.* 354) 442
Coracoid process, (*Fig.* 301) 382
Cord, spermatic, 122
Cornea
  haemorrhage at margin of, 329
  innervation of, 357
Corneal anaesthesia, 358
Corniculate cartilage, 177
Cornu of hyoid, 176
Coronary artery
  bypass graft, 280
  development of, 275
  disease of, 284
  left, (*Fig.* 217) 282–283
  right, (*Fig.* 216) 281–282
Coronary circulation, (*Figs.* 216–217) 280–284
Coronary ligament, (*Fig.* 31) 38, 520
Coronary sinus, 267, 274, 281
  origin of left coronary artery from, 284
  ostium, (*Fig.* 215) 277
Coronary vein, 16, 82, 281
  in portal hypertension, 85
Coronoid process, 187
  fracture of, 457
Corpora cavernosa, 324
Corpus spongiosum, 324
Corti, spiral organ of, 369
Cortical plates of mandible, blood supply to, 181
Cosmesis, 429
Costal cartilage, 2, 137
Costochondral junction, prominence at, 138
Costoclavicular ligament, 411
Costocoracoid membrane, 166
Cough reflex, 332
  reflex contraction of anal sphincters associated with, 66
Cowper's gland, (*Fig.* 256) 324
  palpation of, 77
Coxa valga, 501

Coxa vara, (*Fig.* 413) 499
Cranial fossa, 357
  anterior, 352
  middle, (*Fig.* 156) 187
  trigeminal nerve approached through, 358
Cranial ganglia, (*Fig.* 173) 217–218
Cranial nerves, (*Figs.* 280–294) 352–375
  epineurium of, 341
  palsy of, 352
Craniocleidodysostosis, affecting membrane bones, 422
Craniopharyngeal canal, (*Fig.* 263) 333
Craniopharyngiomas, 336
Craniosacral outflow, 207
Craniotomy, 330
Cranium, blood sinuses of, 342
Creases of hand, (*Fig.* 400) 489–490
Cremasteric artery, 121
Cremasteric fascia, 119
Cremasteric reflex, 120
Cribriform plate, 352
Cribrosa fascia, 130
Cricoid cartilage, 2, 5, 177
Cricopharyngeus muscle, 3, 5–6
Cricothyroid ligament, lymph nodes associated with, 195
Cricothyroid muscle, 177, 203
  innervation of, 372
Crista galli, 342
Crista terminalis, 278
Crista urethralis, 321
Crohn's disease, causing extrasphincteric fistula, 76
Cruciate ligaments, (*Figs.* 431–433) 517–520
Crus of diaphragm, 153
  congenital defect in, 158
  oesophagus in relation to, (*Fig.* 5) 6
  splanchnic nerve perforating, 215
Crux cordis, 281
Cryotherapy, 358
Cryptorchidism, 120
Crypts of tonsils, 190
CSF rhinorrhoea, 352
CT scan, of oesophagus, 10
Cubital vein, median, (*Fig.* 191) 249
Cubitus valgus, (*Fig.* 364) 454, 457
Cubitus varus, (*Fig.* 364) 454
Cuboid, making up foot arch, 539

Cuneiform bones, making up foot arch, 539
Cuneiform cartilage, 177
Curvature nodes, 10
Cusp of mitral valve, (*Fig.* 214) 276
Cyanosis, associated with posterolateral hernia, 157
Cyst(s)
  associated with Rathke's pouch, 333
  branchial, 177, 179
  epidermoid, 329
  of breast, 164
  of common bile duct, (*Fig.* 84) 91–92
  of epididymis, 136
  of kidney, 298
  of oesophagus, 1–2
  of osteitis fibrosa, (*Fig.* 340) 424
  of umbilicus, (*Fig.* 33) 40
  of urachus, 316
  pseudopancreatic, 104
  thyroglossal, (*Fig.* 163) 199–200
Cystic artery, 85, (*Fig.* 85) 92–93
Cystic dilatation of common bile duct, (*Fig.* 84) 91–92
Cystic duct, 78, 88, 90, (*Fig.* 86) 94–95
  absence of, 91
  in gallbladder removal, 97
Cystic enlargement, behind testicle, 136
Cystic node, 17
Cystic vein, 82
Cystocele, 397
Cystogastrocolic band, 32

Dartos muscle, 121, 124
Deafness, fracture of cranial fossa causing, 369
Deep veins, 258
  of leg, venous hypertension in, 263
  thrombosis of, 249, 258
Defaecation
  mechanism of, 66
  pain on, 63
Deglutition, 7
Deltoid ligament, (*Fig.* 442) 530
  of ankle joint, 540
Deltoid muscle, 436
Denonvilliers' fascia, 50, (*Fig.* 250) 317
Dens, 553

Dentate line, (*Fig.* 55) 62
  lymphatic drainage, 63
Descendens cervicalis nerve, 379
Descendens hypoglossi nerve, 374, 379
Descending aorta
  approach to, 239
  coarctation of, 288
  joined to ductus arteriosus, 286
  operations on, 289
  rupture of, 289
Descending colon
  relation to ascending colon, (*Fig.* 39) 47
  resection for cancer of, (*Fig.* 49) 57
Detrusor muscle, 320
Dextrocardia, 280
  associated with posterolateral hernia, 157
Diabetes, amputation associated with, 430
Diaphragm, (*Figs.* 132–137) 152–161
  crus of, *see* Crus of diaphragm
  development of, (*Fig.* 132) 152–154
  distribution of phrenic nerve, (*Fig.* 131) 151
  drainage by mediastinal nodes, 147
  errors in gut rotation due to hernia of, 28
  eventration of, 159
  hernia of, (*Figs.* 135–137) 157–161
  incision of, 151
  injury to, 159
  kidney in relation to, 291
  lung in relation to, 141
  muscle of, 153–155, 159
  nerve supply, 152, 154
  nodes of, 10, 147
  oesophagus in relation to, (*Fig.* 3) 4
  openings in, (*Fig.* 133) 155–156
  passage of thoracic duct through, 269
  pulsion diverticulum situated above, 7
  radicular arteries in relation to, (*Fig.* 278) 349
  relations of, 154
  shoulder pain referred from, 154
  veins of, in portal hypertension, 85
Diaphragma sellae, (*Figs.* 266, 268) 337, 338, 341
Diaphysial aclasia, 422
Diaphysis, (*Fig.* 322) 407
  of short long bones, affected by tuberculosis, 423
Diarrhoea, postvagotomy, 21

Digastric muscle, 176, 183, 188
Digital joints, (*Figs.* 390–393) 479–481
Digital nerve, 494
  block, 493
  pain associated with, 547
Dilator muscle of iris, 355
Dilator pupillae muscle, (*Fig.* 282) 359
  fibres to, 211
Diplopia
  associated with abducens nerve paralysis, 363
  caused by pituitary tumour, 338
Discs, intervertebral (*see* Intervertebral discs)
Discography, 556
Dislocations (*see under* individual joints)
Disse, space of, (*Fig.* 71) 79
Distal convoluted tubule, (*Fig.* 229) 297
Diverticulitis, 39
Diverticulum(a)
  acquired, of thoracic oesophagus, 7–8
  congenital, of common bile duct, (*Fig.* 84) 91–92
  congenital, of oesophagus, 1–2
  due to traction, 8
  hepatic, 78
  pharyngeal, (*Fig.* 4) 5
Dopamine, tumours secreting, 313
Dorsal aorta, 286
Dorsal mesentery, 153
Dorsal motor nucleus, 209
Dorsal spaces of hand, (*Fig.* 396) 488–489
Dorsum sellae, 233, (*Fig.* 267) 337
Douglas' pouch, 51, 323, 397
Drainage tubes, insertion of, 114
Drop-wrist, (*Fig.* 305) 386
Drowsiness, associated with pituitary tumour, 339
Duct(s)
  ectasia, 164
  hepatic (*see* Hepatic ducts)
  of Gartner, (*Fig.* 248) 315
  of Santorini, joining duodenum, 104
  papilloma of, 164
Ductus arteriosus
  branchial arches in relation to, (*Fig.* 218) 286
  left-sided, 287
  patent, 287
Ductus deferens, 121, (*Fig.* 246) 315

Ductus deferens, absence of, 298
  ureter in relation to, (*Fig.* 235) 301–302
  veins of, 136
Ductus venosus, 82, 275
Duodenocolic isthmus, 24, 29
Duodenojejunal flexure, 33
Duodenojejunal fossae, (*Fig.* 26) 33–34
Duodenojejunostomy, 104
Duodenum, (*Figs.* 23–28) 30–35
  annular pancreas of, 104
  bile flow into, 89
  bulb of, (*Fig.* 24) 32
  common bile duct in relation to, 90
  congenital diverticulum of, 32
  congenital obstruction of, 37
  development of pancreas from, 102
  fossae, (*Figs.* 25–28) 33–35
  mobilization of, 35
  movement during development, 26–28
  papilla of, 89
  relations of, 31
  Santorini's duct joining, 104
  stenosis, 1, 104
  ulcers, 20, 31
Dupuytren's contracture, 456, 468
Dural sac, 342
Dural sheath, 341
  pierced by retinal vessels, 352
Dura mater, (*Fig.* 271) 340–342
  nerve supply to, 333
Dysphagia
  associated with retrosternal hernia, 158
  due to spasm of oesophagus, 7
Dysphagia lusoria, due to right subclavian artery, 287
Dysplasia, 499
Dyspnoea, associated with posterolateral hernia, 157
Dystrophia adiposogenitalis, 333

Ear
  bleeding from, 341
  inner, 369
  macrostomia, 174
  middle (*see* Middle ear)
  sinus on helix of, 180
  speculum, stimulation of auricular branch of vagus by, 322

Ectasia, duct, 164
Ectopia testis, 120
Ectopia vesicae, 327
Ectopic anus, (*Fig.* 63) 68
Ectopic kidney, (*Fig.* 231) 300
Ectopic thyroid tissue, 199
Ectopic ureteric orifice, (*Fig.* 237) 304
Edentulous jaw, (*Fig.* 161) 197–198
Ediner–Westphal nucleus, 208
Efferent autonomic nerve fibres, 208–209
Ejaculation
    affected by removal of lumbar ganglion, 221
    interference with, 319
    into bladder, 322
    nerves involved in, 65
Ejaculatory duct(s), 322
    additional ureter opening into, 304
    opening into urethra, 319, 324
    traversing prostate, 320
    ureter in relation to, (*Fig.* 235) 302
Ejaculatory fluid, prevention of reflux into bladder, 319
Elbow, (*Figs.* 363–368) 454–460
    blood supply to, 456
    collateral supply, 232
    extension, motor loss, 385
    joint, Langenbeck's method for exposure of, (*Fig.* 368) 459
    nerve supply to, 457
    operative procedures, (*Figs.* 366–368) 458–460
Embolism, air, following hepatic vein injuries, 87
Emissary vein, (*Fig.* 260) 328, 332
Encysted inguinal hernia, (*Fig.* 114) 127
Endo-abdominal fascia, 160
Endocrine changes, associated with pituitary tumour, 339
Endocrine gland, thyroid, 200
Endoneurium, (*Fig.* 295) 375
Endoprosthesis, 512
Endoscopy, oesophageal landmarks during, 6–7
End plate, of vertebrae, 554
Enophthalmos, 385
Enteratoma, (*Fig.* 33) 40
Enterocele, 397
Enterocystocoele, (*Fig.* 33) 40
Enterogenous cysts of oesophagus, 1–2

Enterotomata, (*Fig.* 33) 40
Epicondyle of femur, 516
Epicranial aponeurosis, 328, 329
Epidermoid cysts, 329
Epididymis, 121, 122, 123
    cystic enlargement associated with, 136
    hydrocele associated with disease of, 135
Epidural anaesthetic, 222
Epidural space, 342
Epigastric artery, 129, 131, 229
    haemorrhage from, 116
Epigastric pain, 226
    associated with pancreas, 104
Epigastric vein, 84, 255
Epileptic fits, shoulder dislocation following, 448
Epineural repair, 376
Epineurium, (*Fig.* 295) 375
    of cranial nerves, 341
Epiphysial cartilage, (*Fig.* 322) 408
Epiphysial centres, (*Fig.* 459) 550–551
Epiphysial vessels, 414
Epiphysis, (*Fig.* 322) 407
    disease of, 423
    fracture separation of, 423
Epiploic arcade, in greater omentum, (*Fig.* 11) 16
Epiploic artery, (*Fig.* 10) 15
Epispadias, 327
Epithelium, of oesophagus, 1
Eponychium, (*Fig.* 402) 491
Epoöphoron, (*Fig.* 248) 315
Erb's paralysis, 384
Erb's point, (*Fig.* 302) 380
Erection of penis, nerves involved in, 65
Ethmoid bone, 352
Eustachian tube, 179, 369
Eustachian valve, 277
Eventration of diaphragm, 159
Ewing's tumour, (*Fig.* 340) 424
Excretory urogram, 71
Exomphalos, 24, 28
Exostosis, cartilage-capped, 422
Exstrophy of bladder, 327
Extensor digitorum communis, (*Fig.* 384) 472
Extensor digitorum longus, (*Fig.* 444) 533
    sheath of, (*Figs.* 446–448) 536

Extensor hallucis longus, (*Fig.* 444) 533
  sheath of, (*Figs.* 446–448) 536
Extensor indicis tendon, 463
Extensor pollicis longus tendon, 463
Extensor retinaculum tendon, 463
Extensors of wrist, (*Fig.* 395) 484
External carotid artery, 330
  formation of, 285
External genitalia, in male, (*Fig.* 258) 326
External jugular vein, (*Fig.* 196) 253, (*Fig.* 262) 331
External occipital protuberance, 342
External sphincter
  of bladder, 319
  of urethra, 324
Extra-adrenal secretory tumours, 312–313
Extradural abscess, 403
Extradural space, 342
Extrasphincteric abscess, (*Fig.* 70) 75–76
Extrasphincteric fistula, causes of, 76
Extravasation of urine, (*Fig.* 113) 124, (*Fig.* 257) 325
Eye
  black, causes of, 329
  formation of, (*Figs.* 145–146) 172
  lymphatic drainage of, 194
  signs, produced by pituitary tumours, 338
Eyeball
  injury to, 329
  innervation of muscles of, 355
  movement affected by abducens nerve paralysis, 363
  sunken, 385
Eyelid
  drooping of, 355, 385
  elevation of, 360
  engorgement associated with proptosis, 338
  haemorrhage into, 329
  lymphatic drainage of, 194
  muscles, innervation of, 355
  paralysis of, 360
  upper, innervation of, 357

Face
  developmental anomalies of, (*Figs.* 145–148) 171–174

Face, lines of developmental fusion, (*Fig.* 148) 172–173
  paralysis of muscles in, 367
  rare malformations of, 174
Facet joints, (*Fig.* 462) 552, 555
  degenerative changes in, 563
Facial artery, lymph node around, 194
Facial canal, (*Fig.* 289) 365
Facial defects, covered by myocutaneous flap, 248
Facial deformities, maxillary osteotomies for correction of, 182
Facial lymph nodes, (*Fig.* 159) 193–194
Facial muscles, 176
Facial nerves, 176, 184, 332, (*Figs.* 287–291) 363–368, (*Fig.* 320) 402
  branchial groove anomalies in relation to, 179
  in radical neck dissection, 197
  lesions of, (*Fig.* 291) 367–368
  mandibular branch of, 367
  parotid gland in relation to, 367
Facial pain, due to trigeminal neuralgia, 358
Facial vein, (*Fig.* 196) 253
  anterior, (*Fig.* 262) 331
  common, (*Fig.* 262) 331
Faecal continence, 68
Falciform ligament, 37, (*Fig.* 73) 80–81, 115
  umbilical vein in, 82
  veins associated with, 83–84
Fallopian tubes, 399
Fallot's tetralogy, 277, 284
False capsule of prostate, (*Fig.* 254) 322
False capsule of thyroid, 201, 207
Falx cerebelli, 341
Falx cerebri, 341
Falx inguinalis, 126, 129, 130
Fascia
  axillary, 163
  cribrosa, 130
  iliaca, (*Fig.* 117) 129
  lata, 124, 129
  lunata, (*Fig.* 65) 72
  of Camper, 123–124
  of Colles, (*Fig.* 113) 123–125
  of Denonvilliers, 50, (*Figs.* 250–251) 318, 323
  of rectum, 50

Fascia, of Scarpa, (*Fig.* 113) 123–125
  of Sibson, (*Fig.* 134) 156
  of Waldeyer, 50
  perineal, 124
  space infections of, 493
  spermatic, 127
  transversalis, 98, 119, 125, 126, 129, 160, 293
Fascial tent, axillary, 166–167
Fasciculi, (*Fig.* 295) 375
Fat, subcutaneous, at birth, 405
Fat pad, infrapatellar, 524
Fatty acids, absorption, 78
Fauces
  pillars of, 190
  tonsils situated at isthmus of, 189
Feet (*see* Foot)
Femoral artery, (*Fig.* 117) 129
  occlusion of, 229, 234
Femoral canal, 129, (*Fig.* 119) 130–131
Femoral condyles, (*Fig.* 426) 513
  hypoplastic lateral, 524
Femoral hernia, (*Figs.* 117–120) 129–132, (*Fig.* 122) 134–135
  coverings, 131–132
  distinguished from inguinal hernia, 126
  strangulated, 131
Femoral nerve, (*Fig.* 118) 130, 506
Femoral ring, 130
Femoral sheath, (*Fig.* 117) 129
Femoral triangle, site of ectopic testis, 120
Femoral vein
  in repair of femoral hernia, 134–135
  saphenous vein entering, 255
  thrombi in, 258
Femoral vessels, exposure of, 244
Femoropopliteal graft, 245
Femur (*see also* Thigh)
  angle of neck of, (*Fig.* 412) 499
  blood supply of head of, (*Fig.* 420) 505–506
  congenital dislocation of head of, 501
  epicondyle of, 516
  excision of head of, 511
  fracture of, 499
  measurement of, (*Fig.* 334) 417
  necrosis of head of, 506
  sarcoma of, 513
  surgical approach to, (*Fig.* 343) 427–428
  uniting of epiphyses, 411

Fenestra vestibuli, (*Fig.* 289) 365
Fetus
  circulation in, 275
  development of branchial arches, (*Fig.* 218) 285
  umbilical vein of, 82
Fibrinogen test, radioactive, 258
Fibro-adenoma, in breast ducts, 164
Fibrosarcoma, periosteal, (*Fig.* 340) 424
Fibrosis
  of breast tissue, 170
  traction diverticulum due to, 8
Fibrous ankylosis, 432
Fibrous capsule of knee joint, 515
Fibrous dysplasia, 499
Fibrous skeleton of heart, (*Fig.* 214) 276
Fibrous tendon sheaths of hand, 477–478
Fibrous trigone, 276
Fibula
  ligaments arising from, (*Fig.* 428) 515
  measurement of, (*Fig.* 337) 420
  perforating vessels associated with, 261
  surgical approach to, 428
  tibulofibula ligament, (*Fig.* 441) 530
Fibular collateral ligament, 516
Filum terminale, 347
Finger(s)
  affected by injury to median nerve, 387
  affected by prolapsed cervical disc, 560
  amputation of, (*Figs.* 408–411) 496–497, 499
  creases of, (*Fig.* 400) 489–490
  incisions, (*Figs.* 405–407) 494–496
  joint dislocation, (*Fig.* 391) 479
  motor loss in flexors of, 385
  Raynaud's disease affecting, 218–219
  tips, gangrene of, 384
First rib, (*Fig.* 303) 383
Fissure-in-ano, 63
  sentinel pile associated with, 68
Fistula
  anal, (*Figs.* 67–70) 74–77
  branchial, (*Fig.* 151) 177–179
  extrasphincteric, causes of, 76
  from bowel, 68
  of lactiferous duct, 170
  tracheo-oesophageal, 1, (*Fig.* 1) 2
Fits, uncinate, associated with pituitary tumours, 339
Flaps, free, 248

Flat bones, blood supply of, 415
Flat foot, 544–545
Flexor carpi radialis, 242
  motor loss of, 385
Flexor carpi ulnaris, 242, (*Fig.* 369) 460
  tendon of, 420
Flexor digitorum longus, sheath of, (*Fig.* 447) 536
Flexor digitorum profundus tendon, (*Fig.* 378) 469
Flexor digitorum sublimis, 455
Flexor digitorum superficialis, 469
Flexor hallucis brevis, sesamoid bones in, 420
Flexor hallucis longus, sheath of, (*Fig.* 447) 536
Flexor pollicis brevis, 392
Flexor profundus, 470
Flexor retinaculum, (*Fig.* 394) 482–484, 534
Fontanelles, (*Fig.* 318) 401–402
Foot (feet)
  accessory navicular in, (*Fig.* 338) 421
  affected by Raynaud's disease, 218–219
  affected by root compression, 559
  arches of, 538–539
  congenital deformities of, 543
  excessive sweating of, 219
  flat, 544–545
  movements of, 538
  muscles of, 392, 542
  pain in, 547
  sole of, 538
Foot-drop
  associated with injury to common peroneal nerve, 394
  associated with injury to sciatic nerve, 392
Foramen(ina)
  caecum, 199, (*Fig.* 163) 200, 342
  incisive, (*Fig.* 147) 172–173
  intervertebral, (*Fig.* 457) 548, 558, 562
  lacerum, veins of, 332
  magnum, 341, 351, 553
  of Langer, 163
  of Luschka, 344
  of Magendie, 344
  of Monro, closed by pituitary tumour, 339
  of Morgagni, hernia through, 157

Foramen(ina), of Winslow, 101
  ovale, 275, 279, 280, 332, 357
  rotundum, 357
  transversarium, 549
  Vesalii, veins of, 332
Forearm
  amputation of, 432
  compartmental syndrome affecting, 238
  fistulae in, 250
  movements of, 454–456
  muscles of, affected by injury, 456
  sensory loss in, 385
  tingling in, 384
Forearm space, (*Fig.* 399) 488
Forefoot, pain in, 547
Foregut
  incomplete division of, tracheo-oesophageal fistula associated with, 1
  rotation of, 22, 23
Forehead, innervation of, 357
Forequarter amputation, 433
Fossa(e)
  duodenal, (*Figs.* 25–28) 33–35
  ileocolic, (*Fig.* 36) 44
  iliac, attachment of small intestine to, 36
  in relation to caecum, (*Fig.* 36) 44–45
  intersigmoidea, relation of ureter to, (*Fig.* 233) 301
  ischiorectal, (*Figs.* 65–66) 71–74
  navicularis, 324
  ovalis, 129, 255, 278
Fractures (*see under structures involved*)
Free flaps, 248
Fröhlich's syndrome, 333
Froin's syndrome, 346–347
Froment's sign, 470
Frontal bone, 401
Frontalis muscle, 329, 401
Frontal lobe
  anosmia due to tumour of, 352
  mental dullness due to pressure on, 339
Frontal sinus
  at birth, 403
  veins of, 332
Frontonasal process, (*Fig.* 145) 172
Frozen shoulder, 446
Fundic gland
  area, 13
  mucosa, 21

Fundus, (*Fig.* 8) 12
Funicular inguinal hernia, (*Fig.* 114) 127
Furuncle, 490
Fused kidney, unilateral, (*Fig.* 231) 299
Fusion (*see also* Arthrodesis)
  of elbow, 459
  of hip, (*Fig.* 425) 512

Gag reflex, 369
Galea aponeurotica, 328, 329, 332
Gallaudet's fascia, 115
Gallbladder, (*Figs.* 86–88) 94–99
  absence of, 95
  anatomy of, (*Fig.* 86) 94–95
  cystic artery in relation to, 92
  development of, 78, (*Fig.* 87) 95–96
  ducts from liver to, 90
  Kocher's incision for approach to, 97
  lymphatics of, 96
  mucus glands of, 96
  removal of, 97
  structure of, 96
  veins of, 96
Gall stones, entering common bile duct, 91
Ganglion(ia), 210–224
  block, sympathetic, (*Figs.* 175–176) 222–224
  cells, myenteric, 7
  congenital absence of, 71
  Gasserian, 357, (*Fig.* 284) 360
  hypogastric, 319
  impar, 210
  Langley's, (*Fig.* 286) 362
  nodosum, (*Fig.* 244) 313
Ganglionectomy, 219
Gangrene, 225, 226
  of gut, 52
  of midgut, 228
  transmetatarsal amputation due to, 430
Gasserian ganglion, 357, (*Fig.* 284) 360
Gastrectomy
  transverse colon in, 45
  vein ligature in, 86
Gastric artery, (*Fig.* 9) 14
  ligature of, 86
  passage through diaphragm, 156
  right, 85
Gastric nodes, 10, (*Fig.* 12) 17

Gastric vein, 16
Gastrocnemius muscle, relation to popliteal artery, 245
  flap, 248
Gastrocolic ligament, 18, 113
Gastrocolic omentum, 113
Gastroduodenal artery, 14–15, 85, 94
  bleeding due to erosion of, 32
Gastro-epiploic artery, (*Fig.* 10) 14–15
Gastrohepatic omentum, portal vein in, 82
Gastrojejunostomy, 20
Gastrolienal ligament, (*Fig.* 13) 18
Gastro-oesophageal junction, displaced into chest, 159
Gastro-oesophageal reflux, 160–161
Gastro-oesophageal sphincter, 160
Gastrosplenic ligament, (*Fig.* 13) 18, 100, 110
Geniculate body, lateral, 353
Geniculate ganglion, 362
Genioglossus muscle, 181
  lymph vessels associated with, 196
Geniohyoid muscle, 181
  nerve supply to, 374
Genital ridge, 119
Genital tubercle, (*Fig.* 258) 326
Genitalia
  external, in male, (*Fig.* 258) 326
  plexus supplying, 216
Genitofemoral nerve, 74, 215, 221
  ureter crossing, 300
Genu valgum, 522
  causing flat foot, 544
Genu varum, 522
Giant-cell tumour, benign, (*Fig.* 340) 424
Gibbus, 565
Gigli saw, 431
Gimbernat ligament, 134
Gingivae, innervation of, 357
Giraldès, organ of, (*Fig.* 112) 123
Girdlestone operation, 511
Glans penis, 324
  at birth, 407
  formation of, 326
Glenohumeral joint, (*Fig.* 346) 433, (*Figs.* 347–351) 434–440
  capsule, 435
  ligaments of, 435
  movement of, (*Fig.* 348) 437
  muscles of, 435

Glenohumeral joint, nerve supply to, 436
Glenoid fossa, 187, 435, 439
Glenoid labrum, 435, 448
Glomerular capsule, (*Fig.* 229) 297
Glomerulus, (*Fig.* 229) 297
Glomus intravagale, 311
Glomus jugulare, (*Fig.* 244) 311
Glomus tympanicum, 311
Glossopharyngeal nerve, 176, 191, 212, 332, (*Fig.* 292) 369
  lesions of, 369
  neuralgia, 370
  taste sensation via, 362
Gluteal artery, supplying head of femur, 505
Gluteus maximus, 72
  bursae under, (*Fig.* 418) 505
  flap, 248
Gonadal veins, collateral circulation through, 266
Gonadotrophins, controlling testis descent, 119
Goose's foot, 367
Gracilis flap, 248
Graft(ing)
  bypass, for arterial occlusion, 234
  femoropopliteal, 245
  nerve, 376
  vein, 256
Grassi, nerve of, 20, 21
Graves' disease, 360
Greater occipital nerve, (*Fig.* 261) 332
Greater omentum
  accessory pancreatic tissue in, 104
  attachment to transverse colon, 45
Great lymph ducts, (*Figs.* 208–211) 268–272
Great lymph trunks, termination of, (*Fig.* 210) 271
Great radicular artery, (*Fig.* 278) 348
Great vessels, (*Figs.* 218–219) 285–289
  embryology of, (*Fig.* 218) 285–286
Groin, (*Figs.* 111–123) 118–137
  hernia repair, 126, (*Figs.* 121–122) 132–135
  swelling in, 256
Guanethidine, in peripheral sympathetic block, 222
Gubernaculum testis, 119
Gums, lymphatic drainage of, 194

Gut
  cancer of, resection for, (*Figs.* 47–54) 56–61
  deficient fixation of, 30
  ischaemia of, 52
  rotation of, (*Figs.* 17–22) 22–30

Haematoma
  of anus, 67
  of posterior fossa, 363
  subdural, 342
Haemodialysis, 248
Haemolytic anaemia, 107
Haemopoietic cells, 78
Haemoptysis, from enlarged bronchial vessels, 146
Haemorrhage
  into oesophagus, 83
  intracranial, 356
Haemorrhoidal nerve, (*Fig.* 66) 73
Haemorrhoidectomy, sphincter muscle in, 64
Haemorrhoids, (*Figs.* 60–61) 66–68, 84
  external, 67–68
  false external, 67–68
  formation near dentate line, 63
  formed from anal cushions, 62
  internal, 66–67
  strangulation of, (*Fig.* 61) 67
Hair follicles, absence on foot, 538
Haller, organ of, (*Fig.* 112) 123
Hallux valgus, 430, 543, (*Fig.* 454) 545–546
Hamate bone, (*Fig.* 369) 460
Hamstrings, affected by injury to sciatic nerve, 392
Hamulus, pterygoid, 182
Hand, (*Figs.* 376–411) 466–498
  affected by prolapsed cervical disc, 560
  amputations of, (*Figs.* 408–411) 496–498
  anomalous blood supply to muscles of, 392
  blood supply of tendons, (*Fig.* 389) 478
  creases of, (*Fig.* 400) 489–490
  digital joints, (*Figs.* 390–393) 479–481
  dorsal spaces of, (*Fig.* 396) 488–489
  excessive sweating of, 219
  fascial spaces of, (*Figs.* 396–399) 485–489

Hand, incisions in, (*Figs.* 405–407) 494–496
  infections of, (*Figs.* 401–404) 490–493
  interossei of, (*Figs.* 382–386) 471–475
  ligaments, (*Figs.* 376–377) 466–469
  midpalmar space of, (*Figs.* 396–398) 485–486
  muscles of, (*Figs.* 378–386) 469–475
  nerve supply of, 387
  numbness of, 384, 388
  position of arthrodesis, (*Fig.* 393) 481
  position of immobilization, (*Fig.* 392) 481
  Raynaud's disease affecting, 218–219
  skin, 466
  tendon sheaths, fibrous, 477–478
  tingling in, 384
Hard palate (*see* Palate)
Hare-lip, (*Fig.* 149) 173–174
Hartmann's pouch, 95
Head
  collateral system to, 230
  detection of movement of, 369
  infant's, 401
  injuries, causing anosmia, 352
  lymph tissue of, (*Figs.* 157–161) 189–198
  lymph trunks from, 270
  movement of, 553
  sympathetic nerve supply to, 213
Headaches, occipital, 333
Heart (*see also* Cardiac...), (*Figs.* 212–217) 273–285
  conduction system, (*Fig.* 215) 277–278
  congenital abnormalities of, 277, 279–280
  coronary circulation, (*Figs.* 216–217) 280–284
  displacement of, 157, 289
  embryology of, (*Fig.* 212) 273–275
  failure of, 277, 288
  fibrous skeleton of, (*Fig.* 214) 276
  penetrating wound of, 284
  septation failure in, 279
Heel, pain in, 537
Heel pad, ulceration of, 431
Heller's cardiomyotomy, 8
Hemianopia
  bitemporal, 334, (*Fig.* 269) 338, 353
  homonymous, 354
  nasal, 353
  quadrantic, 354

Hemiarthroplasty, 512
Hemicolectomy, resulting in damage to ureter, 304
Hemiparesis, 356
Hemiplegia, following carotid artery ligation, 233
Hemivertebra, 550
Henle's loop, (*Fig.* 229) 297
Henry's incision, for exposure of humeral shaft, (*Figs.* 341–342) 425
Hepatic...(*see also* Liver)
Hepatic artery, 78, 85–86, (*Fig.* 85) 92–93
  accessory, 86
  interruption of, 86
  relation to duodenum, 31
Hepatic diverticulum, 78
Hepatic ducts, 88, 90
Hepatic flexure, resection for cancer of, (*Fig.* 48) 57
Hepatic injuries, Pringle's manoeuvre following, 97
Hepatic nodes, 10, (*Fig.* 12) 17
Hepatic resections, (*Fig.* 81) 87–88
Hepatic sinusoids, 78
Hepatic triad, 79
Hepatic tumour, route for treatment of, 83
Hepatic vein, (*Fig.* 80) 86–87
  injuries, 87
  ligation of, 87
  obstruction of, 83
Hepatocytes, 79
Hepatoduodenal ligament, 97
Hepatorenal pouch, 100, (*Fig.* 224) 290–293
Hernia
  abdominal, 113
  acquired diaphragmatic, (*Figs.* 136–137) 159–161
  acquired hiatal, (*Fig.* 136) 159–160
  Bochdalek's, 157
  congenital diaphragmatic, (*Fig.* 135) 157–159
  congenital oesophageal, (*Fig.* 135) 158
  diaphragmatic, 28
  femoral, (*Figs.* 117–120) 129–132, (*Fig.* 122) 133–135
  groin, repair of, 126, (*Figs.* 121–122) 132–135
  incisional, 44
  inguinal (*see* Inguinal hernia)

Hernia, Littre's, 40
  posterolateral, 157
  retrosternal, 157–158
  rolling, (Fig. 135) 158
  sliding, (Fig. 120) 132, (Fig. 136) 159–160
  traumatic, 159
  umbilical, 24
Hernial sac, congenital, 135
Hernioplasty, 133
Herniorrhaphy, 133
Herniotomy, 133
Hesselbach, triangle of, (Fig. 116) 128
Hiatus hernia
  acquired, (Fig. 136) 159–160
  secondary hypertrophy following, 14
Hibernating gland, 405
Hilar nodes, 10
Hill antireflux operation, 6
Hilton's law, 436, 462
Hindgut
  in development of bladder, (Fig. 245) 314
  in relation with entodermal cloaca, 68
  rotation of, 22, 23–24
Hindquarter amputation, 432
Hip, (Figs. 412–425) 498–513
  amputations involving, 512–513
  bursae around, (Figs. 418–419) 504–505
  capsule and ligaments of, (Figs. 415–416) 502
  congenital dislocation of, 501
  dislocation of, sciatic nerve affected by, 392
  fusion of, (Fig. 425) 512
  injury to, 513
  joint replacement of, 512
  nerve supply to, 506
  ossification of, (Fig. 326) 411
  surgery of, (Figs. 422–425) 507–513
  traumatic dislocations of, 501–502
  Thomas' test, 507
  Trendelenburg's test, (Fig. 421) 506
Hirschsprung's disease, 71
Homonymous hemianopia, 354
Hormones
  antidiuretic, 335
  changes, due to micro-adenomata, 339
  released from hypothalamus, 335
Horner's syndrome, 219, 222, 360, 385

Horseshoe abscess, 74
Horseshoe kidney, (Fig. 230) 298–299
Humero-ulnar joint, (Fig. 363) 454
Humerus
  measurement of, (Fig. 330) 416
  surgical approach to, (Fig. 341) 424–425
  ulnar nerve affected by fracture of, 389
  uniting of epiphyses, 411
Hump on back, 566
Hunchback, 565
Hunter's canal, 262
Hydatid of Morgagni, 123, (Fig. 248) 314
Hydrocele, (Fig. 123) 135
Hydrocephalus, 350
  pituitary tumour and, 339
  spina bifida and, 351
Hymen, meconium from vagina above, 68
Hyoglossus muscle, 184
  lymph trunks associated with, 196
Hyoid arch, 176
Hyoid bone, 176
  relation of thyroid gland to, (Fig. 162) 199
  swelling below, (Fig. 163) 199–200
Hypercalcaemia, 207
Hyperhidrosis, 219
Hyperplasia, of parathyroids, 207
Hypertension
  due to coarctation of aorta, 288
  portal, 83–85, 113
  produced by tumour, 312
  venous (see Venous hypertension)
Hyperthyroidism, tarsal muscle in, 360
Hypertrophic pyloric stenosis, 13–14
Hypogastric ganglia, 319
Hypogastric nerve, relation of ureter to, (Fig. 234) 302
Hypogastric plexus, (Fig. 172) 216–217, 218, 319
Hypoglossal canal, veins of, 332
Hypoglossal nerve, 212, (Fig. 286) 362, 374
  in radical neck dissection, 197
Hyponychium, (Fig. 402) 491
Hypoparathyroidism, postthyroidectomy, 207
Hypopharynx, 5
  nerve fibres to, 211
Hypophysectomy, (Fig. 270) 339–340
Hypophysial fossa in relation to cavernous sinus, (Fig. 281) 356

Hypophysis (*see also* Pituitary body)
  errors in development, 333
  optic chiasma in relation to, 352
Hypoplastic lateral femoral condyle, 524
Hypospadias, 326
Hypothalamus, 207
  arterial supply to, 334
  sympathetic fibres arising in, 355
Hysterectomy, 399–400
  damage to ureter caused by, 305

Ileocaecal fossa, (*Fig.* 36) 44
Ileocaecal intussusception, (*Fig.* 40) 46–47
Ileocaecal segment of gut, volvulus of, 30
Ileocaecal valve, 39, 46
Ileocolic artery, (*Fig.* 43) 52
Ileocolic fossa, (*Fig.* 36) 44
Ileocolic vein, 47
Ileum, (*Fig.* 29) 35–36
  blood supply to, 415
  fossae in relation to, (*Fig.* 36) 44–45
Iliac apophysis, 411
Iliac artery, (*Fig.* 178) 227
  internal, 228
  nerves along, 216
  supplying ureter, (*Fig.* 236) 303
Iliac bifurcation, 264
Iliac crest, in determining site for lumbar
    puncture, (*Fig.* 275) 346
Iliac fossa, attachment of small intestine
    to, 36
Iliac lymph nodes, 319
Iliac spine, (*Fig.* 417) 503
Iliac surgery, 243–244
Iliac vein, 49, 255
  congenital absence of valve in, 262
Ilio-coccygeus muscle, (*Fig.* 315) 396
Iliofemoral ligament, relation of subpsoas
    bursa to, (*Fig.* 419) 505
Iliofemoral ligament of hip joint, (*Fig.* 416)
    502
Iliofemoral muscles, 506
Iliohypogastric nerve
  in appendicectomy, 44
  kidney in relation to, 291
Ilio-inguinal nerve, 74
  in appendicectomy, 44
  kidney in relation to, 291

Iliopubic tract, 126
Iliotrochanteric muscles, 506
Impotence
  associated with aorto-iliac disease, 229
  following pelvic surgery, 218
Incisional hernia, 44, 113, 115
Incisions
  laparotomy, (*Figs.* 105–110) 114–118
  through abdominal wall, (*Figs.* 104–110)
    113–118
Incisive foramen, (*Fig.* 147) 172–173
Incisive nerve, 183
Incisor teeth
  in early development, 172
  innervation, 183
Incisura angularis, (*Fig.* 8) 12
Incongruous joint, 434
Incontinence, 397
  associated with ectopic ureteric orifice,
    304
  faecal, 77
  prevention of, 66
Incus, 176
Index finger, amputation of, (*Fig.* 408)
    496–497
Infant, anatomy of, (*Figs.* 318–321) 401–
    407
Infantile hydrocele, 135
Infantile inguinal hernia, (*Fig.* 114) 127
Inferior fascicle, (*Fig.* 215) 277
Inferior mesenteric artery, 22
Inferior mesenteric vein, (*Fig.* 74) 81
Inferior oesophageal sphincter, receptors
    in, 7
Inferior phrenic artery, 8
Inferior thyroid artery, 8
Inferior thyroid veins, 8
Inferior vena cava, 82, 275, (*Fig.* 215) 277
  anomalies of, (*Figs.* 206–207) 266
  blood diverted to, 85
  double, (*Fig.* 207) 266–267
  embryology of, (*Fig.* 204) 263–264
  entry of hepatic veins, 86–87
  opening into diaphragm, (*Fig.* 133) 155
Inferior vesical arteries, 319
Infertility, male, cause of, 137
Infiltrative ophthalmopathy, 360
Inflammatory retraction of nipple, (*Fig.*
    144) 169–170
Infraclavicular nodes, 166

Infrahyoid lymph nodes, 195
Infra-inguinal approach, for femoral
    hernia, 134–135
Inframastoid lymph nodes, 192
Infra-orbital canal, 181
Infra-orbital lymph node group, 194
Infra-orbital nerve, 187
    neurapraxia of, 186
Infrapatellar pad of fat, 524
Infrarenal radicular artery, (*Fig.* 278) 349
Infraspinatus muscle, (*Fig.* 347) 435
Infratemporal fossa, lymphatic drainage
    of, 194
Infundibular artery, 281
Infundibular recess, (*Fig.* 264) 335
Infundibulum, 279, 334, (*Fig.* 265) 336,
    (*Fig.* 268) 338
Inguinal canal, 44, 125–126
    formation, 119
    veins from labia majora through, 256
Inguinal hernia, 44, (*Fig.* 114) 126–127
    direct, (*Fig.* 116) 128–129
    distinguished from femoral hernia, 126
    incision for, (*Fig.* 121) 132–133
    interstitial, (*Fig.* 115) 127–128
    strangulated, 127
    types of, (*Fig.* 114) 127
Inguinal ligament, 124, 125, (*Fig.* 117) 129,
    132, 244
    sutured to Cooper's ligament, 135
    sutured to pectineal ligament, 134
Inguinal lymph nodes, drainage to, 63
Inguinal ring, abdominal, 119, 125
Inion, 342
Inner ear, 369
Innominate vein, at birth, 404
Inokuchi shunt, 85
Interbronchial lymph nodes, (*Fig.* 130)
    147–148
Intercondylar notch, 513
Intercostal arteries, (*Fig.* 277) 348
    enlarged, due to coarctation of aorta,
    288
Intercostal lymph node, 147
    draining to thoracic duct, 270
Intercostal muscle, detachment, 150
Intercostal nerve, 115
    block, 151–152
Intercostal respiration, 405

Intercostal space
    lymph nodes in, 147
    width, 137
Intercostal veins, (*Fig.* 468) 560
    as collaterals, 235
Interdigital ligament, 466
Interfascicular repair, 376
Interlobular septa, of liver, 79
Intermaxillary segment, 172
Intermesenteric plexus, 216
Internal arteriovenous fistulae, 250
Internal carotid artery, 190, 330, (*Fig.* 267)
    337, 353
    cavernous sinus in relation to, (*Fig.* 281)
    356
    formation of, 285
    optic chiasma in relation to, 353
    vagus nerve in relation to, (*Fig.* 293) 371
Internal iliac artery, 228, 319
Internal iliac lymph nodes, 319
Internal jugular vein, (*Fig.* 196) 253–254
    oesophagus in relation to, (*Fig.* 2) 3
Interosseous ligaments, 542
Interosseous nerve, (*Fig.* 395) 484
    posterior, compression of, 457
Interphalangeal creases, 489
Interphalangeal joint, collateral ligaments
    of, 479
Intersphincteric abscess, (*Fig.* 67) 74
Intersphincteric space, 65
Interspinous ligaments, 555
Intertracheobronchial lymph nodes, (*Fig.*
    130) 147–148
Intertransverse ligaments, 555
Intervalvar septum, (*Fig.* 214) 276, 279
Interventricular artery, posterior descend-
    ing, 281
Intervertebral disc(s), 547, (*Fig.* 457) 548,
    (*Fig.* 460) 551, (*Fig.* 463) 553–555
    ballooning of, (*Fig.* 465) 557
    degeneration of, 550–557
    lesions of, (*Figs.* 464–467) 556–560
    lumbar, protrusion of, (*Figs.* 466–467)
    558–559
    narrowing of canal, 561
Intervertebral foramina, (*Fig.* 457) 548,
    558, 562
Intestinal lymph trunk, 268
Intestine
    large (*see* Large bowel)
    lymph trunk collecting from, 268

Intestine, obstruction associated with Meckel's diverticulum, 39
small (*see* Small intestine)
Intracranial pressure, 347, 402
raised, 356
Intracranial venous drainage, 234
Intracuticular abscess, 490
Intraorbital nerve, (*Fig.* 155) 186
Intraparotid lymph nodes, 188
Intravenous infusions, 249
Intussusception, ileocaecal, (*Fig.* 40) 46–47
Iris
dilator muscle of, 355
radial muscle of, 355
Ischaemia, 225
associated with abdominal incisions, 114
following lumbar sympathectomy, 222
of abdominal viscera, 226
of arm, 231
of gut, 52
of leg muscles, 238
of lesser curvature, 16
of nerve roots, 561
of spinal cord, 349
relieved by profundoplasty, 229
Ischial spine, relation of pudendal nerve to, (*Fig.* 66) 73–74
Ischio-coccygeus muscle, (*Fig.* 315) 396
Ischiorectal fossa, (*Figs.* 65–66) 71–74
abscess in, (*Fig.* 68) 75
anal canal in relation to, 61
supporting rectum, 51
Ischium, relation of levatores ani to, 65
Islet cells, in accessory pancreatic tissue, 104
Isthmal coarctation of aorta, (*Fig.* 219) 288
Isthmus, stress fracture of vertebral arch in region of, 563
Ivalon sponge, 52
Ivory osteoma, 422

Jackson's membrane, (*Fig.* 38) 46
Jaundice
associated with choledochal cysts, 92
associated with hepatic duct anomaly, 91

Jaw
accessory ligaments of, 188
dislocation of, 188–189
edentulous, (*Fig.* 161) 197–198
in early facial development, 172
opening of, 188
sensory nerve supply to, (*Figs.* 153–155) 182–187
spread of cancer to, 197
Jejunum, (*Fig.* 29) 35–36
Joint(s) (*see also individual joints*)
contracture of, affecting amputation, 429
disease of, 436
Jugular bulb, 212
carotid body on, 311
Jugular lymph trunk, 148, 196
draining to thoracic duct, 270
termination of, (*Fig.* 210) 271
Jugular vein, 202, (*Fig.* 165) 203, (*Fig.* 262) 331
anterior, (*Fig.* 196) 253, (*Fig.* 262) 331
cannulation of, (*Fig.* 197) 254
cephalic vein connected to, 250
collateral flow after ligation of, 234
compression of, 347
drainage from sinuses into, 342
great lymph trunks in relation to, (*Fig.* 210) 271
internal, 198, (*Fig.* 196) 253–254
jugular lymph trunk entering, 196
lymph nodes associated with, 194, 195
oesophagus in relation to, (*Fig.* 2) 3
relation of great lymph trunks to, (*Fig.* 210) 271
subclavian vein connecting to, 252
used as shunt, 350
Jugulodiagastric lymph node, 195
Jugulo-omohyoid lymph node, 195–196
Juxtaductal coarctation of aorta, 288

Keratitis, neurotrophic, 358
Kidney(s) (*see also* Renal...), (*Figs.* 220–231) 289–300
at birth, 406
blood supply to, (*Fig.* 227) 295–296
ectopic, (*Fig.* 231) 300
horseshoe, (*Fig.* 230) 298–299

Kidney(s), incisions to expose, (*Figs.* 238–240) 306–307
  lymphatics of, 296–297
  nerve supply to, 296
  polycystic, 298
  relations, (*Figs.* 220–226) 290–294
  segments of, (*Fig.* 227) 295
  stones, 295
  transplantation, 295
  unilateral fused, (*Fig.* 231) 299
Klippel–Feil syndrome, 447
Klumpke's paralysis, 385, 392
Knee (*see also* Knee joint)
  alignment, (*Fig.* 435) 522
  articular anastomosis around, 230
  defect, covered by myocutaneous flap, 248
  deformities, (*Fig.* 435) 522
  knock, 522
  perforating veins of, 262
  veins around, 255
Knee joint (*see also* Knee), (*Figs.* 426–440) 513–530
  affected by surgical approach to femur, 427
  amputation through, 530
  aspiration of, (*Figs.* 439–440) 526–527
  bursae around, (*Figs.* 437–438) 524–526
  dislocation of, 526
  ligaments of, (*Figs.* 428–433) 515–520
  locking of, 513, 521
  menisci, (*Fig.* 434) 520–522
  movements at, (*Figs.* 426–427) 513–515
  pain in, 524
  Q angle, (*Fig.* 436) 523
  semilunar cartilages of, (*Fig.* 434) 520–522
  stability of, (*Figs.* 432–433) 519–520
  surgical approaches to, 530
  valgus angle of, (*Fig.* 435) 522
Koch, triangle of, 277
Kocher's incision, (*Fig.* 88) 97–98
Kocher's manipulation, 448
Kocher's method, for exposure of elbow joint, (*Fig.* 367) 458
Kugel's artery, 284
Kuntz, nerve of, (*Fig.* 171) 214
Kupffer cells, 78, (*Fig.* 71) 79
Kyphos, 565

Kyphosis, 556

Labia
  branch of perineal nerve, 73
  minor salivary glands, innervation of, 183
  majora, anaesthesia of, 74
  majora, veins from, 256
  mucosa, blood supply to, 181
  mucosa, innervation of, (*Fig.* 155) 186
  swelling of, 256
Labioscrotal folds, overfusion of, 68
Labioscrotal swellings, (*Fig.* 258) 326
Labour, obstructed by 5th lumbar vertebra, 563
Labrum, glenoid, 435, 448
Labyrinthine artery, 364
Lachman test, 519
Lacrimal gland, 360, 361, (*Fig.* 291) 368
Lacrimation, 368
Lactiferous duct fistula, 170
Lacunae of Luschka, (*Fig.* 249) 316
Lacunar ligament, 130
Ladd's bands, 37
Lamellae, 408
Laminal arch, 547
  joints and ligaments uniting, 555–556
Langenbeck's method, for exposure of elbow joint, (*Fig.* 368) 459
Langer, foramen of, 163
Langley's ganglion, (*Fig.* 286) 362
Laparotomy, 87
  incisions, (*Figs.* 105–110) 114–118
Large bowel (*see also* Colon), (*Figs.* 37–54) 45–61
  blood supply to, (*Figs.* 43–45) 52–55
  lymph drainage of, (*Figs.* 46–54) 54–61
  muscles of, 41
Laryngeal nerves, 202, (*Figs.* 166–167) 203–205, 372
  damage to, affecting voice, 373
  oesophagus in relation to, (*Fig.* 2) 3
  recurrent, in relation to branchial arches, (*Fig.* 218) 286
Laryngitis, in infants, 404
Laryngopharyngeal nerve, 213
Laryngotracheal diverticulum, 1
Laryngotracheal tube, 1

Larynx
  at birth, 404
  cancer of, 195
  innervation of, 372, 373
  intrinsic muscles of, 177
  lymphatic drainage of, 195
  nerve fibres to, 211
Lasegue's test, 559
Lata, fascia of, 124
Latarjet, nerve of, (*Fig.* 14) 19
Lateral collateral ligament, (*Fig.* 443) 531
Lateral geniculate body, 353
Lateral ligament of rectum, 51
Lateral oesophageal nodes, (*Fig.* 7) 10
Lateral rectus muscle, motor nerve to, 363
Lateral sinus, 342
Lateral sympathetic chain, 319
Latissimus dorsi, 150
  flap, 248
Lax tissue, separating tonsil capsule, 192
Leg
  muscle compartments of, (*Fig.* 184) 237–238
  muscles, affected by injury to sciatic nerve, 392
  pain in, 238
  paralysis of, 238
  sensory loss in, 559
  sympathetic denervation, 221
  venous system of, (*Figs.* 198–203) 254–263
Leontiasis, 422
Lesser occipital nerve (*see* Occipital nerve)
Leugart's ledge, 8
Leugart's pouch, 8
Levator ani, 48, (*Fig.* 52) 60, 63, (*Fig.* 59) 65
  attachment of anal canal, 61
  extension of abscess through, (*Fig.* 68) 75
  forming pelvic diaphragm, 396
  nerve supply to, 65
  relations in female peritoneum, (*Fig.* 250) 317
  supporting rectum, 51
Levator palati muscle, 177, 182
Levator palpebrae superioris, 355, 360
Levator prostatae, 322
Levator scapulae, (*Fig.* 351) 440
  paralysis of, 384

Lienorenal ligament, (*Fig.* 13) 18, 100, 109
  relation to pancreas, 104
Ligament(s) (*see also* Ligamentum...)
  attachment to bones, 408
  Cooper's, 126, 130, 134, (*Fig.* 139) 164, (*Fig.* 144) 170
  cruciate, (*Figs.* 431–433) 517–520
  Gimbernat, 134
  glenohumeral, 435
  inguinal, 125
  lacunar, 130
  median arcuate, 6
  of ankle joint, (*Figs.* 441–442)
  of malleus, 176
  of rectum, 50
  of spleen, (*Fig.* 101) 109–110
  of Treitz, 33
  pectineal, 134
  phreno-oesophageal, (*Fig.* 135) 158, (*Fig.* 137) 160-161
  Poupart's, 126
  sphenomandibular, 176, 183, 188
  stylohyoid, 176
  stylomandibular, 188
  temperomandibular, 187
  Thompson's, 126
  thyrothymic, 205
  umbilical, 129
Ligamentum...(*see also* Ligaments)
Ligamentum arteriosum, rupture of aorta in region of, 289
Ligamentum denticulum, (*Fig.* 272) 343, 373
Ligamentum flavum, 555, 557
Ligamentum nuchae, 439, 555
Ligamentum patellae, 524
Ligamentum teres, 80, 82
Ligamentum venosum, 80, 82
Light reflex, consensual, 353
Limb(s) (*see also* Arm; Leg)
  artificial, 433
  long bones of, *see* Long bones
  measurement of, (*Figs.* 330–337) 416–420
  upper, sympathetic denervation of, 219–220
Linea alba, 115
Linea aspera, 427
Linea splendens, 343
Lingual lymph nodes, 196

Lingual mucosa, innervation of, (*Fig.* 153) 183–184

Lingual nerve, (*Fig.* 153) 183, 366
  injection of, (*Fig.* 154) 185
  submandibular ganglion suspended from, (*Fig.* 286) 362
  swelling of axons of, 363

Lingual plate, 184

Lingual tonsil, (*Fig.* 157) 189

Lingual vein, (*Fig.* 196) 253

Lingula, 183

Lingular artery, 145

Lip(s)
  cancer of, 196
  formation of, (*Fig.* 148) 172
  lower, sensory innervation of, 183, 184
  lymphatic drainage of, 194, 196
  median cleft of, 174
  philtrum of, 172
  upper, sensory innervation of, 357

Lipoma, accessory breast tissue confused with, 163

Little finger, amputation of, (*Fig.* 411) 499

Littre's hernia, 40

Liver (*see also* Hepatic...) (*Figs.* 71–81) 78–88
  adhesion to transverse colon, (*Fig.* 91) 101
  arteries of, in relation to bile ducts, (*Fig.* 85) 92–93
  at birth, 406
  blood supply to, (*Figs.* 74–81) 81–87, 105
  development of, affecting rotation of gut, 24
  ducts to gallbladder from, 90
  embryology, 78
  formation of, 32, 37
  histology, (*Fig.* 71) 78–79
  Kocher's incision for approach to, 97
  lobes and segments, (*Figs.* 72–73) 80–81
  lobule, 79
  lymphatic drainage from, 79, 268
  needle biopsy of, 98
  portal hypertension (*see* Portal hypertension)
  portal vein, *see* Portal vein
  relation of kidney to, 292
  resections, 87–88
  spaces around, 100

Liver, transplantation, bile duct affected by, 93

Lobular veins, 206

Local anaesthetic
  injected into epidural space, 342
  technique, for operations on upper teeth, 186

Loculation syndrome, 346–347

Long bones, 411
  after growth is complete, 409
  blood supply to, (*Fig.* 327) 413
  measurement of, (*Figs.* 330–337) 416–420
  surgical approach to, (*Figs.* 341–343) 424–428

Longitudinal ligaments of spine, (*Fig.* 461) 551
  infolding of, 557
  irritation of, 558
  sensory nerve fibres in, 554

Longitudinal sinus, 332

Long plantar ligament, (*Fig.* 451) 541

Long saphenous vein, (*Figs.* 198–199) 255–256

Longus colli muscle, 211, 241

Loop colostomy, 53

Loop inversion of testis, (*Fig.* 111) 122

Lordosis, 553
  lumbar, 507, 562

Lotheissen operation, 133

Louis, angle of, 137

Lower limb amputations, (*Figs.* 344–345) 430–432

Lower oesophageal sphincter, 3

Lumbago, 558

Lumbar curve, of spinal column, 547

Lumbar disc protrusion, (*Figs.* 466–467) 558–559

Lumbar ganglia, 215, 221
  block, 223

Lumbar lordosis, 553, 562

Lumbar lymph nodes, draining to thoracic duct, 270

Lumbar lymph trunk, 268

Lumbar nerve, (*Fig.* 272) 343

Lumbar puncture, (*Figs.* 274–275) 345–346

Lumbar scoliosis, 562

Lumbar spine
  nerves, 216
  stenosis in, (*Fig.* 469) 561

598 INDEX

Lumbar sympathectomy, (*Fig.* 174) 221–222, 229

Lumbar sympathetic trunk, 214, 215–216

Lumbar vertebrae, 549, 563
  sacralization of transverse process of, (*Fig.* 470) 562

Lumbocostal arch
  directing flow of tuberculous pus, (*Fig.* 473) 565
  relation of kidney to, 291

Lumbosacral pedicles, defective, 563

Lumbricals, (*Fig.* 381) 470–475, 480
  sheaths, 486

Lunate bone, (*Fig.* 369) 460

Lungs (*see also* Pulmonary...) (*Figs.* 125–128) 138–144
  abscess, following aspiration, 139
  accessory lobes of, 141–142
  bronchial vessels, 145
  bronchopulmonary circulation, 145–146
  cancer, lymphatic spread of, 149
  collapse, due to lymph accumulation, 271
  compressed by diaphragmatic hernia, 157
  drainage of, (*Fig.* 130) 146–148
  fissures of, 138–139
  hilum, calcified nodes near, 141
  left, 143
  lobes of, (*Fig.* 125) 139–143
  lymphatic drainage from, 148
  oesophagus in relation to, 3
  right, (*Fig.* 125) 139–142
  segments of, (*Fig.* 125) 139
  tuberculosis of, 140
  venous system, 145

Lunula, (*Fig.* 402) 491

Luschka
  joints of, (*Fig.* 462) 551–552
  lacunae of, (*Fig.* 249) 316

Luxatio-erecta dislocation, 448

Lymph (*see also* Lymphatic drainage)
  accumulation in chest, 271
  plexus of Sappey, 167
  route from breast into chest, (*Fig.* 143) 169
  tissue, of head and neck, (*Figs.* 157–161) 189–198

Lymph nodes (*see also under structures involved*)
  axillary, (*Fig.* 140) 165–166
  calcified, 141
  diseased, near oesophagus, 8
  interbronchial, (*Fig.* 130) 147–148
  intercostal (*see* Intercostal lymph nodes)
  intertracheobronchial, (*Fig.* 130) 147–148
  intraparotid, 188
  jugulodigastric, 195
  lumbar, 270

Lymphadenitis, 141

Lymphatic drainage (*see also* Lymph)
  from dentate line, 63
  of bladder, 319
  of breast, (*Figs.* 141–143) 167–169
  of gallbladder, 96
  of kidney, 296–297
  of large intestine, (*Figs.* 46–54) 54–61
  of liver, 79
  of lungs, 148
  of oesophagus, 9–10
  of pancreas, 106
  of rectum, (*Fig.* 52) 60
  of scalp, 193–194, 333
  of stomach, (*Fig.* 12) 16–17, 268

Lymphatic ring, Waldeyer's, (*Fig.* 157) 189, 192–193

Lymphatic spread of lung cancer, 149

Lymphatic spread of malignant tumours from lower rectum, 63

Lymphatic tissue of neck, removal of, (*Fig.* 161) 197–198

Lymphatic watersheds of skin, (*Fig.* 211) 272

McEvedy operation, (*Fig.* 122) 133–134

Mackenrodt's ligament, (*Fig.* 314) 395, 400

Macrostomia, 174

Macula lutea, 355

Male infertility, varicocele causing, 137

Malignant tumours (*see also under Tumours*)
  importance of dentate line for spread of, 63

Malleus, 176
  ligament of, 176

Mammary... (*see also* Breast)

Mammary artery, 229
Mammary cancer
  spread of, 167
  surgical excision of, 171
Mammary nodes, 146–147, 167, 206
Mammary vessels, ligation of, 137
Mammillary body, (*Fig.* 264) 335
Mandible, (*Figs.* 153–156) 181–189, 407
  at birth, 404
  avascular necrosis of bone, 181
  blood supply, 181, 415
  fracture of, 184
  injection of, 184
  lymph nodes of, 194, 196
  ossification of, 410
  osteomyelitis of, 184
  removal in cancer of mouth, 197
  resection of, (*Fig.* 161) 197–198
  sensory innervation of, (*Fig.* 153) 182–183
Mandibular arch, 176
Mandibular branch of facial nerve, 367
Mandibular canal, 183
  spread of cancer to, 197
Mandibular foramen, 183
Mandibular nerve, 176, 182, 357, 369
Mandibular process, (*Figs.* 145–146) 172
  microstomia involving, 174
Manubrium, 137
  lymph nodes behind, 168
  thymus gland behind, 205
Marginal artery, (*Fig.* 43) 52, 53 (*Fig.* 178) 227
Marshall, oblique vein of, 274
Masseter, lymph nodes in front of, 194
Mastectomy, 171
Mastication, muscles of, 176
Mastoid air cells, (*Fig.* 319) 402
Mastoid lymph nodes, scalp drainage, 333
Mastoid process, (*Figs.* 319–320), 188
  lymph nodes beneath, 192
Mastoid vein, 332
Maxilla, (*Figs.* 153–156) 181–189
  blood supply to, 181–182
  innervation of, (*Fig.* 155) 186, 357
  orthognathic surgery to, 186
Maxillary antrum, (*Fig.* 284) 360
  at birth, 404
Maxillary artery, 181, 188
  formation of, 285

Maxillary nerve, 359
  cavernous sinus in relation to, (*Fig.* 281) 357
  supplying upper jaw, (*Fig.* 155) 185–187
Maxillary osteotomy, 186
  for correction of facial deformities, 182
Maxillary process, (*Figs.* 145–146) 172
  microstomia involving, 174
Maxillary teeth, blood supply to, 181
Maxillary vein, (*Fig.* 262) 331
Mayo, vein of, 13, 19, 21
Mayo–Robson incision, (*Fig.* 109) 116
Meckel's cave, 357
Meckel's diverticulum, (*Fig.* 33) 39–40
  accessory pancreatic tissue in, 104
Meckel's ganglion, (*Fig.* 284) 360
Meconium, 68
Medial collateral ligament, (*Fig.* 442) 530
Medial longitudinal arch, in flat foot, 544
Medial popliteal nerve, injury to, 393–394
Median arcuate ligament, 6, 226
Median cubital vein, (*Fig.* 191) 249
Median nerve, 425, 426
  axillary artery in relation to, (*Fig.* 301) 382
  compression of, 457
  injury to, (*Fig.* 307) 386–388
  paralysis of, 385
  supplying hand muscles, 473
  supplying wrist, 462
Median sternotomy, 150, 239
Mediastinal lymph nodes, 10, 147, 206
  connections to thoracic duct, 270
Mediastinal tumour, 2
Mediastinoscopy, cervical, 149
Mediastinotomy, 207
Mediastinum, (*Figs.* 124–131) 137–152
Medulla oblongata, (*Fig.* 273) 345
Medullary bone of mandible, blood supply to, 181
Medullation of autonomic nerve fibres, 208
Megacolon, congenital aganglionic, 71
Membrana tectoria, 553
Membrane bones, 407
  pathology of, 422
Membranous urethra, 324
  relation of ureter to, (*Fig.* 235) 302
  ruptured, 325
Membranous ventricular septum, (*Fig.* 215) 277

Meningeal veins, 332
Meninges, (*Figs.* 271–272) 340–344
Meningitis, 333
 tuberculous, anosmia due to, 352
Meningocele, (*Fig.* 279) 351
 traumatic, 384
Meningomyelocele (*see also* Spina bifida), (*Fig.* 279) 351
Meniscectomy, 522
Menisci, of knee joint, 513, 514, (*Fig.* 429) 516, (*Fig.* 434) 520–522
 tears, 517
Menopause, 398
Mental dullness, due to pressure on frontal lobes, 339
Mental foramen, 183, 197
Mental nerve, (*Fig.* 153) 183
Mentalis muscles, 181
Mesenteric artery, 22, (*Fig.* 43) 52–53, (*Fig.* 178) 227
 hepatic artery in relation to, 93
 inferior, damage to ureter following ligation of, 304
 oesophagus in relation to, (*Fig.* 5) 6
Mesenteric collaterals, (*Fig.* 178) 226–228
Mesenteric vein, (*Fig.* 74) 81
Mesentericoparietal fossa of Waldeyer, (*Fig.* 28) 34–35
Mesentery
 dorsal, 153
 of large gut, (*Figs.* 37–40) 45–47
 to ascending colon, (*Figs.* 39–40) 46–47
Mesoappendix, (*Fig.* 36) 44
Mesocolon
 pelvic, 46
 transverse, (*Fig.* 37) 45
Mesojejunum, fossa of Waldeyer situated in, 34
Mesomesenteric artery, 228
Mesonephric duct, (*Fig.* 229) 297, (*Fig.* 245) 314
Mesonephros, development of testis in relation to, 119
Mesoneurium, (*Fig.* 295) 375
Metacarpal ligament, deep transverse, 468
Metacarpals
 sensory loss over, 386
 tuberculosis of, 423
Metacarpophalangeal creases, 489

Metacarpophalangeal joint, (*Fig.* 384) 472
 collateral ligaments of, (*Fig.* 390) 479
 dislocation of, (*Fig.* 391) 480
Metanephric cap, (*Fig.* 229) 297
Metanephric diverticulum, 297
Metaphysial osteomyelitis, 435
Metaphysial vessels, 414
Metaphysis, 408
 osteomyelitis affecting, 423
Metastatic carcinoma of bone, (*Fig.* 340) 424
Metastatic tumours, causing portal hypertension, 83
Metatarsals
 binding together, 542
 first, deformity of, 543
 making up foot arch, 539
 sesamoid bones associated with, 420
Metatarsus adductus and varus, congenital, 543
Metatarsus primus varus, 543
Metopic suture, 410
Micro-adenomata, hormonal changes due to, 339
Microstomia, 174
Micturition
 difficulty due to narrowing of canal, 561
 muscle control of, 318
Midcarpal joint, (*Fig.* 369) 460
Midcolic veins, 47
Middle ear, 365, 369
 infection of, 403
 tympanic cavity of, 179
Middle finger, amputation of, (*Figs.* 409–410) 497
Midgut
 gangrene of, 228
 loop, malrotation of, 159
 rotation of, 22, 24
Midpalmar space of hand, (*Figs.* 396–398) 485–486
Midtarsal joint, 538
Migraine, basilar, 355
Milk ducts, (*Fig.* 144) 170
Milk ridge, (*Fig.* 138) 162
Miosis, 385
Mitral annulus, (*Fig.* 214) 276
 affected by rheumatic heart disease, 277
Mitral atresia, 280
Mitral valve, (*Fig.* 214) 276, 279
 development of, 274

Moderator band, (*Fig.* 215) 277
Molar teeth, 188
  at birth, 404
  innervation of, 183
  mandibular, 182
  maxillary, blood supply to, 181
  removal of impacted, 184
Mönckeberg's sclerosis, 277
Mondor's disease, 165
Morgagni
  foramina of, hernia through, 157
  hydatid of, 123
Morison's pouch, 100, (*Fig.* 224) 290–293
Morton's metatarsalgia, 547
Mouth
  asymmetry of, 367
  cancer of, 197
  impairment to opening of, 187
  innervation of, (*Fig.* 153) 183, 357, 362
  lymphatic drainage of, 194
  macrostomia, 174
Mucoperiosteum, 197
Mucus glands, of gallbladder, 96
Müllerian duct, 123
Multiple exotoses, 422
Muscles (*see also individual muscles*)
  close to kidneys, 291
  flat, incisions involving, 118
  in amputation, 429
  involved in abdominal incisions, 113
  ischaemic pain in, 225
  leg, veins associated with, (*Fig.* 202) 259–260
  of anal canal, 63
  of anus, (*Fig.* 55) 62, 65–66
  of bile duct, 89
  of bladder, 318–319
  of diaphragm, 153–155, 159
  of facial expression, 176
  of foot, 392, 542
  of forearm, affected by injury, 456
  of glenohumeral joint, 435
  of large intestine, 41
  of mastication, 176, 181
  of oesophagus, 7, 8
  of palate, 174
  of pyloric sphincter, 13
  of rectum, (*Fig.* 55), 62
  of scrotum, 124
  of toes, in pes cavus, 545

Muscles, of urogenital diaphragm, nerve supply to, 73
  of ventricle, 279
  spasm, 436
  tone, poor, causing flat foot, 544
Muscular compartments, (*Fig.* 184) 237–238
Musculi pectinati, 278
Musculocutaneous nerve, 385
Myasthenia gravis, 206
Myelin sheath, (*Fig.* 295) 375
Myelocele, (*Fig.* 279) 351
Myelomeningocele (*see* Meningo-myelocele)
Myenteric ganglion cells, 7
Mylohyoid muscle, 176, 181, 183, 184
Myocardium
  bridging, 282
  impeded growth of, 280
  injury to, 284
  ischaemic, 280
Myocutaneous flaps, 247–248
Myodesis, 429
Myoplasty, 429
Myxoedema, 388

Nail fold infection, (*Fig.* 402) 492
Nasal... (*see also* Nose)
Nasal cavity, innervation of, 357
Nasal concha, 352
Nasal hemianopia, 353
Nasal pits, development of, (*Fig.* 145) 172
Nasal processes
  bifid nose due to incomplete fusion of, 174
  in facial development, 172
Nasal route to pituitary gland, (*Fig.* 270) 340
Nasal septum, 352
  development of, 172
  failure to fuse, (*Fig.* 149) 174
Nasion, (*Fig.* 273) 345
Nasolacrimal duct, 172
  exposed, 174
Nasolacrimal groove, (*Figs.* 145–146) 172
Nasopalatine nerve, 185, 361
Nasopharynx
  innervation of, 357

Nasopharynx, lymphatic drainage of, 194
Natal cleft, pilonidal sinus in, 77
Navicular bone
  accessory, (*Fig.* 339) 421
  making up foot arch, 539
Neck
  aortic arch extending into, 287
  at birth, 404
  collateral system to, 230
  defects, covered by myocutaneous flap, 248
  lymph nodes of, (*Figs.* 159–160) 193–197
  lymph tissue of, (*Figs.* 157–161) 189–198
  lymph trunks from, 270
  pain in, 560
  radical dissection of, (*Fig.* 161) 197–198
  rigidity of, 333
  sympathetic nerve supply to, 213
  webbed, 447
  wounds, 239
Nélaton's line, (*Fig.* 336) 418
Neonatal emergency, associated with tracheo-oesophageal fistula, 1
Nerve(s) (*see also individual nerves*)
  blocks, 151–152, 493
  damage to, associated with dislocations of shoulder, 448
  entrapment syndromes, involving elbow, 457
  fibres, 208–209
  grafting, 376
  in amputation, 429
  repair, 376
  roots, ischaemia of, 561
Nerve supply
  affected by abdominal incisions, (*Fig.* 104) 114
  to bladder, 319–320
  to breast, 165
  to diaphragm, 152, 154
  to external sphincter of bladder, 319
  to glenohumeral joint, 436
  to jaws, (*Figs.* 153–155) 182–187
  to oesophagus, 7–8, 211
  to pancreas, 106
  to temperomandibular joint, 188
  to testis, 119
Nervous system
  autonomic (*see* Autonomic nervous system)

Nervous system, parasympathetic, (*Fig.* 168) 207–208, (*Fig.* 173) 218
  sympathetic (*see* Sympathetic nervous system)
  transmitter substances in, 209–210
Nervus cutaneous colli, (*Fig.* 298) 378
Nervus erigentes, 51, 216, 218, 320
Nervus intermedius, 362, (*Fig.* 287) 363
Neural arches, 555
  fusion of, 561
Neural crest
  cells of, failure to migrate, 71
  paraganglion cells derived from, 311
Neuralgia
  glossopharyngeal, 370
  trigeminal, 358
Neurapraxia, 184, 375
  of infra-orbital nerve, 186
Neuritis, traumatic ulnar, 390
Neuroblastoma, 313
Neurocentral synchondrosis, (*Figs.* 458–459) 549
Neurogenic claudication, 561
Neurohypophysis, (*Fig.* 264) 335
Neurotmesis, 184, 375
Neurotrophic keratitis, 358
Nipple
  congenital retraction of, (*Fig.* 144) 169
  development of, 162
  inflammatory retraction of, 169–170
  lymphatic drainage of, 167
  rudimentary, 163
  supernumerary, 163
Nissen fundoplication, 161
Nodal artery, 278
Node biopsy, prescalene, 149
Node of Ranvier, (*Fig.* 295) 375
Non-chromaffin paraganglia, (*Fig.* 244) 311
  non-secretory tumours arising from, 313
Noradrenaline, 209
  secreted by paragangliomas, 313
  secreted by phaeochromocytomata, 312
Nose (*see also* Nasal...)
  bifid, 174
  bleeding from, 341
  innervation of, 357
  lymphatic drainage of, 194, 195
  veins of, 332, 342
Nuchal lines, 329

Nucleus ambiguus, 217
Nucleus pulposus, 554
Nutrient artery, (*Fig.* 327) 413
Nutrient foramina, 411

Oblique popliteal ligament, (*Fig.* 428) 515, 519
Oblique vein of Marshall, 274
Obturator lymph nodes, 319
Obturator nerve, 506
Occipital artery, 232, (*Fig.* 261) 330
Occipital bone, 401
Occipital condyles, 553
Occipital cortex, 353
  lesions of, (*Fig.* 280) 354
Occipital headaches, 333
Occipitalis muscle, 401
  innervation of, 366
Occipital lobes
  bilateral ischaemia of, 355
  tentorium in relation to, 341
Occipital lymph nodes, scalp drainage into, 333
Occipital muscle, 329
Occipital nerve, (*Fig.* 261) 332
  lesser, (*Fig.* 298) 378
Occipital protuberance, external, 342
Occipital sinus, 341
Occipital vein, (*Fig.* 196) 253, (*Fig.* 262) 331
Occipito-atlanto-axial articulation, 553
Occlusion of arteries, 225–238
Ocular muscles, 357
Oculomotor nerve, (*Fig.* 268) 338, 355, 359
  cavernous sinus in relation to, (*Fig.* 281) 356
Oculopupillary nerve fibres, 213
  division of, 219
Odontoid process, 549, 553
Oesophagus, 3–10
  arteries supplying, 8
  indented by right subclavian artery, 287
  inferior sphincter of, receptors in, 7
  lungs in relation to, 3
  lymph nodes of, (*Fig.* 7) 9–10
  muscles of, 7, 8
  nerve supply to, 7–8, 211
  plexus of, 211

Oesophagus, relations, 4
  smooth muscle of, 7
  spasm of, 7
  sphincter of, 5–6
  subclavian vein in relation to, (*Fig.* 193) 251
  thoracic duct in relation to, (*Fig.* 209) 269
  tumours of, 3, 10
Oestrogen, tissue sensitivity to, 397
Olfactory bulb, 352
Olfactory cells, 352
Olfactory nerve, 352
Olfactory tracts, 352
Omentum, in infancy, 406
Omohyoid muscle, (*Fig.* 165) 203
Omovertebral bone, 447
Ophthalmic artery, 330
Ophthalmic nerve, 359
  cavernous sinus in relation to, (*Fig.* 281) 357
Ophthalmic veins, 332
Ophthalmopathy, infiltrative, 360
Opponens muscle, 469
Optic canal, relation to cavernous sinus, (*Fig.* 281) 356
Optic chiasma, (*Fig.* 267) 337, 352
  pressure on, 334, 336
Optic disc, 352
Optic foramen, 352
Optic nerve, (*Fig.* 280) 352–355, 341
  ciliary nerves associated with, 360
Optic radiation, 353
  lesion of, (*Fig.* 280) 354
Optic tract, 353
Orbital ciliary body, 311
Orbital fissure, superior, 356
Orbital plate, fracture of, 329
Organ of Zuckerkandl, (*Fig.* 243) 312
Os acetabuli, 411, 503
Os tibiale externum, (*Fig.* 338) 421
Os trigonum, (*Fig.* 339) 421
Ossification, (*Figs.* 324–326) 410–412
  centres, 407
  of vertebrae, (*Figs.* 458–460) 549–551
Osteitis fibrosa, cyst of, (*Fig.* 340) 424
Osteo-arthritis, 332, 388, 522
  cervical, 384
  of metatarsophalangeal joint, 546
Osteoma, ivory, 422

Osteomyelitis, (*Fig.* 340) 424
  acute pyogenic, affecting membrane bones, 422
  affecting long bones, 423
  metaphysial, 435
  syphilitic, 423
Osteophytes, 561
  formation of, 552, 556
Osteoporosis, 499, 557
Osteotomy, of hip, 511
Otic ganglion, 217, (*Fig.* 285) 361–362, 369
Ovarian fossa, relation of ureter to, 301
Ovariectomy, damage to ureter caused by, 304
Oxytocin, 335

Pacchionian bodies, 343
Paget's disease, 561
Pain
  at site of previous injury or operation, 219
  due to fractured rib, 151–152
  due to nerve entrapment at elbow, 457
  epigastric, associated with pancreas, 104
  facial, due to trigeminal neuralgia, 358
  in arm, due to cancer of axillary nodes, 160
  in back (*see* Backache)
  in bladder, 320
  in calf, 263
  in forefoot, 547
  in heel, 537
  in knee joint, 524
  in leg, 238
  in neck, 560
  in region of umbilicus, 119
  in shoulder, 96–97, 154, 436, 445
  in sole of foot, 394
  in testes, 123
  in tip of shoulder, 96–97
  joint disease associated with, 436
  referred from diaphragm, 154
  referred from kidney, 290
  referred from oesophagus, 7
  relief, by sympathectomy, 219
  rest, 225
  somatic, 209

Pain, spring ligament associated with, 544
  visceral, 209
Painful arc syndrome, (*Fig.* 358) 445
Palatal mucosa, blood supply to, 182
Palate
  blood supply to, 182
  formation of, (*Fig.* 147) 172
  innervation of, (*Fig.* 155) 186, 357, 373
  muscles of, 174
  soft, relations of tonsils to, 190
Palatine arteries, 182
Palatine foramina, 182
Palatine nerves, 186
Palatine processes, 172
Palatine tonsil, (*Fig.* 157) 189
Palatoglossus muscle, 182
  relation of tonsils to, 190
Palatopharyngeus muscle, 178, 182
  relation of tonsils to, 190
Palm, sensory loss in, 385
Palmar aponeurosis, (*Fig.* 376) 467
Palmar creases, 489
Palmar fascia, (*Figs.* 376–377) 467–468
Palmar skin, 466
Palmaris longus tendon, 465, 467
Palsies, caused by pituitary tumour, 338
Pampiniform plexus, in spermatic cord, 136
Pancreas, (*Figs.* 92–95) 102–106
  accessory tissue, 104
  annular, 104
  arterial supply to, (*Fig.* 94) 105
  cancer of, pain in, 106, 166, 209
  damaged during splenectomy, 104
  embryology of, (*Fig.* 92) 102–103
  fistula involving, 104
  lymphatic drainage from, 106, 268
  nerve supply to, 106
  relations, 30, 104
  transverse mesocolon suspended from, (*Fig.* 37) 45
  venous drainage of, 106
Pancreas divisum, (*Fig.* 93) 103–104
Pancreatectomy, necrosis following, 105
Pancreatic duct, (*Fig.* 86) 94–95
  accessory, 103
  congenital anomalies of, (*Fig.* 93) 103–104
  drainage of, 105
  junction with bile duct, 92

Pancreatic duct, reflux of bile up, 90
  sphincter of, (*Fig.* 82) 90
  union with bile duct, 89
Pancreaticoduodenal artery, 105, 227
Pancreaticoduodenal vein, 82
Pancreaticoduodenectomy, complications
    associated with, 106
Pancreaticolienal nodes, (*Fig.* 12) 17
Pancreatitis, 104
  biliary, 90
  pain associated with, 106
  pain relief from, 219
Papilloedema, 353
Papilloma, duct, 164
Para-aortic glands, 268
Para-aortic lymph nodes, 296, 309
Paracardial nodes, 10
Paradidymus, 123
Paraduodenal fossa, (*Fig.* 25) 33
Paraganglia
  non-chromaffin, (*Fig.* 244) 311
  tumours arising from, 311–313
Paragangliomas, (*Fig.* 244) 313
  intravagale, (*Fig.* 244) 313
Paraganglion system, 311
Paralysis (*see also* Paraplegia)
  abducens nerve, 363
  Erb's, 384
  involving eyelid, 360
  Klumpke's, 385, 392
  of face muscles, 367
  of leg, due to compartmental pressure,
    238
  of pelvic floor, 71
  of sternomastoid muscle, 374
  of superior oblique muscle, 357
  of tendon of inguinal canal, 44
  pituitary tumour associated with, 339
Paramesonephronic duct, 123
Paranasal sinuses, 360
Paraplegia (*see also* Paralysis)
  following abdominal aortic surgery, 349
  following embolization of bronchial sys-
    tem, 146
  following operations on aorta, 289
Parasympathetic nerve supply of bladder,
    320
Parasympathetic nervous system, (*Fig.*
    168) 207–208, (*Fig.* 173) 218
  transmitter substances in, 209–210

Parasympathetic pupilloconstrictor fibres,
    355
Paratenon, 477, (*Fig.* 389) 478, 536
Parathyroid artery, 207
  innervation of, 213
Parathyroid glands, 202, 203, 204, 206–207
  blood supply to, 207
  innervation of, 213
Paratracheal lymph nodes, 10, 195, 206
  biopsy of, 149
Paravertebral gutter, 152
Paravertebral sympathetic trunk, 208
Paresis, associated with pituitary tumour,
    339
Parietal emissary vein, 332
Parietal lymph nodes of thorax, 146–147
Parietal pleura
  biopsy of, 152
  oesophagus in relation to, 3
Parona's space, (*Fig.* 399) 489
Paronychial abscess, (*Fig.* 402) 491
Paroöphoron, (*Fig.* 248) 315
Parotid gland, 188, 194, 369
  branchial cyst in, 179
  facial nerve in relation to, 367
  fistulous track through, 179
  innervation of, 362
Parotid lymph nodes, (*Fig.* 159) 193–194
  scalp drainage by, 333
Pars, of pituitary body, (*Fig.* 264) 335
Pars interarticularis, defect in, (*Fig.* 471)
    563
Patella, (*Fig.* 436) 523–524
  dislocations of, 524
  ossification in, 420
Patella alta, 524
Patellofemoral joint, 523
Patent ductus arteriosus, 287
Patent urachus, (*Fig.* 249) 316
Patent vitello-intestinal duct, 39
Patulous anus, 77
Peau d'orange, due to blockage of lympha-
    tics in breast, 170
Pectineal ligament, sutured to inguinal
    ligament, 134
Pectineus, 130
Pectoral muscles, 137
  absence of, 162
  axillary artery in relation to, (*Fig.* 301)
    382

Pectoral muscles, major, flap, 248
  minor, (*Fig.* 140) 165
  pathway of breast lymphatics through,
    (*Fig.* 142) 168
Pelvic abscess, 48–49, (*Fig.* 68) 75
Pelvic colon, 41
  resection for cancer of, (*Fig.* 49) 57
Pelvic course of ureter, (*Fig.* 234) 301–302
Pelvic diaphragm, (*Fig.* 59) 65, (*Fig.* 315)
    396
Pelvic fascia
  lymphatic drainage between, (*Fig.* 52)
    60
  supporting rectum, 51
Pelvic floor, paralysis of, 71
Pelvic fracture, causing ruptured urethra,
    (*Fig.* 257) 325
Pelvic infection, 75
Pelvic mesocolon, 46
Pelvic splanchnic nerves, 216
Pelvirectal space, abscess in, 74–75
Penile hypospadias, 326
Penile urethra, 324
Penis, 324
  abnormal urethral orifice on, 326
  Colles' fascia over, 124
  connection to dartos muscle, 124
  development of, 326
  dorsal nerve of, 73
  dorsal vein of, 322, 323
  nerves involved in erection of, 65
  site of ectopic testis, 120
Peptic ulcer
  associated with Meckel's diverticulum,
    40
  causing secondary hypertrophy, 14
Percutaneous transluminal angioplasty,
    280
Perforating veins, (*Fig.* 201) 258, (*Figs.*
    201–203) 259–262
  incompetence of, 263
Peri-anal area
  abscess, 74
  fat, 63–64
  inspection of, 77
  veins, rupture of, 67–68
Pericardial sac, oesophagus in relation to,
    4
Pericardiocentesis, 285
Pericardium, bleeding contained by, 285

Pericranium, (*Fig.* 260) 328, 332, 341
Perineal...(*see also* Perineum)
Perineal anaesthesia, 74
Perineal body, anal canal in relation to, 61
Perineal defects, covered by myocutane-
    ous flap, 248
Perineal ectopic anus, (*Fig.* 63) 68
Perineal fascia, 124
Perineal nerve, (*Fig.* 66) 73
Perineal prostatectomy, 323
Perineal skin, rupture of abscess on to, 75
Perineoscrotal hypospadias, 326
Perineum (*see also* Perineal...)
  fasciae of, 123–125
  incomplete migration of anus along,
    (*Fig.* 63) 68
  nerve supply to, 74
  shotgun, (*Fig.* 63) 70
  site of ectopic testis, 120
  swelling of, 256
  trauma causing abscess, (*Fig.* 70) 75–76
  varices of, 84
Perineurium, (*Fig.* 295) 375
Peri-oesophageal nodes, (*Fig.* 7) 10
Periosteal elevator, 150
Periosteal fibrosarcoma, (*Fig.* 340) 424
Periosteal vessels, 414
Periosteum, (*Fig.* 323) 409
  innervation of, 185
  of skull, 341
  stripping of, 181
Periostitis, affecting membrane bones, 422
Peripheral nerves, (*Figs.* 295–313) 375–
    395
  anatomy of, (*Fig.* 295) 375
  lesions of, 386
Peripheral vascular disease, 218–219
Perirenal fat, at birth, 406
Perisinusoidal space of Disse, (*Fig.* 71) 79
Peristalsis, 7
  interference with, 296
Peritoneum
  around mesenteries, 41
  pelvic, (*Figs.* 250, 251) 317–318
  rectum in relation to, (*Fig.* 41) 48–49
Peritonitis, 32
Peritracheobronchial lymph nodes, (*Fig.*
    130) 147–148
Perivascular space, 343
Peroneal nerve, 533

Peroneal nerve, common, 394, 428
  injured by knee dislocation, 526
Peroneal retinacula, (*Fig.* 445) 534–535
Peroneal tendons, recurrent dislocation of, 535
Peroneal vein, 258, 262
Peroneus tertius, (*Fig.* 444) 533
  sheath of, 536
Perthe's test, for varicose veins, 263
Pes anserinus, 367
Pes cavus, 545
Petrosal nerve, (*Fig.* 284) 360, 364
  superficial, 369
Petrosal sinus, inferior, (*Fig.* 196) 253
Petrous bone, 364
Pfannenstiel's exposure, 320
pH, of blood, chemoreceptors responding to, 311
Phaeochromocytoma, 310, 311, 312
Phalanges
  making up foot arch, 539
  terminal, (*Figs.* 402–404) 491–493
  tuberculosis of, 423
  vincula of, (*Fig.* 389) 478
Pharyngeal...(*see also* Pharynx)
Pharyngeal constrictor, inferior, 203
Pharyngeal diverticulum, (*Fig.* 4) 5
Pharyngeal plexus, 213, 332
Pharyngeal pouch, (*Fig.* 150) 177, 179, 189
Pharyngeal tonsils, (*Fig.* 157) 189
  lymph drainage from, 192
Pharyngeal veins, (*Fig.* 196) 253
Pharyngo-oesophageal pouch, (*Fig.* 4) 5
Pharynx (*see also* Pharyngeal...)
  bleeding from, 341
  constrictors of, 177
  formed from branchial arches, (*Fig.* 150) 174–177
  inferior constrictor of, 5–6
  innervation of, 373
  lymphatic drainage of, 194, 195
  lymphoid tissue at entrance to, 189
  primitive, 1
Phenol
  injected to destroy ganglion, 219
  used in lumbar ganglion block, 223
Philtrum, of upper lip, 172
Phlebitis, of superficial veins of breast, 165

Phrenic arteries, 86
  inferior, 8
Phrenic nerve, 154, (*Fig.* 193) 251
  accessory, 252
  affecting supraclavicular nerve, 96–97
  in diaphragmatic incision, (*Fig.* 131) 151
  in radical neck dissection, 197
  on scalenus muscle, 149
  thoracic duct in relation to, (*Fig.* 209) 269
Phrenic vein, adrenal vein draining into, 310
Phrenicocolic ligament, 110
Phreno-oesophageal ligament, 20, (*Fig.* 135) 158, (*Fig.* 137) 160–161
Phrygian cap, 96
Pia mater, (*Fig.* 272) 343–345
Piles, (*Figs.* 60–61) 66–68
  sentinel, 68
  strangulated, (*Fig.* 61) 67
  thrombotic, 67
Pilomotor nerve fibres, 211
Pilonidal sinus, in natal cleft, 77
Pinna
  formation of, 179
  lymphatic drainage of, 193–194
  sensory fibres to, 369
Pinpoint meatus, 328
Pisiform bone, 242, 420, 460
Pituitary body (*see also* Hypophysis) (*Figs.* 263–270) 333–340
  anosmia due to tumour near, 352
  errors in development of, 333
  histology of, 335
  hypophysectomy, 339
  radioactive pellets inserted into, 339
  relations of, (*Figs.* 265–268) 336
  removal by trans-sphenoidal operation, (*Fig.* 270) 339
  tumours of, 336–339, 353
Pituitary fossa, 334, (*Fig.* 267) 337
  deepened, 339
Pituitary hormone, excess of, 339
Pituitary stalk, (*Fig.* 264) 335
Placenta, 82, 273
Plantar aponeurosis, (*Figs.* 451–452) 541
  fibrous bands to, 538
  retinaculum attached to, 533
Plantar calcaneonavicular ligament, (*Fig.* 451) 540

Plantar ligaments, (*Fig.* 451) 541
Plantar pad, 542
Plate, tarsal, (*Fig.* 283) 360
Platysma, fistula passing through, 178
Pleura
    mammary vessels on, 137
    oesophagus in relation to, 3
Pleural cavity
    aspirating lymph from, 271
    division of, 141
Pleural effusion, associated with perfora-
        tion of oesophagus, 3, 4
Pleural sacs, 137
Pleural septum, 141
Pleural space, entry to, 150
Pleuroperitoneal membranes, 153
Plica semilunaris, 190, 191
Plica triangularis, 190, 191
Pneumonitis
    septic, site of, 140
    suppurative, 139
Pneumothorax, avoidance during cannu-
        lation of subclavian vein, (*Fig.* 195)
        253
Poirier, space of, 482
Polycystic kidneys, 298
Polymastia, 162
Polythelia, 163
Polyvinyl alcohol sponge, 52
Pons, 362, (*Fig.* 287) 363
    emergence of trigeminal nerve from,
        357
Popliteal artery
    atherosclerotic stenosis of, 245
    exposure of, (*Fig.* 188) 244–245
    occlusion of, 230
Popliteal fossa, 258
Popliteal ligaments, (*Fig.* 428) 515, 519
Popliteal nerve, medial, injury to, 393–394
Popliteal vein, 258
    thrombi in, 258
Popliteus, (*Fig.* 429) 516
Porta hepatis, 78, 82, 87
    accessory bile duct leaving, 90
Portal hypertension, 9, 83–85
    metastatic tumours causing, 83
    surgery for, 85
    thrombosis causing, 83
    treatment of, 113
    varices associated with, 84

Portal vein, 78, (*Figs.* 74–78) 81–85
    blood pressure, 83
    duodenum in relation to, 31
    gallbladder vein into, 96
    preduodenal, 38, (*Fig.* 76) 83
Portasystemic shunts, (*Fig.* 79) 86
Portohepatography, route for, 83
Portosystemic anastomoses, (*Fig.* 77) 83
Postcardinal vein, 264
Posterior auricular artery, (*Fig.* 261) 330
Posterior auricular vein, (*Fig.* 262) 331
Posterior communicating artery, (*Fig.* 267)
        337
Posterior spinal artery, (*Fig.* 276) 347–348
Posterolateral hernia, 157
Posterolateral thoracotomy, 150
Posteromedial vein, of leg, (*Fig.* 199) 258
Postprandial epigastric pain, 226
Postthyroidectomy   hypoparathyroidism,
        207
Postvagotomy diarrhoea, 21
Pouch of Douglas, 51, 323, 397
Pouch of Hartmann, 95
Poupart's ligament, 126
Pre-auricular lymph nodes, 188
Pre-auricular sinuses, 178, 179–180
Pre-auricular skin tags, 179–180
Preduodenal portal vein, 38, (*Fig.* 76) 83
Preganglionic autonomic nerve fibres, 208
Pregnancy
    location of appendix in, 43
    vulval varicosities during, 255
Prelaryngeal lymph nodes, 195
Premature infants
    delayed closure of ductus arteriosus, 287
    undescended testis in, 119
Premaxilla, 172
Premolars
    innervation of, 183
    maxillary, blood supply to, 181
Prepatella bursa, 526
Prepuce
    at birth, 407
    deformity of, 326
Presacral nerve, 319
Presacral plexus, 216
Prescalene node biopsy, 149
Pressure gradient across site of occlusion,
        225

Pretracheal fascia, 201
  incision for mediastinoscope, 149
Pretracheal lymph nodes, 195
Pretracheobronchial lymph nodes, (*Fig.* 130) 147–148
Prevertebral fascia, 211
Prevertebral nerve plexuses, 208, 211
Primary palate, (*Fig.* 147) 172
  cleft of, (*Fig.* 149) 173–174
Primitive pharynx, 1
Pringle's manoeuvre, 97
Processus vaginalis, 119, 121
  failure of obliteration of, 126
  fluid in, 135
Procidentia, (*Fig.* 42) 50–51
Profunda femoris artery, 229, 244
Profundoplasty, 229
Profundus tendon, test of, (*Fig.* 378) 469
Prolapse (*see under individual structures*)
Promontory of cochlea, (*Fig.* 289) 365
Pronator muscle, compressing median nerve, 457
Pronator teres muscle, 242, 385
Proptosis, 338, 360
Prostate, (*Fig.* 246) 315, (*Fig.* 252) 318, (*Figs.* 253–255) 320–324
  abdominal incision for exposure of, 320
  bladder in relation to, (*Fig.* 251) 318
  carcinoma of, 319, 321
  fascia of Denonvilliers in relation to, 50
  fascial relations, (*Fig.* 254) 322
  lobes of, (*Fig.* 253) 320–321
  palpation of, 77
  projecting into urethra, 321
  rectum in relation to, 322
  seminal vesicle in relation to, (*Fig.* 253) 321
  sympathetic nerve supply to, 319
  ureter in relation to, (*Fig.* 235) 302
  urogenital diaphragm in relation to, 321
Prostatectomy, 322
  causing backflow of ejaculatory fluid into bladder, 319
  retropubic, 323
  transurethral, 324
Prostatic fascia, ureter in relation to, (*Fig.* 235) 302
Prostatic urethra, (*Fig.* 246) 315, (*Fig.* 252) 318, (*Fig.* 253) 321, (*Fig.* 254) 322, 324
  additional ureter opening into, 304

Prostatic urethra, removal of, 322
  ruptured, 325
Prostatic utricle, 324
Prostatoperitoneal fascia, (*Fig.* 251) 323
Prosthesis, 433
Pseudopancreatic cysts, 104
Psoas muscles, (*Fig.* 117) 129, 215
  kidney in relation to, 291
Pterygoid canal, (*Fig.* 284) 360
Pterygoid hamulus, 182
Pterygoid muscle, 182–183, 188
  lateral, (*Fig.* 156) 187
  relation of facial nodes to, 194
Pterygoid plexus, 332
Pterygopalatine fossa, 357
Pterygopalatine ganglion, 217, (*Fig.* 284) 360, 186
Ptosis, 355, 385
  due to deficient fixation of gut, 30
Pubic crest, relation to inguinal ring, 126
Pubis
  attachment of puborectal muscle to, (*Fig.* 57) 63–64
  incisional hernia above, 115
Pubocervical ligament, (*Fig.* 314) 395
Pubococcygeus muscle, (*Fig.* 315) 396
Pubofemoral ligament, (*Fig.* 416) 502
  relation of subpsoas bursa to, (*Fig.* 419) 505
Puboprostatic ligaments, 322
Puborectalis muscle, (*Fig.* 55) 62, 63, 65, (*Fig.* 315) 396
  sling, 68, (*Fig.* 69) 75–76
Pudendal canal, (*Fig.* 65) 72–73
Pudendal nerve, (*Fig.* 65) 72, (*Fig.* 66) 73–74, 324
  block, 73
  branches of, 73–74
  incontinence resulting from damage to, 66
  perineal branch to bladder, 319
  rectal branch of, 63
Pudendal vein, 255
  enlargement of tributaries from, 256
Pulmonary annulus, (*Fig.* 214) 276
Pulmonary artery, (*Fig.* 124) 138, 144–145
  formation of, 286
Pulmonary atresia, 280
Pulmonary embolism, 258
Pulmonary glomus bodies, 311

Pulmonary trunk, formation of, 285
Pulmonary valve, 279
Pulmonary veins, 145, 278
    formation of, 274
Pulmonary vessels, (*Fig.* 129) 144–146
Pulp space infection, (*Fig.* 403) 492
Pulps of teeth, innervation of, 185
Pulse
    absent in lower limbs, 229
    in ankle, 245
Pulsion diverticulum, 7–8
Pupil
    bilateral fixed dilated, 356
    constrictor muscles of, 355
    contraction of, 385
    innervation of, 359
    sympathetic nerve supply to, 213
Pupillary reflex, 353
Pupilloconstrictor fibres, 355
Pyloric antrum, (*Fig.* 8) 12
Pyloric canal, (*Fig.* 8) 12
Pyloric gland area, 13
Pyloric outlet, partial obstruction of, 32
Pyloric sphincter, 13
Pyloric stenosis, hypertrophic, 13–14
Pyloric vein, 82
Pyloroplasty, 20
Pylorus, (*Fig.* 8) 12
Pyramidal lobe, of thyroid gland, 199,
    (*Fig.* 163) 200, 201
Pyramidal tract in crus, pituitary tumour
    interfering with, 339

Q angle, (*Fig.* 436) 523
Quadrantic hemianopia, 354
Quadratus muscle, 291, 367
Quadriceps muscle, 515
    patella in relation to, (*Fig.* 436) 523
Quadriceps tendon, 420
Queckenstedt's test, 347
Quinsy, 192

Rachischisis, 351
Radial artery, (*Fig.* 375) 466
    exposure of, 242
    fistula involving, 250

Radial bursa, 477
Radial collateral ligament, 455
Radial muscle of iris, 355
Radial nerve, 424, 425, 426
    axillary artery in relation to, (*Fig.* 301)
        382
    compression of, 457
    injury to, (*Figs.* 305–306) 386
    supplying wrist, 462
Radicular arteries, (*Fig.* 277) 348
    infrarenal, (*Fig.* 278) 349
Radioactive pellets inserted into pituitary,
    339
Radiocarpal joint, 460
    aspiration of, 463
Radio-ulnar joint, 454
Radius, (*Fig.* 369) 460, (*Fig.* 395) 484
    measurement of, (*Fig.* 331) 416
    surgical approach to, 426
    uniting of epiphyses, 411
Ramstedt operation, 14
Ramus communicans, (*Fig.* 169) 210
Ranvia, node of, (*Fig.* 295) 375
Raphe, median, of tongue, (*Fig.* 160) 196–
    197
Rathke
    folds of, 68
    pouch of, (*Fig.* 263) 333
Ray excision of toe, 431
Raynaud's disease, effects increased by
    overactivity of sympathetic ner-
    vous system, 218–219
Receptaculum chyli, (*Fig.* 208) 268
Rectal...(*see also* Rectum; Rectus...)
Rectal agenesis, 68
Rectal artery, 51, (*Fig.* 43) 52, (*Fig.* 178)
    227, 228
Rectal atresia, 68
Rectal bleeding, due to haemorrhoids, 66
Rectal examination, 63, 77–78
Rectal ligaments, damage to ureters
    caused by division of, 306
Rectal nerve, 73
Rectal plexus of veins, haemorrhoids
    associated with, 66
Rectal pouch, gas in, 70
Rectal stalk, 51, 54
Rectal vein, 49
Rectocele, 397
Rectopexy, posterior, 51

Rectosigmoid junction, 48
Recto-urethral fistula, 68
Recto-urethralis muscle, 51, (*Fig.* 251) 318, (*Fig.* 255) 323
Recto-uterine pouch, 48, 398
  palpation of tumour in, 78
Rectovaginal examination, 399
Rectovaginal fistula, (*Fig.* 64) 68
Rectovesical fascia, relation of ureter to, (*Fig.* 235) 302
Rectovesical fistula, 68
Rectovesical pouch, 48
Rectum (*see also* Rectal...; Rectus...), 41
  absence of ganglia from, 71
  anomalies of, (*Figs.* 62–64) 68–71
  carcinoma of, causing extrasphincteric fistula, 76
  course of, 48
  development of, (*Fig.* 62) 68–69
  fascia of, 50
  intersphincteric excision of, 65
  junction with sigmoid colon, 48
  lateral ligament, 51
  lymphatic drainage of, (*Fig.* 52) 60
  lymphatic spread of tumours from, 63
  muscles of, (*Fig.* 55) 62
  palpation of, 77
  pelvic abscess draining into, 48
  plexus supplying, 216
  prolapse of, (*Fig.* 42) 50–51, 397
  prostate in relation to, 322
  resection for cancer of, (*Fig.* 51) 58
  supports of, 50–51
  sympathetic nerve supply to, 319
  tumours of, 48, 59, 77
  urogenital diaphragm attached to, 51
  uterine ligaments in relation to, (*Fig.* 314) 395
  varices of, 84
  venous drainage of, 49
  X-rays of, 70–71
Rectus femoris, sesamoid of, (*Fig.* 417) 503
Rectus muscle, (*Fig.* 122) 134
  involved in abdominal incisions, 114
  lateral, motor nerve to, (*Fig.* 281) 363
  nerve supply to, 98
Rectus sheath, (*Fig.* 122) 134
Recurrent nerves, 372
  laryngeal, (*Fig.* 166) 203, (*Fig.* 218) 286
  lymph nodes associated with, 195

Recurrent nerves, thoracic duct in relation to, (*Fig.* 209) 269
Reflex
  consensual light, 353
  gag, 369
  pupillary, 353
  sensory fibres, 209
  sympathetic, (*Fig.* 169) 210
Reflux, gastro-oesophageal, 160–161
Regurgitation, 6
Renal...(*see also* Kidney)
Renal agenesis, 298
Renal anomalies, Sprengel's deformity associated with, 447
Renal artery, 295, (*Fig.* 278) 349
  occlusion of, renal failure due to, 229
  supplying ureter, (*Fig.* 236) 303
Renal carcinoma, affecting testicular vein, 136
Renal failure, 298
  due to occlusion of renal arteries, 229
  establishment of fistulae in forearm, 250
Renal fascia, (*Fig.* 225) 293
Renal plexus, 215
Renal vein, 113
  anomalies of, 265
  blood diverted to, 85
  ligation of, 266
  origin of, 264
  relation to testicular vein, 136
Renal vessels, multiple, 300
Resections
  for cancer of gut, (*Figs.* 47–54) 56–61
  hepatic, (*Fig.* 81) 87–88
Resectoscope, 324
Rest pain, 225
Retina, 341, 352
  blood vessels, 352
Retinacula, around ankle joint, (*Figs.* 444–445) 532–535
Retro-achilleal bursa, (*Fig.* 449) 537
Retro-aortic left renal vein, 265
Retrocaecal fossa, (*Fig.* 36) 44–45
Retrocalcaneal bursa, (*Fig.* 449) 537
Retrocaval ureter, (*Fig.* 237) 304
Retropharyngeal lymph nodes, 195
Retroportal artery, 94
Retropubic prostatectomy, 323
Retrosphincteric space, 61
Retrosternal hernia, 157–158

Retzius, space of, 115
Rheumatic heart disease, 277
Rheumatoid arthritis, synovial swelling associated with, 388
Rhinorrhoea, CSF, 352
Rhomboid fossa, of clavicle, (*Fig.* 325) 411
Rhomboid ligament, 411
Rhomboid muscles, 384, (*Fig.* 351) 440
Rib(s)
  blood supply to, 415
  cervical, (*Figs.* 303–304) 383–384
  first, (*Fig.* 303) 383
  fractured, splenic injury associated with, 108
  kidney in relation to, (*Fig.* 223) 292
  pain due to fractured, 151–152
  removal of, 150
  thoracic ganglia in relation to, 214
  thoracic vertebrae in relation to, 549
  unequal growth of, 138
Rib spreader, 150
Rickets, 499
Ring of Vieussens, 281
Riolan, arch of, 228
Rolling hernia, (*Fig.* 135) 158
Rotator cuff, (*Fig.* 347) 435
  action of, (*Fig.* 349) 438
  blood supply to, (*Fig.* 357) 444
  lesions involving. (*Figs.* 357–358) 444–446
  tears, 446
Rutherford Morison's incision, 116

Saccule, 369
Sacral...(*see also* Sacrum)
Sacral agenesis, 71
Sacral curve, supporting rectum, 51
Sacral ganglia, 216, 221
Sacral nerve, 73, 216
  fibres, 209
  injury to, 50
  spinal, 218
Sacralization of transverse process of 5th lumbar vertebra, (*Fig.* 470) 562
Sacrococcygeal ligament, 65
Sacro-iliac joint, pain associated with, 558
Sacrospinalis muscle, 306
Sacrospinous ligament, (*Fig.* 66) 73

Sacrotuberous ligament, 72, (*Fig.* 66) 73
Sacrum (*see also* Sacral...), 547
  connection with transverse process of 5th lumbar vertebra, (*Fig.* 470) 562
  palpation in rectal examination, 78
Sagittal sinus, 332, 342
Salivary glands
  buccal, innervation of, 182
  labial minor, innervation of, 183
  nerve fibres to, 211
  parotid, 188, 369
  secretion, 368
Salivary nucleus, 208
Santorini's duct, (*Fig.* 92) 103, 104
Saphenofemoral junction, varicose vein at, 262, 263
Saphenous nerve, 255, 533
  injury to, 528
Saphenous opening, 129
Saphenous vein, 245, (*Figs.* 198–199) 254–262
  accessory, 255
Sarcoidosis, biopsy to investigate, 149
Sarcoma (*see also* Cancer)
  of femur, 513
  osteogenic, (*Fig.* 340) 424
Scalene muscles, 156, (*Fig.* 209) 269
  nodes, 10
  phrenic nerve on, 149
  relation to thoracic duct, (*Fig.* 209) 269
Scalenus medius, plexuses on, (*Figs.* 296–304) 376–385
Scalp, (*Figs.* 260–262) 328–333
  blood vessels of, (*Figs.* 261–262) 330–332
  defect, covered by myocutaneous flap, 248
  innervation of, 357
  layers of, (*Fig.* 260) 328
  lymphatic drainage of, 193–194, 333
  nerves of, (*Fig.* 261) 332–333
  wounds, 330
Scaphoid bone, (*Fig.* 369) 460
  fracture of, (*Fig.* 371) 462–463
Scapula
  blood supply to, 415
  congenital anomalies of, 447
  development of, 411
  nerve, 380
Scapulothoracic linkage, (*Fig.* 346) 433

Scar hernia, 113
Scarpa's fascia, (*Fig.* 113) 123–125, (*Fig.* 257) 325
 site of testis, 120
Schmorl's nodes, (*Fig.* 464) 556
Sciatic nerve, 221, 506
 damage to, 502
 injuries to, (*Fig.* 312) 392–393
 pudendal nerve in relation, 73
Sciatica, 561, 563
Sclerema neonatorum, 405
Sclerosing adenosis, of breast, 164
Scoliosis, 550, 557, 565–566
 disc protrusion associated with, (*Fig.* 467) 559
 lumbar, 562
 structural, 411
Scrotal branch of perineal nerve, 73
Scrotum, (*Figs.* 111–112) 118–137
 Colles' fascia over, 124
 corrugations of skin, 124
 dimpling of, 122
 formation of, 326
 muscle of, 124
 temperature effect on, 124
 unfused, 327
 varicocele affecting temperature of, 137
Sebaceous glands, absence on foot, 538
Secondary palate, (*Fig.* 147) 172
 cleft of, (*Fig.* 149) 174
Secondary sexual characteristics, absence associated with dystrophia adiposogenitalis, 333
Secretory nerve fibres, 211
Secretory tumours, 312–313
Sella turcica, 334
 changes in, 339
Semicircular canals, 369
 lateral, (*Fig.* 289) 365
Semilunar cartilages, of knee joint, (*Fig.* 434) 520–522, 524
Semilunar ganglion, 233
Semimembranosus, tendon of, (*Fig.* 429) 516, 519
Seminal fluid, flow into bladder, 221
Seminal vesicle, (*Fig.* 246) 315
 additional ureter opening into, 304
 palpation of, 77
 peritoneal relations, (*Fig.* 251) 318
 peritoneum reflected onto, 48

Seminal vesicle, prostate in relation to, (*Fig.* 253) 321
 sympathetic nerve supply to, 319
 ureter in relation to, (*Fig.* 235) 302
Seminiferous tubules, 119
Sensory nerve fibres, afferent, 209
Sentinel pile, 68
Septal cusp, (*Fig.* 215) 277
 of tricuspid valve, (*Fig.* 214) 276
Septation, failure of, in heart, 279
Septic arthritis, 435
Septum transversum, 78, 152–153
Sequestra, 423
Serratus anterior muscle, 150, (*Fig.* 350) 439, 440
 paralysis of, 384
Sesamoid bones, 420–421, 460
 attachment of plantar aponeurosis, 542
 of rectus femoris, (*Fig.* 417) 503
Sex cells, primordial, 119
Shock, Pringle's manoeuvre following, 97
Shotgun perineum, (*Fig.* 63) 70
Shoulder, (*Fig.* 346) 433–434
 abduction of, (*Figs.* 349–351) 437–440
 arthrodesis, (*Fig.* 362) 453
 aspiration of joint, 449
 dislocation of, 447–449
 drop, associated with removal of spinal accessory nerve, 197
 frozen, 446
 pain, 96–97, 154, 436, 445
 subluxation, 447–449
 surgical approaches to, (*Figs.* 359–361) 449–453
 transacromial approach to, (*Fig.* 361) 451–453
Shoulder strap incision, (*Fig.* 359) 450
Shunt
 portasystemic, (*Fig.* 79) 86
 splenorenal, 113
Shunting procedures, for hydrocephalus, 350
Sibson's fascia, (*Fig.* 134) 156, 220
Sigmoidal arteries, (*Fig.* 43) 52, (*Fig.* 178) 227
Sigmoid colon, resection for cancer of, (*Fig.* 51) 59
Sigmoid loop, 48
Sigmoid sinus, 342
Singing, affected by damage to laryngeal nerve, 373

Sino-atrial node, 274, (*Fig*. 215) 277
Sinus
  branchial, 177
  cervical, (*Fig*. 150) 177
  of cranium, blood supply to, 342
  pre-auricular, 178, 179–180
  venosus, (*Fig*. 212) 273, 274
  vitelline, (*Fig*. 33) 40
Sinus node artery, 281
Sinusoids, 79
Sinuvertebral artery, (*Fig*. 457) 548
Sinuvertebral nerve, (*Fig*. 457) 548, 554
Situs inversus abdominalis, 38
Skeletal tuberculosis, (*Fig*. 473) 563–565
Skin
  cancer, removal of plexus on deep
    fascia, 272
  flaps, in amputation, 429
  lymphatic watersheds of, (*Fig*. 211) 272
  necrosis, complicating arterial grafting,
    256
  of breast, lymphatic drainage of, 167
  of neck, lymphatic drainage of, 195
  pilomotor fibres to, 211
  tags, pre-auricular, 179–180
Skull
  accumulation of cerebrospinal fluid in,
    350
  at birth, 401
  centres of ossification, 410
  fracture of, 329
  metopic suture mistaken for fracture,
    410
  occipital condyles of, 553
  periosteum of, 341
  sinus bleeding following fracture of, 342
Sliding hernia, (*Fig*. 120) 132
  repair of, 161
Small intestine, (*Figs*. 29–33) 35–41
  accessory pancreatic tissue in, 104
  anastomosis, (*Fig*. 30) 36–37
  arteries, arrangement, (*Fig*. 29) 36
Smell
  loss of sense of, 352
  sensation of, due to pituitary tumour,
    339
Smooth muscle
  oesophageal, 7
  of internal sphincter of bladder, 318

Soft palate
  blood supply to, 182
  tonsils in relation to, 190
Soleal sinuses, 258
  as site for initiation of varicose veins,
    262
Soleal thrombosis, 262
Soleal venous sinuses, 262
Sole of foot, 538
  pain in, 394
Somatic collateral system, 229
Somatic fibres, 211
Somatic pain, 209
Space of Disse, (*Fig*. 71) 79
Space of Poirier, 482
Space of Retzius, 115
Spasm
  of oesophagus, 7
  of stomach, 14
Speech, affected by cleft palate, 174
Spermatic cord, 123, (*Fig*. 117) 129
  inguinal ring in relation, 126
  pampiniform plexus in, 136
  torsion of, 122
Spermatic fascia, 119, 121, 127, 129
Spermatocele, 136
Spermatogenesis, temperature effect on,
    124
Sperm count, low, associated with varico-
    cele, 137
Sphenoid bone, site of pituitary body, 334
Sphenoidal sinus, 336, (*Fig*. 268) 338, (*Fig*.
    281) 356
  sella turcica bulging into, 339
Sphenoid bone, site of pituitary body, 334
Sphenomandibular ligament, 176, 183, 188
Sphenopalatine artery, 181–182
Sphenopalatine nerve, supplying hard
    palate, (*Fig*. 155) 186
Sphincter
  incontinence resulting from damage to,
    66
  of ampulla, (*Fig*. 82) 90
  of anus (*see* Anal sphincter)
  of bladder, 318–319
  of common bile duct, (*Fig*. 82) 90
  of Oddi, 89, (*Fig*. 82) 90
  of oesophagus, 5–6
  of pancreatic duct, (*Fig*. 82) 90
  of urethra, 304
  vesical, (*Fig*. 253) 321

Sphincterotomy, sphincter muscle in, 64
Sphygmomanometer cuff, 388
Spina bifida (see also Meningomyelocele), (Fig. 279) 350–351
cystica, 351
occulta, (Fig. 279) 350–351
Spinal accessory nerve, 193, (Fig. 294) 373
in radical neck dissection, 197
Spinal anaesthetic, 222
Spinal arteries, 289, (Figs. 276–277) 347–348
Spinal canal, 547
acquired narrowing of, 561
congenital narrowing of, (Fig. 469) 561
incomplete closure of, 350
Spinal column, (Figs. 456–473) 547–566
at birth, 405
components of, 547
curves of, (Fig. 456) 547
intervertebral discs (see Intervertebral discs)
laminal arches united by joints and vertebrae, 555–556
sacralization of transverse process of 5th lumbar vertebra, (Fig. 470) 562
scoliosis, see Scoliosis
spondylolisthesis (see Spondylolisthesis)
tuberculosis of, (Fig. 473) 563–565
vertebrae uniting joints and ligaments, (Figs. 461–463) 551–555
vertebral venous system, (Fig. 468) 560
Spinal cord, 547
at birth, 405
blood supply to, 289, (Figs. 276–278) 347–350
relationship to spinal column, 558
vascular branches from bronchial system, 146
Spinal dura, 342
Spinal nerve, 210, 211, (Fig. 457) 548, 554
relationship to spinal column, 558
roots, 342
Spine
lateral curvature of, 550
lumbar (see Lumbar spine)
Spinous process, 547
Spiral organ of Corti, 369
Splanchnic arteries, supplying kidneys, 297
Splanchnic nerve, 211, 215, 216, 296, 320

Splanchnic nerve, block, (Fig. 176) 224
in relation to diaphragm, 156
supplying adrenal glands, 309
supplying pancreas, 106
Spleen (see also Splenic...), (Figs. 95–103) 106–113
accessory, (Fig. 97) 107
arteries of, 110–111
blood supply to, 18, (Figs. 102–103) 110–112
collateral supply to, 232
embryology of, (Figs. 95–96) 106–107
hilum of, accessory pancreatic tissue in, 104
injury to, 108
ligaments of, (Fig. 101) 109–110
lymph trunk collecting from, 268
relations, 104, (Fig. 98) 107–108
removal of, 107
rupture of, 112
transplantation of, 112
veins of, 111
Splenectomy, 18, 109, 112–113
damage of pancreas during, 104
infection following, 106
Splenic...(see also Spleen)
Splenic artery, 18, 113, (Fig. 178) 227, 232
lymph nodes along, 17
Splenic flexure, resection for cancer of, (Fig. 48) 57
Splenic vein, (Fig. 74) 81–82, 106, 113
Splenorenal ligament, (Fig. 13) 18
Splenorenal shunt, 113
Splenosis, 112
Spondylolisthesis, (Figs. 471–472) 562–563
causing narrowing of canal, 561
Spondylolysis, 563
Spondylosis, 556
Sprengel's deformity, 447
Spring ligament, (Fig. 451) 540
affected by flat foot, 544
Stapedial artery, formation of, 285
Stapedius muscle, 176
innervation of, 365
Stapedius reflex, 368
Stapes, 176
Steal phenomenon, 221, 230, (Fig. 179) 231
Stellate ganglion, (Fig. 171) 213–214, 219
block, (Fig. 175) 222–223

Stenosis
  abnormal fusions of endocardial valves
    associated with, 280
  duodenal, 1, 39, 104
  in vertebral canal, (*Fig.* 469) 561
Sterility, following prostatectomy, 322
Sternal defects, covered by pectoralis
    major flap, 248
Sternal notch, 137
Sternoclavicular joint, (*Fig.* 346) 433,
    (*Figs.* 355–356) 442–443
Sternohyoid muscle, 202
Sternomastoid muscle, (*Fig.* 159) 193–195
  branchial cysts along, 179
  branchial sinus situated along, 177
  ganglia displaced into, 220
  lymph nodes beneath, 192
  paralysis of, 374
  spinal accessory nerve in relation to,
    (*Fig.* 294) 373
  thyroid in relation to, 201
Sternothyroid muscle, 202
Sternotomy, 239
  median, 150
Sternum
  in diagnosis, 137
  splitting of, 115
Stomach, 10–22
  blood vessels of, (*Fig.* 9) 14–16
  formation of, 23
  herniated, 158–159
  lymph drainage of, (*Fig.* 12) 16–17, 268
  oesophagus in relation to, (*Fig.* 3) 4
  peritoneal reflections of, (*Fig.* 13) 18
  relation of pancreas to, 104
  subdivision of, (*Fig.* 8) 12
  veins of, 16, 83
  wall, accessory pancreatic tissue in, 104
Stomadeum, (*Fig.* 145) 171–172
Stones, kidney, 295
Strangulated femoral hernia, 131
Strangulation, of haemorrhoids, (*Fig.* 61)
    67
Streptococcus, haemolytic, 493
Stress fracture, of vertebral arch, 563
Stress incontinence of urine, 397
Striated muscle, of external sphincter of
    bladder, 319
Stridor, 404
Stylohyoid ligament, 176
  ossification in, 192

Stylohyoid ligament, tonsils in relation to,
    190
Stylohyoid muscle, 176
Styloid process, 176
Styloids of radius and ulna, determining
    levels of, (*Fig.* 333) 416
Stylomandibular ligament, 188
Stylomastoid foramen, emergence of facial
    nerve from, (*Fig.* 290) 366
Stylopharyngeus muscle, 176, 369
Subaponeurotic space, accumulation of
    fluid in, 329
Subarachnoid space, 341, 343, 352
  circle of Willis in, 232
Subcaecal fossa, 45
Subcalcaneal bursa, (*Fig.* 449) 537
Subcardinal veins, 264
Subcarinal lymph nodes, 10, (*Fig.* 130)
    147–148
  position in thorax, (*Fig.* 124) 138
Subcervical glands of Albarran, 321
Subclavian artery(ies), 203, 232, (*Fig.* 193)
    251, (*Fig.* 303) 383
  aberrant right, 287
  approach to, 239
  compression of, 384
  formation of, 286
  occlusion of, 231
  plexus to, 213
Subclavian lymph trunk
  draining to thoracic duct, 270
  termination of, (*Fig.* 210) 271
Subclavian steal syndrome, (*Fig.* 179) 231
Subclavian vein, (*Figs.* 193–196) 251–253,
    (*Fig.* 303) 383
  cannulation of, (*Fig.* 194) 252–253
  great lymph trunks in relation to, (*Fig.*
    210) 271
  jugular lymph trunk entering, 196
Subclavicular dislocation, 448
Subclavius muscle, indenting axillary
    vein, (*Fig.* 192) 250–251, 381
Subclavius nerve, 381
Subconjunctival haemorrhage, 329
Subcoracoid dislocation, 448
Subcutaneous abscess, 490
Subcutaneous fat, at birth, 405
Subcuticular infection, 490
Subdeltoid/subacromial bursa, (*Fig.* 353)
    440

Subdural haematoma, 342
Subdural space, 342
Subglenoid dislocation, 448
Subgluteal bursae, (*Fig.* 418) 505
Subinguinal lymph nodes, (*Fig.* 211) 272
Sublingual gland, 362
Submandibular ganglion, 184, 217, (*Fig.* 286) 362, 366
Submandibular lymph nodes, 194
Submandibular salivary glands, 184, 194
Submental lymph nodes, (*Fig.* 159) 193–194, 196
Subphrenic abscess, (*Figs.* 90–91) 99–102
Subphrenic spaces, (*Fig.* 90) 100
Subpsoas bursa, (*Fig.* 419) 505
Subpyloric nodes, (*Fig.* 12) 17
Subscapular nerve, 436
Subscapular vein, (*Fig.* 140) 165
Subscapularis muscle, (*Fig.* 347) 435
Subtalar joint, 538
Subtrigonal glands, 321
Subtrochanteric amputation, 432
Suction-socketed limb, 433
Suctorial pad, at birth, 404
Sulcal artery, (*Fig.* 276) 347
Sulcus, buccal, 186
Superficial femoral artery occlusion, 229
Superficial temporal artery, (*Fig.* 261) 330
Superficial temporal vein, (*Fig.* 262) 331
Superior mesenteric artery, 22
 oesophagus in relation to, (*Fig.* 5) 6
Superior mesenteric vein, (*Fig.* 74) 81
Superior oblique muscle
 innervation of, 356
 paralysis of, 357
Superior orbital fissure, 356
Superior sagittal sinus, 342
Superior vena cava, (*Fig.* 193) 251, (*Fig.* 196) 253, 267, 275, (*Fig.* 215) 277
 anomalies of, 267
 embryology of, 263–264
 obstruction of, (*Fig.* 182) 235–236
 position in thorax, (*Fig.* 124) 138
Superior vesical artery, 319
Supernumerary bones, (*Fig.* 338) 421
Supernumerary bronchus, 144
Supracardinal veins, 264
Supraclavicular nerve
 affected by phrenic nerve, 96–97
 descending, (*Fig.* 298) 378

Suprahumeral articulation, (*Fig.* 346) 433, 440
Supralevator anomaly, 71
Supramandibular lymph node group, 194
Supraorbital artery, (*Fig.* 261) 330
Supraorbital nerve, (*Fig.* 261) 332
Supraorbital vein, (*Fig.* 262) 331
Suprapatella bursa, 526
Suprapleural membrane, (*Fig.* 134) 156
Suprapyloric nodes, 10
Suprarenal aneurysm, 243
Suprascapular nerve, 381, 435
Suprasphincteric abscess, (*Fig.* 69) 75–76
Supraspinatus muscle, (*Fig.* 347) 435
Supraspinatus tendon, (*Fig.* 357) 445
Supraspinous ligament, 555
Supratrochlear artery, (*Fig.* 261) 330
Supratrochlear nerve, (*Fig.* 261) 332
Supratrochlear vein, (*Fig.* 262) 331
Sural nerve, 256
 grafting of, 376
Sutural bones, 410
Sutural membrane, 341
Swallowing, 5
 difficulty with, 8, 370
Sweat glands
 nerve fibres to, 209
 secretory fibres to, 211
Sweating
 lack of, 385
 sympathectomy to reduce, 219
Sylvian system, 342
Syme's amputation, 431
Sympathectomy
 lumbar, (*Fig.* 174) 221–222
 surgical, (*Fig.* 174) 218–222
 upper thoracic and cervical, 219–220
Sympathetic denervation, affecting development of collaterals, 226
Sympathetic ganglion block, (*Figs.* 175–176) 222–224
Sympathetic nervous system, (*Fig.* 168) 207–208, (*Figs.* 169–171) 210–216
 pelvic part of, 216
 supply to bladder, 319
 supply to veins, 249
 sympathectomy, 218–222
 transmitter substances in, 209
Sympathetic reflex arc, (*Fig.* 169) 210
Sympathetic trunks, (*Fig.* 169) 210–211

Symphysial cartilage, 410
Symphysis, absence of, 327
Symphysis menti, at birth, 404
Symphysis pubis, (*Fig.* 58) 64
  peritoneal relations, (*Fig.* 251) 318
  uterine ligaments in relation to, (*Fig.* 314) 395
Synapses, autonomic nerve, transmitter substances in, 209–210
Synovial fluid, 521
Synovial swelling, 388
Synovial tendon sheaths of hand, (*Fig.* 387) 476–477
Synovium, 524
Syphilitic osteomyelitis, affecting epiphysis, 423

T lymphocytes, 106
Taeniae coli, 41, 43
Talocalcaneal joints, 538
Talofibular ligament, (*Fig.* 443) 531
Talonavicular joint, 538
Talus
  accessory, (*Fig.* 339) 421
  making up foot arch, 539
  ossicle fused with, (*Fig.* 339) 421
Tamponade, 284
Tarsal muscle, 355, (*Fig.* 283) 359–360
  nerve fibres to, 211
  paralysis of, 385
Tarsal plate, (*Fig.* 283) 360
Tarsal tunnel, 538
  syndrome, 394
Taste (*Fig.* 291) 368
  buds, innervation of, 366
  fibres of tongue, 184
  lesions of olfactory nerve affecting, 352
  loss of sensation of, 369
  nerve pathway for, 362
Technetium scan, for ruptured spleen, 112
Tectorial membrane, 551
Teeth
  blood supply to, 181
  extraction of, 186
  incisor (*see* Incisor teeth)
  innervation of, (*Fig.* 153) 183, (*Fig.* 155) 185–186, 357
  rudiments at birth, 404

Teeth, upper, anaesthetic technique, 186
Tegmen tympani, (*Fig.* 289) 365
Tela choroidea, 343
Temporal artery, 188
  superficial, (*Fig.* 261) 330
Temporal bone, (*Fig.* 156) 187, 188
  facial nerve in, 364
Temporal fossa, lymphatic drainage of, 194
Temporal lobe
  abscess, 403
  pituitary tumour causing pressure on, 339
Temporal vein, superficial, (*Fig.* 262) 331
Temporalis muscle, 182, 188
Temporomandibular joint, 181, (*Fig.* 156) 187–189
Temporomandibular ligament, 187
Tendinitis
  calcific, 445
  of biceps tendon, 446
Tendo Achillis, 532, (*Figs.* 447, 449) 536–537
  rupture of, 538
  short, causing flat foot, 544
  spur associated with, 546
Tendo calcaneus, 536
Tendon(s)
  cartilaginous centres in, 420
  of inguinal canal, 44
  of Todaro, (*Fig.* 214) 276, 277
Tendon reflex of biceps, affected by prolapsed cervical disc, 560
Tendon sheaths
  around ankle joint, (*Figs.* 446–449) 535–538
  of hand, (*Figs.* 387–388) 476–478
  infections, 493
Tenosynovitis, 493
  in fingers, 476
Tensor palati, 176, 182
  innervation of, 362
Tensor tympani, 176
  innervation of, 362
Tentorial coning, reversed, 363
Tentorial herniation, resulting in abducens nerve paralysis, 363
Tentorium cerebelli, 341, 345, 356
Teres major muscle, 241
  relation of axillary vein to, 250

Teres minor muscle, (*Fig.* 347) 435
Terminal phalanges, (*Figs.* 402–404) 492–493
Testicle (*see also* Testis)
  connection of dartos muscle to, 124
  cystic enlargement behind, 135
Testicular artery, 121, 136
  supplying ureter, (*Fig.* 236) 303
Testicular atrophy, 136
Testicular veins, 136
Testis (*see also* Testicle)
  appendix, (*Fig.* 112) 123
  descent of, 119–120
  development of, 119–120
  ectopia, 120
  gubernaculum, 119
  inguinal hernia in relation to, 127
  injury to, 119
  inversion of, (*Fig.* 111) 121–122
  pain in, 123
  retractile, 120
  swelling of, 123
  torsion of, 122
  tunica vaginalis, fluid in, 135
  vestigial structures in connection with, (*Fig.* 112) 123
Testosterone, controlling testis descent, 119
Tetralogy of Fallot, 277, 284
Thalamus, lateral geniculate body in, 353
Thenar space, (*Figs.* 396–398) 486–488
Thermocoagulation of roots of trigeminal nerve, 358
Thigh (*see also* Femur)
  blood diverted to, 221
  claudication in, 229
  fascia of, 124
  perforating veins of, 262
  swelling in, (*Fig.* 473) 565
  varices of, 84
  veins in, 255
Third occipital nerve, (*Fig.* 261) 332
Third ventricle
  development of hypophysis from, (*Fig.* 263) 333
  drowsiness due to pressure on, 339
Thomas' hip flexion test, 507
Thompson's ligament, 126
Thoracic... (*see also* Thorax)
Thoracic aorta, rupture of, 289

Thoracic disease, procedures used to investigate, 149
Thoracic duct, (*Fig.* 193) 251, (*Fig.* 209) 269–271
  anomalies of, 270
  drainage into, 147
  injury to, 270, 271
  jugular lymph trunk entering, 196
  passage through diaphragm, 156
Thoracic ganglia, 213–214
  block, 223
Thoracic nerve, relation of kidney to, 291
Thoracic oesophagus, (*Fig.* 3), 3–4
  acquired diverticula of, 7–8
Thoracic radicular artery, (*Fig.* 278) 348–349
Thoracic sympathectomy, 219–220
Thoracic sympathetic trunk, 214–215, 219
Thoracic vertebrae, 549
  collapse of, 565
  position of, 137
Thoraco-abdominal incision, 150–151
Thoracolumbar outflow, 207
Thoracotomy
  left anterior, 240
  posterolateral, 150
Thorax (*see also* Thoracic...)
  at birth, 405
  lymph nodes, (*Fig.* 130) 146–148
  lymph trunks from, 270
  penetrating wounds of, 137
  position of heart in, (*Fig.* 213) 275
  surgical access to, (*Fig.* 131) 149–152
Three vessel disease, 284
Thrombophlebitis, affecting anal skin, 68
Thrombosis
  associated with bronchial artery, 146
  axillary vein, (*Fig.* 192) 250–251
  bronchial artery, 146
  causing portal hypertension, 83
  deep vein, 249, 258
  in appendicitis, 41
  infected, passage into cranial cavity, 332
  subclavian artery, 384
  venous, due to torniquets, 239
Thrombotic pile, 67
Through-arm amputation, 432

Thumb
    affected by injury to median nerve, 387
    affected by prolapsed cervical disc, 560
    amputation of, 496
    small muscles of, 469–470
Thymectomy, 206
Thymoma, 206
Thymus, 205–206
    at birth, 406
    behind manubrium, 205
    parathyroid glands associated with, 206
    tumours, 206
Thyroglossal duct, (*Figs.* 162–163) 199–
        200
Thyrohyoid membrane, lymph nodes on,
        195
Thyrohyoid muscle, nerve supply to, 374
Thyroid artery, (*Figs.* 164–166) 202–204,
        207, 211, 232
    inferior, 8
Thyroid cancer, 205
Thyroid cartilage, 177, (*Fig.* 162) 199, 200,
        (*Fig.* 167) 205
    fibres arising from, 5
Thyroid gland, (*Figs.* 162–167) 198–205
    agenesis, 200
    blood supply to, (*Figs.* 164–165) 202–203
    cancer of, 205
    close surgical relations of, 203–204
    congenital anomalies of, (*Fig.* 163) 199–
        200
    development of, (*Fig.* 162) 198–199
    ectopic, 199
    innervation of, 213
    lobes of, 199, (*Fig.* 163) 200, 201
    lymph drainage of, 195, 205
    oesophagus in relation to, (*Fig.* 2) 3
    parathyroid glands associated with, 206
    relations to muscles, 201
    veins, 8, 202, 206, (*Fig.* 196) 253
Thyroidea ima artery, 203
Thyroidectomy, 203, 207
    nerve damage due to, 372
Thyropharyngeus, 5
Thyrothymic ligament, 205
Tibia
    attachments of upper surface of, (*Fig.*
        431) 518
    measurement of, (*Fig.* 337) 420
    perforating vessels associated with, 261
    subluxation of, 519

Tibia, surgical approach to, 428
    tibulofibular ligament, (*Fig.* 441) 530
    uniting of epiphyses, 411
Tibial arteries, 229
    exposure of, 247
Tibial collateral ligament, (*Fig.* 430) 516–
        517
Tibial condyles, 513
Tibial nerve
    exposure of, 246
    injury to, 393–394, 526
Tibial plateau, 514
Tibial spines, (*Fig.* 431) 518
Tibial syndrome, anterior, 394
Tibial tubercles, 513
Tibial vein, (*Fig.* 201) 258, 262
Tibialis anterior
    extensor retinaculum in relation to, (*Fig.*
        444) 533
    sheath of, (*Figs.* 446–448) 536
Tibialis posterior, sheath of, (*Fig.* 447) 536
Tibulofibular ligament, (*Fig.* 441) 530
Tic douloureux, 358
Toe(s)
    affected by root compression, 559
    amputation of, 430
    clawing of, 392, 545
    muscles, in pes cavus, 545
    Ray excision of, 431
Toe-to-finger transplant, 248
Tongue
    basal vessels of, 196–197
    cancer of, 194, 197
    ectopic thyroid tissue in base of, 199
    foramen caecum of, 199
    innervation of, 184, 357, 362, 366
    lingual tonsil, 189
    lymphatic drainage of, 194, 195, (*Fig.*
        160) 196–197
    muscles, innervation of, 374
    sensory fibres to, 369
    taste (*see* Taste)
Tonsil(s) (*Figs.* 157–158) 189–193
    adherent, 192
    blood supply to, (*Fig.* 158) 191
    cerebellar, herniation of, 351
    development of, 189–190
    lymph nodes, 193, 195
    lymphatic drainage into, 192
    relations, 190

Tonsillar artery, (*Fig.* 158) 191
Tonsillar fossa, 177, 189
  bleeding from, 192
Tonsillectomy, 190
Tooth (*see* Teeth)
Torniquet(s)
  causing venous thrombosis, 239
  test, for varicose veins, 263
Trachea, 1
  at birth, 404
  bifurcation of, 137
  lymphatic drainage of, 195
  nerve fibres to, 211
  oesophagus in relation to, (*Fig.* 2) 3,
    (*Fig.* 3) 4
  subclavian vein in relation to, (*Fig.* 193)
    251
  thoracic duct in relation to, (*Fig.* 209)
    269
  thyroid gland astride, 200
Tracheitis, in infants, 404
Tracheo-oesophageal fistula, 1, (*Fig.* 1) 2
Tracheo-oesophageal folds, 1
Tracheo-oesophageal groove, 204, 205
Traction diverticulum, 8
Tragus
  pre-auricular nodes in front of, 193
  sinus in front of, 180
Transacromial approach to shoulder, (*Fig.*
    361) 451–453
Transfemoral amputation, 431
Translabyrinthine lesion, (*Fig.* 291) 368
Transmetatarsal amputation, (*Fig.* 344)
    430
Transmitter substances in autonomic
    nerve synapses, 209-210
Transrectus incision, 97
Trans-sphenoidal operation to remove
    pituitary, (*Fig.* 270) 339
Trans-sphincteric abscess, (*Fig.* 68) 75
Trans-sphincteric fistula, 75
Transtrochanteric amputation, 512
Transurethral prostatectomy, 324
Transverse arch of foot, (*Fig.* 450) 539
Transverse colon, 41
  adhesion to liver, (*Fig.* 91) 100
  resection for cancer of, (*Fig.* 48) 57
Transverse ligament, 553
Transverse mesocolon, (*Fig.* 37) 45
Transverse metatarsal ligament, 542

Transverse process, of 5th lumbar verte-
    bra, sacralization of, (*Fig.* 470) 562
Transverse sinus, 332
Transverse tarsal joint, 538
Transversus abdominis, relation of kidney
    to, 291
Transversus muscle, 126
Transversus thoracis muscle, 137
Trapezius bone, (*Fig.* 369) 460
Trapezius flap, 248
Trapezius muscle, (*Fig.* 350) 439
  spinal accessory nerve supplying, 373
Trapezoid bone, (*Fig.* 369) 460
Trapezoid ligament, (*Fig.* 354) 442
Traumatic hernia, 159
Traumatic meningocele, 384
Traumatic ulnar neuritis, 390
Trefoil canal, (*Fig.* 469) 561
Treitz, ligament of, 33
Trendelenburg hip test, (*Fig.* 421) 506
Trendelenburg operation, (*Fig.* 200) 255
Triangle
  of Calot, 97
  of Hesselbach, (*Fig.* 116) 128
  of Koch, 277
Triceps
  affected by prolapsed cervical disc, 560
  brachial artery in relation, 242
  bursae in relation to insertion, (*Fig.* 365)
    456
Tricuspid annulus, (*Fig.* 214) 276
Tricuspid atresia, 277, 280
Tricuspid valve, (*Fig.* 214) 276, 279
  development of, 274
Trigeminal artery, 233
Trigeminal cave, 357
Trigeminal ganglion, (*Fig.* 173) 218
  removal of, 363
Trigeminal nerve, 182, 211, 355, (*Figs.*
    282–286) 357–363
  nerves of scalp derived from, 332
  thermocoagulation of roots of, 358
Trigeminal neuralgia, 358
Trigone of bladder, 314
  additional ureter opening into, 304
  fibrous, 276
Triquetral bone, (*Fig.* 369) 460
Trochanter of femur, bursae on, (*Fig.* 418)
    505

Trochlear nerve, (*Fig*. 268) 338, (*Fig*. 281) 356–357
Truncal vagotomy, 20
Truncus arteriosus, (*Fig*. 212) 273, 280, 285
Tuber cinereum, (*Fig*. 264) 335
Tuberculosis
  causing middle-lobe collapse, 141
  of hip, 507
  of short long bones, 423
  of spine, (*Fig*. 473) 563–565
  of vertebrae, 423, 563
  site in lung, 140
Tuberculous meningitis, anosmia due to, 352
Tuberosity of calcaneus, weight bearing on, 539
Tubular coarctation of aorta, 288
Tumour(s) (*see also individual tumours and under tissues and structures involved*; *see also* Cancer; Carcinoma; Fibrosarcoma; Sarcoma)
  affecting circulation of cerebrospinal fluid, 347
  arising from paraganglia, 311–313
  bronchogenic, 149
  catecholamine content of, 311
  causing spondylolisthesis, 563
  cells, in vertebrae, 560
  mediastinal, 2
  metastatic, causing portal hypertension, 83
  non-secretory, 313
  secretory, 312, 313
Tunica vaginalis, 120, 122
  fluid in, 135
Tympanic antrum, (*Fig*. 319) 402
Tympanic cavity, 179, (*Fig*. 289) 365
  lymphatic drainage of, 194
Tympanic membrane, innervation of, 371
Tympanic nerve paragangliomas, (*Fig*. 244) 313
Tympanic plexus, 369

Ulcer
  ankle, 259
  duodenal, 20, 31
  peptic (*see* Peptic ulcer)
  stomach, 16

Ulcer, venous, 259
Ulcerative colitis, palpation of rectum for, 77
Ulna, (*Fig*. 369) 460, (*Fig*. 395) 484
  measurement of, (*Fig*. 332) 416
  surgical approach to, 426
  uniting of epiphyses, 411
Ulnar artery
  exposure of, 242
  fistula involving, 250
Ulnar bursa, 476
Ulnar claw-hand, (*Fig*. 308) 389
Ulnar collaterals, 232, 455
Ulnar nerve, 242, 380, (*Figs*. 308–311) 389–392, 425, 470
  compression of, 457
  injury to, (*Figs*. 308–309) 389–390
  paralysis, 385
  supplying hand muscles, 473–474
  supplying wrist, 462
  transposition of, (*Fig*. 310) 391
Ulnar neuritis, traumatic, 390
Ultrasonography
  in biliary tract disease, 89
  in treatment of subphrenic abscess, 102
Umbilical hernia, 24
Umbilical ligament, 129, 314
Umbilical ring, 29
Umbilical vein, 24, 82, (*Fig*. 212) 273, 275
Umbilicus
  discharge of intestinal contents at, 39
  incisions involving, 115
  urine discharging at, 316
  veins of, 84
Uncinate fits, associated with pituitary tumours, 339
Uncovertebral joints, (*Fig*. 462) 551–552
Upper limb amputation, 432–433
Urachus, 314
  congenital abnormalities of, (*Fig*. 249) 315–317
  cyst, (*Fig*. 249) 316
  patent, (*Fig*. 249) 316
  relations in female peritoneum, (*Fig*. 250) 317
Ureter, (*Fig*. 229) 297, (*Figs*. 232–239) 300–307
  arteries used to replace damaged section of, 319
  bladder in relation to, (*Fig*. 252) 318

Ureter, blood supply to, (*Fig.* 236) 303
  bud, (*Fig.* 229) 297, (*Fig.* 245) 314
  congenital abnormalities of, (*Fig.* 237)
    304
  double pelvis of, (*Fig.* 237) 304
  incisions to expose, (*Figs.* 238–240) 306–
    307
  nerve supply, 302
  ovariectomy causing damage to, 304
  prostate in relation to, (*Fig.* 235) 302
  seminal vesicle in relation to, (*Fig.* 235)
    302
  surgical damage to, 304–306
  sympathetic trunk in relation to, 215
Urethra
  congenital abnormalities of, (*Figs.* 258–
    259) 326–328
  congenital valves in, 328
  formation of, (*Figs.* 246–247) 314
  groove of, 326
  male, (*Figs.* 256–259) 324–328
  membranous, 324
  opening of ejaculatory ducts into, 319
  orifice on ventral surface of penis, 326
  penile, 324
  prolapse of female, 398
  prostate projecting into, 321
  prostatic, additional ureter opening
    into, 304
  rupture of, (*Fig.* 113) 124–125, (*Fig.* 257)
    325
  sphincter of, 304
  valves in, 328
Urinary infection, 304
Urinary organs, development of, 297
Urinary sphincter, paralysis associated
    with spina bifida cystica, 351
Urine
  congenital causes of obstruction to out-
    flow of, (*Fig.* 259) 327
  discharging at umbilicus, 316
  extravasation of, (*Fig.* 113) 124, (*Fig.*
    257) 325
  meconium stained, 68
  outflow obstruction, 321
Urogenital diaphragm, 72, (*Fig.* 251) 318
  attachment of rectum to, 51
  nerve supply to, 73
  prostate in relation to, 321
Urogenital fold, (*Fig.* 258) 326

Urogenital sinus, primitive, (*Fig.* 245) 314
Urogram, excretory, 71
Urological abnormalities, 71
Urorectal septum, 68, (*Fig.* 245) 314
Uterosacral ligament, (*Fig.* 314) 395
  infiltration by tumour tissue, 78
Uterus
  arteries of, 301, 305
  ligaments of, 305, (*Fig.* 314) 395
  palpation of, 77
  position of, (*Fig.* 316) 397
  prolapse of, (*Figs.* 314–316) 395–398
  relations in female peritoneum, (*Fig.*
    250) 317
  supports of, (*Fig.* 315) 396–397
  sympathetic nerve supply to, 319
Utricle, 369
Uvula
  cleft of, 174
  innervation of, 357
  muscle of, 182
  vesicae, 321

Vagal trunk branches, 372
Vagina
  additional ureter opening into, 304
  damage to ureters caused by application
    of clamps to, 305
  examination of, (*Fig.* 317) 398–399
  formation of, 314
  fornix, drainage of pelvic abscess
    through, 48
  hydrocele, (*Fig.* 123) 135
  hysterectomy, 400
  inguinal hernia, (*Fig.* 114) 127
  ischial spine palpated through, 74
  meconium from, 68
  pelvic abscess draining into, 48
  position of, (*Fig.* 316) 397
  prolapse of, (*Figs.* 314–316) 395–398
  smear, 398
  ureter in relation to, 301
Vagotomy, 20–21
Vagus nerve, (*Fig.* 166) 203–204, 212, 217,
    (*Fig.* 293) 370–373
  abdominal course, 18–21
  anterior, (*Fig.* 14) 19
  auricular branch of, 332, 366

Vagus nerve, branchial arches in relation to, (*Fig.* 218) 286
  glomus intravagale on, 311
  in radical neck dissection, 197
  laryngeal branch of, 177
  lesions of, 372–373
  oesophagus in relation to, (*Fig.* 2) 3, 7
  passage through diaphragm, 156
  posterior, (*Fig.* 15) 19–20
  supplying pancreas, 106
Valgus angle, of knee joint, (*Fig.* 435) 522
Valsalva, aortic sinuses of, 277
Valves
  cardiac, formation of, 274
  in leg veins, 254
  in urethra, 328
  in vein grafts, 256
  in veins, 249, (*Fig.* 201) 258, 262–263
  of foramen ovale, 275
Valvular atresia, 280
Varices, anorectal, 84
Varicocele, 136–137
  operation for, 136–137
Varicose veins, 248, 261
  aetiology of, 262–263
  diagnosis, 263
  portal obstruction associated with, 83
  recurrent, 255
Vas aberrans, (*Fig.* 112) 123
Vasa brevia, 18
Vasa recta, 36, 53
Vascular access, (*Figs.* 191–197) 249–254
Vascular approach, (*Figs.* 185–190) 239–248
Vascular disease, peripheral, 218–219
Vascular reflexes, sensory fibres of, 209
Vasoconstrictor nerve fibres, 211
Vasodilatation by sympathectomy, 218
Vasospastic conditions, relieved by sympathectomy, 218-219
Vastus intermedius, 427
Vastus lateralis, 427, 515
Vastus medialis, 515
Veins (*see also* Venous…; *see also specific veins and under structures involved*), (*Figs.* 191–207) 248–267
  deep (*see* Deep veins)
  grafts, 234, 248, 250
  smooth muscle in, 248

Veins, sympathetic innervation of, 249
  valves in (*see* Valves in veins)
  varicose veins, *see* Varicose veins
Vena azygos major, passage through diaphragm, 156
Vena cava
  anomalies of, (*Figs.* 206–207) 266–267
  blood flow to, 83
  inferior (*see* Inferior vena cava)
  position in thorax, (*Fig.* 124) 138
  superior (*see* Superior vena cava)
Vena comitans, 250
Venepuncture, 249, 250
Venous…(*see also* Veins)
Venous catheter, 250
Venous collateral mechanisms, 234
Venous hypertension, 261
  in upper saphenous system, 262
  transmission in saphenous veins, 258
Venous infarction, colonic, 47
Venous sinuses, intracranial, (*Fig.* 271) 340–341
Venous thrombosis, due to torniquets, 239
Venous ulceration, 259
Ventral mesentery, persistence of, 37
Ventricle, (*Fig.* 212) 273, 279
  left, (*Fig.* 215) 277, 279
  muscle of, 279
  right, (*Fig.* 215) 277, 279
  third, drowsiness due to pressure on, 339
Ventricular septum, (*Fig.* 214) 276
  defect of, 277, 279
Ventriculo-atrial shunt, 350
Ventriculography, 350
Ventriculoperitoneal shunt, 350
Ventriculosubarachnoid shunt, 350
Vertebrae
  blood supply to, (*Fig.* 329) 414
  joints and ligaments uniting, (*Figs.* 461–463) 551–555
  ossification of, (*Figs.* 458–460) 549–551
  position of, 137
  prominens, 549
  regional characteristics of, 549
  structure of, 547
  subluxation of, 556

Vertebrae, transverse process of, (*Fig.* 470) 562
  tuberculosis of, 423, 563
  tumour cells in, 560
Vertebral arch, (*Fig.* 458) 549, 550
  defect of, 563
Vertebral artery, (*Fig.* 179) 231, 232, (*Fig.* 267) 337, (*Fig.* 278) 348–349, 549, 553
  approach to, 239
  innervation of, 213
  osteophytes from uncovertebral joints affecting, (*Fig.* 462) 552
Vertebral bones, overgrowth of, 561
Vertebral canal
  longitudinal ligament in, (*Fig.* 461) 551
  stenosis, (*Fig.* 469) 561–562
Vertebral displacement, 563
Vertebral venous system, (*Fig.* 468) 560
Vertebrobasilar insufficiency, 552
Vertical vein, (*Fig.* 468) 560
Verumontanum, 321, (*Fig.* 256) 324
Vesical arteries, 319
Vesical sphincter, (*Fig.* 253) 321
Vestibular anus, 68
Vestibular nerve, 369
Vestibule, formation of, 314
Vestibulocochlear nerve, (*Fig.* 287) 363, 369
Vieussen's ring, 283
Villi, arachnoidal, 343
Vincula of phalanx, (*Fig.* 389) 478
Visceral autonomic nerve fibres, block of, 224
Visceral collateral system, 229
Visceral lymph nodes of thorax, 147–148
Visceral nerve fibres, 211
Visceral pain, 209
  relief by sympathectomy, 219
Visceral reflexes, sensory fibres of, 209
Vision, loss of, 355
Visual cortex, 354–355
Visual fibres, 353
Visual field
  affected by pituitary tumours, 337–338
  defect, 353
Vitelline cysts, 40
Vitelline sinus, (*Fig.* 33) 40
Vitelline system, (*Fig.* 33) 40

Vitelline vein, 83, (*Fig.* 212) 273, 275
Vitello-intestinal duct, remnants of, 38
Vocal cords, 203
  affected by thyroidectomy, 372
  at birth, 404
Voice
  affected by damage to laryngeal nerve, 373
  pitch of, 203
Volar approach to wrist joint, (*Fig.* 374) 465
Volar ligaments, 468, 482, 483
Volar plate, (*Fig.* 390) 479
Volar zig-zag incision, (*Fig.* 406) 494
Volkmann's ischaemic contracture, 456
Volvulus
  due to deficient fixation of gut, 30
  neonatorum, 30, 37
  of caecum, 46
Vomiting of blood, 83
Vulva
  inspection of, 398
  labia (*see* Labia)
  varicosities of, 255–256
Vulval anus, 68

Waldeyer
  fascia of, 50
  fossa of, 34
  lymphatic ring of, (*Fig.* 157) 189, 192–193
  mesentericoparietal fossa of, (*Fig.* 28) 34–35
Warren shunt, (*Fig.* 79) 86
Weber's syndrome, 356
Willis, circle of (*see* Circle of Willis)
Wirsung's duct, 103
Wormian bones, 410
Wrist (*Figs.* 369–375) 460–466
  binding bands, (*Figs.* 394–395) 482–485
  collateral ligaments of, 482
  creases, 489
  motor loss in flexors of, 385
  movements of, (*Fig.* 370) 461–462
  surgical approach to, (*Figs.* 372–375) 463–466

X-rays
  magnification factor, 89
  of rectum, 70–71
Xanthochromia, 346
Xiphoid process, excision of, 115

Zone of calcification, 409
Zuckerkandl, organ of, (*Fig.* 243) 312
Zygomatic arch, 187, 329
Zygomatic bone, 182
  fractures of, 186–187
Zygomaticofacial nerve, 187
Zygomaticotemporal nerve, 187, (*Fig.* 261) 332